The Complete Spa Book *for* Massage Therapists

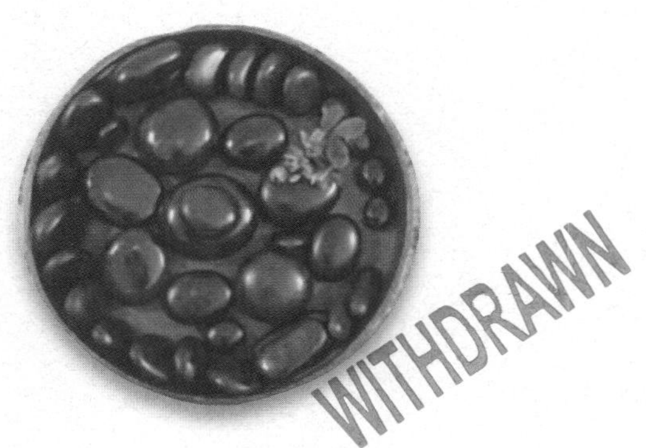

The Complete Spa Book for Massage Therapists

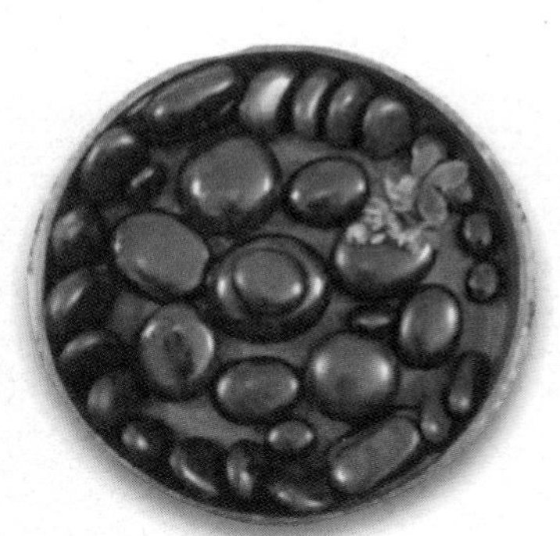

Steve Capellini

Photography by Yanik Chauvin

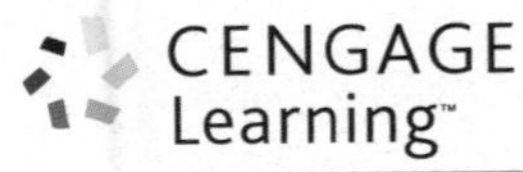

Australia • Brazil • Japan • Korea • Mexico • Singapore • Spain • United Kingdom • United States

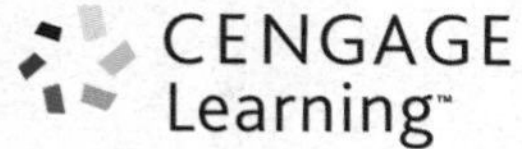

The Complete Spa Book for Massage Therapists
Steve Capellini

President, Milady: Dawn Gerrain

Publisher: Erin O'Connor

Acquisitions Editor: Martine Edwards

Senior Product Manager: Philip Mandl

Editorial Assistant: Maria Hebert

Director of Beauty Industry Relations: Sandra Bruce

Senior Marketing Manager: Gerard McAvey

Production Director: Wendy Troeger

Senior Content Project Manager: Nina Tucciarelli

Senior Art Director: Joy Kocsis

For product information and technology assistance, contact us at
Professional & Career Group Customer Support, 1-800-648-7450
For permission to use material from this text or product,
submit all requests online at http://**cengage.com/permissions**
Further permissions questions can be e-mailed to
permissionrequest@cengage.com

Library of Congress Control Number: 2009935191

ISBN-13: 978-1-4180-0014-1

ISBN-10: 1-4180-0014-0

Milady
5 Maxwell Drive
Clifton Park, NY 12065-2919
USA

Cengage Learning products are represented in Canada by Nelson Education, Ltd.

For your lifelong learning solutions, visit http://**milady.cengage.com**

Visit our corporate website at http://**cengage.com**

Printed in United States
1 2 3 4 5 XX 13 12 11 10 09

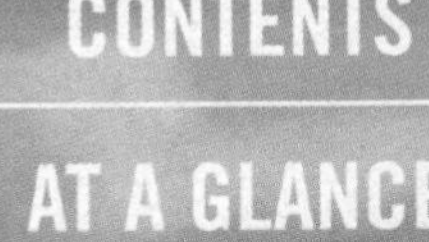

CONTENTS AT A GLANCE

CONTENTS

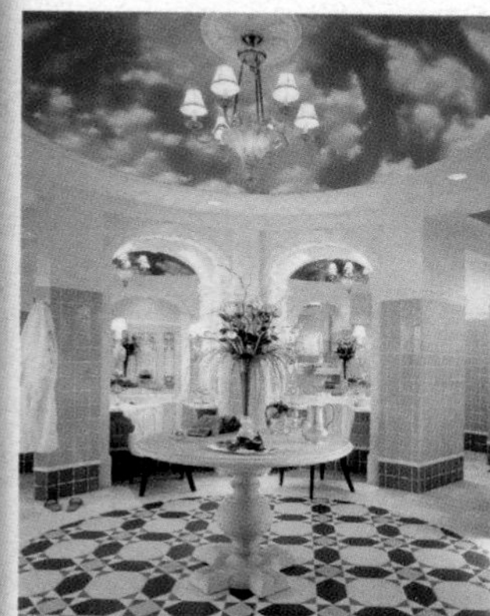

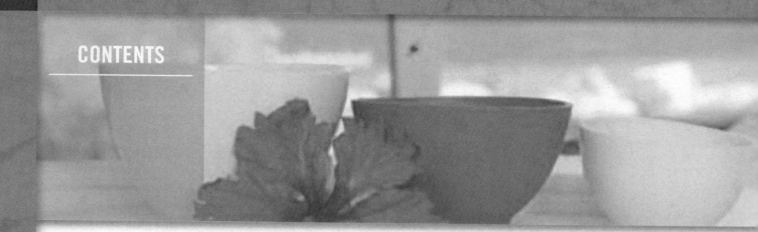

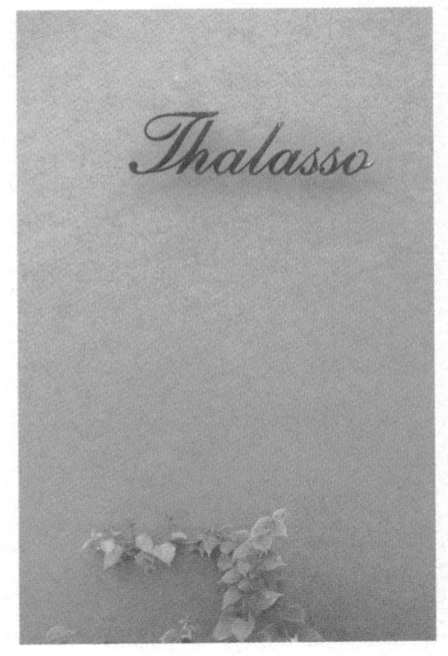
Thalasso

PART 2 HYDROTHERAPY FOR THE 21ST CENTURY: WATER-BASED SPA TREATMENTS

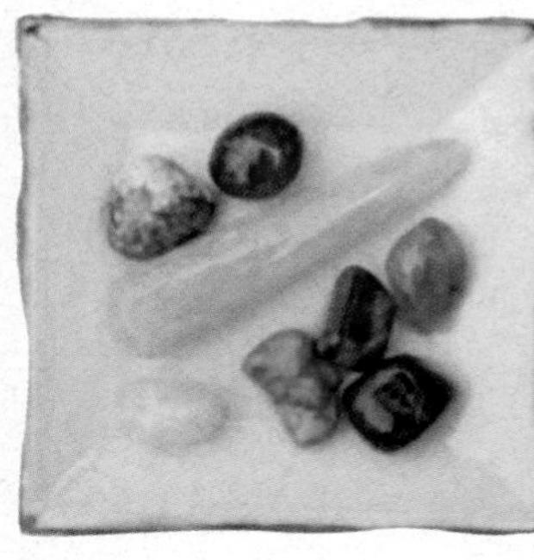

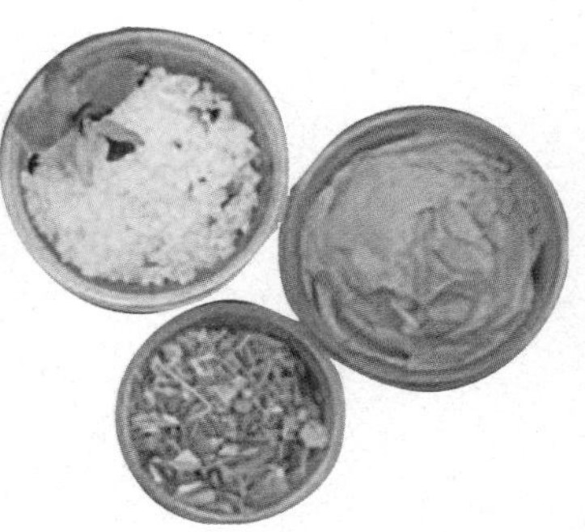

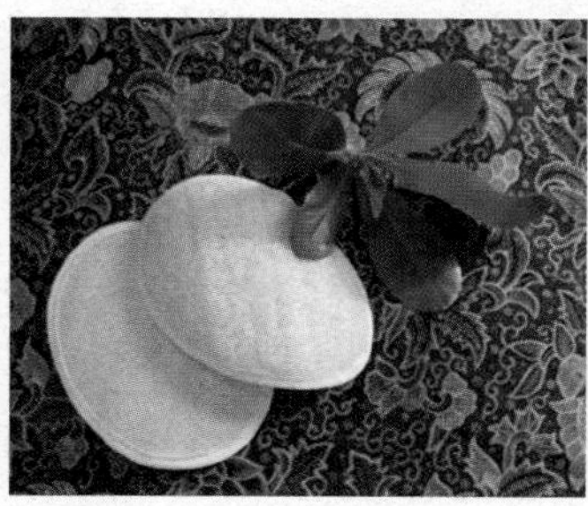

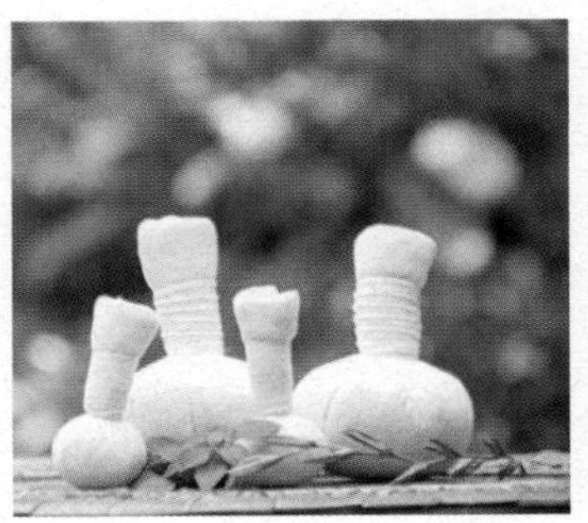

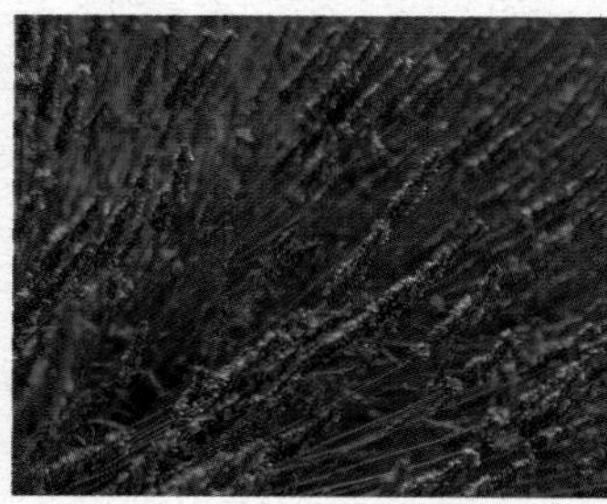

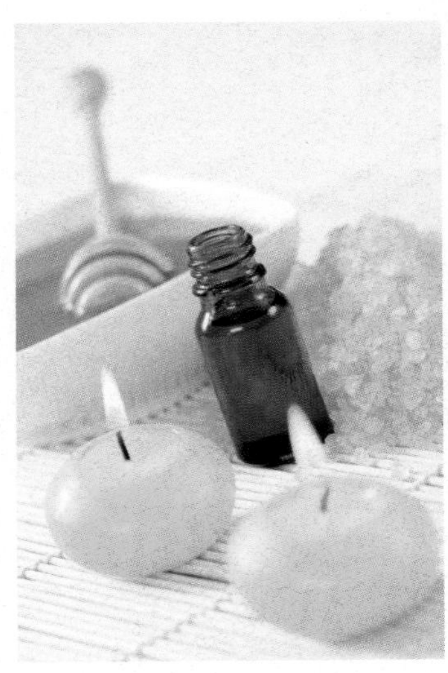

PART 3 SPA CAREERS

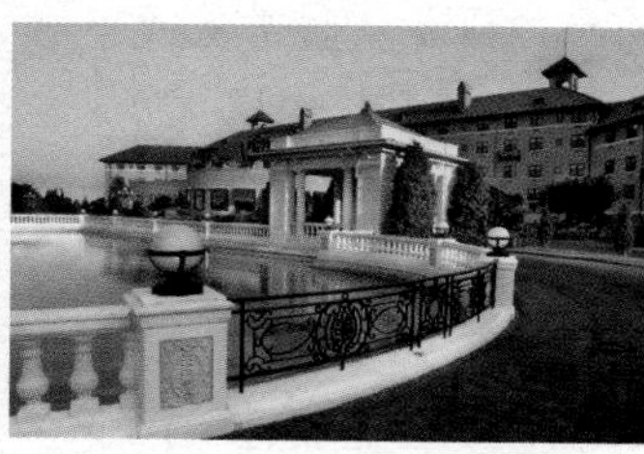

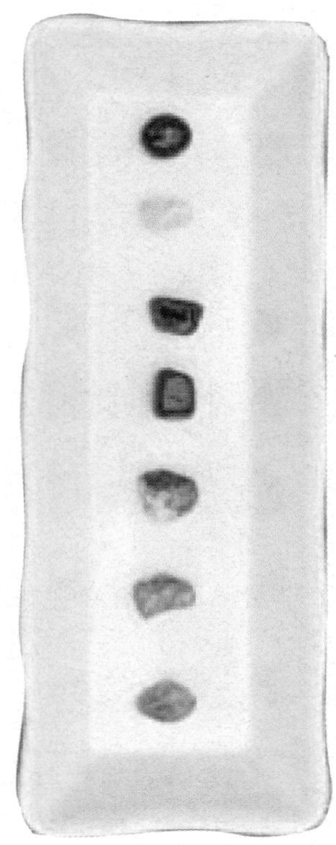

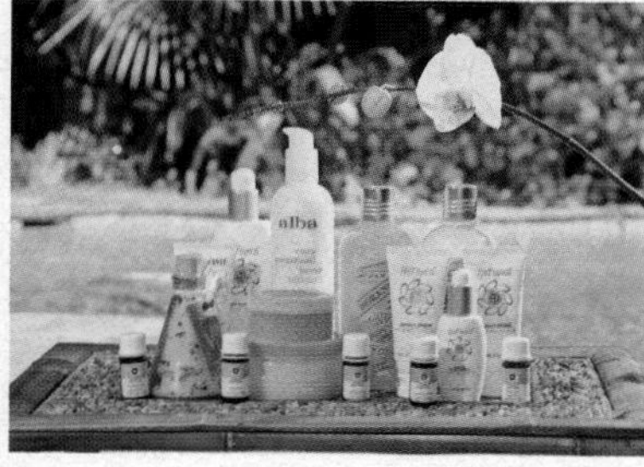
alba

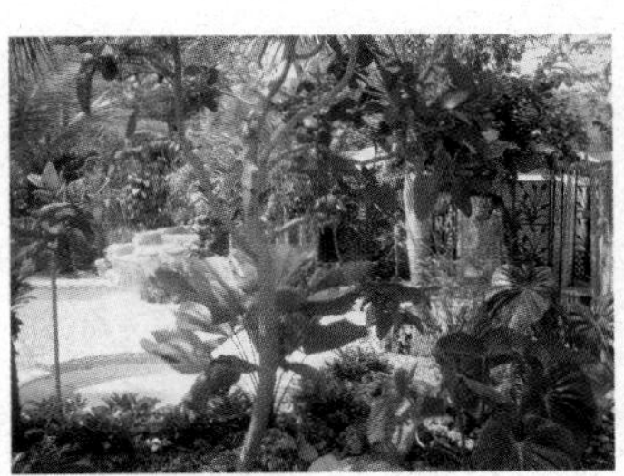

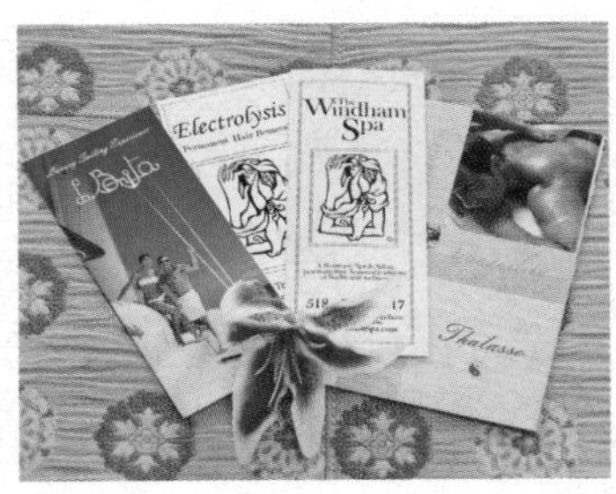
Electrolysis
Windham Spa
Thalasso

PREFACE

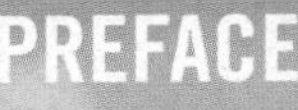

Maybe you are a single parent. Maybe you are fresh out of school. Maybe you have reached a place somewhere in the middle of your life and you felt a change was needed. Whatever your particular situation, a career move into the spa industry can be vastly rewarding. In this field, you will help people feel better, look better, and actually *be* better through an emphasis on therapeutic wellness and stress relief.

The environments where you may find yourself working include some of the most beautiful in the world. The clients you will meet and interact with are often influential, well-known, creative individuals whom you can help and get to know. Many spa therapists travel far and wide, see the world, and make new friends. This can become your life, if you have the education and the tools to be successful at your new endeavor. That is what this book is all about. In these pages, you will learn more about spas than you perhaps realized was possible. In the first section, you will discover the rich history of spa cultures from around the world and how they have developed into the modern spas where so many therapists have found rewarding and fulfilling work. In Section 2, you will come to understand the intricacies of hydrotherapy and the ways it is actually applied by working therapists in the modern world. You will learn how to safely perform specialized spa bath and shower treatments, and understand how to master the powers of heat and cold to balance and soothe your clients. You will find out how human skin is regenerated through a myriad of exfoliations, and you will discover the many healing potentials found in our oceans. In Section 3, you will come to know the therapeutic properties of herbs, muds, clays, and other natural products from the Earth. You will learn what makes a spa massage different from a massage given in any other environment, and how you can make your own spa massages the best they can possibly be. You will work with heated basalt stones, learning how to safely apply them during a spa massage. You will be introduced to the most popular essential oils used in spa settings and be shown how to incorporate them into simple yet effective aromatherapy protocols.

Beyond learning about spa modalities and hydrotherapy, you will also find out what it takes to be a successful member on a top-notch spa team. In Section 4, you will learn the ins and outs of finding and securing the best spa jobs, and then providing the best possible customer service once you have done so. You will come to appreciate the importance of selling therapeutic spa products to clients and how you can increase your own prosperity by doing so. And if you are one of the many therapists who hope to open spas of their own one day, you will find plenty of information here to get you started.

Throughout your studies in this text, you will be given many opportunities to both give and receive dozens of therapeutic (and luxurious) spa treatments. In fact, by the time you are through with your spa studies, you will have experienced more spa services than all but the most seasoned spa goer. Each and every protocol features detailed step-by-step instructions, as well as a full-featured set of information about products needed, room setup, benefits, contraindications, and much more.

Sprinkled within each chapter are many notes of interest in the form of tables, sidebars, and profiles of working spa professionals who will help inspire you on your quest for knowledge and skill in this field. You will also find SPA TIP callouts, SPA CAUTION callouts and SPA ETIQUETTE callouts to help draw your attention to those points deserving particular attention.

Throughout the book, you will notice that the instructions and examples are gender-neutral, meaning that some of them will use the "he" pronoun and some will use the "she" pronoun. Though there are more female therapists working in the spa industry than males, both genders are held in equally high regard by spa owners and guests, and no intentional favor is given to either in the following pages.

The new skills you gain through your study of spa therapy will make you a highly portable professional, sought after by many employers, with a repertoire of skills that has grown much richer and deeper. There is much to know if you want to successfully join the thousands of people who are making places for themselves in the spa world. So, let's get started . . .

EXTENSIVE TEACHING AND LEARNING PACKAGE

A number of ancillary materials accompany *The Complete Spa Book for Massage Therapists.* These materials are designed to support student learning and to provide instructors with everything they need to successfully teach the concepts in the core textbook.

Workbook

The Complete Spa Book for Massage Therapists – Student Workbook provides various review tools with both individual exercises—matching questions, word scrambles, crossword puzzles, true or false, and fill-in-the-blanks—and group activities like role-plays, hangman, and even a quiz fashioned after the *Jeopardy!* game show. Other features like Mental Portrait, Spa Tips/Techniques, Be Prepared, and Self-Searching allow students the opportunity to test their comprehension and place themselves in real-life situations. Plus, all important step-by-step spa procedures are reinforced by the use of detailed rubrics, allowing students precise self-assessments of skill performance and level of development.

Course Management Guide on CD-ROM

The purpose of *The Complete Spa Book for Massage Therapists Course Management Guide* is to give educators strong support in providing the highest-quality instruction in the discipline of spa therapies for the massage therapist, given the wide range of teaching institutions, course lengths, classroom facilities, and local licensing issues involved. It is designed to serve as your partner in making spa education effective, interesting, and fun, while also helping your students develop their mental, ethical, and therapeutic skills.

The comprehensive *Course Management Guide* has been created specifically to support spa therapy education in the massage school environment. Your students deserve the best possible education, and the public deserves competent, enthusiastic, and knowledgeable therapists to work on them. This material was developed with those goals in mind. The spa industry continues as a major force in the hiring and development of massage therapists. As educators, our primary focus is to support students in their growth and to prepare them for successful careers by providing inspiring yet realistic training and training materials. Because spa education for massage therapists in North America does not yet have any universally accepted standards, this Course Management Guide and *The Complete Spa Book for Massage Therapists* text, along with the companion workbook, strive to be as comprehensive and non-exclusionary as possible. In some states and regions, parts of the material may not apply to massage therapists, yet all of the information is important for therapists to understand and master if they are going to be well-rounded spa professionals, even if they are called upon to perform Swedish massage exclusively and no other services.

We are well-aware of the diverse learning environments present in massage schools and the wide range of needs as far as spa therapy education is concerned. For this very reason, Cengage Learning has not set this spa therapy training curriculum in stone but rather presents it as a range of options that are, then, further customizable according to your needs. The three main options, for which comprehensive lesson plans and support materials have been developed include:

Short "Weekend" Spa Course (16–24 Hours)

If your school is operating on a tight schedule with very little extra time for spa therapy training available, you could implement the short course, which can be taught over a weekend if necessary. This will give students an idea of what to expect if they were to pursue spa therapy training further, making it possible for them to decide if this is the right choice for them before investing a large amount of time or effort in their studies. This course is similar to what a professional massage therapist would experience as part of a continuing education program, and over the years, it has proven quite useful. Many therapists, after having taken this level of training, have been able to successfully perform several spa modalities and even develop a spa therapies specialty in their own practices. Because of the short duration of this course, only a fraction of the material in *The Complete Spa Book for Massage Therapists* can be delivered in the classroom itself. Thus, many supplementary learning exercises and activities are suggested for students' self-guided learning after the class is over.

Mid-Length Spa Course (36–60 Hours)

For those students who know they want to pursue work in the spa field, but where time or other constraints do not allow the school to offer a full spa track, the mid-length course affords the opportunity to review the entire core text, with discussions and exercises in the classroom that reinforce learning. Lectures and hands-on experiences are limited to key points and major modalities, with an abundance of suggestions for self-directed study both during the course and after its completion. Students who pass this course will have a firm grasp of the basic skills and knowledge needed by therapists seeking a career in the spa industry. Graduates will feel confident in approaching spas when seeking employment. In addition, they will know how to set up and maintain a spa practice or small spa facility of their own.

Long Spa Course (78–130 Hours)

The long spa course can be implemented as a full post-graduate track, such as many schools provide along with tracks in sports massage or Eastern therapies, for example. This program is for the school that has seen a growing need among the student body for comprehensive, in-depth spa therapy training. All modules, modalities, exercises, and activities in *The Complete Spa Book for Massage Therapists* are covered, with guided lectures to elucidate each part of all 18 chapters. Students who successfully graduate from this program will have a thorough understanding of what it takes to work in the modern spa industry. They will be among the most knowledgeable and highly trained of all their peers seeking career opportunities in this field.

Customizable Learning

Any of the three main curriculum choices can be modified to fit the particular time frames and educational needs of your school. In shorter versions of any of the curriculums, educators can recommend that students experience many of the exercises and activities on their own, while limiting class time to core knowledge development and direct hands-on experiences. In longer versions of each curriculum, educators can take full advantage of the extensive support materials and educational tools provided in the text and in this guide. For the mid-length and long courses, one hour of hands-on documented practice time on spa modalities should be completed outside of class per each lesson provided. Alternatively, this documented practice can be carried out in the school's spa clinic, if such a clinic is available.

Course Management Guide Support Materials

Upon determining the length of the spa curriculum that you are offering at your school, you can choose the appropriate set of lesson plans from this guide. All three of the curricula are supplemented with a number of documents:

- syllabi
- sign-in sheets
- activity worksheets
- forms

- checklists
- academic progress evaluations
- hands-on skill level check lists
- theory grade records by course unit

These are found in the support materials section of this guide. The uses for most of these forms will be self-evident. However, the *theory grade records by course unit* may be new. This form is used to record the test grades of each successive test for each student in one location, so that it will not be necessary to file a large number of tests for each class. After the student signs this form, each separate test grading sheet can be recycled. The same form contains a place to keep records of student performance on all of the Hands-On Skill Level Checklists provided throughout the *Course Management Guide*.

Lessons Plans

The lesson plans in each of three curricula are divided into several sections:

1. SIGN-IN SHEET:
   The sign-in sheet contains some of the information from the lesson plan, with the addition of an area for students to sign in on the bottom of the form. This can be printed separately, signed, and filed with the instructor's materials, creating a detailed written record of the subject taught, date, facilities and resources used, student responsibilities, and students in attendance.
2. SUBJECT:
   The section (Part 1, 2, 3, or 4) of *The Complete Spa Book for Massage Therapists* addressed in the lesson.
3. TOPIC:
   Specific topic(s) within the text section covered in the lesson plan.
4. LESSON OBJECTIVES:
   What the students will be able to understand or perform upon completion of the lesson and practice.
5. IMPLEMENTS, EQUIPMENT, & SUPPLIES:
   Items needed by both students and instructors to successfully complete the lesson.
6. TEACHING AIDS:
   Audio/visual equipment, handouts, etc., to be used by the instructor.
7. FACILITY:
   Theory, practical classroom, or both.
8. TIME ALLOTMENT:
   Broad guidance is provided for the time allotted to each lesson. This *Course Management Guide* was written to function effectively in many teaching situations, with a wide variance in required learning hours. The instructor's choice of activities to be included and hands-on protocols to be performed as part of each lesson will greatly impact the time allotment for each lesson.
9. PRIOR ASSIGNMENT:
   What the student needs to have completed prior to the class.

10. EDUCATOR REFERENCES:
    References available to the instructor to further expand his or her knowledge on the subject and enhance the class.
11. NOTES TO THE EDUCATOR:
    Suggestions and reminders to better prepare the educator for the class.
12. LEARNING MOTIVATION:
    Reasons why the material presented in this lesson is relevant and useful to the student. Instructors, of course, can modify and personalize the introduction and motivation for the lesson if they so desire.
13. SPA THOUGHT FOR THE DAY:
    Also found on the first instructor-support PowerPoint slide for each lesson, these quotes set the tone for the class and provide some spa-specific insights on which students can focus as they begin their training each day.
14. SUBJECT OUTLINES & NOTES:
    A two-column format with a brief description of the material on the left side and more in-depth notes on the right side. Instructors can read or paraphrase the information here as they teach the class. Also listed here are supplementary materials that support the instructor's leadership in the classroom.
15. SUMMARY AND REVIEW:
    Includes a summation of the class and answers to chapter review questions.
16. ACTIVITIES TO REINFORCE LEARNING:
    This section lists activities, projects, games, group processes, etc. that instructors can assign to reinforce material covered in the class. Depending upon the time available, these activities can be incorporated into the class or assigned for time outside the classroom. Space is provided for instructors to write in additional activities developed by students or the instructor. These, then, can be used by other instructors at the school in the future.
17. STEP-BY-STEP MODALITY PROTOCOL HANDOUTS:
    Where applicable, step-by-step protocols for spa modalities are provided within the lesson plan so they can be printed out and used by students in the practical classroom environment, removing the need to have the textbook present during potentially messy procedures. These sheets make it easier for the students to keep track of their progress while learning spa treatments.
18. HANDS-ON SKILL LEVEL CHECKLISTS:
    Educators can use these forms to check the progress of students as they learn and master each practical skill. The forms are tied to the practical procedures presented and list specific performance criteria that can be used with the school's practical grading program to determine a student's competency in any given practical skill. These criteria have been provided because various accrediting agencies mandate that practical skills be evaluated on the basis of written criteria established by the school for the purpose of measuring student learning. To be effective, the application of these criteria must be uniform and consistent, and these forms may help you with that.

19. TESTS:
 Multiple-choice tests are provided at the end of every lesson in *The Complete Spa Book for Massage Therapists*, and they are assigned, where applicable, in each lesson plan. For the short and mid-length curricula, where multiple chapters may be discussed in the course of one lesson, modified tests are provided that combine information from the various chapters.
20. TEST ANSWER KEYS:
 Test answers are provided for instructors.

Instructor Support Slides

The Instructor Support Slides use PowerPoint® technology, offering instructors pre-designed presentations to accompany *The Complete Spa Book for Massage Therapists*, making lesson plans simple yet incredibly effective. This chapter-by-chapter CD-ROM has ready-to-use presentations that will help engage students' attention and keep their interest through its varied color schemes and styles. Instructors can use the presentations as-is or adapt them to their own classrooms by importing photos, changing graphics, or adding slides.

ABOUT THE AUTHOR

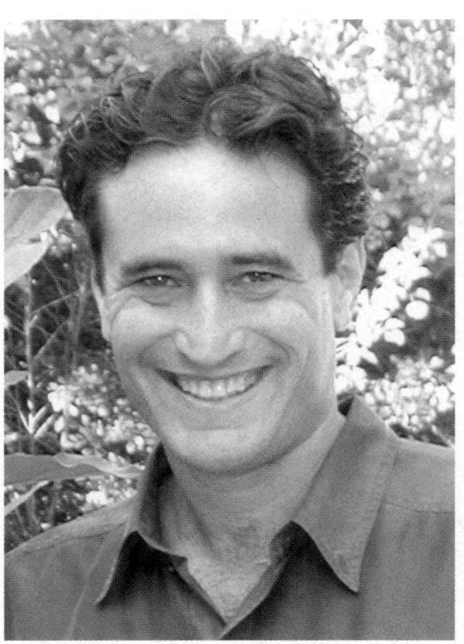

Steve Capellini has been working in the spa industry since 1983, first as a massage therapist, then as a trainer, supervisor, consultant, and writer. He has trained the staffs at several top properties and currently teaches spa workshops to massage therapists, estheticians, and entrepreneurs across the U.S. and Canada. He wrote the monthly Spa Letters column for *Massage & Spa Today*, and he has published four previous books: *The Royal Treatment, Massage Therapy Career Guide, Massage for Dummies,* and *Making the Switch to Being Rich*. He has also published dozens of articles in trade journals and consumer magazines. As a spa spokesperson promoting spa-related products from Glade, Lands End, and others, he has given keynote speeches and appeared on dozens of TV shows and in many magazine articles. He was in charge of developing the spa programs for the Pelican Hill Resort in Newport Beach, California, and the Pritikin Longevity Center in Miami, Florida. He also created the spa training curriculum for East-West College in Portland, Oregon. He travels internationally to learn techniques that he incorporates into custom massage and spa treatments.

ACKNOWLEDGEMENTS

This book has been a collaborative effort over an extended period of time. I would like to gratefully acknowledge some of the many people who have helped to bring it to fruition. Without each of them, this book would not exist. First, my family, who supported my efforts—Atchana, Brandon, Tyler, Lek and Pat, Bob, Joan, and Umpun. Also, our extended Siam Lotus restaurant family who fed me and where the first meeting regarding the creation of this book took place. Thanks to Kalen Connerly and Darcy Scelsi, who shepherded the book through its early incarnation, and to Martine Edwards, Philip Mandl, and their Cengage crew, who have seen it through to completion. Thank you to the "POD," that special group of friends who have endearingly dubbed me "Spa Man" as I've developed this book and my trainings. You know who you are. Thanks to the many school owners who have had me present my spa trainings over the years. This experience has proven invaluable in the creation of this book. Nancy Dail, in particular, offered much support and advice in this regard. Lynda Solien-Wolfe and the folks at Performance Health have always been supportive and interested in my efforts. Thank you for reading early drafts of the manuscript. The International Spa Association (ISPA) has been very helpful in supplying up-to-date information about the modern spa industry, and I thank them for that. Thanks to all the talented professionals who took time out to be interviewed for the profiles in this book—it would not be the same without you. I appreciate the openness of Zoetry Paraiso de la Bonita Resort & Thalasso, who welcomed me and the entire crew in for a week of filming at their gorgeous property. I hope our photos do it justice. And speaking of photos, special thanks to model Kerri Marshburn and to Yanik Chauvin of Touch Photography, who waited more than two years for the photo shoot to finally happen. *Merci, mon ami*. You are a pro.

REVIEWERS

Tracy H. Wright, LMT, NCBTMB, Owner, Massage the Wright Way, and Hydrotherapy Instructor, Educating Hands School of Massage, Miami, FL

Jeff Bockoven, LMT, CRTT, RCP, Director, Iowa Massage Institute, Des Moines, IA

Susan G. Beck, BS, NCTMB, Massage Therapy Program Coordinator/Instructor, Department of Health Occupations, College of Technology, Idaho State University, Pocatello, ID

Deborah Taylor, LMT, Instructor East West College of the Healing Arts, Portland, OR

Jennifer M. DiBlasio, AST, CHT, ACMT, Career Training Academy, New Kensington, PA

Joanne Hunt, LMT, ASMT, BS, MT Program Coordinator Keiser Career College, West Palm Beach, FL

Kelly Zimmerman, BS, NCMT, Massage Therapy Instructor, Clinic Administrator, Miller-Motte Technical College, Cary, NC

Lisa Seguin, BA, LMT, MTI, Corporate Director of Massage Therapy, ATI Career Training Center, Grand Prairie, TX

Lisa Mertz, PhD, LMT, Program Coordinator, Massage Therapy Program, Queensborough Community College/City University of New York, Bayside, NY

Michael J. Konsor, LMT, Instructor, Glendale Career College, Glendale, CA

Cynthia Gill, LMT, Instructor, Body Business School of Massage Therapy, Durant, OK

Samuel Gill, LMT, Instructor, Body Business School of Massage Therapy, Durant, OK

Sarita Kalu, PhD, LMT, Former Owner of Maat Institute, and Mind and Body Spa, St. Louis, MO

Kevin Snedden, LMT, Owner, Holistic Touch Training Center, LLC, Spa Manager/Consultant Argosy Casino Hotel & Spa, Chairman, Missouri State Board of Therapeutic Massage, President, Federation of State Massage Therapy Boards, Kearney, MO

Nan Gillett, BS, LMI, LMT, Massage Therapy Instructor, El Paso Community College, El Paso, TX

Dana Sullivan, LMBT, Instructor, Miller-Motte Technical College, Cary, NC

Ryan Jay Hoyme, Massage Program Coordinator, Minnesota School of Business, Rochester, MN

PHOTOGRAPHY CREDITS

Photography taken on location by Yanik Chauvin, yc@image-y.com.

Additional Photo Credits

Part 1 Opener: Image copyright 2009, Angels at Work. Used under license from Shutterstock.com

Chapter 1 Opener: Image copyright 2009, ChipPix. Used under license from Shutterstock.com

Chapter 2 Opener: Image copyright 2009, Phil Date. Used under license from Shutterstock.com

Chapter 3 Opener: Image copyright 2009, Sklep Spozywczy. Used under license from Shutterstock.com

Part 2 Opener: Image copyright 2009, Terekhov Igor. Used under license from Shutterstock.com

Chapter 4 Opener: Image copyright 2009, Yanik Chauvin. Used under license from Shutterstock.com

Chapter 5 Opener: Image copyright 2009, Vadim Ponomarenko. Used under license from Shutterstock.com

Chapter 7 Opener: Image copyright Paul Whitted, 2009. Used under license from Shutterstock.com

Part 3 Opener: Image copyright 2009, Liv friis-larsen. Used under license from Shutterstock.com

Chapter 8 Opener: Image copyright 2009, Yanik Chauvin. Used under license from Shutterstock.com

Chapter 10 Opener: Image copyright 2009, Faithworks Communications House. Used under license from Shutterstock.com

Chapter 11 Opener: Image copyright 2009, Matka Wariatka. Used under license from Shutterstock.com

Chapter 12 Opener: Image copyright 2009, Image Worx. Used under license from Shutterstock.com

Chapter 13 Opener: Image copyright 2009, János Gehring. Used under license from Shutterstock.com

Chapter 14 Opener: Image copyright 2009, Stephen Coburn. Used under license from Shutterstock.com

Chapter 15 Opener: Image copyright 2009, Yuri Arcurs. Used under license from Shutterstock.com

Chapter 17 Opener: Image copyright 2009, VG Studio. Used under license from Shutterstock.com

Chapter 18 Opener: Image copyright 2009, Dmitriy Shironosov. Used under license from Shutterstock.com

Figure 1-2	Image copyright Matthew Collingwood, 2009. Used under license from Shutterstock.com
Figure 1-3	Image copyright CAN BALCIOGLU, 2009. Used under license from Shutterstock.com
Figure 1-4	Reprinted with permission from Spa Research Fellowship
Figure 1-5	Reprinted with permission from Spa Research Fellowship
Figure 1-7	Reprinted with permission from Spa Research Fellowship
Figure 2-1	Courtesy of Hershey Entertainment & Resorts Company, Hershey, PA
Table 2-1	Courtesy International Spa Association (ISPA)
Figure 2-2	Courtesy International Spa Association (ISPA)
Figure 2-3	Courtesy SpaQuality LLC
Figure 2-4	Courtesy SpaQuality LLC
Figure 2-5	Courtesy SpaQuality LLC
Table 2-3	Courtesy International Spa Association (ISPA)
Table 2-4	Courtesy International Spa Association (ISPA)
Figure 2-6	Image copyright Yanik Chauvin, 2009. Used under license from Shutterstock.com
Table 2-5	Courtesy International Spa Association (ISPA)
Table 2-6	Courtesy International Spa Association (ISPA)
Figure 2-7a	Courtesy International Spa Association (ISPA)
Figure 2-7b	Courtesy of The Day Spa Association
Figure 3-1	Courtesy of Sattva Spa, Denver, Colorado
Figure 3-4	Photo courtesy of Massage Warehouse
Figure 3-5a	Photo courtesy of Massage Warehouse
Figure 3-5b	Photo courtesy of Massage Warehouse
Figure 3-5c	Photo courtesy of Massage Warehouse
Figure 3-14	Photo courtesy of Richard Eidson
Figure 3-25	Courtesy Natural Resources Spa Consulting, Inc.

CHAPTER 1

Spa History

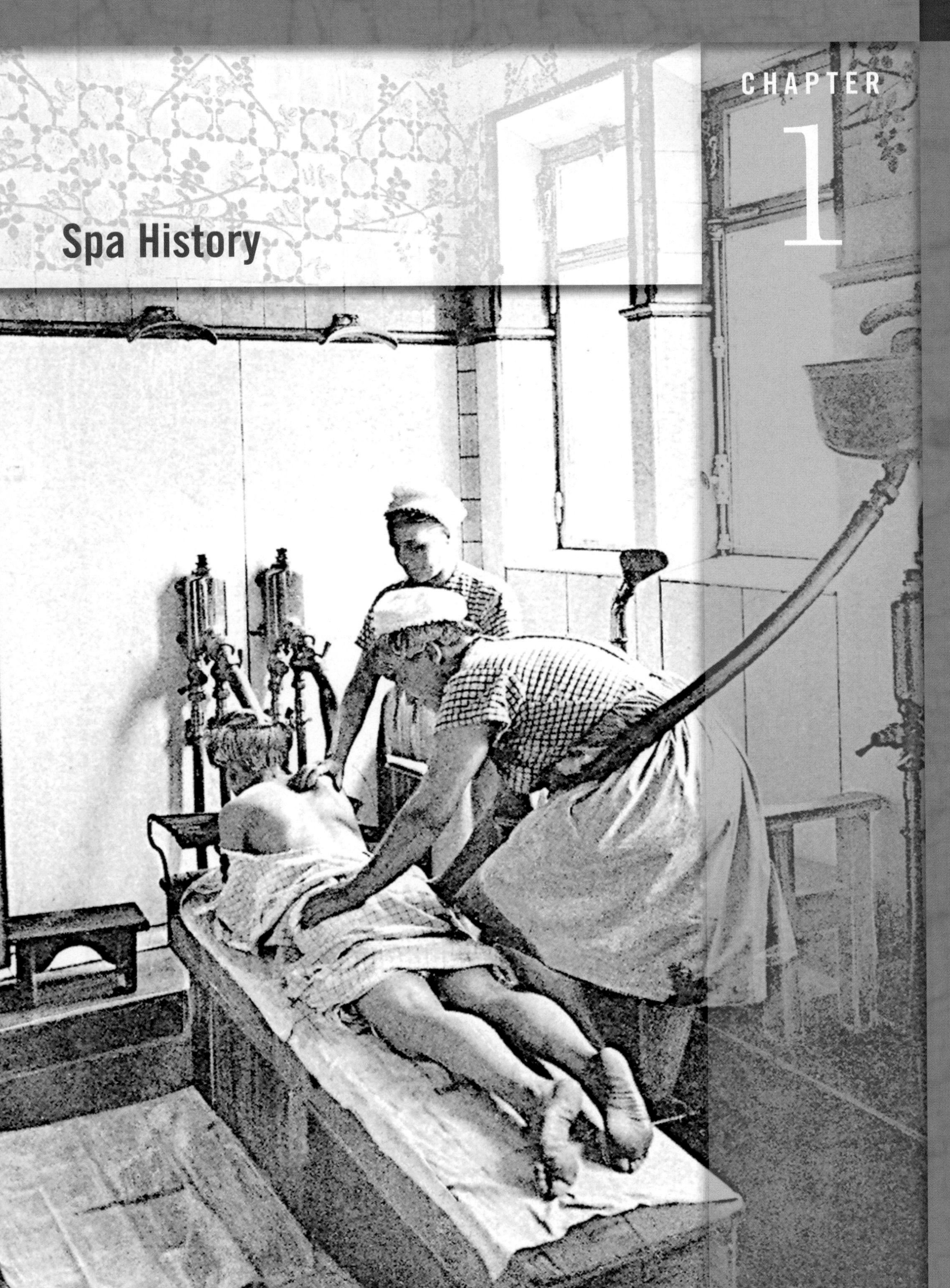

LEARNING OBJECTIVES

1. **Explain the origins of spas and the word *spa* itself.**
2. **Describe the historical roots of Greek and Roman bathing practices.**
3. **Describe spa practices used in ancient Roman baths.**
4. **Describe the layout of ancient Roman baths with specific rooms and their uses.**
5. **Explain the use of hammams in Islamic cultures and describe traditional practices used there.**
6. **Explain the historical role of the massage therapist in various spas around the world.**
7. **Explain the historical development of spas in Europe after the Roman Empire.**
8. **Describe the healing philosophy of the "father of modern hydrotherapy" Sebastian Kneipp.**
9. **Explain the historical development of spa therapies in the Americas.**
10. **Describe features of some historical Asian spas, specifically Japanese.**

INTRODUCTION

Spas have been around for a long, long time. Thousands of years, in fact. Ever since humans developed the technology that made it possible to harness the powers of water for pleasure and therapy, they have done so. And even long beforehand, in the lost recesses of pre-history, people all around the planet surely used natural hot springs, cold rivers, stones, plants, and touch to heal themselves and each other. These were the proto-spas of our race. The spas that we enjoy today did not spring up out of nowhere but rather were born from long experience over hundreds of generations. This is the world you are entering and which you will inhabit as a spa therapist.

You will be working with the accumulated experience and knowledge of those who have gone before you, and thus it is appropriate to take a look, in this first chapter, at the history of spas throughout the ages. Perhaps the most famous historical spas are those in ancient Rome, but they are by no means the only ones. This chapter will also cover spas from Turkey, Greece, Asia, and even the New World, among other areas. You will find many differences among these spas. Some were built for the exclusive use of men. Others were for women only. Still others were for both sexes. Some spas were considered almost sacred and reserved for quiet, contemplative experiences, while others were raucous meeting places filled with commerce, entertainment, sports, and other activities. Whatever their particular characteristics, they all shared a common origin in that most precious and useful of natural resources: water.

IN THE BEGINNING—SPAS' WATERY ROOTS

Water (Figure 1–1) is the essence of many spa services. It is the environment in which much of the healing and rejuvenation at spas take place. We know from archeological studies and written accounts that the earliest spas were often found at the source of a natural spring or, in the case of the ancient Romans for example, at sites to which such water was redirected via aqueducts. So, what exactly does the word "spa" mean? By some accounts, it is an acronym, which is a word formed by putting together the first letters of other words. In this case, they are the words "*sanitas per aqua*" or any of several variations on those Latin words, all of which mean the same thing: "health through water." This belief, however, is somewhat misleading (see Did You Know). Various other stories about the derivation of the word have circulated over the centuries. Some say the term *espa* derived from the Latin verb *spagere,* which means "to sprinkle or flow," like a fountain or spring. Others cite a Belgian spring called Espa, from the Walloon language word for "fountain."

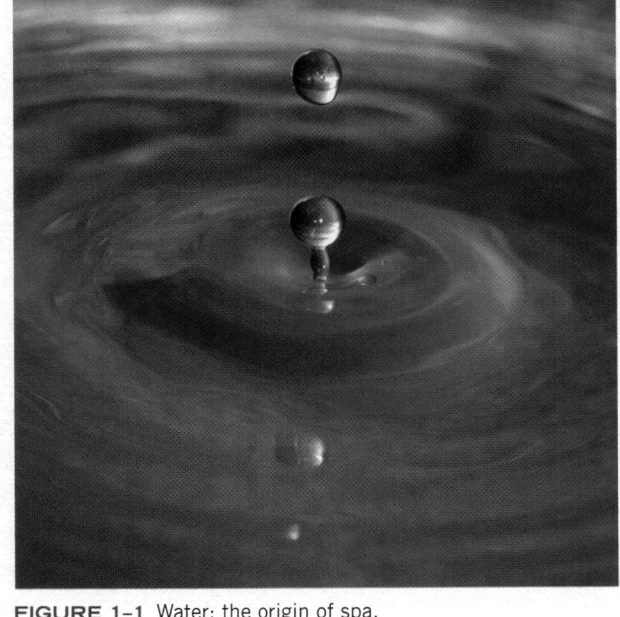

FIGURE 1–1 Water: the origin of spa.

In spite of the folklore and mystery surrounding the origins of the word, it can be stated with certainty that our modern usage of the word "spa" came to us from the Belgian town of the same name, where spring waters rich in iron have been used for centuries to treat various illnesses. In sixteenth-century England, people began using springs medicinally in the same manner. One such spring, the Harrogate Tewit Well, was referred to in 1596 by English physician Dr. Timothy Bright as the "English Spaw." In this manner, the term *spa* began to be used as a general description of a place with healing waters, rather than the one specific place in Belgium alone. The waters at these early spas provided their healing primarily through ingestion, rather than bathing, but over the years both internal and external applications became customary.

Spas have always been all about water. Drinking medicinal waters. Soaking in mineral-laden waters. Inhaling the vapors of steaming water. Gazing at the tranquil waters of a spring-fed pond deep in the forest. Wherever people came together to enjoy these waters and take advantage of their healing properties, the spirit of spa was alive. In many cultures, communal bathing became a part of this

The Spa Acronym Conundrum

Did You Know?

The letters S.P.A. are sometimes said to stand for an acronym of various Latin words, including:

Sanus per aquam
Salus per aqua } health through water
Sanitas per aqua
Solus per Aqua – water in itself

All of these, though, are most likely "backcronyms" rather than acronyms. A backronym is a word thought to be originally coined as an acronym; in reality, its source was different and the acronym was applied later. Acronyms, with one exception, have only been used since the beginning of the twentieth century. The exception, "SPQR," is, not surprisingly, Roman, and stood for *Senatus Populusque Romanus.*

spa experience. Early Mesopotamians, Egyptians, and Minoans sought health and healing through the use of public baths thousands of years ago, but it was not until the Greeks and Romans came along that the art was truly taken to its peaks. The Greeks enjoyed baths as far back as 500 BC. In fact, one of the most famous battles of all times took place on the site of a hot springs that was used as for communal bathing. When the legendary 300 Spartan warriors first arrived at Thermopylae in August 480 BC to defend the narrow passage from invading Persians, they found bathers enjoying the springs and had to advise them to leave prior to the great battle. The word *Thermopylae* itself comes from the Greek for "hot gates." The gates refer to the narrow passage between the sea and the cliffs that existed there at that time, and the heat, of course, refers to the hot springs.

The Greeks enjoyed natural hot springs like those at Thermopylae, and they also partook in more formalized bathing and sweating. Homer, among others, wrote that Greeks developed basic hot water tubs and hot air baths known as **laconica**, named after the region where Sparta was located, and where the idea originated. The laconica were built next to a gymnasium, in a round shape with a high tapering conical roof that could be closed or opened to permit the escape of hot hair and steam. These were basic structures heated with hot coals or hot rocks, and although the ancient Greeks created the foundations for future development in bathing, and they definitely enjoyed the pleasures and purifications that hydrotherapy offered, their efforts were rudimentary compared to those that followed during the days of the Roman Empire.

laconica

hot, dry chambers in Roman baths, similar to today's sauna, named after the more ancient Greek hot air bath (singular **laconicum**)

THE ROMAN BATHS

For at least 200 years prior to the opening of the first grand scale bath, Roman citizens enjoyed smaller-scale baths known as **balnea**, which were inspired by the Greek laconica. Each balneum was designed for use by a particular neighborhood, where they stood five to a block on average in Rome. These modest facilities were so popular that a succession of Roman emperors was inspired to eventually create much larger baths, calling them **thermae**, after the Greek word for heat. It was Marcus Agrippa, Augustus Caesar's trusted friend and general who, in 25 BC, began construction on the first of the larger-scale baths, which bore his name. After that time, thermae became an important part of many an emperor's legacy, and successive leaders seemed to vie with each other for the creation of ever more opulent bathing facilities. Among the most important of these, each named in honor of the emperor who commissioned its construction, were Nero (65 AD), Titus (81 AD), Domitian (95 AD), Commodus (185 AD), Caracalla (217 AD), Diocletian (305 AD), and Constantine (351 AD).

In 33 BC, there were 170 public and private baths in the city of Rome. At the end of the fourth century AD, there were 11 grand thermae and almost a thousand private baths or balnea. The baths of Diocletian alone could hold 3,000 bathers at one time. With the institution of these baths both in Rome and in its far-flung provinces, and the construction of the massive aqueduct system to supply them, the average Roman citizen used 300 gallons of water per day, compared to just 50 gallons per day for the modern American. The baths were very important, not just for cleansing, but for health, fitness, and as a social gathering place.

balnea

smaller neighborhood communal bathing facilities of the Roman Empire, precursor to the much larger and more grand Thermae (singular **balneum**)

thermae

Roman name for their central communal bathing complexes, constructed by emperors, which featured sports halls, restaurants, massage areas, and various types of baths; *thermae* means heat in Greek

The larger baths could accommodate thousands of people, and entrance fees were kept extremely modest so that even the most humble of citizens could enjoy them. Emperors subsidized these colossal projects in order to gain fame and popularity, and the emperors themselves enjoyed the baths as much as anyone else. Some were reported to have bathed several times a day. Poetry was read in the baths. Political discussions were held. Exercise and sport were common, as were the preparation, sale, and consumption of food and drink. And, of course, there was massage.

Although attending the public baths was a big part of daily life for huge numbers of Romans, not every citizen was a big fan of spas. Some people felt that the baths inspired indolence, gluttony, and an overall weakening of health. The famous rhetorician Seneca wrote an unflattering description of a typical bath that he happened to live next to:

> Imagine all these kinds of voices . . . While the sporting types take exercise with dumb-bells, either working hard or pretending to do so, I hear groans; every time they release the breath they have been holding, I hear sibilant and jarring respiration. When I meet some idle fellow content with a cheap massage, I hear the smack of a hand on the shoulders, and, according to if it is open or closed when it strikes, it gives a different sound. If a ball-player appears on the scene and begins to count the scores, I'm finished! Suppose there is also some brawler, and a thief caught in the act, and a man who likes the sound of his own voice while taking his bath. Then there are the bathers who leap into the pool, making a mighty splash. But all these people at least have a natural voice. Just imagine the shrill and strident cries of the attendants who pluck the hair from the bathers' bodies, who never cease their noise except when they are plucking the hair from somebody's armpits and making another scream instead of themselves. Then there are various cries of the pastry cooks, the sausage-sellers, and all the hawkers from the cook-shops, who advertise their wares with a sing-song all their own. (Stobart, 1961, p. 337)

In addition to the noise mentioned by Seneca, the baths also featured poets trying to outdo each other, reciting their poetry aloud in hopes of winning a dinner invitation from a wealthy patron. There was gambling going on, board games being played, philosophy being loudly espoused, prostitution being practiced, and an overall raucousness that is quite dissimilar from what we consider a spa to be today.

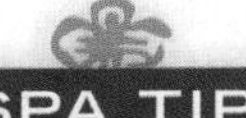

SPA TIP

As proven by the discovery of oil lamps at the baths in Pompeii, night-time bathing was sometimes practiced by ancient Romans.

SPA TIP

"It would be a mistake to assume that the average Roman engaged in strenuous exercise before taking his bath, like the Greek athletes. Roman gymnastics was merely a prelude to bathing, a form of recreation, and not intended as training for competition. The 'athletes' were often elderly and not necessarily in good shape, but they hoped to improve their health and ward off disease through exercise."

from *Baths and Bathing in Classical Antiquity* by Fikret Yegül

apodyterium
changing room in a Roman bath

palaestra
exercise area found at many early Roman bath houses, modeled after the ancient Greek wrestling schools

hypocaust
a hollow space in the floor or walls of ancient Roman spas into which hot air was created by fires for heating a room or bath

tepidarium
coolest of the warmed rooms in a Roman bath, where patrons received massage

Layout of the Roman Bath

When Roman citizens visited the baths, they had a choice of many different environments in which to spend their time. Arriving after the workday was over in the early afternoon, they would often first visit the changing area, or **apodyterium**, where they would leave their clothes under the supervision of bath workers, or, if they were more well-to-do, with their own servants or slaves. It was not wise to leave property unguarded in the baths, which were a notorious haunt of thieves. Many patrons would take advantage of the **palaestra** for some exercise before bathing, perhaps engaging in ball games, wrestling, or boxing. From there, patrons progressed through a series of rooms warmed to varying temperatures by a fire kept raging below the stone floors of the building in a furnace-like room called the **hypocaust**. Each of these rooms had a special name. The **tepidarium**, or warm

Meet the Original Massage Therapist—A Slave

Did You Know?

The typical Roman masseur was a skilled slave. These slaves either belonged to the owner of the bath house, or to a particular wealthy patron who would bring them along to the baths for his own private use. Some Roman citizens even had private baths at their own villas where their slaves would perform massage for them. Various of these slaves also became expert at blending aromatic oils and also at cleansing and exfoliating the skin. Several types of oil were used for massage at this time, including olive, sesame, and almond, and among the most common essential oils added were thyme, lavender, and rose.

Following in the Greek tradition, oils and sand would often be applied to the skin of Roman spa goers, usually before exercise, and this needed to be cleaned off afterwards with water and special instruments called **strigils**, which are described in Chapter 6. Thus, these ancient slaves employed aromatherapy, massage therapy, and hydrotherapy, as well as exfoliation techniques, and in this sense they could be considered very similar to the spa therapists of today.

Not much is known about the actual massage maneuvers employed by these slave therapists, but we know one thing at least: There was extensive and vigorous tapotement involved, at least in some of the massages, as described by a famous chronicler of the time. Suffice it to say that the typical massage given by a masseur/slave was likely to be a rather invigorating experience compared to the tranquil and relaxing spa massages of today.

These ancient therapists could be found working in several areas of the bath, often in the tepidarium. Some texts mention special rooms for offering massage, called **unctorium**, which comes from the Latin *unctio*, which means anointing. Thus, it is likely that these therapists were known as *unctors*. Another word, **aleipterion**, which came from the Greek, was used to describe warm rooms for the application of oil, but eventually, after the time of Augustus Cesar, it came to describe larger portions of the structure or the entire bath, not just the massage area.

strigil

metal scraper used by ancient Romans to exfoliate the skin

unctorium

room for applying oil massage in an ancient Roman bath

aleipterion

warmed room for applying oil in an early Roman bath

caldarium

main hot room in Roman baths

frigidarium

coldest room in the Roman thermae, with cold water plunges, where bathers cooled down after sweating in the other heated chambers

room, is where massage often took place. It also had a large bathing pool. The **caldarium** was much hotter and featured baths of different temperatures as well. The floor was heated to such a degree in this room that Romans needed to wear sandals to walk upon it. The laconica was even hotter and could be compared to a modern-day sauna, where hot, dry air permeated the space and induced profuse sweating. After heating their bodies and building up a good sweat, bathers usually paid a visit to the **frigidarium**, which featured one or more large unheated pools. The modern-day equivalent is the cold plunge featured at many spas. See Chapter 5 for more information about cold plunges. Linen towels were available to vigorously rub the skin dry afterward, leaving patrons refreshed and revitalized.

Romans did not have a set pattern for visiting the bath chambers, and patrons could experience any area they chose in any order they wished. The entire indoor area was kept perpetually warmed. Several days were needed to heat a thermae, and it was not practical to heat them up and cool them down. The hypocausts kept hot air flowing under floors and through walls at all times. The amazing system of Roman aqueducts kept a plentiful supply of water streaming in for use in the baths. All of this activity took place under magnificent vaulted ceilings, and the grounds surrounding the bath buildings themselves were often equally as impressive, with vast gardens, stately libraries, and private meeting rooms.

SPA TIP

The grand opening of a major spa was as important an occasion thousands of years ago as it is today. At the well-preserved thermae in Pompeii, Italy, a still-readable inscription is visible on one wall: "There will be a dedication of the baths and the public is promised a slaughter of wild beasts, athletics, awnings to shade the sun, and perfumed sprinklings."

As Roman civilization spread, so too did the use of the baths. "*Bene lave*" (meaning "have a good bath!") was a familiar greeting for people in the Roman empire stretching from northern Africa all the way to England. Many Roman outposts were built at the site of a spring so that one of their baths could be constructed there. Some of these locations still feature spas today, and some, like Bath in England (Figure 1–2), have undergone extensive recent renovations.

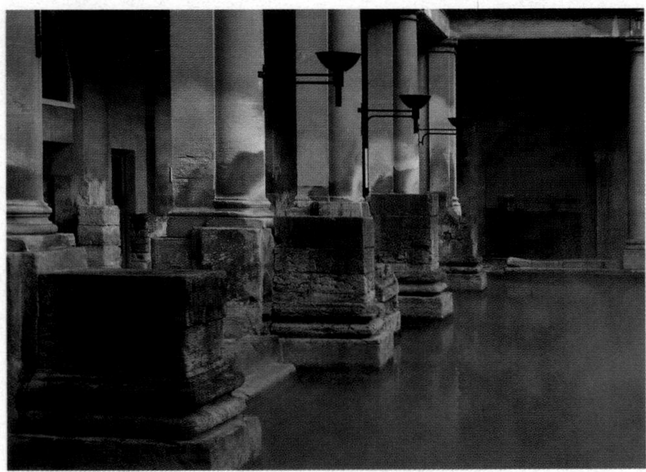

FIGURE 1–2 Roman baths at Bath, England.

THE TURKISH HAMMAM

Descendants of the Roman thermae, **hammams** developed as an integral feature of daily life in the Ottoman Empire (1299–1923). Men and women bathe separately in the hammam, which, besides being a social center of the community, also holds spiritual significance. Often, the atmosphere inside the hot steamy main chamber known as the **sicaklik**, where bathers are scrubbed and massaged, seems more like a church than a spa, with diffused lighting streaming down from small glass windows in the domed ceiling, and silence reigns. Some form of the hammam, which means "heat" in Arabic, has been incorporated into the culture of Arabic peoples for centuries.

hammams

found in Islamic countries, the hammam, called a "Turkish bath" in the West, is a communal bath house, usually quite ornate, with separate facilities for men and women

sicaklik

main heated chamber in a hammam, where the massage and exfoliation take place

Western nations, including England and the United States, have imported the concept of the hammam, which they called Turkish baths, with varying degrees of success. A British diplomat, David Urquhart, first popularized the concept in England in the 1850s. Turkish baths became quite popular, and since that time, over 600 such baths have opened in Britain alone, with many more in other countries, including the U.S., where Dr. Charles Shepard opened the first one in 1863. In spite of such success, the hammam has

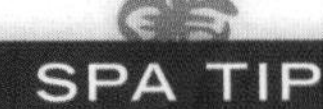

SPA TIP

Although Roman baths are often associated with debauchery and orgies, during most of the Roman Empire, bathing was not a co-ed experience. Women typically came to the baths earlier in the day, and men arrived after noon. Mixed bathing was sometimes practiced in the larger pools, but it was not until near the end of the Empire that these standards were relaxed and licentious behavior between bathers became more common.

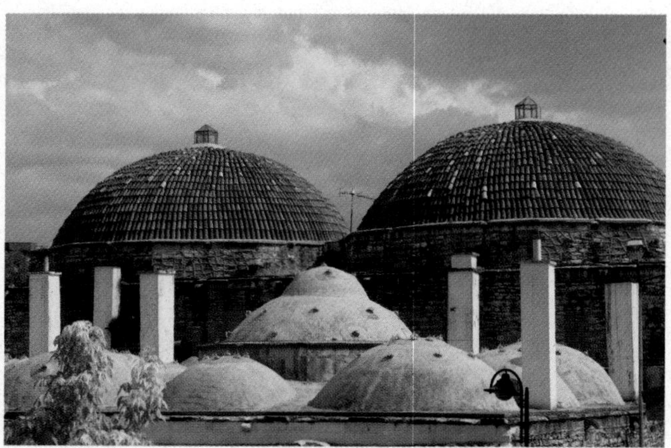

FIGURE 1–3 Islamic hammams were monumental and beautiful structures similar to Roma thermae.

not achieved the widespread use and acceptance elsewhere that it has in Turkey and several other parts of the Islamic world, where it is ubiquitous and tightly interwoven into the daily lives of most people, being used as a social gathering place for many occasions.

As far as the hammam facility itself, very little changed from the system first implemented in the Roman thermae. The original hammams of the Ottoman Empire were, at first, structurally part of mosques, but they quickly evolved into separate facilities and then monumental complexes designed by the greatest architects in the Islamic world (Figure 1–3).

camekan
changing room in a hammam

gobektasi
large heated marble platform found in hammams, upon which scrubbing and massage are performed by tellaks

sogukluk
in a hammam, the cool chamber for relaxing after massage and scrub received in a heated chamber

The typical hammam consists of a changing area, or **camekan**, which is lined with changing cubicles, with a fountain in the center. The sicaklik (similar to the caldarium) is the main heated chamber, and this is where massage and vigorous exfoliation take place atop a large heated marble slab called a **gobektasi**, which means "belly stone." The cool room (similar to the frigidarium), is called the **sogukluk**. This is where patrons can relax, have a cup of tea, and perhaps doze off in a private cubicle.

EUROPEAN SPAS

When the Roman Empire fell, the magnificent thermae crumbled into ruins (Figure 1–4). Over the ensuing years, baths and bathing rose and fell in popularity, reaching a famed nadir in the Middle Ages, when bathing was considered by many to be bad for one's health. Some organized bathing took place even at this time, however, most notably in the court of Charlemagne in the late eighth century. According to the emperor's biographer, one of the main reasons Charlemagne chose Aachen for his court rather than Rome was because he enjoyed swimming in the city's thermal baths, which he visited often with family and guests. So, it can be seen that even during times when bathing was most out of favor, some adherents were still enjoying its healing properties.

SPA TIP

The opulence and grandeur of ancient spas has inspired the creation of many fabulous modern spas. For a list of some of the best spas around today, take a look at *100 Best Spas of the World,* an informative and inspirational book by Bernard Burt and Pamela Joy Price.

The Ottoman Empire, as noted, saw a resurgence in the popularity of the baths with their hammams, which spread into Europe. By the time of the Renaissance, there were several established spa towns across Europe, including Paeffers in Switzerland, Baden-Baden and Karlsbad in Germany, Montecatini and Saturnia in Italy, Bath in England, and, of course, Spa in Belgium. Czechoslovakia, Hungary, Bulgaria, and several other European countries also have a history of spa culture. The first scientific book on the Czech spa treatment regimen for treating disease was published in 1522. The locales where such spas operate are still known today as "spa towns" (Figure 1–5). They owe their existence to the water source and the therapies that were applied there. In addition, the Finns

Did You Know?

Massage Therapists in the Hammam

When you visit a hammam, you experience an intense form of spa therapy consisting of vigorous scrubbing and firm massage strokes, all taking place in a hot steamy chamber. The massage therapist uses a coarse mitten, known as a **kese**, to scrub your skin. Other people are around you, beneath a high domed ceiling. Hot water is poured over your body to wash away the soap and grime from the outside world. You are given a pair of wooden clogs, or **nalins**, so you will not slip on the wet marble floors, and you wear a wrap called a **pesternal** around your body.

Massage workers in hammams are known as **tellaks**. Originally, hundreds of years ago, these were primarily young boys who not only massaged and exfoliated patrons but also often acted as prostitutes for their male clients as well. In fact, a book in the Ottoman archives called *Dellakname-i Dilkusa* (The Record of Tellaks) offers surprising detail about the services performed by these bath workers: their rates, their relative beauty, and their ability to satisfy their customers. Tellaks were recruited from non-Muslim nations under the Turkish Empire, such as Jews, Albanians, Bulgarians, Lebanese, Greeks, and others. The relationships that formed between a tellak and his clients could become very intimate and emotional. Wars were fought over these young massage boys. Moguls and sultans prized their companionship.

After the fall of the Ottoman Empire and the modernization that followed, the tellaks no longer fulfilled this sexual function. Today, hammam therapists are adults who offer spa therapy, not prostitution. Female hammam attendants are known as a **natirs** and work on women. But in spite of this reformation, the term "hammam oglani," or "bath boy," is used in Turkish as a euphemism for a homosexual.

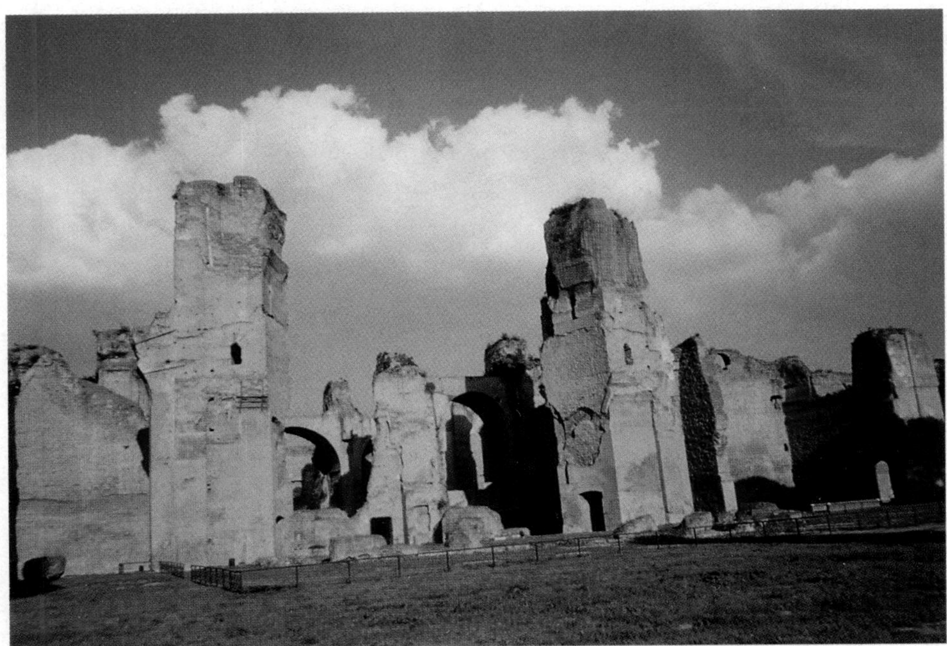

FIGURE 1–4 Ruins of the ancient Roman baths of Caracalla.

kese

a coarse mitten carried in the soap case, it not only scoured the dirt out of the pores, but also served to deliver a bracing massage; it was specially woven out of hair or plant fibers

nalins

the wooden clogs, often ornate, worn in the hammam to help avoid slipping

pesternal

ornate cloth or silk wrap worn around the body while at a hammam

tellaks

hammam workers, providing massage and exfoliation; in ancient times, sexual favors and sometimes close emotional relationships with clients were also a part of the tellak's role

natirs

female versions of the tellaks, traditional hammam workers

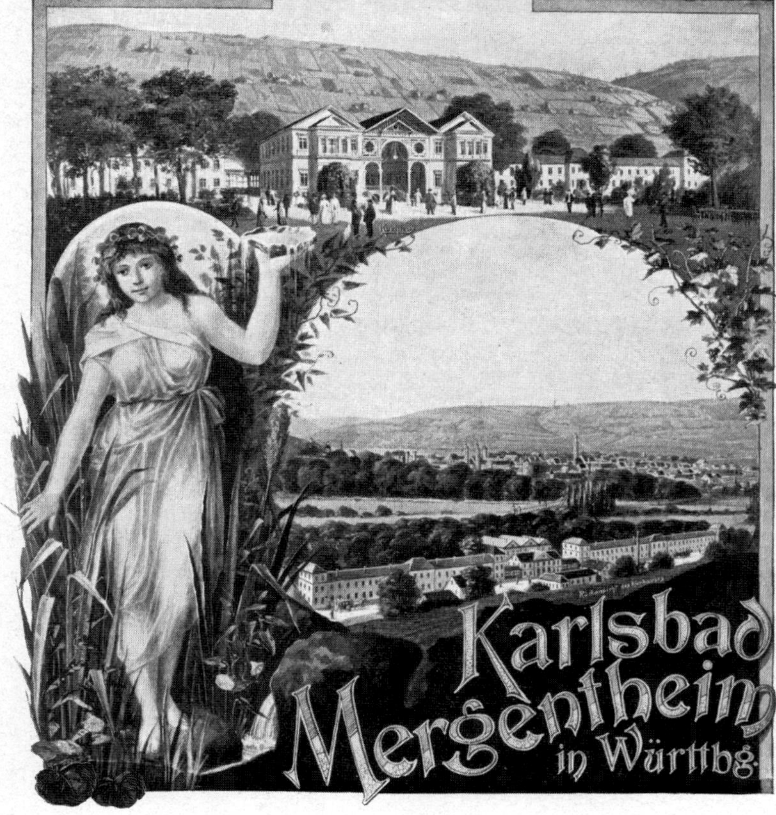

FIGURE 1–5 Advertisement for an early European spa in a typical spa town, Karlsbad, Germany.

banya

traditional Russian communal steam bath

crenotherapy

from the Greek "crene," which means "rising," any treatment incorporating spring water, mud, and vapor

became famous during this period for their saunas, and the Russians for their **banyas** (as will be explained in Chapter 5), but these are not full-fledged spa facilities as we have come to think of them.

For centuries, Europeans have gone to such locations to "take the cure" and undergo **crenotherapy** using the natural mineral waters found there, hoping to stimulate digestion, improve the immune system, and even cure disease. In Europe, to this day, spa philosophy continues to be more remedial and medically oriented than spa philosophy in the New World. Many European health plans pay for spa visits and spa treatments. Spa goers are likely to be prescribed a regime by medical personnel on staff at the spa. This regime may include multiple immersions in therapeutic waters and even the ingestion of mineral-laden spring waters in an attempt to improve physical conditions.

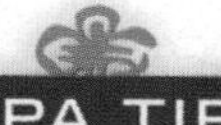

SPA TIP

If you want to pronounce the word "spa" like a native of the town Spa in Belgium does, start with an "sh" sound as if you were going to say "shopping," and then add the "pa" for the slightly Germanic sounding word, "shpa."

SEBASTIAN KNEIPP

Sebastian Kneipp (pronounced "knipe") was a towering figure in the world of hydrotherapy and natural healing. Born in Germany in 1821, he fell ill with tuberculosis at the age of 28 and was able to cure himself by following the advice he found in a little-known manual on hydrotherapy. His primary method for this self-cure was frequent immersions in the frigid waters of the Danube river,

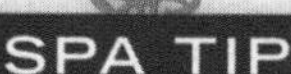

SPA TIP

"Water is not the source of life, it is life"

— Antoine de Saint-Exupéry

which, he believed, would literally shock his body back into health. His plan worked.

Kneipp became a priest and used some of the healing methods he had developed through self-experimentation to treat severely ill people. When some of these people recovered, he gained notoriety, eventually writing a book on the subject. The publication of *My Water Cure* (*Meine Wasserkur* in German) in 1886 became a phenomenon and catapulted him to fame, making him one of the best known people in Germany. He published another book, *The Way You Should Live*, in 1889, cementing his fame and influence. More than simply a treatment method, Kneipp's **kur** entailed an entire lifestyle change centered upon natural living. He claimed that this lifestyle, which he practiced and taught for 42 years in the spa village of Bad Worishofen, Germany, consisted of five main components, or pillars.

kur

German word meaning (course of) treatment, or cure, often used in conjunction with "wasser," meaning water; *Wasserkur* can mean "hydrotherapy" and specifically that type taught by German healer Sebastian Kneipp

The Five Pillars of Kneipp Therapy

Kneipp encouraged people to lead a healthy lifestyle that included physical exercise, wholesome foods, and five specialized practices that can be considered direct precursors to the modern day spa lifestyle. These practices are: hydrotherapy, phytotherapy, exercise, nutrition, and lifestyle.

Hydrotherapy

Sebastian Kneipp was considered by many to be the "father of modern hydrotherapy." He developed over 100 treatments involving the use of water in all its forms: solid, liquid, and steam. You will learn how to perform many of these treatments in Section 2. The powerful effects of water, both hot and cold, proved to be helpful for even the most seriously ill of Kneipp's patients. During his lifetime he became known as the "water doctor" and was known to have cured many people.

SPA TIP

Sebastian Kneipp created certain hydrotherapy treatments that might be considered strange by some people. Some of his more exotic creations include:

Dew Walking: walking barefoot on dew-moistened grass to promote circulation and strengthen the immune system

Water Treading: walking in a body of water filled below the knee, such as large basin, bathtub, fountain, lake, or ocean, to strengthen veins, induce sleep, and stimulate metabolism

Snow Walking: walking barefoot in snow from a few seconds up to three minutes to stimulate the immune system and promote circulation

Phytotherapy

Kneipp proved through his research that certain herbs and plants could support healing, and he developed several products such as teas, ointments, and oils for use in baths, herbal wraps, and other treatments. The use of such products is called **phytotherapy**, and many of his formulations are still used in spas around the world today under the Kneipp brand.

Exercise

Kneipp believed that regular physical exercise stimulates natural bodily functions in the musculoskeletal, cardiovascular, digestive, and nervous systems. He also considered massage to be an important supplement to exercise.

phytotherapy

the use of plants or plant extracts for medicinal purposes, especially plants that are not part of the normal diet

Nutrition

Because he experienced it in his own life, Kneipp knew that many diseases could be avoided or cured through the implementation of a proper nutritious diet consisting of simple foods prepared with care so that their minerals and vitamins were not lost.

kivas

large chambers, often wholly or partly underground, in a Pueblo Indian village, used for religious ceremonies and other purposes, sometimes heated to create a sauna-like environment

temazcal

a native steam-bath that was in general use in Mesoamerican cultures, from the Nahuatl language meaning "bath house" or "house of heat"

Temazcalera

specially trained healer who conducts sessions using heat, herbs, and sometimes massage in the temazcal, or Mexican sweat lodge

Lifestyle

Kneipp taught people to live a balanced lifestyle that was in harmony with the natural environment and the surrounding culture. He also taught people to be self-reliant about their own health and showed them how they could pursue the "five pillars" on their own at home. Kneipp lived to be 76 years old and died in 1897 after a long and productive life made possible by adherence to his own five principles.

AMERICAN SPA ROOTS

In the Americas, hot springs have been revered as sacred healing sites for centuries. Native Americans often set these places apart and agreed not to fight or hunt in them. They also created their own early "spas" by pouring water over heated stones in small enclosures called *sweat lodges*. Southwest Indians such as the Anasazi constructed special ceremonial structures known as **kivas**, in which they performed rites and induced sweats. These rites are still carried out today by modern tribe members and other interested people. Usually a group experience, the sweat lodge was used for purification, worship, and for strengthening social bonds. Often, young men would enter the lodge, which was then heated to extreme temperatures. It was thought that by taking on this suffering, the stronger members of the community could symbolically help relieve the suffering of the older, weaker, or sickly members.

One particular type of early American sweat lodge, the **temazcal** (Figure 1–6), took root in pre-Columbian Mexico, where they could be found in every village, no matter how small or remote. The Nahuatl Indians gave the temazcal its name, meaning "house of heat" or "bath house." These special igloo-shaped dwellings were turned into steam chambers by introducing red-hot volcanic rocks, which were then covered with herbs and water to produce a therapeutic vapor. A specially trained healer, called the **Temazcalera**, directs the experience, using a vent and a fan to control the heat and humidity in the chamber. She chooses herbs to help promote healing of specific conditions, and she can even administer massage when called for. In the Nahuatl culture, the goddess of the sweat bath was Temazcalteci, "the grandmother of the baths," who was worshipped in every temazcal throughout the region. In addition, these bathing chambers were aligned in cosmic directions, with the fire being placed in the East where the sun god rose, and bathers entered the doorway from the South, which was thought to represent entry into and rebirth out of the womb. The Spanish conquistadors, naturally, reacted strongly against this practice, which they considered idol worship. Thus they banned the use of the temazcals and tried to eradicate them, but were never completely successful.

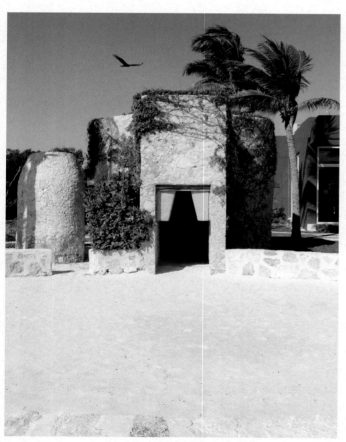

FIGURE 1–6 The Temazcal, an early Mesoamerican spa experience.

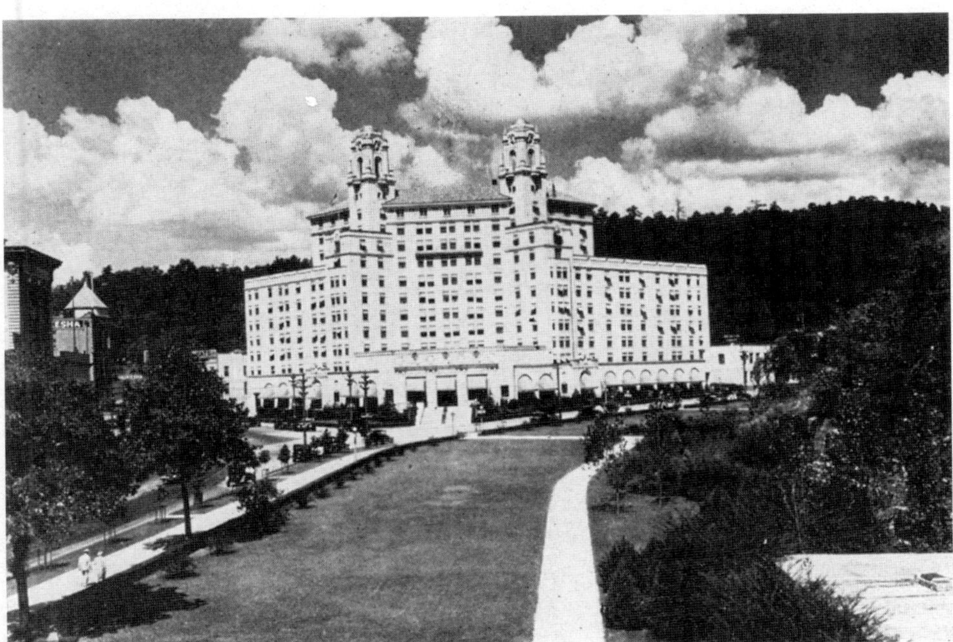

FIGURE 1–7 U.S. health spas or "sanatoriums" like the ones in Hot Springs, Arkansas were popular early in the 20th century and drew thousands of people to fancy new hotels like the Majestic.

During the nineteenth and early twentieth centuries, spa-like health retreats were built in many areas of North America, most notably Hot Springs, Arkansas (Figure 1–7), White Sulphur Springs, West Virginia, and Saratoga Springs, New York. These facilities were often referred to as **sanatoriums** because people visited them when attempting to cure themselves of diseases such as tuberculosis. John Harvey Kellogg opened the Battle Creek Sanatorium in Michigan. Typical treatments administered at these early hot springs health spas always included a soak in the mineral pools, which became very popular. Saratoga Hot Springs, for example, was first introduced in its natural state to white settlers by Native Americans in the 1700s, and by the early 1900s it was accommodating thousands of visitors a day in extensive facilities. Franklin Delano Roosevelt spent much time at Warm Springs, Georgia, where he originally went to help treat his polio, eventually purchasing the land and building a cottage which came to be called the Little White House.

sanatoriums

also spelled *sanitariums*, resorts for improvement or maintenance of health, especially for convalescents, early examples of which, such as the Kellogg Sanatorium in Battle Creek, Michigan, are thought of as precursors to the modern health spa

As the 1900s progressed, older facilities gave way to more modern spa ventures that focused on holistic health, fitness, diet, and overall well-being. The first such spa was the Golden Door in California, which opened in the late 1950s. Since that time, spas have continued to expand and modernize their offerings and facilities. See Chapter 2 for more information about present-day spas.

ASIAN SPA ROOTS

Many Asian cultures have a tradition of massage and hydrotherapy treatments that has been passed down through the ages. In Thailand, for example, these traditions have included the use of heated herbal poultices during massage, which was often performed on temple grounds or other special locations. You will learn more about these poultices and their use in Chapter 8. In Indonesia, ritualistic bathing and massage were developed hundreds of years ago, especially for royalty, and you will learn one example of these practices, the Lulur ritual from Java, in Chapter 12.

onsen

hot springs, and especially the bathing facilities and resorts around them, in Japan

In modern times, many Asian countries have developed thriving spa industries, but the country with the most extensive historical bathing practices in Asia is definitely Japan. Because it is such a volcanically active country, Japan is sprinkled with thousands of hot springs, or **onsen**, which have been used for communal bathing, personal renewal, and meditation for centuries. The word *onsen* has come to signify more than just the spring itself. It also includes the facilities and lodging that have grown up around these sites. So, in a way, the word can be understood as a traditional term for "spa" as we use it today. Onsen are always found in natural outdoor settings, and they feature baths of varying temperature. Treatments at many onsen include massage and hydrotherapy. Some Japanese people regard these sites as more than spa vacation destinations, but rather as spiritual retreats, where specific customs are to be observed.

According to tradition, men and women typically bathed together at the onsen, though this practice has become less common over the years. The onsen, in addition to providing sanitation and therapeutic waters, also became a central fixture of Japanese social life. Family, friends and even coworkers visit them in groups. They are considered to be a retreat from daily life. As such, the atmosphere in most onsen is tranquil. Noise is kept to a minimum, and the surroundings are intentionally beautiful, set in nature, with baths made of cypress, marble, or granite.

SPA PROFILE

Susie Ellis, President, SpaFinder, Inc. and Editor in Chief, SpaFinder.com

The Spa Community

Susie Ellis and her husband Peter purchased the spa-specific travel company, SpaFinder, in 2001. Since that time, they have greatly expanded the business, and it is now the leading media and marketing force in the spa industry, working with over 8,000 spas to provide marketing solutions, customer management technologies, gift certificate programs (SpaFinder and its new gift division, Salon Wish), publications, and research. The company has also used its technological expertise to develop an online booking and management system called SpaBooker. This means that spas have no need to install software on their own computers and that the program can be updated quickly and often. The system is of particular benefit to massage therapists, who can go on the Net to check their appointments and schedule for the day. "We were able to use the latest technology to come up with something truly different and valuable for businesses of all sizes," notes Ellis.

This willingness to embrace new technology and forge so many new directions in the industry has turned SpaFinder into a key player, not just in the U.S. but all around the world. As president of the multi-branched organization, Susie Ellis sits squarely in the hub of the ever-expanding global spa community. "This is exactly what it feels like," says Ellis. "We get to be in a place where we can see what's happening globally in the spa industry. We maintain a database that is quite broad—as there are tens of thousands of spas in the world and dozens of separate spa associations. We work with the industry and media internationally and we are proud to be deeply involved with the development of the Global Spa Summit. All of this activity is marketed via the Internet and through our publications."

Even though SpaFinder is embracing technology and all things new, Ellis puts a strong emphasis on traditional spa values that have been passed down through history. She studies the historical perspective on spas, all the way back to Greece and the Roman Empire, down through European developments and spas in the New World, right up

(Continued)

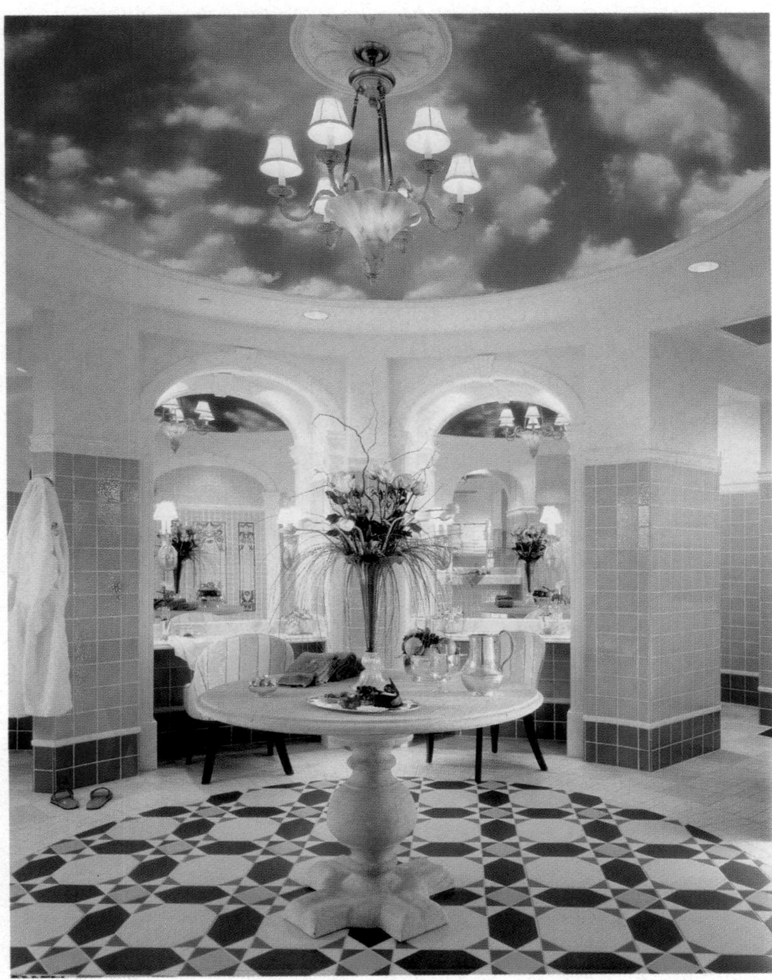

FIGURE 2–1 Some modern spa facilities are lavish.

at all. There are spas that offer psychological counseling, medical screening, shamanic vision-questing, Watsu®, team building, Turkish bathing rituals, rock climbing, tennis clinics, cooking classes, weight loss, skiing, women's retreats, and much more.

In recent years, spas have become specialized, with certain types of spas featuring specific offerings and catering to specific audiences, such as weight-loss spas, outdoor adventure spas, hydrotherapy spas, and others. All of this specialization has made education a priority in the spa industry, for two reasons. First, the public needs to be educated regarding spas in order to make the best choices for themselves when selecting a spa experience. Second, spa employees and potential employees need to be educated on the ever-growing number of modalities and special services available in order to perform them in a safe and effective manner.

THE STATE OF THE SPA INDUSTRY TODAY

The spa industry today is a dynamic and ever-changing segment of the economy that has seen tremendous growth in the late twentieth and early twenty-first centuries. Officially part of the **hospitality industry**, spas provide extremely

hospitality industry
the entire economic sector, including spas, that serves the public through lodging, dining, personal services, and entertainment offerings

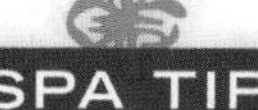

SPA TIP

With approximately 14,000 spas in the U.S. alone, it may seem like the marketplace is already overcrowded and you should not bother joining the industry. But if you divide total approximate spa revenues ($10 billion) by the total number of spas (14,000), you come up with the average income per spa, which is $714,286. Do you think that number makes it worthwhile to explore the spa industry a little further?

specialized services that set them apart from other choices when consumers are deciding where to spend their discretionary income. An increasing number of people are seeing the benefit of these services, as evidenced by the rising tide of spas and spa-going. The total number of U.S. spas almost quintupled during the late 1990s into the early 2000s, rising from under 3,000 to nearly 14,000 (Figure 2–2). People paid a total of 138 million visits to spas in 2007, spending $10.9 billion (Table 2–1).

In the first few years of the twenty-first century, the spa industry experienced a leveling out of its meteoric expansion, and many experts now believe it is entering a phase of moderate growth. The industry has experienced the first year-to-year dip in the number of consumers planning to visit a spa. While the number of facilities is still increasing, overall spa revenues and the total number of spa employees are not exploding any more. Spa owners and directors have begun to catch their collective breath and are now focusing on improving the quality of their workforce and their offerings for an ever more experienced and demanding audience. Accordingly, the need for qualified, well-trained personnel continues to be strong.

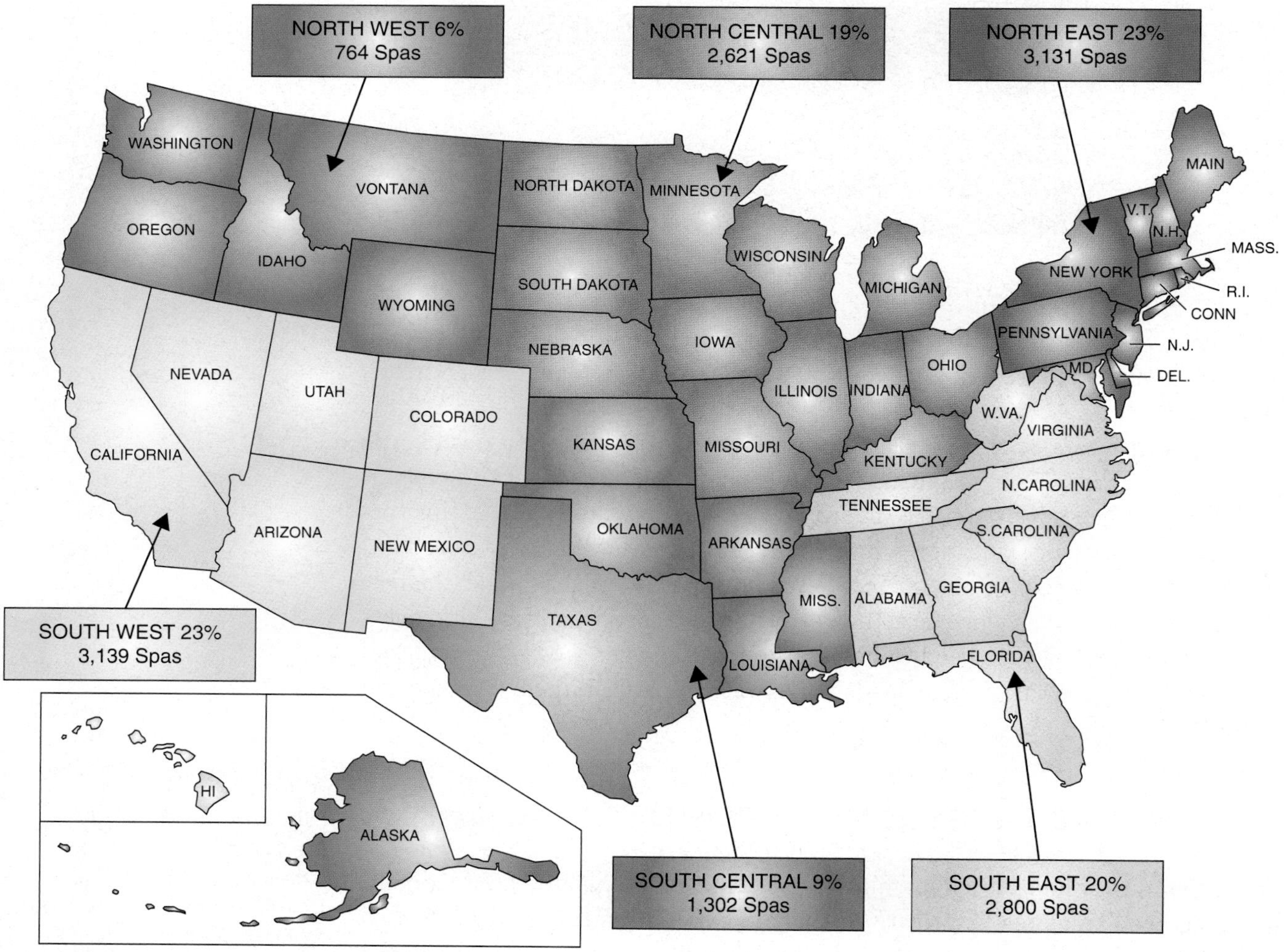

FIGURE 2-2 Distribution of U.S. spas by region.

ISPA 2008 U.S. SPA INDUSTRY UPDATE THE BIG FIVE			
	2006	**2007**	**ANNUAL GROWTH**
Revenue	$9.4 billion	$10.9 billion	16%
Spa Visits	111 million	138 million	25%
	JULY 2007	**JUNE 2008**	**ANNUAL GROWTH**
Locations	14,615	18,089	24%
Total Employees	232,673	303,719	31%
Full-Time	117,067	143,267	22%
Part-Time	73,076	111,973	53%
Contract	42,530	48,479	14%
Square Footage	56.2 million square feet	59.9 million square feet	7%

TABLE 2–1 Overall Size and Growth of the U.S. Spa Industry (courtesy ISPA).

A number of trends continue to shape the character of the spa landscape. According to Susie Ellis, president of SpaFinder, these trends include:

- **Weight Loss:** The number-one reason that people cite for making a visit to a destination spa is to get healthier and slim down.
- **Luxury:** Spas represent the height of luxury, and people are willing to pay for a special luxurious experience at a spa, even if it is once in a lifetime.
- **Mother/Daughter:** People are looking for ways to include friends and loved ones in their spa experiences, and those spas that make it easy with special packages such as mother/daughter retreats can increase their business. Even children and teens are being taught the benefits of spa-going, and it is not unusual to encounter youthful clients in many spas that offer a family emphasis.
- **Men:** Although spas are more popular with women, they are attracting an ever-growing number of men as well. Spas cater to a mere 30 percent male audience, but that still signifies over $3 billion in sales to men per year.

SPA TIP

Spas are the number-one employer of newly graduated massage therapists. No other single industry employs so many therapists or offers them such a wide range of opportunities for growth and success.

Types of Modern Spas

Spas encompass a wide array of businesses, offering their customers many choices, in much the same way that restaurants offer people choices in price, menu, service, and ambience. Although each spa is unique, they can be categorized into six major types: destination spas, hotel/resort spas, day spas, club spas, medical/dental spas, and mineral spring spas.

Spas in all of these categories, of course, are "devoted to enhancing overall well-being through a variety of professional services that encourage the renewal of mind, body and spirit." This is their commonality. Yet they attract a diverse clientele and present a wide range of philosophies and methods. The following two examples, Canyon Ranch Spa and Joy Spring Day Spa, highlight the broad spectrum of offerings.

destination spas

facilities with the primary purpose of guiding individual spa goers to develop healthy habits and achieve lifestyle transformation through a multi-day comprehensive program that includes spa services, physical fitness activities, wellness education, healthful cuisine, dedicated overnight accommodations, and special-interest programming

Many therapists would consider it a dream job to work for Canyon Ranch, one of the best known **destination spas** in the world. The spa was founded in 1979 by Mel Zuckerman, a businessman in Tucson, Arizona. He was successful but overweight and unhealthy, like so many people who lead sedentary, high-stress lifestyles. A trip to a California spa offered him and his wife a new vision, and they hoped to offer that same vision to guests at their new spa. The operation grew rapidly, expanded to a new location in Massachusetts in the 1980s, opened its first SpaClub at the Venetian Resort in Las Vegas in the 1990s, and continues to grow rapidly today, with a Canyon Ranch spa aboard the *Queen Mary II* cruise ship, a healthy lifestyle community in Florida called Canyon Ranch Living, another resort spa near Orlando, and much more. Canyon Ranch has become a global brand, attracting thousands of the most affluent and well-traveled people in the world. Its staff of medical doctors, psychologists, fitness experts, nutritionists, bodyworkers, chefs, and hospitality specialists cater to people who pay thousands of dollars a week. This is definitely the high end of what spas represent today.

Spas need not be grand ventures backed by multimillionaire investors. Tiny spas can offer the same level of service and therapeutic value as large spas like Canyon Ranch. One such spa was Joy Spring. Owned and operated by just one woman, Joy Spring was situated in a trendy California coastal town for many years. The owner has since sold her spa to open another location in Los Angeles, and her future is looking bright. The waiting room at Joy Spring consisted of two chairs and a single bookshelf in an area the size of a closet. But there was a little water fountain there, and a sense of calm. The small selection of books and gift items on the shelf was carefully chosen and arranged in an appealing way. Inside the treatment area was a steam cabinet, a massage table, and not too much else. When clients spent time in that room, however, they felt as if the rest of the world disappeared.

Both of these examples, Canyon Ranch and Joy Spring, have the right to call themselves spas because spas can be so many things to so many people. Regardless of the size of the operation or the breadth of offerings found there, a spa's success or failure will usually be determined by the quality of the therapeutic interaction between one guest and one therapist at a time. Canyon Ranch owner Mel Zuckerman was aware of this, and that is why he signed himself up for a massage and an herbal wrap every day during the first year of business in order to keep the emphasis where it belonged, on the treatments.

What is a modern spa, in its essence? It is certainly different than spas of antiquity or even spas of a generation ago. Today, people expect a lot from spas. When visitors enter, they want to be swept away. Spas in this sense are almost a form of entertainment, and while the best spas certainly strive to enhance customers' lives and offer visible improvements in health and beauty, they must also pay heed to the "experience" they are creating and the feelings their guests go home with after that experience. Each type of spa has a different type of opportunity to do that for its clients. Take a look at Table 2–2 for a description of the six main categories of spas in operation today. Read through the sections which describe the clientele at each type of spa and what you as a massage therapist can do to improve guests' experiences when working there.

TYPE OF SPA	APROX. U.S. #	DESCRIPTION	LOCATION	CLIENTELE	THERAPISTS' GOALS
Destination Spa	71	Facility with overnight accommodations catering exclusively to spa guests, often featuring advanced modalities and elaborate signature services in beautiful surroundings.	Usually a separate building or compound with several buildings set apart from neighboring businesses or residences.	High-discretionary-income individuals or couples willing to spend $2,500 to $6,000 per week on health and wellness.	Therapists working at destination spas should become thoroughly familiar with the spa's mission and overall treatment philosophy so they can enhance guests' experience through allied modalities.
Hotel/Resort Spa	1,218	Spas located within larger encompassing hotel or resort. Spa can be a main feature of the property or simply an "amenity" for guests to use at their leisure, offering a wide array of treatments, some rivaling those at destination spas. Also includes cruise ship spas.	All major resorts and high-end hotels include spas with their new properties or add them to existing properties in order to compete effectively. Spas rated high by consumers on list of requested hotel features.	Families, couples. Medium to high income range, either dedicated spa goers or casual vacationers. Often one partner will spa while the other golfs, plays tennis, etc.	Therapists should strive to learn what each guest needs, whether that be relaxation services or specific work to assist in activities (such as golf, tennis, swimming, etc.) undertaken at the resort.
Day Spa	10,988	A spa where guests visit for a few hours or a day, with no sleepover accommodations available. These spas range from rudimentary one-person operations to full-blown centers offering treatments on a par with the large resorts.	Often situated within a hair salon. Can be a store front, stand-alone building, a single multipurpose room, part of a massage clinic, in a shopping mall, or even in airports.	Day spas cater to a wide array of individuals of many social classes, from low-medium to high income levels who prize proximity, affordability, and personalized service.	Therapists should forge strong client–practitioner bonds with the spa's guests because they will become repeat customers and therefore benefit by ongoing therapy.

TABLE 2-2 Types of Spas. *(Continued)*

TYPE OF SPA	APROX. U.S. #	DESCRIPTION	LOCATION	CLIENTELE	THERAPISTS' GOALS
Club Spa	484	Spas that are part of a larger physical fitness facility, ranging from a minor addition to a major focus of the business.	Many upscale urban fitness clubs consider it essential to include a spa, especially multipurpose lifestyle clubs.	Physically active individuals who prize optimal performance and appearance. Medium to medium-high income range.	Therapists in club spas need to know the fitness goals of each client and how the use of weights and equipment has affected them physiologically.
Medical/Dental Spa	915	Medical/dental spas are either dedicated spa facilities that operate in conjunction with a nearby medical practice or are incorporated into the actual practice, always under the supervision of a medical professional.	Can be located at a wellness retreat center, at a resort, in a stand-alone building, or as part of an existing medical/dental practice.	Ranging from high-income individuals willing to pay extra for personalized medical services in a comfortable environment to everyday patients at medical/dental offices given extra attention with or without spa services in a spa-like setting.	Therapists should have a basic knowledge of the procedures employed at the spa and how they affect the overall health of the clients, especially regarding the skin and muscles affected by these procedures, whether they be invasive or noninvasive.
Mineral Springs Spa	77	Spas located at the actual source of mineral springs and incorporating these waters into their program and treatments.	Can be located at a wellness retreat center, at a resort or in a stand-alone building.	A wide range, from weekend family vacationers at rustic spring sites to five-star hotel goers on gourmet retreats.	Therapists should be familiar with the chemical components of the spa's waters and how they affect health through their chemical, thermal, and mechanical actions.

TABLE 2–2 Types of Spas.

SPA PROFILE SpaQuality

As spas proliferate, an agreed-upon standard of quality becomes necessary. Consumers need to be protected from dangerous, unethical, or unsanitary situations, and spas themselves need a standard against which to judge their progress and relative standing within the industry. They also need tools that will help them improve their businesses and attract more customers. While membership in an organization or placement on a spa travel Web site may be an implied endorsement, it does not certify that the spa has achieved a certain level of quality. Thus, independent agencies have arisen to act as certifying bodies for the spa industry. One popular standard is **SpaQuality** (Figure 2–3).

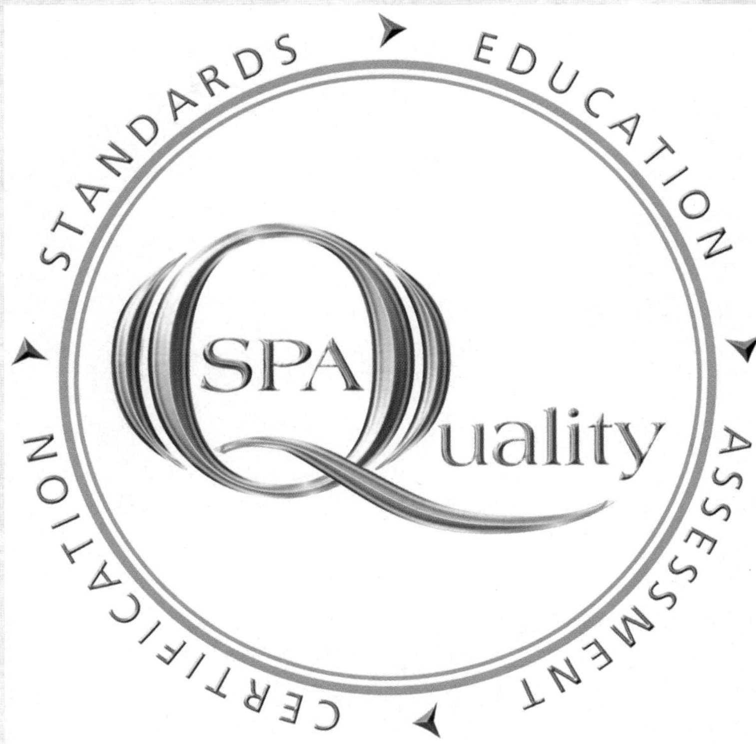

FIGURE 2–3 One popular standard for certifying that spas have achieved a certain level of excellence is SpaQuality.

Julie Register, a journalist and spa industry expert, developed The International Standards of SpaExcellence^{SM} to provide a framework for spa owners, directors, and managers who wish to achieve a sustainable spa business with loyal clients, dependable staff, smooth operations, and financial success. She created this system specifically for the spa industry, building on the foundation of recognized quality management standards such as the Malcolm Baldrige National Quality Award, the International Standards Organization (ISO 9000), Joint Commission on Accreditation of Healthcare Organizations (JCAHO), Occupational Safety and Health Administration (OSHA), and others.

"Rather than reinventing the wheel," says Register, "we decided to examine the standards from other industries and see how we could apply many of them to spas. We basically reorganized the quality assessment process to work within this specialized field, putting things in a language spa professionals could understand. Some spas were already certified by ISO 9000, but we wanted something very specific, just for spas."

The system that Register and her partner Linda Bankoski have created is detailed and in-depth (Figure 2–4). It offers spa owners, operators, and employees a way to truly get to know where they stand: their strengths, their weaknesses, and how they can improve. And attaining higher levels of certification can bring greater success as well.

"One whole section of our Standards focuses on constant improvement," says Register. "We never let them rest! Even when a spa has attained our highest Level of Excellence, we keep coming back to do anonymous assessments to make sure they maintain their standards. Our anonymous guests have been thoroughly trained; it's much more detailed than just a regular **secret shopper**, so our spas really have to be on their toes."

So, what exactly does the SpaQuality process entail? "The intent of the Standards is to describe the common elements of successful spas in an organized framework," says Register. "While the Standards describe what successful spas do, they

(Continued)

SPA PROFILE SpaQuality *continued*

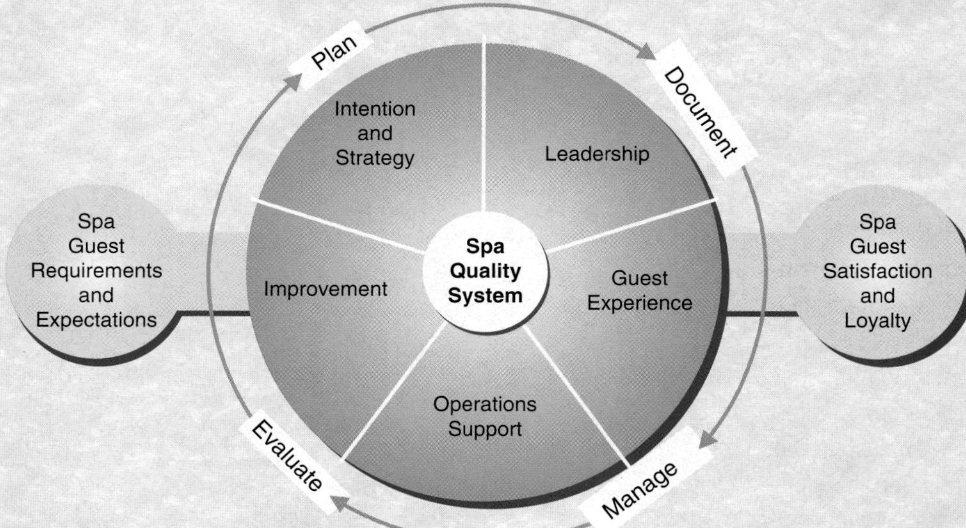

FIGURE 2–4 The analysis involved with certifying the quality of spas is in-depth and comprehensive.

do not describe exactly how the spa must operate nor do they seek to make all spas alike. Basically, we utilize a series of observations, self-evaluations, interviews and on-site anonymous guest assessments to determine whether spas have successfully achieved the next level of SpaExcellence. There are five levels in total, and in the SpaExcellence system, to be successful, spas need to demonstrate that they have achieved the highest level in the following areas: spa management, spa guest experiences, spa operations support and spa improvement."

Register believes the spas that embrace these principles of effective management will promote confidence among spa goers and enhance the public image of the spa industry as a whole. "We provide a comprehensive education, assessment and certification process," she says. "And for those spas that have gone through the process and demonstrated compliance to the standards at a level of excellence 3, 4 or 5, we give the crystal award of SpaExcellence℠." (See Figure 2–5.)

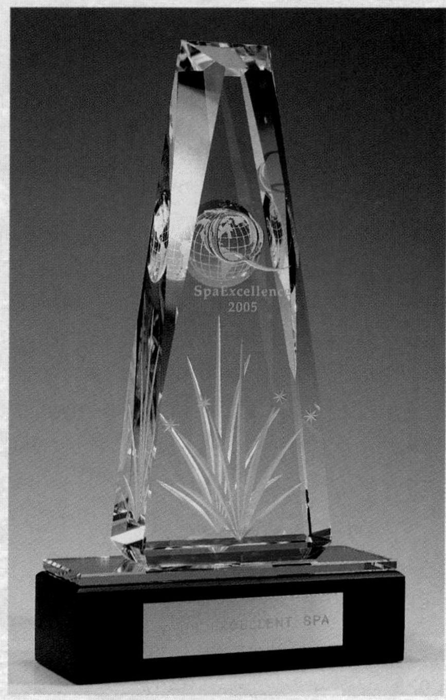

FIGURE 2–5 Spas that have demonstrated compliance to the standards of SpaQuality at a level of excellence 3, 4 or 5 are given the crystal award of SpaExcellence℠.

"Right now we as spa professionals need to get the word out to the rest of the world and help them understand the value spas have to offer. One of the ways to do that is to make sure that there are not so many bad spas out there. We are at a point right now before spas are really going to blast off. There are millions of consumers who are still waiting to feel 100% comfortable about spas before they venture inside. We're all in this together and we're hoping our standards will help."

THE SPA CLIENT

Who, exactly, visits the thousands of spas now in operation and pays all those billions of dollars to receive all those spa services? It is helpful to know more about spa goers for three main reasons:

- **in order to find them:** Statistical information helps spas find potential clients and then develop successful treatment programs and marketing plans to entice them to visit.
- **in order to understand them:** Instead of experiencing a stream of random people flowing through the front door, spas can use **demographic** information to help categorize clients according to their background, needs, and desires.
- **in order to treat them better:** By learning why people visit spas (or do not visit spas) and what keeps them from (or encourages them to) experience new services, spa owners and practitioners can more reliably give high-quality service that guests will appreciate.

The most obvious generalization that could be made about spa goers is that they are primarily women. While this is certainly true, the percentage of female versus male spa goers has been steadily decreasing. Now, nearly one-third of spa goers are men. This is a big change. In the 1980s, male spa visitors made up less than 10 percent of all spa goers.

The average age of spa goers is around 40, so the crowd tends to be a mature one, slightly older than the typical age for those who receive massage therapy outside the spa setting, which is around 30 years old. Income and education are also determining factors, with the average spa goer reporting an income of over $70,000 and over half of them holding college degrees. See Table 2–3 for more detailed information about spa goers.

People visit spas for a wide variety of reasons. For some, it is mere curiosity. For others, it is a life-or-death decision. Many have gone to spas to change their lifestyles completely and try to regain lost health. The data in Table 2–4 highlights the most common reasons people visit spas.

Without a large and increasing number of consumers interested in experiencing spa services, today's spa industry would collapse in short order. It is important, therefore, for therapists to understand these consumers and determine how to best serve them. Although each person is of course unique, spa consumers in general can be classified into five broad categories: Non–Spa Goer, Novice Spa Goer, Opportunistic Spa Goer, Enthusiastic Spa Goer, and Seasoned Spa Goer.

Client Type 1 – Non–Spa Goer

Regardless of how excited you as a massage therapist are about the large numbers of people who visit spas, the reality is that a much larger number do not go to spas. Many, perhaps, never will. Non–spa goers outnumber spa goers approximately three to one. Do these non–spa goers have something wrong with them, then? Do they not understand the stunning benefits, not to mention pleasures, they would receive upon visiting a spa? Is money that much of an issue that they have decided never to check out spas, even one time? Are they that self-conscious

SpaQuality

a popular standard (with multiple tiers of achievement) by which to judge spa businesses, created by an independent agency that acts as certifying body for the industry

secret shopper

individual hired to visit a (spa) business anonymously and be treated as a normal guest in order to report back about the quality of service provided

demographics

the characteristics of human populations and population segments, especially when used to identify consumer markets

SPA TIP

While some spas are successful catering exclusively or primarily to women, many are now finding it wise to cater to men also, or they risk losing a third of their potential business. A few spas have even been successful catering to men only. Whether you work in a spa or open your own spa one day, it is important to make men feel at home.

	U.S.			CANADA		
	TOTAL 100%	MALE 31%	FEMALE 69%	TOTAL 100%	MALE 29%	FEMALE 71%
How long have you been visiting spas?						
Less than 1 year	15%	18%	15%	16%	26%	25%
1–2 years	13%	14%	12%	17%	20%	16%
3–5 years	31%	28%	32%	25%	22%	27%
6–8 years	16%	15%	17%	13%	16%	12%
9–12 years	11%	7%	14%	9%	7%	10%
More than 12 years	13%	18%	11%	10%	9%	11%
First service received on first spa visit						
Massage	68%	84%	61%	45%	75%	33%
Facial	13%	5%	17%	20%	6%	25%
Manicure	6%	3%	7%	10%	1%	14%
Pedicure	4%	1%	5%	9%	3%	11%
Body Scrub/Body Wrap	3%	2%	3%	4%	3%	4%
Hydrotherapy	3%	5%	2%	5%	7%	3%
Hair Removal	2%	0%	2%	4%	1%	5%
Other	1%	1%	2%	4%	4%	3%
Most common treatment received in the past 12 months						
Facial	54%	27%	67%	57%	27%	70%
Manicure	57%	23%	72%	54%	22%	67%
Massage	63%	61%	64%	46%	54%	42%
Pedicure	56%	22%	72%	52%	22%	64%
Sauna/Steam	43%	49%	40%	39%	51%	34%
Deep Tissue Massage	48%	53%	45%	33%	43%	29%
Typical spa partner						
Alone	69%	57%	74%	74%	64%	78%
Close female friend(s)	31%	5%	43%	28%	6%	37%
Spouse or domestic partner	28%	50%	18%	24%	46%	15%
Age						
18–24	11%	8%	12%	10%	9%	10%
25–34	19%	13%	21%	20%	17%	21%
35–44	22%	24%	21%	25%	24%	25%
45–54	24%	24%	24%	20%	23%	19%
55–64	14%	15%	14%	13%	13%	13%
65 and older	10%	15%	8%	12%	13%	12%
Marital status						
Married	60%	64%	59%	51%	59%	48%
Single	19%	17%	20%	18%	20%	17%
In a committed relationship	12%	9%	14%	16%	15%	17%
Widowed/Separated/Divorced	8%	10%	7%	15%	7%	18%
Education						
No college degree	19%	9%	23%	37%	31%	40%
College graduate	40%	40%	40%	38%	36%	40%
Post-graduate schooling	41%	51%	37%	24%	33%	20%
Household income						
Under $50K	15%	9%	18%	34%	26%	38%
$50K–$99K	41%	34%	44%	40%	39%	40%
$100K and over	44%	57%	38%	26%	35%	22%

TABLE 2-3 Characteristics of the Average Spa Goer, abbreviated (courtesy ISPA).

about their bodies? How can they be brought around to the "right" perspective and finally see the true value of spas?

While it is true that some people just need a little education in order to see the benefits of spas, others have pondered the benefits and determined that they are not worth the effort. Some, indeed, are price-conscious and see spa spending as a waste of money. Others are not so price-conscious, but they do not have the time to visit spas. Others simply choose to not make spa-going a priority in their lives.

Regardless of how foreign spas may seem to this majority of people, the possibility still exists that their minds could be changed. Somebody could think up a new spa concept that makes them feel comfortable instead of intimidated. Somebody could begin offering spa services at bargain-basement prices. Thousands of massage therapists could begin offering spa services in people's homes.

These people, the non-spa goers, are the ones paid least attention to by existing spas, simply because the cost of attracting a new client is so much higher than gaining repeat business from an existing one. Some spa professionals have been tempted to conclude that the "masses" who have not yet visited a spa are not worth the effort of attracting and educating, but this would be a mistake. Although a large majority of people have never visited a spa, many need only a few kind words and some brief explanations to understand how safe, fun, and satisfying spa-going can be.

REASON FOR SPA VISIT	PERCENTAGE
Reduce Stress	46%
Soothe Sore Joints/Muscles	38%
Feel Better about Myself	31%
Mental/Emotional Health	28%
Improve My Appearance	22%
Overall Wellness	19%
Opportunity to Socialize	8%
Recovery from Injury	5%
Lose Weight*	4%
Recuperation from Cancer	<1%

TABLE 2–4 Reason for Spa Visits (courtesy of ISPA).

**Note that weight loss is the number-one reason for visits to destination spas, as cited earlier in this chapter, but when all the day spas and resort spas are added to the equation, the percentage of visitors seeking weight loss drops dramatically.*

Client Type 2 – Novice Spa Goer

The novice spa goer has already paid a few visits to spas and found them enjoyable, but she has not decided to make spas an ongoing part of her life. This is somebody who may still feel uncomfortable or intimidated by some aspects of the spa experience. She is not sure if she's "doing everything right." She harbors secret feelings that the other patrons at the spas she visited were more knowledgeable or worldly. She may not have been thoroughly convinced about the true value of spa services and still considers them a luxury.

SPA TIP

A Spa for the Masses

The vast majority of people are non–spa goers, and this is partly so because of real or perceived self-image concerns. "That's just not me," many of these people will say. They cannot imagine themselves inside the typical spa setting, which they may consider "snobbish" or "elitist." Spa owners can make non–spa goers more comfortable by creating more relaxed environments that do not scream "exclusivity." When first-time spa goers finally do pay a visit, massage therapists can make them feel more comfortable in the spa setting by thoroughly explaining the benefits of the therapies and gently educating them about spa etiquette in a helpful tone that is not condescending. Until this industry creates a home for the 75 percent of all consumers who still shun spas, spa business owners and massage therapists have no grounds for complaining about a lack of business.

This client needs ongoing education, and a bit of hand-holding as well. Massage therapists should pay special attention to these clients, because they represent the greatest opportunity for creating positive impressions that will turn occasional spa goers into dedicated fans. Sometimes, spa goers at this stage have the tendency to become loyal to a particular therapist rather than to a particular spa. This is understandable, but it is not recommended. Cultivating star therapists on staff is counterproductive to the ultimate success of a spa business, and while it is sometimes difficult to avoid, it should definitely not be promoted.

Client Type 3 – Opportunistic Spa Goer

This type of client has decided unequivocally that spas are a good thing. He goes to spas (almost always a day spa or medical spa) when he has the time and he remembers to make an appointment, which is usually done on the spur of the moment, the same day or at most one day in advance. He keeps his eyes open for any spa coupons or special offers, and when the time comes for a little self-indulgence, spas are up there on the list with things he would like to do, in addition to sports, entertainment, and other leisure pursuits. Massage therapists need to be aware of clients in this category so they can educate them about the benefits of more consistent spa-going.

Client Type 4 – Enthusiastic Spa Goer

This client frequents spas and yet still feels that she does not have enough time and/or money for all the spa-going she would truly like. She books appointments in advance and keeps up with the largest trends in the spa industry. She may be among the first to want to experience new treatments when they become available. Perhaps subscribing to a consumer spa magazine, she looks for value and excitement in her spa-going, perhaps seeking out new spas. She may even have visited a destination spa once or twice, or a mineral spring spa, paying top dollar for an all-inclusive spa immersion experience.

Massage therapists need to recognize these spa enthusiasts when they arrive because they like to be treated a little special, and they deserve it. Therapists can help them feel cared for by discussing the details of spa products and spa treatments, speaking as if to an equal so as to include the client in the inside world of spa therapy.

Massage therapists working in spas should be aware of the different types of spa clients and adjust their interactions with them accordingly. "I treat all my clients as equals," is a phrase often heard spoken by well-meaning therapists, but this attitude may in fact make certain clients feel less appreciated and less understood. Those therapists who learn to distinguish between non–spa goers, novices, opportunists, enthusiasts, and seasoned spa goers will advance their careers more quickly and do a more admirable job representing the spas that they own or where they work.

Client Type 5 – Seasoned Spa Goer

The seasoned spa goer has the discretionary income necessary to experience all types of spas, often on a consistent basis. She has been to several destination spas, plans her travel and vacations around spa availability, and actively seeks out the latest and greatest facilities, products, and therapists. However, she will often not sign up for seasonal offerings because she realizes they may be more of a trend than a core therapeutic offering. She tends to stick to what works: massages, facials, and a select set of signature treatments.

Massage therapists may find it hard to impress the seasoned spa goer, who may have an "I've seen it all" attitude. Therapists, then, need to treat her with respect and strive to make her a co-creator of her own spa experience. Therapists can ask her about her varied spa background and seek informed input that will help further customize the treatment.

MASSAGE THERAPISTS IN THE SPA SETTING

Without massage therapists, spas would be very different places. The most popular image people have of spas and the one most often used in advertising is that of a woman or man lying on a massage table, head tilted unnaturally to the side, smiling for the camera while getting treated to a massage (Figure 2–6). Spas since Roman times have featured massage, and today, people still expect massage to be front and center on the menu. Yet while it is true that people consider massage an essential part of the overall spa experience, it is not the only thing they value. Also important are ambience, guest service, esthetic treatments, wellness, nutrition, and more. They want the spa to run like a well-oiled machine, with no delays or inconsistencies. In short, while massage is the most important thing to you as a therapist, it is secondary to the overall spa experience for guests. You need to remember this and focus the same amount of energy on becoming a valuable player on the spa's "team" as you do on your own personal therapeutic skills (see the section on Teamwork in Chapter 15).

How many therapists actually work in the spa industry? While the number is in constant flux and impossible to determine exactly, you can estimate the number by referring to Table 2–1 once again. When you consider that the spa industry employs over 300,000 people, and if you assume that approximately 15 percent of the spas' employees are therapists (a conservative number), you can see that spas may easily employ 45,000 therapists. That is a small city filled with nothing but massage therapists working in U.S. spas alone. Imagine what the number must be in the quickly growing international spa community.

A therapist needs no other license or qualification other than a massage license or certification in order to work in the spa industry. However, many therapists feel it is helpful to take a spa training program, either as a part of their schooling or through continuing education. This education makes them more likely to find jobs in the spa industry as it demonstrates seriousness and dedication. Many spas offer their therapists continuing education at a reduced cost, or free, as a benefit of prolonged employment at the spa. Instructors either visit the spas to train the entire staff or the spa pays all or part of the tuition for off-site trainings. Before accepting this type of benefit, therapists must make a firm commitment to the spa by completing a certain period of employment or by signing a contract that makes them liable for the cost of their training if they leave the spa within a specified period of time.

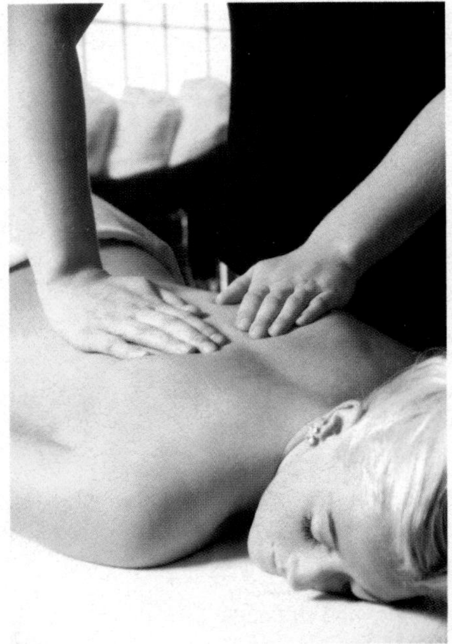

FIGURE 2–6 The most popular image people have of spas and the one most often used in advertising is that of a woman or man lying on a massage table.

Even those therapists who are not directly employed by the spa industry stand to benefit greatly by the popularity of spa modalities. As shown in Table 2–5, the most frequently requested spa offering among consumers is "home visit spa" services. Independent therapists who provide these services and market themselves stand to greatly increase their overall business (see the profile—Succeeding with Home Spa Services—in Chapter 17). Those therapists who wish to provide home spa modalities for their private clients can judge which ones may be most popular by studying the data in Table 2–6, Interest in Particular Types of Spa Services.

INTEREST IN PARTICULAR TYPES OF SPAS	EXTREMELY INTERESTED	VERY INTERESTED	FAIRLY INTERESTED
Home Visit Spa	6%	10%	20%
Family-Oriented Spa	2%	10%	16%
Country Club Spa	3%	5%	12%
Airport Spa	3%	5%	8%
Pet Friendly Spa	2%	5%	6%
Males-Only Spa	2%	4%	6%
Prenatal Spa	2%	3%	4%
Teens-Only Spa			2%
Dental Office Spa			3%

TABLE 2-5 Spa Treatments: Experience and Interest (courtesy of ISPA).

	% OF SPA GOERS WHO HAVE ALREADY EXPERIENCED SERVICE		% OF SPA GOERS VERY INTERESTED IN TRYING IT FOR FIRST TIME	
	U.S.	CANADA	U.S.	CANADA
Massage	72%	53%	11%	16%
Facial	66%	69%	8%	6%
Manicure	66%	63%	5%	5%
Pedicure	63%	59%	5%	7%
Deep Tissue Massage	54%	41%	13%	17%
Sauna/Steam	52%	51%	9%	9%
Body Scrub/Wrap	41%	37%	10%	12%
Aromatherapy	39%	42%	9%	8%
Movement Classes	23%	24%	13%	16%
Hot Stone Massage	22%	18%	28%	26%
Hydrotherapy	17%	19%	8%	13%
Couples Massage	17%	9%	16%	15%
Shiatsu	16%	17%	17%	18%
Energy Work	11%	22%	12%	16%
Lifestyle Classes	10%	17%	13%	12%
Guided Meditation	8%	12%	6%	10%
Thai Massage	8%	8%	17%	20%
Vichy Shower	7%	5%	6%	11%
Tai Chi	5%	10%	8%	12%
Lymphatic Drainage	3%	6%	4%	8%
Ayurvedic Treatments	3%	3%	5%	7%
Watsu	1%	1%	4%	7%

TABLE 2-6 Interest in Particular Types of Spa Services (courtesy ISPA).

Forming Realistic Expectations

The prospect of working in the modern spa industry may seem daunting at first because there are so many variables involved, so many questions to ask. Through the influence of the media, gossip, or sheer lack of information, some massage students and beginning therapists form incomplete or misguided perceptions about what it is like to work in a spa. These perceptions spread through the massage community, making it nearly impossible to tell myth from reality. Some of the most common misperceptions circulating about the spa industry are listed in the Did You Know? sidebar: Spa Myths vs. Spa Realities.

It is important to form realistic expectations about what it will be like working in the spa industry. Some therapists tend to romanticize the idea, while others disparage the idea. The reality is that working in the modern spa industry is quite similar to working in any other modern industry. Challenges and concerns will inevitably arise, many of which you will learn about in Chapter 15. At this stage, it is important to understand three basic realities:

- The spa industry is the largest single employer of massage therapists.
- Competition among therapists for the best spa jobs will continue to grow as higher-quality spa-specific education in massage schools becomes more widely available and a greater number of freshly minted therapists enter the market each year.
- Many opportunities exist in spas for massage therapists to move up to supervisor, manager, director, and other positions.

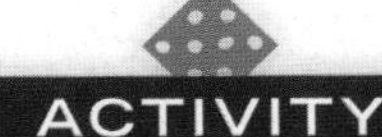

ACTIVITY

Spa Association Membership Application

Write a one-page essay as part of an application for membership in a spa association. Include at least three reasons why you think your participation would benefit the organization. Also, list two or more projects or committees you would like to take part in as a member, and explain why.

THE SPA COMMUNITY

The modern spa community is comprised of three main components: associations, corporations, and individuals. Though each of these is a distinct entity with its own self-interests and goals in mind, they have also come together to form a cohesive industry with a collective voice. Those massage therapists who are serious about entering the spa industry need to learn as much as they can about this community as they seek their own unique places within it, whether that be as employees, private practitioners, or spa owners.

Associations

A number of associations directly or indirectly serve the spa industry (Table 2–7). The associations that have the most impact on therapists working in spas include the **Day Spa Association**, the Medical Spa Association, and ISPA, which is the main professional association of the spa industry (Figure 2–7). ISPA was officially launched in 1991 by a small group of dedicated professionals who had a vision for the future of spas. There were 150 attendees from 10 countries at the first conference, and no trade show floor. Membership included no day spas and very few affiliates. Prior to that time, spas were run by independent business owners with only loose affiliations with each other, if any at all. Sixteen years later, the organization had thousands of members from 75 countries, and the

Day Spa Association

an association of member spas, vendors, and related companies devoted primarily to the successful practices of day spas, as opposed to resort or destination spas; sponsors an annual day spa–specific convention

Spa Myths vs. Spa Realities

Did You Know?

MYTH: As a therapist in a spa, you will be expected to do 10 massages in a row without a break.

REALITY: While a very small number of insensitive spa owners still try to force the maximum work out of their therapists, the trend today is to take care of therapists. A burnt-out staff is not good for customer relations. Five to six massages per day, often with a 10- to 15-minute break between sessions, is the normal maximum. Also, spa modalities such as body scrubs and wraps are not as hard on therapists' bodies.

MYTH: The only kind of massage done in spas is "pampering" massage.

REALITY: Many spas offer advanced bodywork modalities on their menus, including craniosacral, neuromuscular, myofascial, and more. In some cases, training in these techniques is even provided and paid for by the spa.

MYTH: Therapists are always poorly paid in spas.

REALITY: While it is true that spas have high overhead costs and must try to keep their expenses down, therapists still typically make $20 to $40 per hour, with no overhead expenses of their own.

MYTH: Only unmotivated or unskilled therapists work in spas.

REALITY: Many highly motivated and skilled therapists work in spas. Some find it optimal to let the spa take care of business while they focus on therapy, and they are content to remain in that relationship for many years. Others quickly move up to become supervisors, trainers, lead therapists, and directors. Some therapists pursue other goals while working in the spa, using it as a stepping stone.

MYTH: You cannot perform in-depth work over a period of time in spas because the clientele is constantly changing.

REALITY: Roughly three-quarters of all locations are day spas or club spas, with a local, repeat clientele. Even at resort and destination spas, therapists can work with clients repeatedly during their stay or even during return visits.

SPA TIP

The Day Spa Expo is a smaller conference, held in Las Vegas each year, that specializes in helping owners and practitioners who work in day spas as compared to the larger resort and destination spas that receive much of the attention at the ISPA conference. Therapists who work in day spas or plan to open their own day spas will find this conference valuable.

trade show could only be held at the largest conference centers because it was so huge. In addition to providing a forum for growth, commerce, education, and mutual support, ISPA has become in some ways a guiding light for the industry as well, as evidenced in the code of ethics (see Did You Know? sidebar) by which all member spas must abide.

Attending a Spa Tradeshow

If you become serious about pursuing a career in the spa industry in any capacity, it is important to visit events where thousands of other like-minded professionals gather to share knowledge and inspiration, as well as buy and sell products and services. Spa tradeshows can be broken down into two main categories: those organized by associations and those organized by corporations. Though they are not drastically dissimilar at first glance, the association-sponsored events tend to focus more heavily on general education and inspiration, while the corporate

INDUSTRY ASSOCIATIONS			
ASSOCIATION	**ADDRESS**	**PHONE**	**WEB**
Spa			
American Spa Therapies Education and Certification Council (ASTECC)	1014 N Olive Ave West Palm Beach, FL 33401	(800) 575-0518	http://www.asteccse.com
Day Spa Association	310 17th St Union City, NJ 07087	(201) 865-2065	http://www.dayspaassociation.com
International Spa Association (ISPA)	2365 Harrodsburg Rd, A325 Lexington, KY 40504-4326	(888) 651-4772	http://www.experienceispa.com
National Coalition of Esthetic & Related Associations	484 Spring Ave Ridgewood, NJ 07450-4624	(201) 670-4100	http://www.ncea.tv
Leading Spas of Canada	PO Box 157 Sooke, BC VOS 1NO	(800) 704-6393	http://www.leadingspasofcanada.com
Medical Spa			
American Association of Naturopathic Physicians	2366 Eastlake Ave E Ste 322 Seattle, WA 98102	(206) 323-7610	http://www.naturopathic.org
American Holistic Medical Association	4101 Lake Boone Trl, 201 Raleigh, NC 27607	(919) 787-5181	http://www.holisticmedicine.org
International Medical Spa Association	310 17th St Union City, NJ 07087	(201) 865-2065	http://www.medicalspaassociation.org
Medical Spa Society	60 E 56th St New York, NY 10022	(866) MEDISPA	http://www.medicalspasociety.org
National Center for Complementary and Alternative Medicine (NCCAM)	9000 Rockville Pike Bldg 31, Rm 5B-38 Bethesda, MD 20892	(888) 644-6226	http://nccam.nih.gov
The Ayurvedic Institute	PO Box 23445 Albuquerque, NM 87192	(505) 291-9698	http://www.ayurveda.com
Massage & Bodywork			
American Massage Therapy Association (AMTA)	820 Davis St Ste 100 Evanston, IL 60201	(847) 864-0123	http://www.amtamassage.org
Associated Bodywork & Massage Professionals (ABMP)	28677 Buffalo Park Rd Evergreen, CO 80439	(800) 458-2267	http://www.abmp.com
National Association for Holistic Aromatherapy	4509 Interlake Ave N #233 Seattle, WA 98103-6773	(888) ASK-NAHA	http://www.naha.org

TABLE 2–7 Spa-Related Associations.

events focus more heavily on the vendors who supply products and product-specific education. Both are extremely worthwhile for anyone serious about spas. One day spent on a trade show floor and in the classrooms of experienced teachers at these events can supply information it would take months to gather on your own.

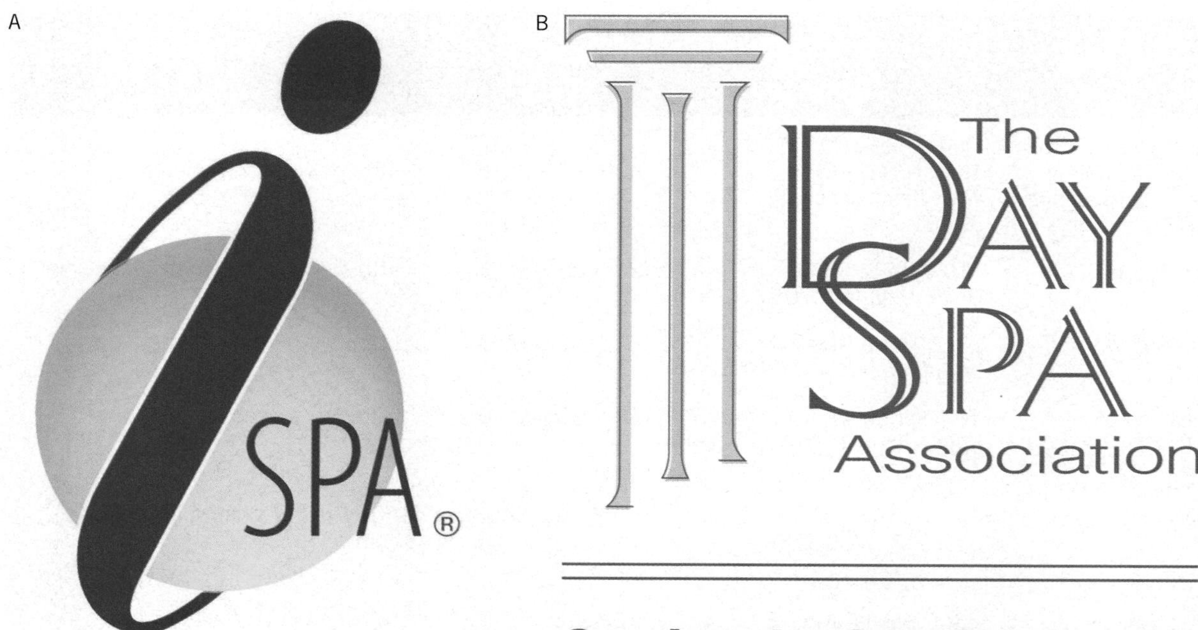

FIGURE 2–7A&B The International Spa Association (ISPA) and the Day Spa Association (DSA) are the main professional associations of the U.S. spa industry.

When attending a spa trade show, keep the following points in mind in order to get the most out of your experience:

- Go with a friend if possible. Even if you don't know anyone who's going, call your local massage school or chapter and see if somebody else from your area will be attending.
- If you want to save money on your trip, suggest sharing a hotel room with another attendee.
- Call the conference headquarters and ask for a list of other people attending alone who are looking for rides or roommates.
- Mingle at luncheons, dinner banquets, and parties, introducing yourself to as many people as you can. People expect to be approached at conferences. No need to be shy.
- Spend a lot of time talking to vendors at the booths in the exhibit hall. They all want to get to know you because you may be a potential customer or business partner. Stroll slowly through the aisles, spending time getting to know each person and their products. Later, when you see them in the hallways or at functions, you'll have a basis for conversation.
- Have fun. Definitely partake of the social agenda created for each one of these events. If people have seen you doing the limbo the night before, they'll be more likely to strike up a conversation the next day.
- If you notice any other people there alone, see if you can offer them a little company.

SPA TIP

Remember to bring *plenty* of business cards to the spa trade show. A commonly heard line goes as follows: "Oh, I just gave out my last card. Sorry." As a general rule, bring three or four times as many business cards as you think you will need.

Did You Know?

ISPA Member Code of Ethics, abridged (courtesy ISPA)

ISPA Spa Member Code of Ethics, abridged (courtesy ISPA)

- Member will be guided in all activities by truth, accuracy, fairness, and integrity.
- Member pledges loyalty to the Association and agrees to pursue and support its objectives.
- Member pledges to keep informed on the latest techniques, developments, and knowledge pertinent to professional improvement.
- Member will help fellow members reach personal and professional fulfillment.
- Member will utilize every opportunity to enhance the public image of the spa industry.

Staff

- Staff, when hired, is provided with a Policy and Procedures Manual that is reviewed and updated annually.
- Staff is provided with and/or given access to constantly updated Treatment Procedure and Product manuals for all treatment modalities, including the spa's menu.
- Staff is given a job/responsibility description upon hiring, followed up with at least one annual evaluation of each individual's job performance.
- All specialized staff such as fitness instructors, personal trainers, massage therapists, estheticians, nail technicians, hairstylists, nutritionists, physiologists, psychologists, and medical technicians comply with applicable international, federal, state, and local regulations with regard to licensing, registration, and appropriate certification.
- During operating hours, there is at least one staff member scheduled on site who has current CPR certification.

Service

- Staff is courteous, helpful, knowledgeable, and articulate.
- Staff is committed to anticipating the guests' needs and serving them.
- Staff believes in the precepts of spa wellness and is willing and able to share these philosophies with guests.
- Staff zealously guards the guest's privacy and modesty.
- Staff is attentive to preserving the spa environment at all times.

See Table 17–3 for a listing of spa trade shows and Table 17–2, Choices in Spa Education, for more information.

Companies Related to the Spa Industry

As the spa industry has grown, a number of companies have grown alongside it. The eight main categories these companies fall under are: spa treatment products, spa/hydrotherapy equipment, exercise equipment, software, apparel/lifestyle, spa travel and recommendation, consulting, and distribution. Within each one of these categories, certain companies have excelled, forming partnerships within the spa industry and capturing a large percentage of sales. At the same time, new companies

vendors

companies or individuals that supply a (spa) business with needed equipment, products, or supplies

are rapidly being formed and entering the spa. These companies, taken as a whole, are often referred to as **vendors**. As a massage therapist in the spa industry, you will need to be familiar with these companies and their products in order to understand spa guests' overall experience. If you know how a specific piece of the spa's exercise equipment works the quadriceps muscles, for example, you will be better-prepared when treating a guest who is complaining about his sore thighs. Table 2-8 lists the eight main categories of spa-related companies with some examples of the most well-known companies within the industry and the reasons

SPA COMPANY CATEGORY	PRIMARY GOODS AND SERVICES	REPRESENTATIVE COMPANIES	IMPACT ON MASSAGE THERAPISTS
Treatment Products	oils, lotions, seaweeds, muds, clays, herbs, cosmetics, esthetic products	Pevonia, Aveda, Spa Tech, Dermalogica, Creative Spa, Jurlique, mdskincare, B. Kamins, Babor, Darphin, Jamu, Tara Spa Therapy	When therapists know more about the products they apply, through vendor training or self-study, they can better serve clients and enhance retail sales
Spa & Hydrotherapy Equipment Manufacturers	saunas, steam baths, Jacuzzis, hydro tubs, specialized showers, treatment chambers, pools, massage tables, wet tables, massagers	Living Earth Crafts, Custom Craft, Touch America, HydroCo, LPG USA, Sanijet	Therapists need to know the contraindications for and health impact created by each piece of equipment on guests. They also need to be extremely familiar with operation for ease of use
Fitness Equipment Manufacturers	treadmills, stationary bicycles, elliptical machines, weight machines, free weights, aerobics equipment	Precor, Cybex, Nautilus, Life Fitness, Gym Source, Nordic Track	Therapists gain knowledge about guests' therapeutic needs by knowing how each piece of equipment affects guests' muscles and overall health
Spa Software Companies	scheduling, inventory, booking, point-of-sale and marketing software, as well as biofeedback and relaxation tools	Spa Soft, Spa Biz, Harms Software, Resort Suite, Wild Divine, Mikal	Therapists who have an understanding of how spa software facilitates booking, scheduling and sales can perform their duties more effectively
Spa Apparel and Lifestyle Companies	books, DVDs, CDs, candles, teas, sport drinks, nutrition products, ingestible herbs, supplements, robes, clothing, fitness wear	Hay House, Silhouette, Jen Morgan, Cypress, Kimbaks, Sensi, Prana	The most effective therapists can recommend products that fit guests' expectations of how to continue the spa experience at home
Travel and Recommendation	Spa ratings and information, travel agent services, gift certificates	SpaFinder, Spa-Addicts, Spa and Salon Wish	Therapists who open their own spas need to know how travel and recommendation services can help grow their businesses
Consulting	Assistance to develop or improve spa businesses	Wynne Business, Resources and Development, Preston Inc., ESPA, JGL, Smith Club & Spa, Blu Spa, Sylvia Planning and Design, Interdesign Spa Consulting	Some therapists become spa consultants and others hire consultants to help them develop their own spa businesses
Distribution	Clearinghouse for many spa product and equipment categories all within one company	Massage Warehouse, Scrip Massage & Spa Supply, Universal Companies, New Life Systems, Relaxus	Distributors streamline the purchase of spa equipment and products for therapists who want a "one-stop spa shop"

TABLE 2-8 Companies Related to the Spa Industry.

why it is important for massage therapists to become well-versed in the products and equipment these companies provide. In addition to the companies working directly in the spa industry, many allied industries have received a boost in sales due to the growth of spas, including architects and designers who have been contracted to help create spas, banking and insurance professionals who have specialized in helping spas do business, and construction firms that have built spas.

Spa Treatment Product Companies

Perhaps the most visible companies in the spa industry are those that provide the products that are actually applied to clients' bodies in the treatment rooms. These companies need to gain the respect and trust of spas in order to provide the products that will come into such intimate contact with their clients. If those clients do not have a positive experience with the products, they will not return to the spa, no matter how beautiful, expensive, or well-run it is. In addition, the products being used in the spa help create the overall ambience through the dispersal of aromas from herbs, seaweeds, clays, and oils (see discussion on "spa smell" in Chapter 17). Guests' most direct, lasting impact at many spas may be created, ultimately, by the product companies, not the spas themselves.

Spa and Hydrotherapy Equipment Manufacturers

Spas acquire much of their pizzazz from the fancy equipment they purchase. Sleek, space-age devices create a sense of exclusivity in high-end spas, and manufacturers who know this create ever more sophisticated and stylish equipment (Figures 2–8, 2–9, and 2–10). At the same time, spa equipment has become much more utilitarian in recent decades as spas moved out of antiquated systems featuring monolithic tubs and slabs upon which to perform **wet treatments** and into custom-designed pieces created with the input of practitioners in mind. See Chapter 3 for a thorough discussion of spa equipment.

wet treatments

spa treatments that involve the use of water, often in specially manufactured showers or baths

Exercise Equipment Manufacturers

Most destination spas and resort spas (and certainly all club spas) feature an array of fitness equipment to supplement the spa lifestyle. Some medical spas also use exercise equipment, often with medical components, such as treadmills with stress test **EKG** devices and body composition analysis machines. Massage therapists who understand the basic uses, contraindications, and effects of this equipment will have a much better grasp of spa clients' needs on the treatment table.

EKG

a graphical recording of the cardiac cycle produced by an electrocardiograph, often used in conjunction with treadmills at medical spas

SPA TIP

Massage therapists who understand the basic uses, contraindications, and effects of exercise equipment in the spa will have a much better grasp of spa clients' needs on the treatment table.

Spa Software Companies

Software is an integral part of most modern spas of any size. Without it, spa business owners would be forced to spend much more time on paperwork and menial tasks. Because software is integrated so thoroughly into most aspects of spa operation, software development companies have had to become conversant in many aspects of the spa business. The representatives who train spa owners and employees on the software, whether in person on site or remotely over the phone, often provide a great deal of help to spas, especially during startup and expansion phases.

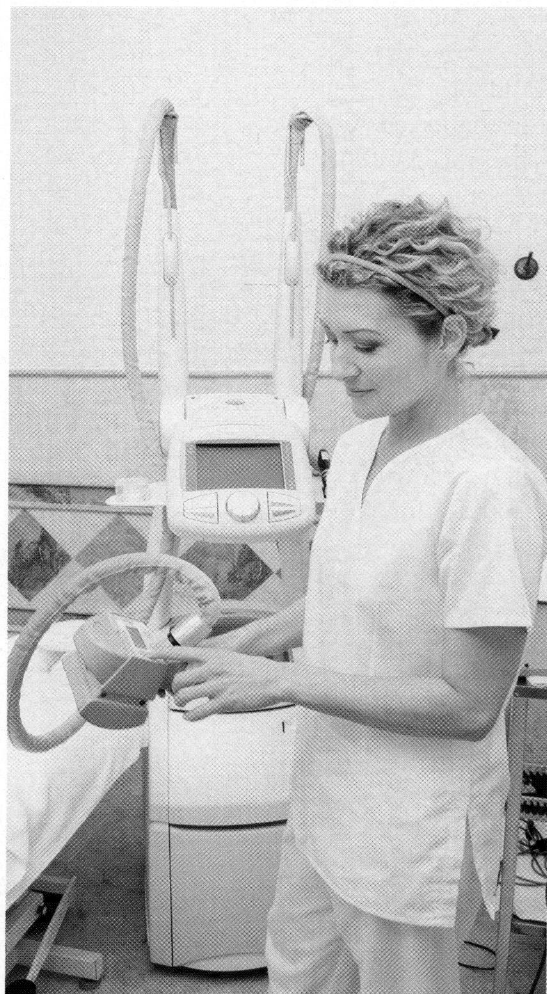

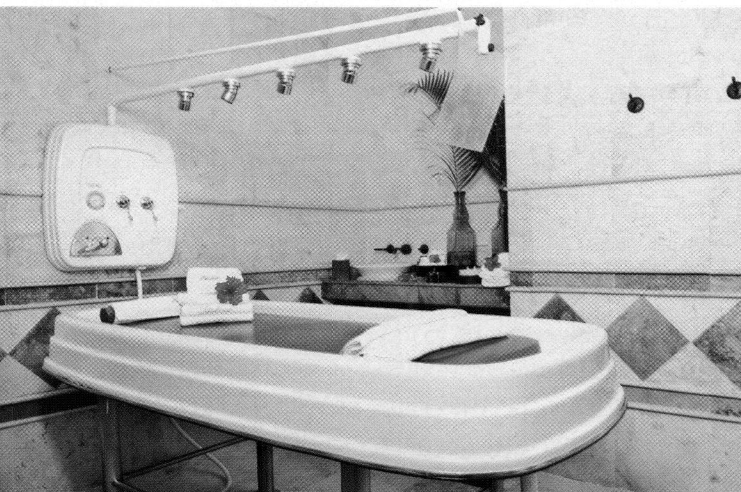

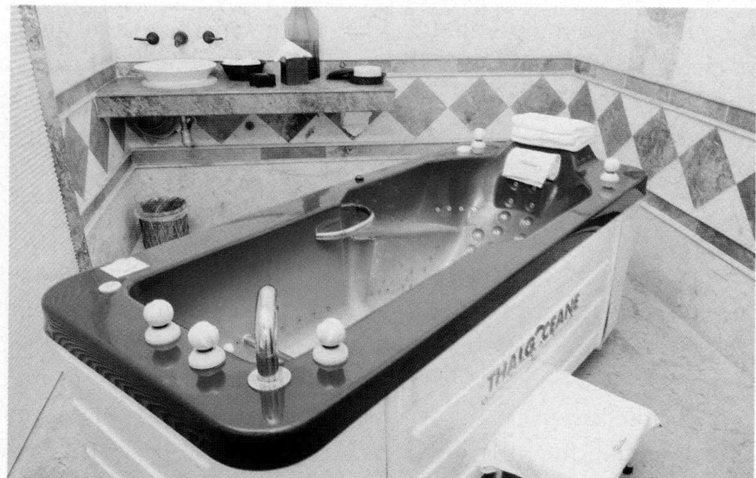

FIGURES 2-8, 2-9, 2-10 High-end spas often feature sophisticated and stylish equipment.

Spa Apparel and Lifestyle Companies

Each spa has its own philosophy. This philosophy is represented not only by the services offered at the spa but also by the products the spa offers its clients to take home. Spa retail shops are filled with lifestyle items such as candles, cards, tapes, books, and apparel. Fitness outfits, loungewear, and spa robes are especially popular. Therapists who wish to be in sync with the spa's philosophy often choose to become customers of these lifestyle companies themselves. They "walk the talk" of the spa lifestyle.

Spa Travel and Recommendation Companies

Consumers seeking recommendations and spa-specific travel services turn to a handful of companies that feature special offers combined with plentiful information. Many of these companies include gift certificate programs that are valid at hundreds or thousands of spas. The top-tier travel companies also produce consumer magazines.

Spa Consultants

Hundreds of individuals and companies offer consulting services in the spa industry. Some specialize in concept and design, others in treatment menu and staffing, and others in finance. A small number provide all of these services, plus ongoing spa management that is outsourced to them by resorts, hotels, and country clubs. The field has become so well-established that some **spa consultants** are even offering training services that certify other people as spa consultants.

spa consultants

professionals with expertise in helping entrepreneurs and practitioners navigate the waters of spa design, development, and management, sometimes doing hands-on work during various stages and at other times offering advice only

Spa Distributors

Several companies have gathered all the items needed by spa operations under one roof. Often, these companies have the economies of scale that make it possible to offer the best pricing, plus reduced shipping costs through consolidation. In addition, distributors have made forays into spa education and consulting as well. These companies will continue to merge and grow as the spa industry matures.

Important Individuals in the Modern Spa Industry

Although the energy and hard work of many people has certainly contributed to the amazing growth of the spa industry, there are certain individuals whose contributions stand out. As someone who will potentially make all or part of your living within the spa industry, it is appropriate and respectful to understand the gift you will be inheriting from those pioneers who have made the modern spa industry what it is today. The following list, though by no means exhaustive, highlights some of the individuals who played key roles in creating and developing modern spas in North America.

Deborah Szekely

Deborah Szekely is often referred to as the *grande dame* of the modern spa industry. Along with her husband Edmond (a Hungarian scholar, author, and philosopher known as "The Professor") she opened the first destination spa, Rancho la Puerta, in Baja California in the 1940s. She then visited Japan to study the traditional Ryokan inns, which were designed to welcome and restore weary travelers. After that trip, she and her husband opened the famed Golden Door Spa in Escondido, California, in 1958. This eventually became the most well-known spa in the United States. The Szekelys' firm belief in fitness, wellness, a healthy, pesticide-free diet, and living close to the land was adhered to by movie stars, moguls, and average individuals from every walk of life. Mrs. Szekely has also been active in the arts, politics, and humanitarian pursuits, having opened a school for the deaf, established a learning center and museum dedicated to immigrants, and even running for Congress. As the years went by, her son Alex Szekely took over the operation of the spas until his untimely death from cancer in 2002. In honor of his contribution to the spa industry, the International Spa Association announced the Alex Szekely Humanitarian Award, which is given each year to individuals who made contributions toward integrative medicine, actively promoting the preventive health and lifestyle behavioral changes that contribute to longevity and quality of life.

Mel Zuckerman

Mel and Enid Zuckerman founded the original Canyon Ranch Health Resort in Tucson, Arizona, in 1979. Canyon Ranch opened in Lenox, Massachusetts, in 1989. The first Canyon Ranch SpaClub opened at The Venetian Resort in Las Vegas, Nevada, in 1999. In 2002, Canyon Ranch opened a SpaClub facility at the Gaylord Palms Resort and Convention Center in Kissimmee, Florida. In January 2004, Canyon Ranch debuted its third Canyon Ranch SpaClub onboard the *Queen Mary II* luxury ocean liner. And Canyon Ranch Living, the company's first healthy living residential community, is now open in Miami Beach, Florida.

Andrew Weil

Though not a spa owner himself, Dr. Andrew Weil has played an important role at the Canyon Ranch Spa in Tucson. He is the director of the Program in Integrative Medicine at the University of Arizona College of Medicine, which receives support from the spa, and he is a past recipient of the Alex Szekely Humanitarian Award. Dr. Weil has also been the keynote speaker for the annual ISPA conference, and penned the forward to *The Canyon Ranch Guide to Living Younger Longer: A Complete Program for Optimal Health for Body, Mind, and Spirit*. Many in the spa industry look to him for leadership and inspiration.

Noel de Caprio

Noel de Caprio is acknowledged throughout the industry as the "Mother of Day Spas". The owner of Noelle Spa for Beauty and Wellness in Stamford, Connecticut, she helped originate the modern day spa concept back in the 1970s. She fought a twelve-year battle against breast cancer, which inspired her to turn her spa into a true healing center that offers private meditation, hypnotherapy, Reiki, shiatsu, and acupuncture, not just pampering services. She also helped create a "Look Good . . . Feel Better" program for cancer patients, and the spa provides a wig service for those undergoing chemotherapy. Mrs. de Caprio passed away in 1998, but her spa and her work still survive.

John and Ginny Lopis

A husband-and-wife team that has been at the forefront of spa development for many years, as consultants and spa directors they have helped create some of the most popular spa facilities and programs in the U.S. and internationally, including Canyon Ranch, the Doral in Miami, and Topnotch in Vermont. Eventually, they became owners of a new destination spa, The Lodge at Woodloch, in northeast Pennsylvania. Their programs take people beyond health, fitness, and relaxation into self-discovery. Honored as visionaries in the industry, they have found ways to attain success and profitability for spas while always maintaining a focus on environmentalism, economic sustainability, and human growth.

RESEARCH

Spa Profile

Complete a two-page profile of an operational spa, either one that you can visit and research in person or one that you can research at a distance on the Internet, in books, or through phone interviews. Include a profile and/or interview of the owner, spa director, manager, treatment supervisor, or staff therapist if possible. Focus on the spa's operating procedures, its competition, its employees, and its clientele. Ask hard questions about what it is really like working in the spa industry day-to-day, such as:

- *What is the turnover rate for staff, and how often do new people need to be hired?*
- *How many staff are full-time or part-time? Does the spa pay benefits?*
- *Does the spa know the cost of acquisition for each new client? What is it?*
- *Is it difficult to adjust staffing for seasonal ups and down in business?*
- *How does the spa target potential clients and market to them? Do they specifically try to attract male clients?*
- *What are the most popular services at the spa? Least popular?*
- *How often does the spa add new services to the menu? How do they train therapists to perform them? Do they pay for therapists' training?*
- *Approximately how many vendors and suppliers does the spa need to keep stocked and open for business? Are all of these relationships positive? Do any vendors supply training for therapists on staff?*
- *Does the spa belong to any industry associations? If so, has membership been helpful? Has anyone at the spa attended industry trade shows?*
- *Does the spa have any quality-control systems in place? Do they follow a specific set of guidelines or code of ethics?*

After you have gathered the real-world information for this profile, ask yourself how it compares to your vision of the spa you would like to create or work in one day.

Bernard Burt

For years, Bernard Burt has kept his finger on the pulse of the spa industry and has kept many people in touch with that pulse through his "Spa-Goer Newsletter" and his widely read books, including *Fodor's Healthy Escapes* and *100 Best Spas of the World*. He took part in the founding of the International Spa Association and has played an important role in creating a cohesive, marketable spa industry to which the general public can relate. Many spa professionals look to him for the latest news and trends.

Sheila Cluff

Sheila Cluff is founder of The Oaks at Ojai Spa in Ojai, California. An internationally known fitness expert, a former board member of ISPA, and a member of the College of Sports Medicine as well as the Intercontinental Hotels Advisory Travel Board, Cluff was the recipient of the ISPA Visionary Award, rewarding her for her dedication to the industry. In May 2002, *Spa* magazine recognized her as a pioneer of the American spa industry with a "Trailblazer" tribute. Cluff introduced "cardiovascular dance," a forerunner of aerobics, to the world in the 1950s. For decades she has helped guests at her spa attain wellness and personal power through healthy living.

ACTIVITY

Your Ideal Spa

Write a one-page description of the ideal spa that you would one day like to work in or own yourself. Who would you like as your boss, or who would you like to hire? What type of spa would it be? What model(s) of previously successful spa(s) would you follow? How many therapists would be on staff? Where would it be located?

SPA ETIQUETTE

When visiting spas in person or calling spas on the phone to gather information for a research project, always identify yourself honestly and state the true nature of your business rather than pretending to be a spa customer and asking lots of probing questions while receiving a treatment.

CONCLUSION

Spas today are some of the most innovative and fast-moving businesses in the world. Although based on ancient techniques and traditions, they are thoroughly modern. Becoming a part of the spa industry offers massage therapists a way to join the fast-paced global economy without sacrificing their dreams and goals of helping other people through massage therapy and other wellness services. In order to play a successful role in this industry, it is helpful to understand how other people forged successful spa careers and how they simultaneously helped many clients and colleagues along the way. It is important to learn and grow with colleagues and mentors in spa associations. And it is crucial to form strong connections with the people who support the industry through their products and knowledge. Without becoming an active member of the spa community, massage therapists will play only a limited role in the industry that supplies more massage jobs than any other.

REVIEW QUESTIONS

1. Name some trends in the spa industry.
2. Approximately how many people were working in the spa industry in 2008?
3. What is the main difference between a destination spa and a day spa?
4. What are the five general categories of spa goers, and how can therapists positively affect their experiences in the spa?
5. Which professional spa associations are most relevant to therapists working in the spa industry? Why?
6. How do those therapists who are not directly employed by the spa industry stand to benefit greatly by the popularity of spa modalities?
7. What are some of the member codes of ethics of the International Spa Association that directly affect massage therapists who work in spas?
8. Why is it important for massage therapists to be familiar with companies that are related to the spa industry?

CHAPTER

3

Spa Equipment, Facilities, and Procedures

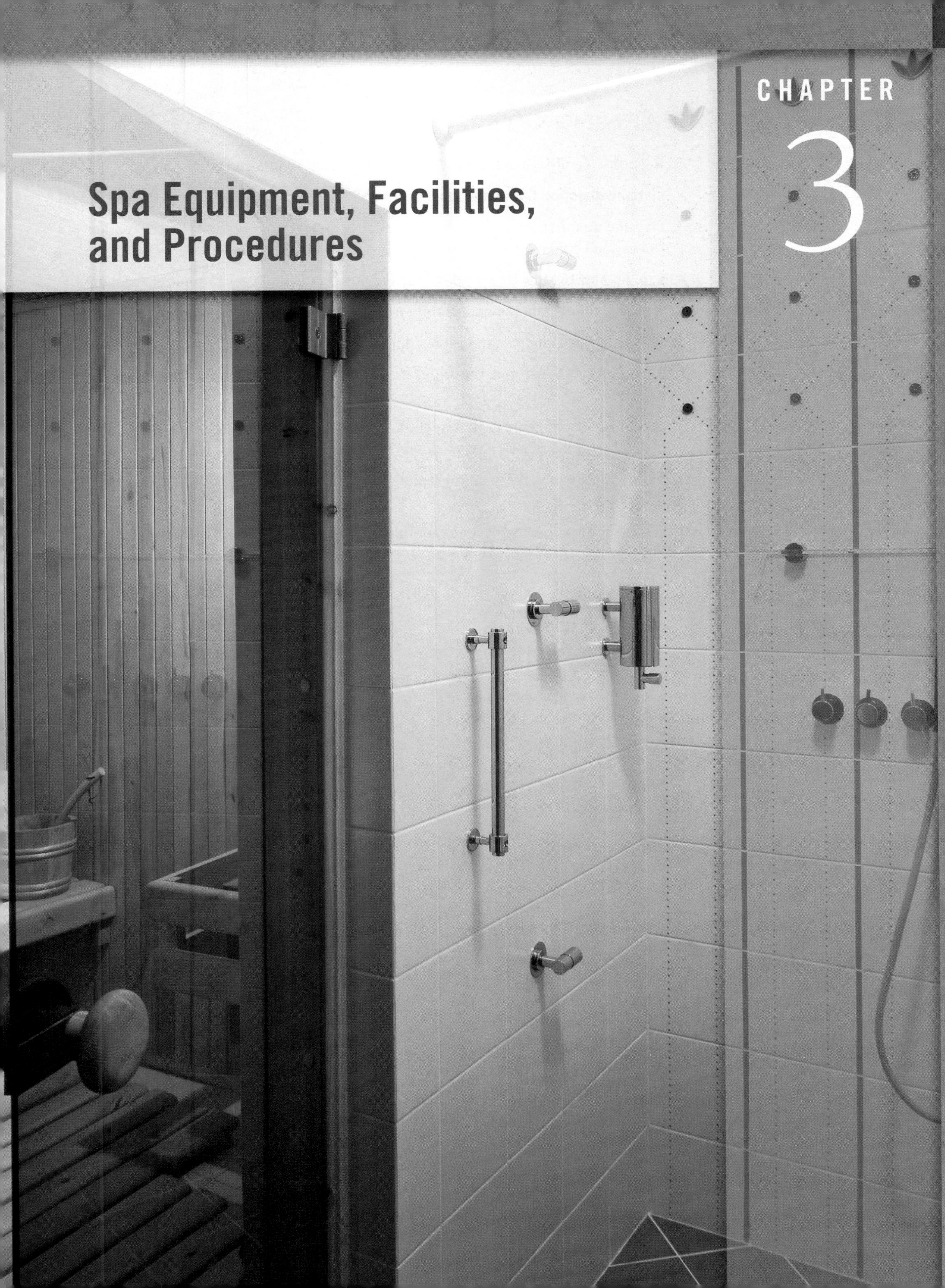

LEARNING OBJECTIVES

1. **Describe the difference between a spa "wet room" and a spa "dry room."**
2. **List and describe the items necessary to set up a spa dry room.**
3. **List and describe equipment used in spa wet rooms, including showers, baths, tables, and chambers.**
4. **Explain how to stock the proper supplies and products for a spa treatment room.**
5. **Identify and explain the main safety issues encountered in the spa environment.**
6. **Define 10 general spa safety rules and explain why they are important.**
7. **Define 10 general spa therapist self-care rules and explain why they are important.**
8. **Define risk management as it applies to the spa therapist, and explain the three main categories of risk management issues faced by spa businesses.**
9. **Define the actions that spa therapists and spa owners can take to improve risk management.**
10. **List the most important issues regarding sanitation and hygiene in the spa.**

INTRODUCTION

As a future spa employee or owner, you need to know everything you can about the fundamental physical reality of spas, especially the equipment and facilities needed to make spas work, yet a surprisingly large number of massage therapy students have never even visited a spa. Imagine you were an aspiring baseball player hoping to join the major leagues, but you had never even seen a baseball game played. Or you were a novice actor hoping to make it big in Hollywood, but you'd never been to the movies. This total lack of knowledge and experience is unthinkable, and yet therapists routinely apply for spa positions with absolutely no idea what spas are like. This is not acceptable. Study this chapter carefully in order to familiarize yourself with the basic realities of spas, including the sanitary and safe use of spa facilities and equipment, and the orderly effective use of spa supplies. The information and activities here will help you develop an appreciation for the environment in which you may soon be spending a good deal of time.

When clients walk through the front door of a luxurious spa, or even a private therapist's small spa treatment practice, what do they experience? What are the impressions created by spas on the senses of spa goers? Every decision made regarding physical spa facilities has a direct impact on the spa's guests as well as the spa's employees. The quality of the facility and equipment is of the utmost importance. This by no means implies that only expensive facilities and equipment are appropriate. As long as they are safe, sanitary, effective, and attractive, even the most basic facilities can create a fabulous spa experience. The key to this type of experience lies in an intense attention to detail regarding every aspect of the physical spa itself. This chapter addresses those details.

ACTIVITY

Go to a Spa!

Go visit a spa! In Chapter 14 you will be assigned the activity of visiting a spa and receiving a treatment in order to evaluate the experience. For now, simply visiting a spa is enough. You need not spend any money or take any risks. Simply stop by a spa and ask for a menu of services. If it is available, ask for a tour of the spa facilities as well. Take close note of the equipment, furniture, and fixtures. Are there lockers? Changing rooms? Hydrotherapy equipment? Are any "back of the house" areas visible, or is there a seamless façade of tranquility and beauty? Are any guests visible? Do they look comfortable and secure, or vulnerable and uncertain? Upon returning from your visit, write a paragraph outlining your overall impression of the spa, giving your gut reaction as to what it felt like to be there.

DRY ROOM VERSUS WET ROOM

The very first distinction that must be drawn when describing spa treatment facilities is that between a **wet room** and a **dry room** (Figures 3–1 and 3–2, Table 3–1). As a spa therapist, you will be operating in either a dry room or wet room for much of your time on the job. It is important, then, for you to understand how these rooms function, how to clean, maintain, and stock them correctly, which treatments can be best performed in each, and how to properly use each for the benefit of your clients.

wet room

a spa treatment room that is usually tiled and has a source of water (showers, bath, wet table, etc.) and drainage for the application of hydrotherapy treatments and cleansing of spa products from clients' bodies

dry room

a spa treatment room that does not have a source of water (showers, bath, wet table, etc.) or drainage, requiring the use of moist towels, insulated containers, heating elements, and other supplies to recreate a full spa experience

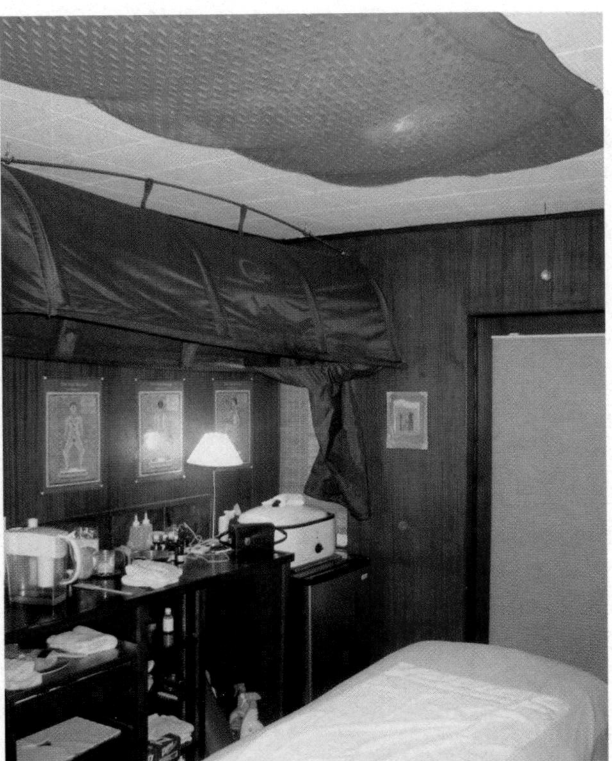

FIGURE 3–1 A spa dry room can be a regular massage room, even with carpeting on the floor. Notice the heater/insulator units to keep products, towels, etc., warm.

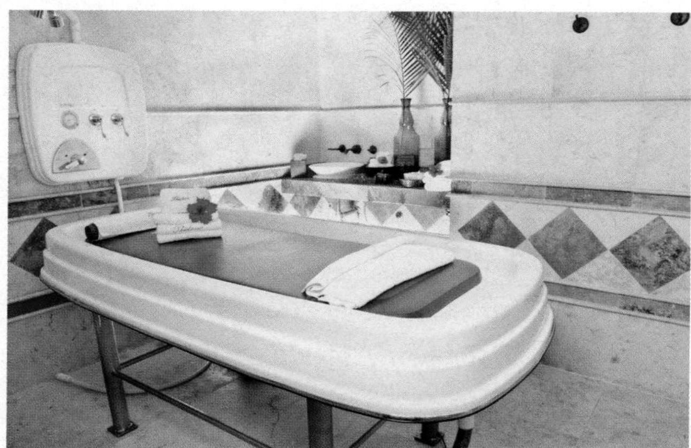

FIGURE 3–2 A spa wet room includes plumbing and usually a high-end table or hydrotherapy equipment.

A dry room can be defined simply as a spa treatment room that does not have a source of water. There is no shower, no bathtub, no hydrotherapy tub, no wet table, no drain in the floor, and usually no tiles on the floor or walls. A dry room can be a normal massage room, even if it has carpeting on the floor and no sink. A source of water somewhere nearby is necessary, however. Dry rooms require the use of moist towels, insulated containers, heating elements, and other supplies to recreate a full spa experience, but all of these can be purchased for much less than the cost of installing the plumbing and spa equipment needed for a wet room.

A wet room can be defined as a spa treatment room, usually tiled, that has a source of water in it such as a shower, a bathtub, a **hydrotherapy tub** or a wet table with **Vichy shower**. Also, by definition, it requires drainage for the water. This is where hydrotherapy treatments take place, and also where many spas perform their body wraps and exfoliation services. The advanced shower systems (see Chapter 4) found here aid in the cleansing of spa products from clients' bodies as well.

hydrotherapy tub

technician-operated soaking tub with computerized zone-specific jet systems and underwater massage hose

Vichy shower

a horizontal bar with multiple down-facing nozzles along its length, suspended above a wet table used to shower clients lying below

Until the late 1980s, wet rooms were often tiled from floor to ceiling and featured a monolithic tiled slab in the center of the room upon which clients lay to be slathered with copious amounts of product and sprayed with forceful bursts from hoses attached to the wall. This is no longer the case. Modern wet rooms feature tables with built-in drains that make tiling on the walls and ceiling (and sometimes even the floor) unnecessary (Figure 3–3). Spa products can be washed from the skin and sent directly into the drain, doing away with the

	WET ROOM	VS	DRY ROOM
Infrastructure	plumbing, plumbed treatment table, drain, tiled floors and perhaps walls as well		regular massage room without shower or tub or even sink needed in room, but a source of water is needed nearby
Equipment	treatment table (called a wet table), shower(s), optional hydrotherapy tub		massage table, insulating container to keep products and towels hot
Supplies	blanket, sheets, towels, thermal blanket, plastic body wrap, exfoliants, muds, clays, seaweeds, massage lubricants, essential oils		blanket, sheets, towels, thermal blanket, plastic body wrap, exfoliants, muds, clays, seaweeds, massage lubricants, essential oils
Advantages	perceived as high-end and luxurious, fast and effective hydrotherapy, quick washing of product from skin, immersive hydrotherapy benefits for clients		inexpensive to build, can be included in any massage practice with little alteration, clients often enjoy luxury of more intense hands-on care by therapist
Disadvantages	expensive to build, perceived as "cold" by some clients, uses large amount of water, underused if not equipped for regular massage treatments		difficult to clean certain spa products from clients' skin, cannot provide high-tech hydrotherapy baths and shower treatments
Safety Issues	slips on wet tile floors, potential electrical hazards, copious use of hot water makes burning a concern		the need to heat towels and product can create a burn hazard

TABLE 3–1 Wet Room/Dry Room Comparison.

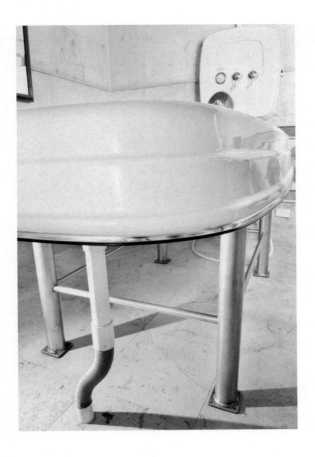

FIGURE 3–3 Modern wet tables have built-in drains.

need for extra cleanup. This also serves to keep therapists dry as well. In the past, many therapists donned bathing attire to perform wet treatments.

The Spa Classroom

Although a growing number of massage training facilities have built spa-specific classrooms that may include wet rooms with showers, wet tables, and hydrotherapy equipment, the majority do not have such amenities. While it is unique and enjoyable to learn in an environment that closely simulates a spa wet room, it is not absolutely necessary. Spa owners and directors repeatedly state that the most important aspects of spa training are in fundamental knowledge, modality familiarization, basic hands-on technique, appropriate team-oriented attitude, and customer service skills. Ability to operate specific pieces of spa equipment is not on the list. If you do have the opportunity to study in a wet room environment at your school, enjoy the experience, but also be aware that you will likely need more equipment-specific training when you begin work, because the brand, model, and procedure may differ from property to property. Even if your school has the latest wet room equipment, it will benefit you to learn dry room procedures as well to round out your skill set and make you a more valuable all-around spa professional. In addition, if you open a spa yourself one day (see Chapter 17) you might choose to offer dry room treatments at first because infrastructure costs to build out a wet room are high. The spa treatment protocols described in Chapters 4 through 13 in this book will be clearly marked as to whether they are dry room–specific or not.

SPA ETIQUETTE

A regular massage room in a spa is not referred to as a "dry room" unless it is equipped to perform spa treatments in addition to massage. Do not make this classic squares-and-rectangles error. Every dry room can be used as a massage room, *but* not every massage room can be used as a dry room.

SPA TIP

Resourceful therapists can perform a large number of spa treatment modalities in a dry room with the use of hot wet towels to remove product and cleanse the skin. Paradoxically, clients sometimes prefer this technique because of the added personal attention. High-tech showers and tubs are great, but the simple act of having the skin cleansed by a caring therapist can be just as luxurious, and sometimes more so.

Wet Room Confusion

Did You Know?

Therapists are sometimes confused as to whether they need to develop an expertise in wet room procedures in order to become full-fledged spa therapists or to open their own day spa. Several basic questions arise from this confusion. Answers to these questions are listed below.

Q: Are there any spa treatments that cannot be administered in a dry room as compared to a wet room?

A: Yes. A Vichy shower, for example, cannot be administered in a dry room because, by definition, it includes a shower. The same applies to a hydrotherapy bath. However, all body wraps and exfoliation services performed in spa wet rooms can be modified for application in a dry room setting.

Q: Will clients still visit a spa if it does not include a wet room?

A: Definitely yes. Some guests may expect a wet room at larger spa facilities, but the majority of guests are quite happy receiving massages, esthetic services, and body treatments in a dry room.

Q: In order to compete with other spas, is a wet room necessary?

A: Only if the spa is a large, high-end facility, usually a resort or destination spa. Smaller day spas with dry rooms can compete with larger wet room–outfitted spas in the same area, especially if they offer a better price and/or equal or better service.

Q: Isn't it better to have a wet room because massage treatments can be offered in them as well, and that way the room will be used more?

A: Not necessarily. The extra costs associated with building and maintaining a wet room may outweigh the benefits of having the extra space available. Also, some clients prefer not to receive massage treatments in a wet room because they feel, rightly or wrongly, that it is too cold or impersonal.

Setting Up the Spa Dry Room

Later in this chapter you will find descriptions and explanations regarding the spa wet room and equipment specific to it. For now, we will concentrate on the dry room, how it works, and how to prepare it. How big does a spa dry room need to be? In general, the answer to that is, approximately the same size as a massage room, but preferably a little bigger to accommodate the extra equipment, supplies, and linens needed to perform spa treatments. At the very least, spa dry rooms need extra storage space compared to typical massage rooms. The equipment you will need to perform spa services in a dry room is listed in the sections below.

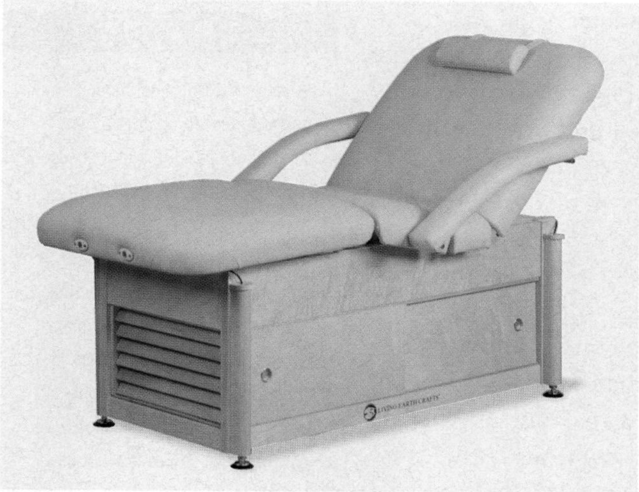

FIGURE 3–4 The multipurpose treatment table is the centerpiece of an effective spa dry room. (Photo courtesy of Massage Warehouse.)

Treatment Table

The centerpiece for any successful spa dry room is the treatment table. Ideally, this should be a multipurpose table, meaning it can be used for a number of spa services plus massage in a manner that is comfortable for clients and ergonomically effective for therapists (Figure 3–4). A multipurpose table costs more than a typical massage table, but the benefits far outweigh the extra cost. These tables make it easy to lift clients' upper bodies for face treatments or raise the knees for foot treatments, and some even include foot basins for soaking during these procedures.

SPA TIP

A spa dry room should be slightly larger than a normal massage room (ideally a minimum of 10" × 14") in order to accommodate the extra equipment and supplies.

Water Source

As we learned in Chapter 1, the word *spa* has come to stand for water (*sanitas per aqua*), and so it will come as no surprise to you that water is a needed ingredient for your spa services, even in a dry spa room. However, it is important to note that the water source need not be within the room itself. A sink down the hall or in a nearby bathroom is sufficient. This source is used to moisten towels, wash clients' skin, warm products, and steep herbs. Water can be brought into the dry treatment room in various kinds of containers, including hydrocollators and roasters.

Heating Units

Most dry spa rooms contain heating units of one kind or another. Although it is possible to offer spa services using hot water from the tap to heat products and towels, it is difficult and inefficient. The three most popular heating units used in dry spa rooms are hydrocollators, hot towel cabbies, and roasters (Figure 3–5).

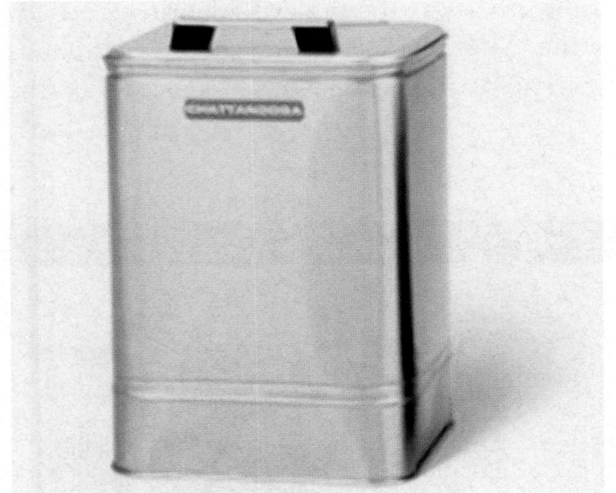

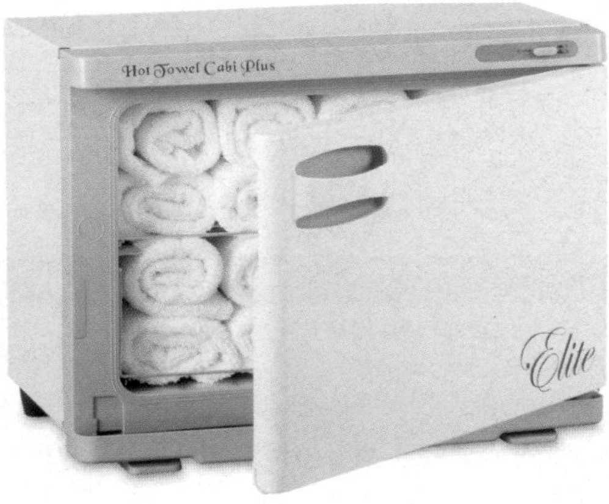

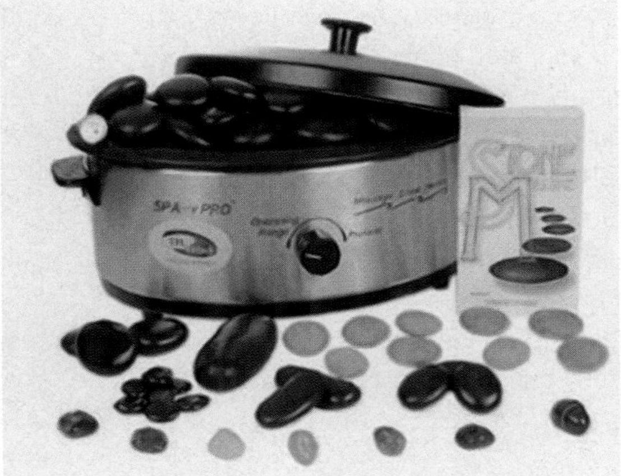

FIGURE 3–5 These three options are the most popular heating units used in dry spa rooms. (Photos courtesy of Massage Warehouse.)

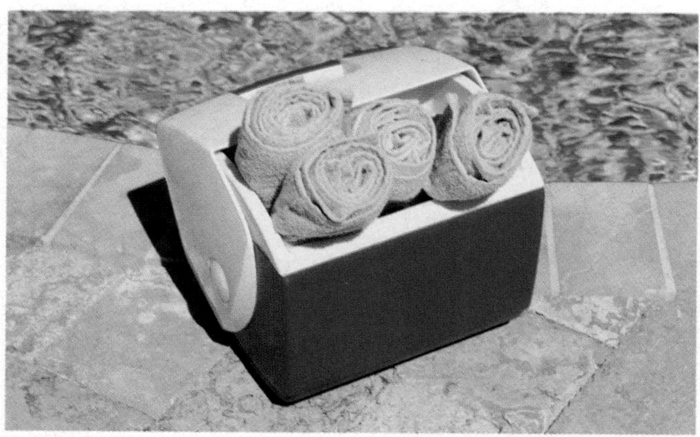

FIGURE 3–6 Ice chests, also known as Spa Thermal Units, can be used to keep towels and spa products hot in the dry treatment room.

Insulated Containers

Even the most luxurious and well-equipped spas use insulated containers in their treatment rooms to keep products, towels, sheets, and sometimes stones hot while in transport or while waiting to be applied to the client's body. Often, these are simply ice chests, plastic bus trays or other readily available containers, repurposed for use in the dry room (Figure 3–6). When used in this capacity, an ice chest is referred to by some therapists as a **Spa Thermal Unit (STU)**. When kept in such containers, towels and products remain hot throughout the duration of a treatment so that, for example, a therapist can wring out towels in hot water and place them in the STU at the beginning of an exfoliation service to have them available to cleanse products from the body during a full half-hour.

Spa Thermal Unit (STU)

an ice chest or other insulated container repurposed for use in a spa dry room to keep towels and products hot prior to treatment

cocoon

another term for spa body wrap, so called because the client is tucked inside the surrounding sheets and blankets like a chrysalis

Blankets

Blankets are used extensively in spa treatments to wrap clients, creating a layering effect for warmth and protection which is sometimes referred to as a **cocoon** (Figure 3–8). Specific types of blankets have been favored in different areas at different times. At one point, wool was the preferred fabric because it was thought to be the best insulating material. However, spas today employ a wide range of materials for use in wrapping. The blanket layer is usually on the

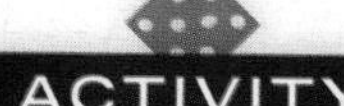

ACTIVITY

Hot Towel Safety

Because hot towels are used so extensively in dry spa rooms, and potentially in your classroom as well, become familiar with their use by practicing this simple procedure. First, fold a high-quality hand towel in half twice, roll it up, then dip it into very hot water—165°F maximum, 120°F minimum—and wring it out. Make sure to wring out every drop of moisture you can, using protective gloves (Figure 3–7). Place the towel in an insulated container or hot towel cabbie, then have a partner lie on the massage table, face down. Take the towel out, unroll it and air it out for a moment, then place it gently on your partner's back, letting the heat soak into the pores. Make sure to check the temperature of the towel on the skin of your own inner forearm first. Slide the towel slowly over your partner's back, as if you were cleaning spa products from the body. Many people find the sensation of being "washed" in this way by another person is more enjoyable than simply taking a shower to clean off spa products.

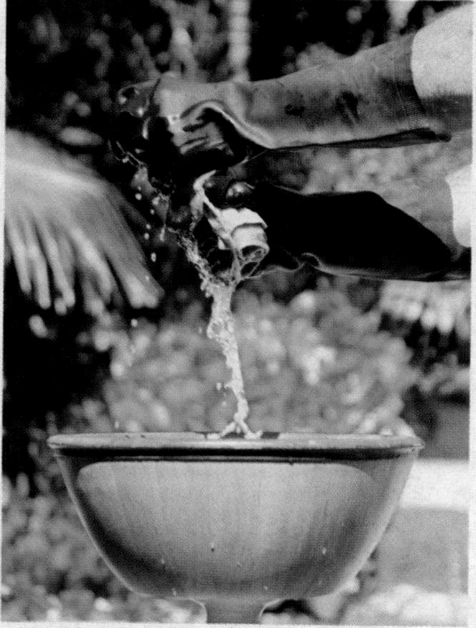

FIGURE 3–7 People find the sensation of hot towels being applied quite enjoyable.

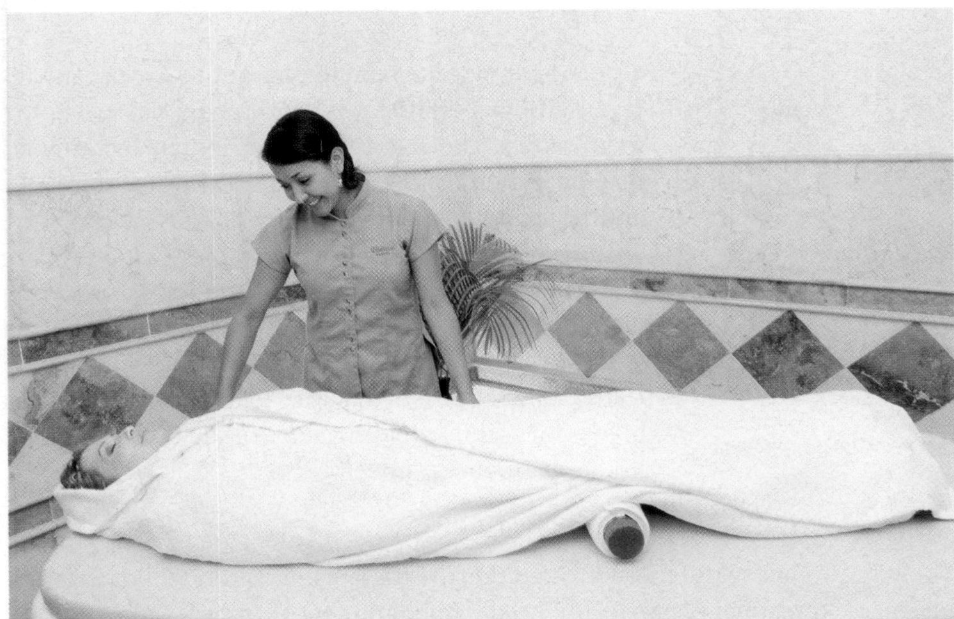

FIGURE 3–8 Being wrapped in blankets during a spa treatment is sometimes referred to as a "cocoon."

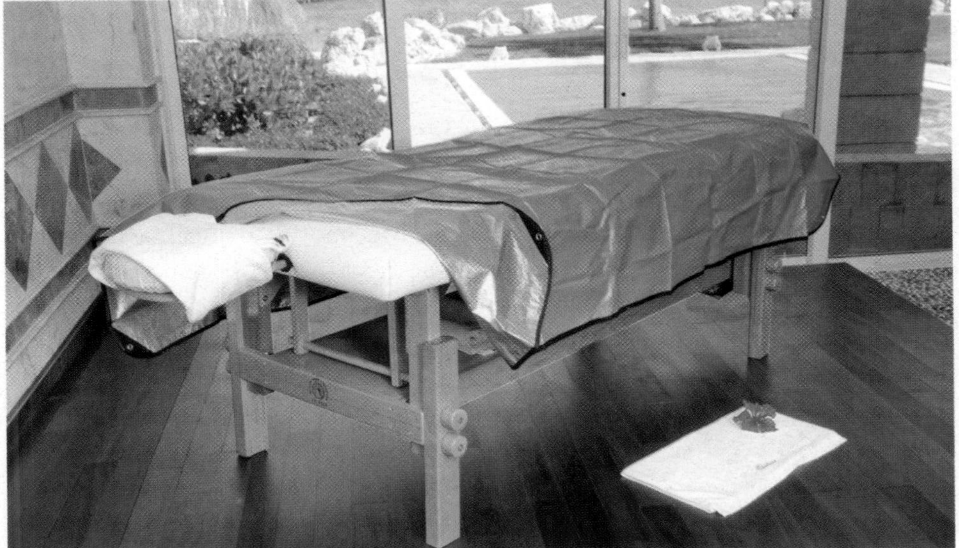

FIGURE 3–9 Thermal blankets play a role in insulating clients during spa treatments.

SPA CAUTION

It is not recommended that you use a microwave oven to warm up towels for spa treatments. Microwaves heat objects unevenly, and towels heated in this manner may have patches you do not notice that are too hot to safely apply to clients' skin.

bottom closest to the treatment table and consists of the outermost layer in any wrapping procedure.

The **thermal blanket** (Figure 3–9), also referred to as a **space blanket**, is made from a special material first developed by NASA in 1964 to help protect delicate space ship parts. It is also used by outdoor enthusiasts to remain warm in harsh conditions. It reduces bodily heat loss by reflecting 80 percent of it off a silver metallic surface back to the wearer. These blankets are constructed by layering a precise amount of pure aluminum vapor onto a thin, durable film substrate. In spa dry rooms (and wet rooms, as we shall see), these blankets often form an extra insulating layer around clients' bodies when they are wrapped. They can also be used to protect massage treatment tables from water and spa products.

thermal blanket

metallic blanket often used by outdoor enthusiasts to remain warm in harsh conditions, repurposed for body wraps in the spa setting and also for protection of massage treatment tables from water and products

space blanket

see *thermal blanket*

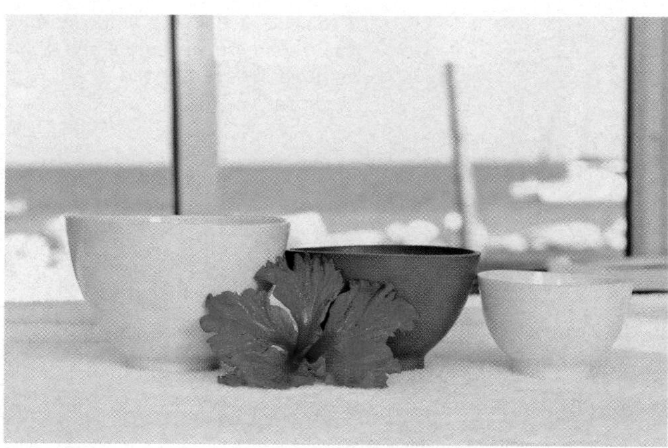

FIGURE 3–10 Spa bowls are used by therapists to keep products warm and easily accessible.

Spa Bowls

Spa bowls were originally developed for use as the mixing bowls dentists use to prepare the paste for tooth molds. They are rubberized, extremely durable, usually brown or green in color, and prized for their ability to retain the heat of any spa product placed within them (Figure 3–10). Therapists use them for seaweeds, muds, clays, exfoliants, and other products, often floating the bowl in hot water or nestling it next to hot towels in a cabbie or roaster. Another attractive feature of spa bowls is that they tend to wobble instead of overturn, thus avoiding a multitude of messy spills in the spa room.

spa bowls

rubberized bowls used to hold and to warm spa products during treatments, prized for their insulation, sturdiness, and stability

Wheeled Stool

Many spa rooms feature a small stool for the therapist to sit on while performing specific treatments, especially head, hand, and foot treatments, that require extended periods focusing on one part of the body. It is best if this stool is on wheels for easy movement from one side of the treatment table to the other (Figure 3–11). Comfortable stools with high-quality, quiet wheels are most suitable for the spa room.

Face Cradle

Face cradles are not used as often in spa rooms as they are in massage rooms, for one main reason: Traditional spa wet rooms featured treatment slabs instead of tables, and there was no way to attach a face cradle to these slabs. Over the years, as specialized spa treatment tables became more popular, they usually lacked face cradles, like the slabs, even though face cradles could have readily been added to the spa treatment table. Then, as practitioners began using regular portable massage tables for spa services in dry rooms, this tradition continued, and most dry spa services were applied without face cradles, too. Now, however, spa therapists have realized that face cradles are acceptable, easily adaptable, and actually preferable for spa treatments, and they are incorporating them into most, if not all, services (Figure 3–12). You will notice that many protocols in this book feature face cradles. If you see protocols anywhere that do not feature the cradles, you can adapt the protocol for use with them.

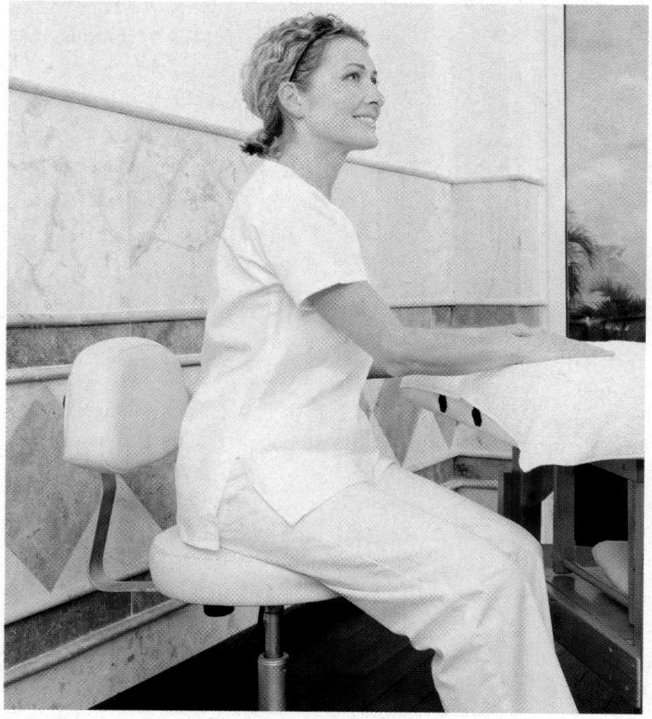

FIGURE 3–11 A comfortable wheeled stool is a great tool for the spa treatment room.

Optional Dry Room Equipment

In addition to the basic supplies and equipment needed to perform most services, dry spa rooms can feature a wide range of optional devices to enhance the therapeutic outcome of the treatments rendered. Some of these devices add an element of heat to spa therapy, either through immersion in a hot medium such as wax or steam, or through general heating of the treatment space with infrared lighting or other means. Optional equipment is sometimes devoted to the organizing or streamlining of the treatment space as well. See Chapter 17, under "A Consciously Created Environment," for more detailed information about optional supplies and décor to enhance the spa room. The items listed below are commonly found in dry rooms.

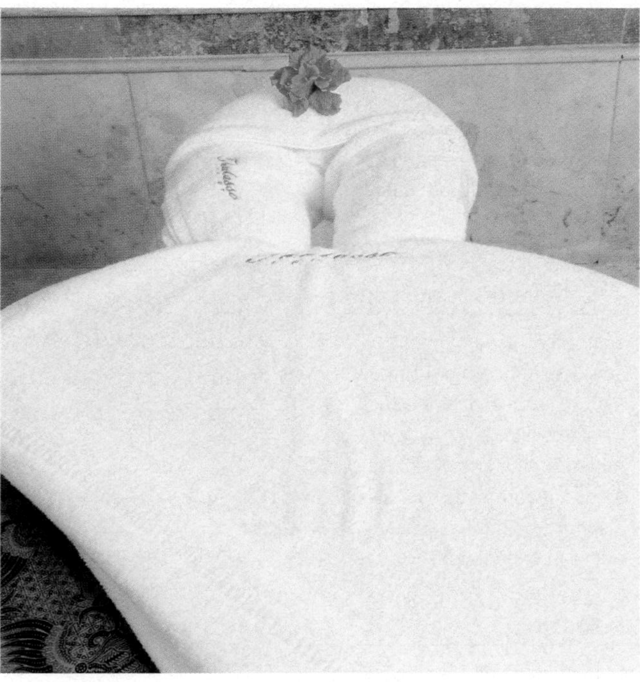

FIGURE 3–12 Face cradles can be used for almost all spa treatments.

Paraffin Wax

Estheticians and cosmetologists have used therapeutic paraffin wax in the spa setting for many years, and more recently, massage therapists have begun applying it as well, with good results. The wax is heated to approximately 129°F in electric basins that are usually kept on a counter or table in the treatment room. These basins vary in size and shape depending on the intended use (Figure 3–13). Detailed information about the therapeutic application of paraffin can be found in Chapter 5.

treatment bar

console (often wheeled) with various heated bins for storage and easy access to spa products and supplies

Treatment Bar

With all of the extra products and supplies needed to apply spa services in the confined space of a treatment room, some spas elect to consolidate these items in one console called a **treatment bar**. These consoles allow an economical use of space by providing multiple heated bins for items such as rocks, towels, sheets, oils and body muds, and they also have storage space below the bins.

Steamy Wonder™

the brand name for a steam canopy that fits over treatment tables, allowing therapists to apply heat treatments in a limited space

Steamy Wonder™

Steamy Wonder™ is the brand name for a steam canopy that can be placed over the treatment table (Figure 3–14). Clients recline on the table as usual, and the canopy is lowered over them. Steam generated in a crock pot is fed into the

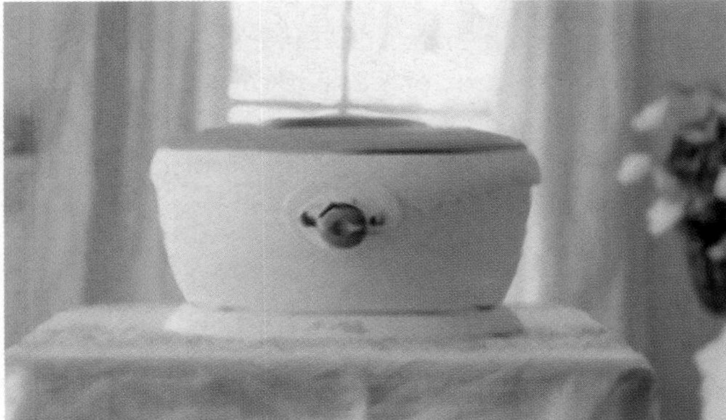

FIGURE 3–13 Paraffin heating basins are a common sight in spa treatment rooms as therapists become more well acquainted with their use.

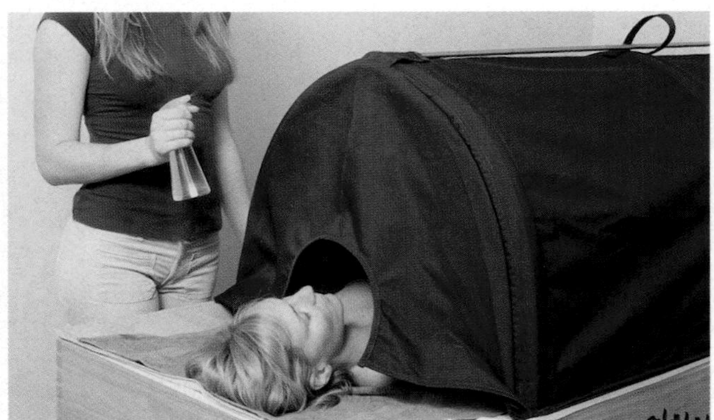

FIGURE 3–14 The Steamy Wonder™ is used effectively by many therapists when space or budget does not allow for a full steam room or sauna.

Russian steam cabinet

small, usually fiberglass chamber in which a person sits, head outside, while bathed with steam generated from a unit in the base

laser skin resurfacing

sometimes used in medical spas, the process of using laser light to remove damaged or wrinkled skin, layer by layer, to minimize fine lines, especially around mouth and eyes, and also for treating facial scars or uneven pigmentation

Botox®

trademark name for a highly purified preparation of botulinum toxin Type A, injected under the skin to smooth wrinkles and to treat certain muscle conditions

microdermabrasion

technique using a high-pressure stream of abrasive crystals against the skin for exfoliation, usually performed only on the face by licensed estheticians

facial machines

piece of equipment used by estheticians to treat clients' skin, usually combining several instruments including steam generator, brushes, magnifying lamp, vacuum, galvanic current, and others

wet area

that part of a spa devoted to services using water including baths, showers, sprays, wet tables, etc.; can include both private treatment rooms and public spaces; often broken down into separate male and female areas

canopy with a fan, heating the client's body quickly and effectively with minimal residual moisture and no damage to the table. These steam canopies are appropriate for use in small dry rooms with minimal space available. Some spas hang a canopy from the ceiling and lower it for the appropriate treatments. The steam tents are especially useful before herbal wraps and other heat treatments.

Infrared Lamp

Spa rooms can and do become cold. It is especially important to keep clients warm when they are wet or when they have spa products applied to their skin. Therefore, many spas incorporate supplemental heating units to warm the air around the treatment table. The most common heaters are infrared lights. These can be recessed in the ceiling or mounted on a stand. Some stands are on wheels so they can be moved to the area of the spa room most needed.

Russian Steam Cabinet

Another option for applying steam heat to spa clients in an enclosed dry space is the **Russian steam cabinet**. This device opens in the front and has a seat inside upon which the client sits. The cabinet is closed and a small generator in the base emits steam, creating moist heat. The client's head remains outside of the unit throughout the treatment, which helps avoid sensations of claustrophobia in most clients.

Saunas

Saunas are a staple at many larger spas, but in smaller spas and dry rooms they are less common, if not completely unknown (see Chapter 5 for more detailed information about saunas and steam baths). One exception is the infrared sauna, which uses radiation to heat the client rather than hot rocks to heat the air inside the sauna. Infrared saunas can be plugged into a normal wall outlet, and the smaller units only take up a few square feet of floor space.

Foot Bath

Some spa dry rooms have foot baths that can be filled in a preparation area and brought in for treatments. These can be simple basins or electric models that feature heat, vibration, and water jets.

Other Equipment

Many spas, of course, also feature other equipment such as **laser skin resurfacing** systems, syringes to inject **Botox®**, **microdermabrasion** machines, and **facial machines**. The use of these and other pieces of equipment found in the spa will not be described in this book, because treatments performed with them are outside the scope of practice for massage therapists.

SPA WET ROOM EQUIPMENT

The equipment used in spa wet rooms or **wet areas** can be broken down into four main categories: showers, tubs, tables, and chambers (Figures 3–15 through 3–17). Each category features several variations, and equipment manufacturers have all come up with their own version of each one of these variations, leading

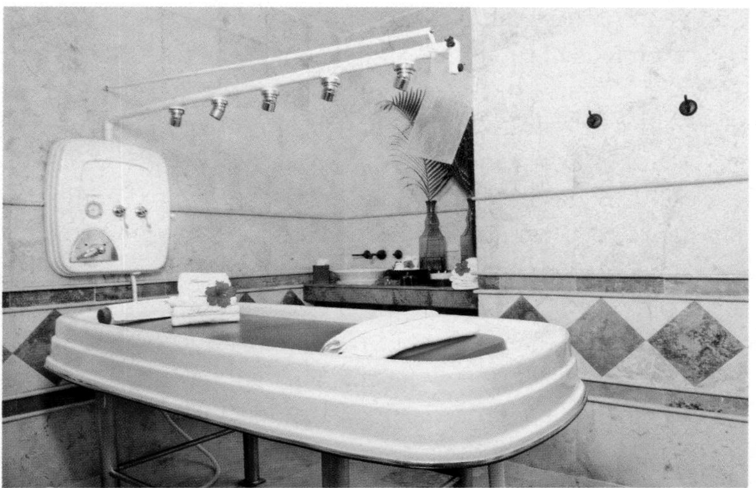

FIGURE 3–15 Vichy showers are a key feature in many spa wet areas.

SPA CAUTION

The Russian steam cabinet is comfortable for most people because the head remains cool outside the heating chamber. Even so, some clients report intense claustrophobia inside these devices. Clients should never be left alone when entering a Russian steam cabinet for the first time.

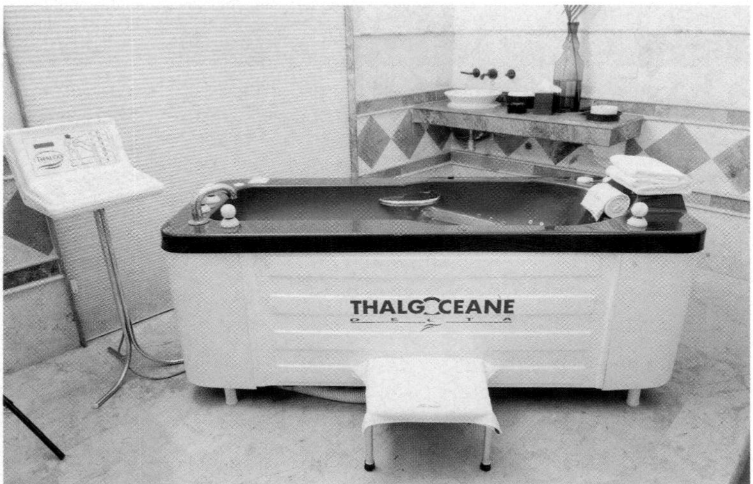

FIGURE 3–16 Hydrotherapy tubs offer a great deal of adjustability for the operator and a comprehensive treatment for the client, including therapeutic ingredients and targeted percussive action from multiple water jets.

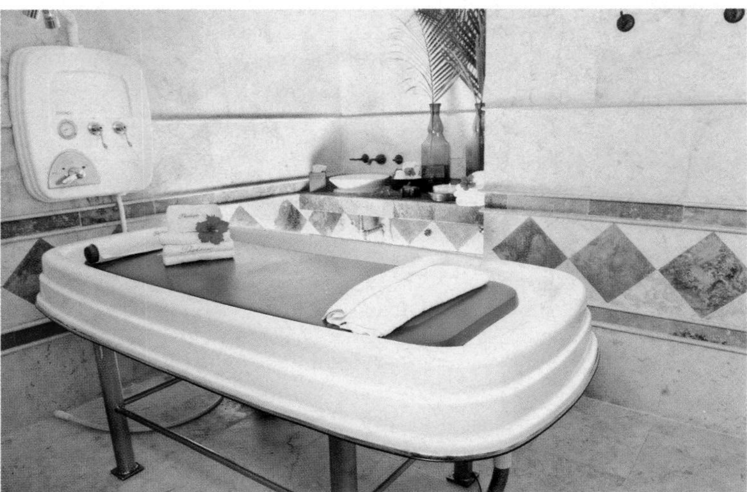

FIGURE 3–17 Modern wet tables contain most if not all excess water and product during spa treatments, keeping the area neat and clean.

to a wide array of products. Wet room equipment is often expensive, costing thousands or even tens of thousands of dollars for one unit. These units can be the centerpiece of a room which has been designed specifically for them, or they can be combined with one or more other pieces of equipment to create a spa suite or dedicated wet treatment area.

Because each spa has its own unique array of wet room equipment, newly hired therapists are not generally expected to know how to operate them all. Training is offered on operations, sanitation, and precautions for each. It is beneficial, however, for therapists to have a conceptual knowledge of how each piece of equipment works, its intended therapeutic outcomes, and a brief background or history of how it was developed. The following chapters will introduce you to the use of this equipment in detail. For now, familiarize yourself with the data in Table 3–2 to gain a preliminary understanding of wet room equipment and its purpose.

WET ROOM EQUIPMENT				
CATEGORY	SUBCATEGORY	DESCRIPTION	USE	POPULARITY
Showers	Hot/Cold Shower	regular shower at hot or cold temperature	washing off product, heating body, closing pores	most common option, but has the least therapeutic applications
	Vichy Shower	multiple showerheads on horizontal bar extending over table	washing off product, relaxation, hot/cold contrast therapy, luxurious	popular in many high-end spas, but clients need to be educated on use; sometimes underused
	Swiss Shower	multiple showerheads in large stall pointing at clients from all directions	washing off product, stimulating circulation, hot/cold contrast	installed in traditional European-concept spas, not as popular in modern facilities
	Scotch Hose	powerful spray jet aimed at standing client	forceful stimulation of circulation and skin	popular in traditional seaside thalassotherapy centers, less so in modern spas
Baths	Hydrotherapy Tub	technician-operated computerized zone-specific jet systems and underwater massage hose	targeted stimulation of multiple zones on client's body plus powerful water-pressure massage	very popular in destination and resort spas, less so in day spas
	Jacuzzi/Whirlpool/ Hot Tub	tub with non-programmed jets	relaxation prior to massage or spa treatment	very popular, common in spas with wet areas
	Soaking Tub	non-jetted tub for soaks, usually with therapeutic ingredients	relaxation and absorption of therapeutic ingredients	popular in spas with a focus on natural therapeutic ingredients and/or seawater
	Mud/Enzyme Bath	tub or vat filled with therapeutic mud, peat, sawdust, etc.	absorption of therapeutic ingredients, relaxation, detoxification	popular but only in specialized resort spas with nearby natural mud, enzymes, etc.

TABLE 3–2 Wet Room Equipment. *(Continued)*

WET ROOM EQUIPMENT				
CATEGORY	**SUBCATEGORY**	**DESCRIPTION**	**USE**	**POPULARITY**
Tables	Wet Table	waterproof table with built-in drainage, usually with shower mounted overhead or on nearby wall	easy cleansing of spa products from skin, ability to drain large amount of water (as from Vichy shower) without mess	very popular, most spas with a wet room invest in a wet table, though a shower and regular massage table suffice
	Treatment Pedestal	solid structure built to waist height upon which clients lay for wet treatments	washing of spa products from skin	common in older traditional spa setups, not common in modern spas
	Soft Pack Table	rubberized cover atop a platform that lowers into liquid medium	cushions and supports clients during body wraps	rare, expensive, but highly prized by therapists and clients who experience it
Chambers	Steam Chamber	tiled room with adjacent steam generator to produce moist heat	open pores prior to treatment for effective absorption of spa products	very popular in spas with wet areas
	Rasul Chamber	ornately tiled room of Middle Eastern design for multiple clients to experience steam and mud application	creates a specialized ritual for application of products, opens pores, promotes group experience of spa service	popular in high-end spas, especially in Europe
	Hammam	Turkish style treatment room with moderate steam and treatment table for exfoliation and massage	recreation of Turkish bath experience in modern spa setting, cleansing of skin, purification, relaxation	creates an exotic spa environment which is increasing in popularity
	Spa Suite	private room(s) meant for one guest or private party at a time with a range of wet room equipment available (showers, baths, tables, etc.)	provides clients with privacy while receiving spa wet treatments and massage	popular in exclusive spas with clients who want to pay for privacy and exclusive use of equipment for a period of time

TABLE 3–2 Wet Room Equipment.

Spa designers and builders need to keep many details in mind while installing wet room equipment, and they go through considerable expense to get them running properly. As a spa therapist, you need to understand this. Owning and operating this equipment is expensive. It requires skill, hard work, and a professional focus on safety and sanitation issues (see sections later in this chapter) to provide wet room services. The spa therapist is part of a team that makes the offering of these services possible.

SPA TIP

The successful operation of spa equipment requires the cooperation of the equipment manufacturer, spa designer, installation expert, trainer, and finally the hands-on therapist who will perform the treatment. If you develop a healthy respect for the entire team of individuals who make the treatment possible, you will become a more professional therapist.

Stocking and Storage in the Spa Room

Spa rooms require a larger capacity for stocking and storing supplies and equipment than a simple massage room. Consider the amount of towels and sheets alone that you will need to perform multiple spa treatments each day, and you will understand that provisions must be made for extra storage space either in

SPA ETIQUETTE

Wet Room Temperature

In the spa wet room, temperature control is of the utmost importance. At many points during wet room services, clients will be vulnerable to getting chilled. This occurs when you moisten a client's skin with water or product, and when you unwrap clients who have been warmly cocooned for a time, exposing them to cooler air than that inside the wrap. The general rule for wet rooms is to keep the temperature warmer than you as a therapist might prefer; 80°F to 82°F seems to be ideal for most spa wet rooms. Though you may sweat a bit while working in such conditions, it is the client's comfort that comes first.

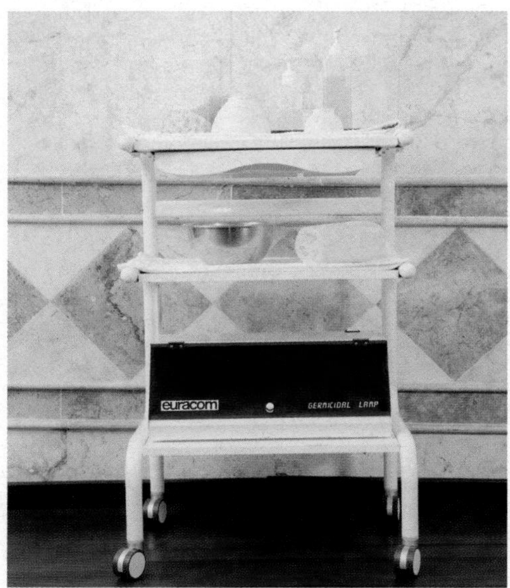

FIGURE 3–18 Wheeled carts are valuable in the spa room to store supplies and keep ingredients handy for treatments performed in different parts of the room.

the spa room or nearby. This extra storage is normally carved from unused areas such as under treatment tables and along walls near the ceiling. Often, extra cabinets, drawers, and shelving are added to spa rooms in order to increase storage capacity.

Available counter space in the spa room is valuable real estate for the storage and display of **back bar** products, heating units, music players, tabletop fountains, mixing bowls, and other supplies. A wheeled cart (Figure 3–18) is helpful when performing treatments in the spa room because it allows you to easily move needed supplies close to your side for easy access during a face, foot, hand, or full-body service.

Spa rooms, unlike massage rooms, need a **staging area** or **prep area** in which to mix ingredients, heat towels, wring sheets, and also store products and supplies. Ideally, this takes place out of the client's view, either in a curtained-off area within the treatment room itself or in a separate area outside the room. The treatment area that is visible to the client should be stocked neatly with all products, equipment, and supplies necessary to perform each procedure.

back bar

refers to the larger (compared to retail) spa product jars and bottles kept on the shelf and used in the spa treatment room, originally an esthetician's term

staging area

(same as prep area)

prep area

space in which to mix ingredients, heat towels, wring sheets, and also store products and supplies, either inside the treatment room, ideally curtained off, or outside the room in a hallway, closet, etc. (same as staging area)

Towels and Laundry

Spas generate an inordinate amount of laundry. It is not unusual for one treatment to require four hand towels, three bath towels, and a full-sized sheet. Multiply that by six treatments a day in a modest number of treatment rooms (four, say), and the amount of linens washed on a daily basis easily soars into the hundreds. When dealing with laundry in the spa treatment area, it is important, therefore, that spa therapists observe the following guidelines:

- Whenever possible, hide laundry concerns from clients. Use a hamper or other receptacle in the room, preferably out of sight.
- Wash linens in hot water for sanitation reasons (see section on sanitation later in this chapter).
- Use storage wisely, keeping as many linens as possible in the treatment room itself and easily accessible, with a backup supply in a nearby storage area.
- Conserve on the number of towels and sheets used in each service. Do not use extra linens unnecessarily.

For those towels and sheets that come into direct contact with muds, seaweeds, and other products, spas often choose darker earth-tone colors to mask

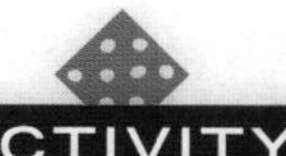

ACTIVITY

A Clean and Organized Work Area

When practicing spa treatments in your classroom, it is important to keep the treatment area clean and organized for two main reasons. First, you will be learning how to present an attractive and professional environment to the clients who will enter your spa treatment room one day, and second, you will learn how an organized work area allows you to quickly find whatever product or equipment you need while performing a treatment. Professional spa therapists share in the responsibility for keeping treatment areas organized and clean, and you as a spa therapy student need to become accustomed to this task.

As a group activity for the whole class, spend time cleaning the treatment area, folding towels and sheets neatly, refilling bottles with oils, etc., replenishing the back bar, polishing equipment, stocking all products and supplies in appropriate spaces, sweeping the floor, and disinfecting all surfaces.

When working at an actual spa, you may not be required to clean and organize the treatment space to this degree, but this "basic training" will help you build your spa skills from the ground up, much as professional chefs do while in culinary school.

potential staining and create a more natural look. Blue, green, and brown shades are popular. White is sometimes used because these linens can be bleached. Blankets of any color can be used as they do not come into direct contact with spa products during normal use.

SAFETY ISSUES IN THE SPA

Regarding safety, spa therapists require an especially high level of vigilance for two main reasons: risk to clients and risk to themselves. As far as clients go, spas pose a specific combination of risks found in few other work environments. These risks are caused primarily by the pervasive use of heat and water, which can lead to a number of potential dangers, including fainting, heart attacks, slips and falls, drowning, burns, and scalds. In addition, there are potential issues with products due to allergic reactions. All safety issues and contraindications for each treatment will be covered as part of the hands-on instruction in the following chapters. In Table 3–3 you will find some general safety rules that apply to all treatments and the spa environment in general.

SPA CAUTION

If a client has an allergic reaction to a spa product, therapists should follow the spa's written procedures for such an incident. If no such written procedures exist:

1. Remove product from client's skin, rinsing it off with soap if necessary.
2. Make sure the client is comfortable, with no immediate threat to health or well-being.
3. If a severe allergic reaction takes place, call medical authorities.
4. Let spa management know about the reaction.
5. Document the incident in writing, using an incident report if one is available at the spa.

SAFETY RULE	DESCRIPTION
#1 Keep surfaces dry.	Any surface in the treatment room that becomes slippery can potentially create a problem, even if the surface is high, such as a countertop, and does not normally come into contact with clients. Spilled products can drip onto floors where people can slip on them.
#2 Self-test product temperatures.	Before applying products or hot towels, rocks, etc., to clients' skin, test them on your own skin first to make sure they are not too hot. The most typical area for this kind of self-testing is the inner forearm, which has thin, sensitive skin (Figure 3–19).
#3 Use non-slip floor coverings.	Wherever a potentially slick floor surface exists in the spa, such as tiles, linoleum, wood, slate, etc., have non-slip covers where clients are likely to walk. In the case of a sudden unexpected spill, throw a towel down over the area to absorb the mess and then make sure it is cleaned up immediately.
#4 Post warning signs where appropriate.	Place cautionary signage wherever it might be necessary in addition to the lawfully required warning signs near hot tubs, pools, saunas, etc.
#5 Assist clients when exiting heat treatments.	Clients may become lightheaded at any time in the spa, especially when exiting heat treatments such as baths and wraps. Always provide support and assistance at these times.
#6 Keep water temperatures in safe range.	Whenever water is being used for application to clients directly or to heat other spa products or equipment, monitor the temperature with a thermometer or digital readout.
#7 Fully wring out sheets and towels that come into contact with clients.	Wet towels and sheets that are applied to clients' skin need to be wrung out thoroughly to avoid the possibility of scalding. The material itself will not scald clients, but the moisture in the material may, making it important to get as much moisture out as possible.
#8 Use intake forms and ask about allergies.	Many spas use intake forms that ask about allergies, medical conditions, or pregnancy in order to more safely treat clients. If the spa does not use an intake form or if a client refuses to sign one, problems can arise (see sidebars).
#9 Communicate with clients.	If a client appears disoriented or distressed at any time in the spa, immediately communicate your concern. Have the client sit down. Offer to bring a glass of fresh water. If it is necessary, contact a nurse or other health care practitioner or call 911.
#10 Document everything.	Whenever a safety issue arises, a client is hurt, you are hurt, or any complaint is made, communicate this with your superiors and write down any pertinent facts. Some spas provide **incident reports** for this purpose (see Figure 18–15).

TABLE 3–3 General Spa Safety Rules.

incident report

official written, signed document outlining the details of an event that may potentially be cause for litigation or disciplinary actions

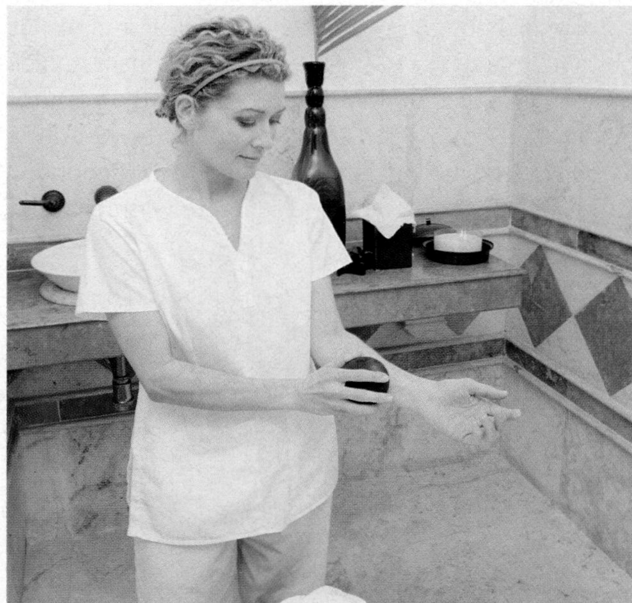

FIGURE 3–19 Test hot products, towels, rocks, etc., on your own skin before applying them to clients. The sensitive skin of the inner forearm works well for this testing.

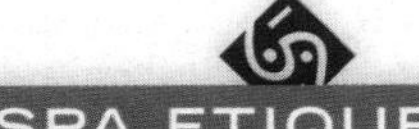

SPA ETIQUETTE

One of the most basic safety tips in spas involves the traditional custom of offering water to clients after a massage or body treatment. It is important that clients stay hydrated, and some therapists believe that drinking water after treatments helps with the elimination of impurities. So, offering clients a glass of water is not only good for their health, but a gracious gesture as well, perfectly suited for spas. Some spas make this offering into a special ritual (Figure 3–20).

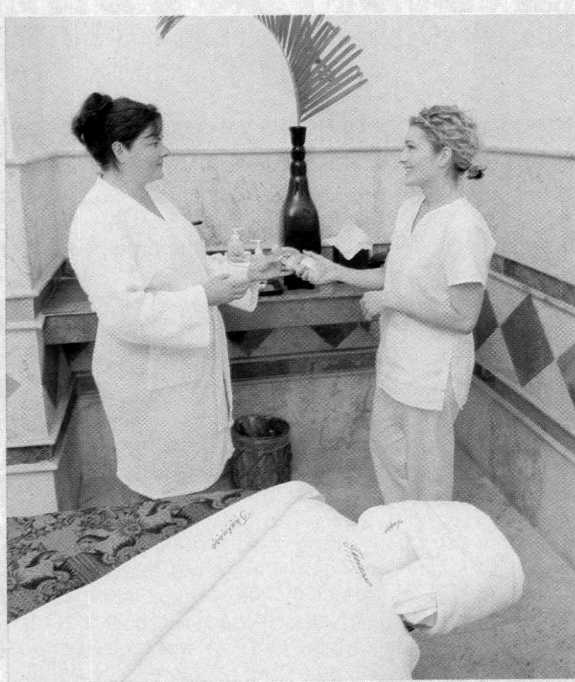

FIGURE 3–20 Offering clients a glass of water after massage and body treatments helps keep them healthy, and it is a gracious gesture.

SELF-CARE FOR THE SPA THERAPIST

As a working professional massage therapist, you will always be faced with the challenge of avoiding **burnout** and maintaining your own health. When you work as a spa therapist, these challenges will be magnified by two primary factors:

burnout

the fatigue or injury suffered by therapists as a result of an excess workload

1. Spa therapists typically work non-stop for many consecutive hours. They are often called upon to do more back-to-back treatments, including massage and other modalities, than those therapists who perform massage therapy alone. Their hours may be longer as well.
2. Spa therapists work in conditions that are somewhat dangerous due to slippery surfaces, an abundance of water, the presence of heat, and the use of heavy equipment.

Many hardworking spa therapists have had their careers cut short by repetitive stress injuries, accidents, and just plain fatigue. Even though it may appear to an outside observer that spa therapists' work is done in slow motion, in tranquil environments, with very little chance for injury, you will eventually find the job physically challenging. In order to minimize these risks, follow the self-care rules for spa therapists described in Table 3–4.

Indisputably, self-care is central to the long-term health of all spa therapists, and the warnings mentioned here should be taken seriously. Yet, at the same time, it is interesting to note that regarding self-care, therapists who perform spa treatments hold two key advantages over those who perform massage therapy alone:

1. The products, hydrotherapy and heat that spa therapists apply to clients have an equally therapeutic effect on their own bodies. Thus, performing spa therapy is therapeutic for the therapist.
2. Many spa modalities require less effort on the part of therapists, such as body wraps, during which clients are covered for much of the allotted treatment time and the therapist has little or no work to perform.

SELF-CARE RULE	DESCRIPTION
#1 Identify and consistently engage in proper body mechanics.	You need to follow the same guidelines for proper body mechanics during spa therapy as you do for massage therapy. See the tip for Spa Therapists' Body Mechanics below and also refer to the body mechanics guidelines supplied with the protocols for each treatment in the following chapters.
#2 Manage your time wisely.	Spa therapists have only short periods of time between treatments for breaks. Use this time wisely. Have products and supplies prepared beforehand so breaks can be used for rest.
#3 Organize the treatment area.	Spa therapy entails the use of many more products than massage therapy. If all of these products, plus the equipment and supplies needed to prepare them, are within easy grasping distance in the treatment room, this will eliminate the need to reach, bend, and lift unnecessarily.
#4 Get a good floor mat to walk on around the treatment table.	The back and legs can become extremely sore and tired while working all day in a spa treatment room. Rubberized padding or a thick rug or carpet beneath the table takes some of the strain off. Floor mats should be of the anti-fatigue variety, with enough cushioning to relieve foot, leg, and low back stress. Wraps, scrubs, and many other spa treatments can be performed in a carpeted dry room. For wet rooms, drainage mats along with floor drains are best. If mats are pulled up frequently for cleaning, small interlocking mats are lighter than one big mat. Mats should have beveled edges to reduce tripping hazards. If you need permission from a manager, director, or owner to purchase floor mats, enlist the aid of fellow therapists on staff to convince them these mats are necessary.
#5 Exercise between treatments.	After an hour or more of performing precise, contained movements, spa therapists benefit by some larger movements between treatments or at the end of the day. Just a minute of jumping jacks or jogging in place will stimulate circulation, invigorate muscles, and combat fatigue (Figure 3–21).
#6 Stretch between treatments.	Spa therapists' muscles and joints can become stiff during a full day's work, and it is important to occasionally stretch them out. You can use the treatment table as a prop for these stretches (Figures 3–22 through 3–24).
#7 Truly relax.	While between treatments or at the end of the day, use progressive relaxation, visualization, meditation, or similar techniques to deepen rest and hasten recuperation from long days of work. Even a short (20 minutes) nap, if possible, may help with energy levels.
#8 Get back in touch with nature during the day.	Even the most beautiful spa room can feel claustrophobic after a time. Take the opportunity to step outside for a moment whenever possible, breathe some fresh air, step on the Earth, and gaze at the sky.
#9 Consider giving your body a break.	During days off, consider not doing private clients. Even though you may lose some income in the near term, you may extend your career in the long run.
#10 Eat right.	Light meals or snacks taken throughout the day while working in the spa will improve energy levels and performance.

TABLE 3–4 Spa Therapist Self-Care Rules.

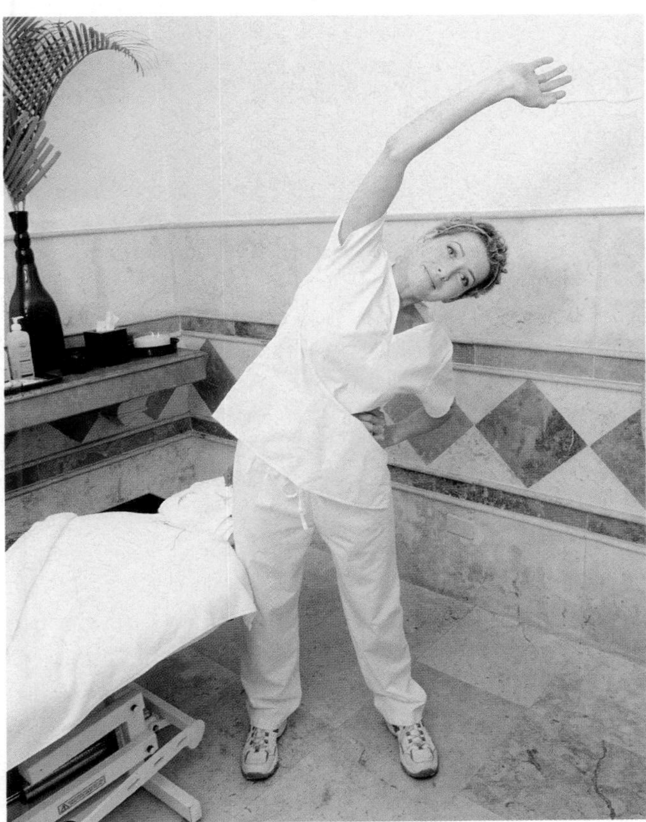

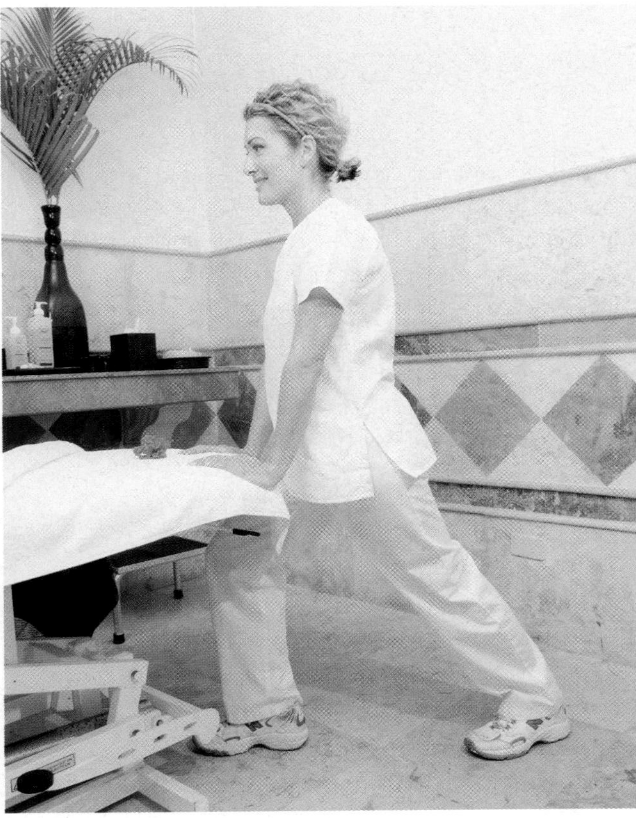

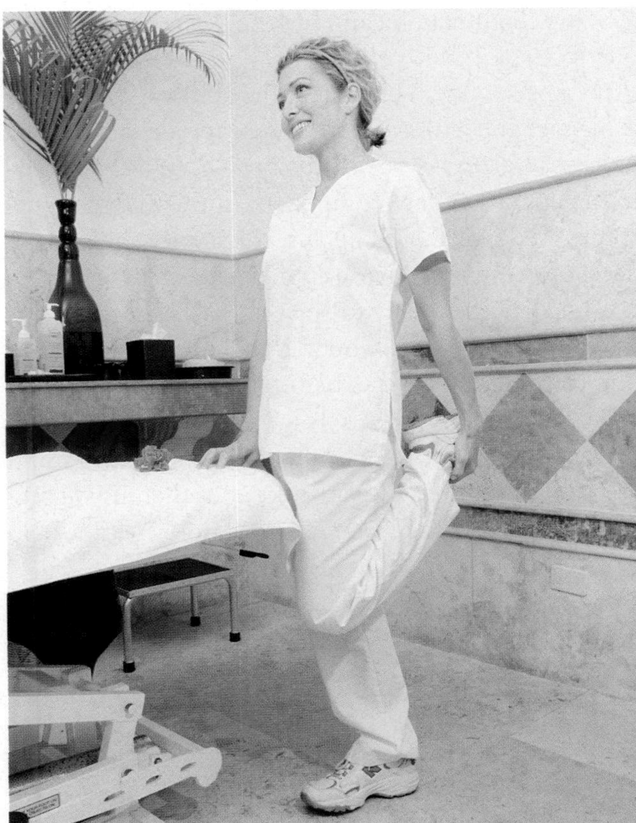

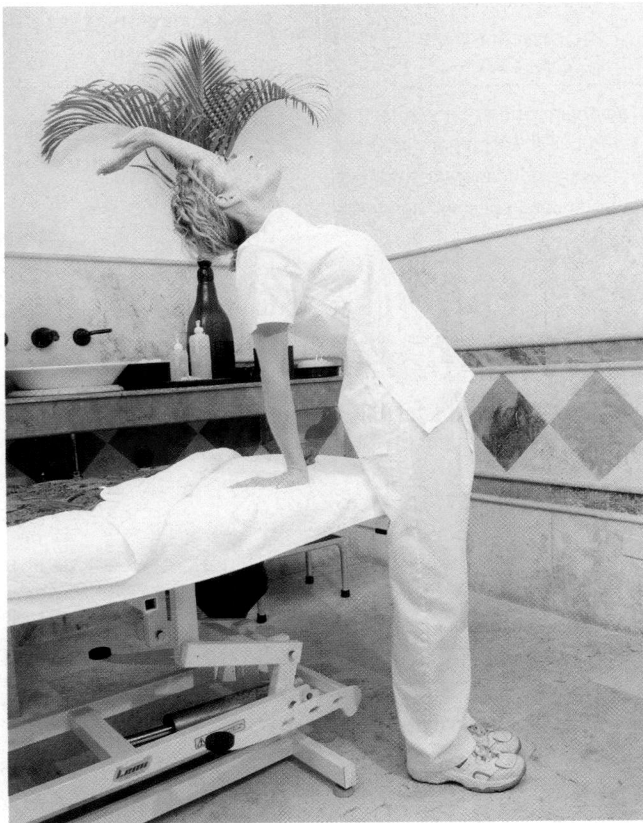

FIGURES 3–21, 3–22, 3–23, 3–24 It is important for spa therapists to occasionally stretch muscles and joints that are stiff from a long day's work.

SPA CAUTION

You Need a Break

What should you do when management at the spa where you work offers insufficient breaks? What if all the therapists you work alongside grumble and complain? What if one of your colleagues, or more than one, comes down with a repetitive stress disorder? This is a tricky problem. As an employee who has accepted the conditions of employment offered by an employer, you are bound to follow the rules or suffer the consequences. On the other hand, if you risk the chance of injury, is it worth it to keep your job? Complaining to an outside authority will do little good because the spa is probably not breaking any laws. You can complain to members of the local massage community and attempt to lower the spa's reputation, but this is counterproductive if you want to continue working there. The best advice is to ask about the length and quantity of breaks before you accept a job. If it is possible, ask current employees how they feel about the spa's policies on this topic. If you accept a certain set of rules, only to complain about them later, you are not being fair to yourself or your employer. Check about break times and similar policies that will affect your health *before* accepting a job offer.

The successful spa therapist ideally maximizes the advantages inherent to spa work while also following the self-care rules. In this manner, the choice to follow the path of spa therapy may actually extend the number of years a therapist can perform his or her art. Some therapists choose to practice spa therapy later in their careers, when they realize the toll that massage is taking on their bodies. Other therapists alternate back and forth between performing straight massage therapy and spa therapy, interspersing the two modalities during the week or even during the day. This combination can offer the best of both worlds to both clients and practitioners.

Commission on Massage Therapy Accreditation (COMTA)

an organization that grants credit and recognition for massage education institutions that maintain certain standards

While working as a spa therapist, you will benefit by the ability to self-assess your own level of stress and manage that stress with the appropriate techniques. The **Commission on Massage Therapy Accreditation (COMTA)** requires certified massage schools to include a self-care component in their educational offerings. They recommend that students should be able to identify the physiological and psychological effects of stress, and choose appropriate stress reduction techniques to address them. This applies equally to spa therapists. Accordingly, the very first step in using appropriate self-care while on the job at the spa is to become skilled at identifying the causes of stress before they become painful problems. The very best advice you can follow, then, is to "take care of yourself." While working in a spa, monitor your own state of health and your state of mind consistently. Follow the safety rules and the self-care rules, but then if you still notice stress creeping into your work life, take immediate action. Ask for help from a coworker or supervisor.

SPA TIP

Body Mechanics for the Spa Therapist

As a general rule, therapists should use the same body mechanics while performing spa treatments that they use for massage treatments. However, treatment-specific body mechanics apply to several spa modalities, and these will be discussed along with the protocol for each treatment in the following chapters.

LIABILITY AND RISK MANAGEMENT FOR THE SPA THERAPIST

As spas become more popular, they are also more frequently targeted for lawsuits. This is unfortunate but unavoidable, an inevitable result of spas' skyrocketing popularity. The richer spas get, the more people are likely to target them, and the more vulnerable they are to other types of losses such as those caused

SPA PROFILE

Save Your Hands!

Lauriann Greene and Rick Goggins

Like many massage therapists, Lauriann Greene experienced job-related injuries that made it difficult for her to work. But her case was more troubling than most, with an earlier onset. "I became injured while I was still in massage school," she recalls. "I was able to pass my state boards and get my license, but I was too injured to be able to continue my career as a hands-on massage therapist. Instead, I decided to do specialized research to understand why massage therapists get injured as a result of the work they do. I started giving workshops on injury prevention and self-care across the U.S. and Canada, and I used my training as an MT and the experience of working with hundreds of MTs in these workshops to write *Save Your Hands! Injury Prevention for Massage Therapists*, a comprehensive self-care guide for massage therapists. In my own life, I wish there had been information like this available to me while I was a student that could have helped me prevent my own injury. So I learned the hard way how important self-care and injury prevention really is."

Over the years, Lauriann's book has been successful in helping many therapists avoid injury, which prompted her to write a new edition. *Save Your Hands!* was first published in 1995, and the second edition, co-authored with Rick Goggins, CPE, LMP, has been greatly expanded to include extensive information about ergonomics, which is an essential component of injury prevention and self-care. Rick Goggins has been an ergonomist for over 15 years. He also attended massage school in order to learn more about the musculoskeletal system. Shortly after graduating, he began working with Lauriann on a survey of massage therapists' musculoskeletal health issues. "I had experienced some upper extremity symptoms during massage school myself," states Rick, "but recognizing them for what they were and getting the appropriate treatment right away kept me from having a more serious condition. I had read *Save Your Hands!* during this time, so of course I was interested in working with Lauriann. After we wrote an article on the survey results (which found a high rate of symptoms and injury among experienced MTs), Lauriann asked if I would be interested in working with her on the second edition of the book. It seemed like a natural fit for my experience, so I agreed."

Lauriann and Rick agree on several key points that can help those therapists who work in spas enjoy longer and more productive careers. "Therapists need to establish clear expectations when they go to work for someone else," says Lauriann, "how many massages are reasonable in one day, what is the length of breaks between sessions, are deep tissue sessions alternated with lighter treatments, etc. Good treatment room ergonomics, self-care, body mechanics, conditioning exercises, etc. are critical in high workload situations, but even they may not be enough if therapists regularly exceed their capabilities, become fatigued and increase the likelihood of injury."

Ergonomist Goggins echoes these concerns. "Drainage mats and good footwear (non-slip soles) are important for working on slippery wet room floors," he says. "Good mats can also help with fatigue from standing all day. Spas need to use the right kind of tile in treatment rooms with a lot of water. Glazed tile can become too slippery. Floor drains in key areas can also help to prevent a lot of standing water. In addition, wet linens should be handled carefully, and not wadded up and thrown into one large, heavy basket. Small bundles of linens placed into several smaller baskets or mesh bags can lighten the load for lifting. Next to lifting, spending long periods of time bent over at the waist is one of the main causes of low back injury. When possible, therapists should place a hand down for support. A folded up towel on the edge of the hydro tub could form a chest support for short periods of bending over."

(Continued)

SPA PROFILE Save Your Hands! *continued*

Lauriann points out that spas may present opportunities for self-care that can be more difficult to find in other massage therapy work. "It is always helpful when you can incorporate a number of different modalities into any one treatment session," she says. "Different techniques and modalities allow the therapist to use different parts of the body to perform the treatment, and to build periods of recovery into their sessions to allow them to rest. Some techniques such as body wraps do give practitioners an opportunity to rest once the client is fully wrapped. Some spas may require therapists to do some form of hands-on massage, such as face or foot massage, during these treatments. This massage should be done while seated (as a break from standing) and with a very light touch."

But what should spa therapists do if they start to notice the beginning of injuries creeping in, yet they still need to keep working hard to keep their job? "The key is for spa therapists to adopt good injury prevention practices in the first place so that injury doesn't interrupt their work life," states Lauriann. "If injury does happen despite your best efforts, early, effective treatment is absolutely essential. Once you're injured, you will have to make adaptations to your work, reduce your workload or take some time off to allow the injury to heal, otherwise you can end up with a chronic injury that can be debilitating. All the more reason to prevent injury before it ever happens!"

The work that Rick and Lauriann do through their books and workshops focuses on a multifaceted approach to preventing injury. "Since there are many different aspects of a massage therapist's work and life that contribute to injury," states Rick, "using one single method to prevent injury, like just using good body mechanics, is rarely effective. Spa therapists can most effectively avoid injury by applying the principles of ergonomics and good body mechanics to their work, developing the physical conditioning necessary to do their work, avoiding certain techniques and adapting others to cause less stress, avoiding unhealthy attitudes about work, applying injury prevention principles to life outside of work, and maintaining their general health. All of these topics are covered in the second edition of *Save Your Hands: The Complete Guide to Injury Prevention and Ergonomics for Manual Therapists*."

Through their writings, workshops, ergonomic evaluations, and their consulting work at schools and spas, Rick and Lauriann continue to spread the gospel of injury prevention for massage therapists, a topic that is especially relevant for those therapists who work long hours in spas everywhere. Therapists seeking more information can visit the Web site at http://www.saveyourhands.com.

risk management

the technique of assessing, minimizing, and preventing accidental loss to a (spa) business through the use of insurance and safety measures

tort liabilities

the responsibility for compensation a (spa) business potentially has for any injury suffered by a client while under the spa's care or while on the spa's property

by natural disasters. When spa owners, managers, therapists, and other personnel attempt to minimize the chance of losses to the business and to formulate a plan for dealing with them when they arise, they are engaging in a process called **risk management**. Some spas have a risk management program in place, while others operate day to day, hoping that disaster will not strike. It is best, of course, to understand what can be done to minimize risk and what plan of action should be followed in the event of a crisis.

The risk management issues faced by spa businesses can be broken down into three main categories: employment issues, sexual harassment issues, and **tort liabilities** issues.

1. **Employment issues**
   These include wrongful firing, breach of contract, partnership problems, discrimination, overwork, immigration, licensing, and more.

Employment lawsuits can flow in either direction. Some are instigated by disgruntled employees who feel the spa is mistreating them. Others are filed by employers who feel they have been wronged by therapists or other employees.

2. **Sexual harassment issues**
   These issues arise most commonly when a spa therapist is accused of harassing a client. Of course, there are other types of sexual harassment cases, including cases when clients are accused of making inappropriate advances toward therapists, and when one employee accuses another of harassment.
3. **Tort liabilities issues**
   These issues are not limited to spas alone, but the very nature of the spa environment exacerbates the potential problems, due primarily to the use of heat (sauna, steam, hydrotherapy), water, and complicated equipment, as mentioned earlier in this chapter. Included in this category are slips, falls, burns caused by hot rocks, baths or showers, product liability, allergic reactions, faulty equipment, improper use of equipment, and more.

Each individual who works at a spa of any size, from large resort spas to therapist-owned day spas, should take a proactive approach when it comes to avoiding potential problems, whether they be employee issues, sexual harassment issues, or tort liability issues. While working as a spa therapist, you will be part of a team whose every member needs to understand and comply with a set of self-imposed guidelines that help spa businesses avoid lawsuits and complaints whenever possible and respond to them appropriately when they do occur. In order to most effectively fulfill this role, all spa therapists should be prepared to take certain actions, listed below. Spa owners need to be prepared to take action as well and to work with lawyers and other professionals to create the spa's risk management program.

Actions spa therapists can take to improve risk management in the spa:

- Study all guidelines, standard operating procedures, employee manuals, equipment instruction manuals, and job descriptions carefully prior to or at the commencement of employment in the spa. Too often, these materials are not read thoroughly enough.
- Follow these guidelines conscientiously during your everyday work at the spa.
- When an incident of any kind occurs, report it to supervisors immediately (see example of an incident report in Chapter 18).
- Volunteer for advanced training on all spa equipment, even if you are not typically responsible for using it to administer treatments.
- Willingly attend all employee meetings and ask questions about any risk management issues about which you may be uncertain.
- If it is allowed by spa management, practice safe and proper use of equipment and facilities during off hours with coworkers to become more familiar and comfortable with them.
- Learn CPR and other life-saving techniques that might be needed in an emergency situation.

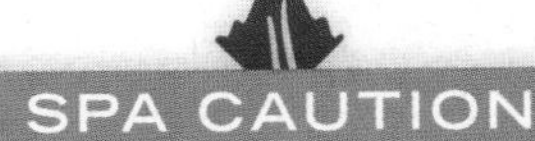

Providing spa services without a signed intake form may create unnecessary liability for the spa. In some spas, if a client refuses to fill out an intake form, it is the right of the therapist to refuse service. Therapists need to confirm this with spa management prior to refusing service, however.

THERAPEUTIC DAY SPA

INTAKE FORM

Therapeutic Day Spa
1234 Main Street
Any Town, NY 02101

Name:________________________________ Birthday:____/____ Wedding Anniversary____/____

Mailing Address:____

Telephone: Home ____________________ Work ____________________ Mobile __________________

City:______________________ State:______ Zip:__________ E-Mail Address: ______________________

How did you hear about our spa? ____

The following information is needed to ensure your well-being while enjoying spa services. All information will be kept confidential.

- ☐ Yes ☐ No Do you bruise easily?
- ☐ Yes ☐ No Have you been in an accident or suffered any injuries in the past 2 years?
- ☐ Yes ☐ No Do you have tension, soreness, or sensitivity to pressure?
- ☐ Yes ☐ No Do you have any allergies?
  To what? ____
- ☐ Yes ☐ No Have you had surgery in the past 5 years?
  Please explain____
- ☐ Yes ☐ No Do you have other medical conditions or take any medication we should know about?
  Please explain____
- ☐ Yes ☐ No Are you currently applying any topical medications that might affect your skin?
- ☐ Yes ☐ No Are you pregnant or trying to become pregnant?

Please circle any of the following conditions listed below that apply to you:

Contact Lens	Chronic Fatigue	Osteoporosis Arthritis
Rheumatism	Headache/Migraines	Anxiety Attacks
Epilepsy/Seizures	Fibromyalgia	Allergies
Numbness/Chronic Pain	Blood Clots	Claustrophobia
High Blood Pressure	Tuberculosis	Kidney or Liver Disease
Diabetes	Asthmas	Varicose Veins
HIV/AIDS	Lymphoma	Cardiac Problems
Herpes	Hepatitis	Skin Irritation
Cancer	Bursitis or Gout	Tendonitis
Joint Sprain or Dislocation	Ulcers	Neck Pain or Back Pain

What is your goal for this session? (circle the one most applicable)
Sooth Aching Muscles Stress Reduction General Health Enhance Sport Training Injury Recovery

What type or pressure do you prefer? (choose one or more)
Very Deep Deep Firm Light Not Sure

FIGURE 3–25 Spas without a comprehensive intake form run a higher risk for liability (courtesy Natural Resources Spa Consulting, Inc.). *(Continued)*

Please describe any particular issues you are having with your body such as pain, stiffness or injury that your therapist should be aware of. Do you have any areas that need more work? ______________________________
____

I understand that the massage and spa treatments I receive are provided for the purpose of relaxation, well being and relief of muscular tension. If I experience any pain or discomfort during this session, I will immediately inform the practitioner so that the pressure and/or technique may be adjusted to my level of comfort. I understand that if I forego the opportunity to communicate my needs with the practitioner and continue the treatment, I am liable for payment of the scheduled appointment.

Because massage/bodywork, esthetic services and spa treatments should not be performed under certain medical conditions, I affirm that I have stated all my known medical conditions and answered all the questions honestly. I agree to keep the practitioner updated as to any changes in my medical profile and understand that there shall be no liability on the practitioner's part or Therapeutic Day Spa's part should I fail to do so.

I also understand that any illicit or sexually suggestive remarks or advances made by me will result in immediate termination of the session, and I will be liable for payment of the scheduled appointment.

Client Signature

X ______________________________________ Date ________________

FIGURE 3–25 Spas without a comprehensive intake form run a higher risk for liability (courtesy Natural Resources Spa Consulting, Inc.).

Actions spa owners can take to improve risk management in the spa:

- Call the local state bar to find an attorney to work with.
- Establish a relationship with this attorney prior to problematic situations arising. The attorney should conduct a review of the spa and make a site visit to assess potentially dangerous or risky situations that may expose the spa to liability.
- The attorney should also review the client **intake/disclaimer/waiver form** or create one for the spa if it does not already exist (Figure 3–25).
- Post all necessary signage in the spa, such as warnings about hot tub or steam/sauna use.
- Place non-slip mats on the floor and take other safety precautions
- Become familiar with the guidelines issued by OSHA regarding spa workplaces and ensure that all of them are being followed.
- Fully train all staff regarding proper procedures and document their training in order to avoid risk issues.

intake form

a series of questions related to health, allergies, spa experience, and general information (address, birthday, etc.) asked of clients when they first visit the spa; sometimes includes a waiver or disclaimer

disclaimer

statement clients are asked to sign releasing a (spa) business from responsibility for injuries or damages incurred while undergoing specific procedures

waiver

a form clients sometimes sign at spas that relinquishes their right to claim damages caused by certain procedures (see disclaimer)

SPA ROOM SANITATION

Spa treatment rooms, of course, need to be kept spotlessly clean, and beyond the surface appearance, they also need to be as sanitary and germ-free as possible. By their nature, spa rooms can become breeding grounds for unhealthy organisms, including molds and bacteria. The abundance of steam, damp towels, pooled water, organic muds, freshly reconstituted seaweeds, pure oils, and other

SPA ETIQUETTE

You may find a job at a spa and be overjoyed at first, only to find out quickly that the spa owner's or director's vision is not therapeutically aligned with our own. The spa's focus may be on pampering rather than therapy, and they may not even require clients to fill out intake forms prior to their first treatment. What should you do if you feel strongly that clients should fill out such a form, but the spa has no plans to use one? You have four choices:

1. Keep your thoughts to yourself and carry on with your job, thankful you are receiving a paycheck.
2. Keep your thoughts to yourself and start looking for work elsewhere.
3. Politely let the spa owner or director know your feelings, but stay on the job regardless of the outcome.
4. Politely let the spa owner or director know your feelings, and state your intention of leaving if an intake form is not used at the spa.

Each of these options is viable. You have to search your own heart and judge the overall value of working in the spa. How much does it mean to you? Are your coworkers an inspiration to be with? Do you feel your career is being enhanced by working there? Make an informed decision before acting. One action that is never advisable is to confront the owner or director angrily and demand that an intake procedure be instituted. A self-righteous therapist has very little power in such a situation and will most likely end up without a job, having accomplished nothing for the spa's clients.

natural products all combine to make vigilant sanitation procedures an absolute necessity in the spa setting.

In general, all spa equipment, from the smallest brush to the largest hydrotherapy tub, should be sanitized after each and every treatment. Spa equipment manufacturers are well aware of how sensitive spa owners, therapists and clients are to hygiene issues, and they provide the industry with items that are easy to sanitize and maintain. New innovations have made spas safer and more germ-free than ever. For example, new "pipeless" tubs make it possible to offer hydrotherapy treatments without pumping water through pipes where it can potentially stagnate and create breeding grounds for bacteria. The water in these units is circulated through self-contained pumps, creating the bubbling and water pressure found in traditional tubs but without the need for pipes (Figures 3–26 and 3–27).

In larger facilities, the cleanliness and safe functioning of the spa is often the responsibility of employees such as spa technicians or locker room attendants. Even if this is not part of your job description as a spa therapist, however, you can create a "mental checklist" for safety and sanitation to review while on the job. Quickly going over such a list in your mind at the beginning of each shift will help ensure the spa's smooth, safe operation, and it will engender a greater sense of participation on your part. This is especially important when starting to work at a new spa where the facilities and procedures are still unfamiliar. Take a look at the Therapeutic Day Spa Safety & Sanitation Checklist (Figure 3–28) and keep it, or something like it, in mind when you are on the job.

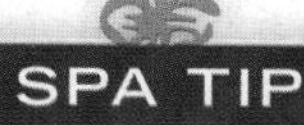

SPA TIP

Spa therapists sometimes mistakenly use the term autoclave when referring to a germicidal cabinet. While autoclaves are used extensively in medical and dental laboratories, medical spas, and nail salons, they are less common in resort spas, day spas, or destination spas, where germicidal cabinets are more widely used.

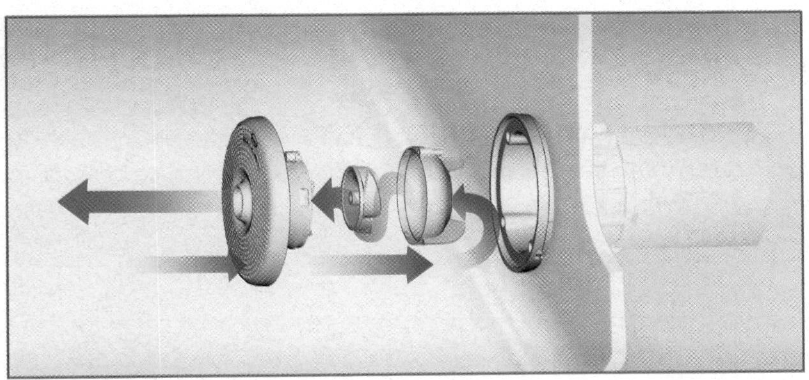

FIGURE 3–26 Spa equipment manufacturers devise new ways to make spa treatments hygienic such as the "pipeless" blower for hydrotherapy tubs and foot baths (courtesy Sanijet).

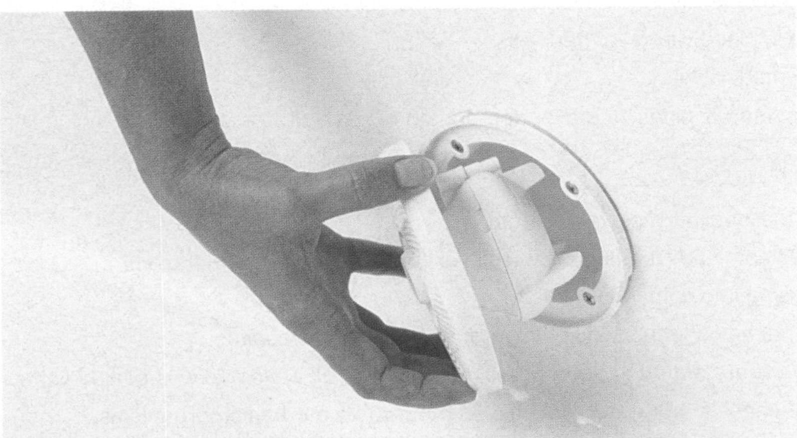

FIGURE 3–27 Sanijet pumps and blowers are easily removed for cleaning and have no pipes that can become infected with germs (courtesy Sanijet).

Many smaller implements that come into contact with clients, such as hair brushes, skin brushes, and combs, are reused, but they first need to be sterilized. Most spas use a **germicidal solution** for this purpose, dipping these implements into it in order to kill bacteria. Then, once the implements are sterilized, they are often stored in a box on a treatment room countertop. This box, called a **germicidal cabinet**, features an always-on ultraviolet light that provides a clean, germ-free environment for storage. It is important to note that although the cabinet does provide a sterile environment, it does not actually sterilize implements itself. Either a germicidal solution or an **autoclave** is used for actual sterilization. Autoclaves are vessels in which water is heated above its boiling point in order to completely sterilize whatever is put inside them. Tools used in day spas, resort spas, and destination spas are sometimes sterilized this way, but autoclaves are more common in medical spas and nail salons.

An attractive option to sterilizing small spa implements is to give them away as part of a spa treatment. Guests are usually delighted to take something home, and the low per-unit cost of these items can be built into the price of the treatment. Typical items that are given away in this manner include loofah mitts and gloves. Specific suggestions for this technique will be suggested in the treatment protocols for each appropriate modality.

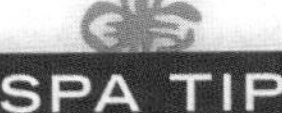

SPA TIP

Most muds and seaweeds wash out of linens. However, the majority of spas feature blue, green, or earth-toned linens in treatment rooms in case any minor staining or discoloring does occur over time. White linens can be bleached, but then the bleached material would come into contact with clients' skin during wraps and other occasions when their pores are open, which is thought to be inappropriate at many facilities.

RESEARCH

Using spa magazines, spa books, or the Internet, research safety and sanitation measures used in spas, athletic clubs, public pools, hot springs, and similar facilities. Choose one measure in particular and write a one-page paper on its purpose, uses, effectiveness, cost, client acceptance, and popularity.

germicidal solution

liquid used to prevent spread of infection through spa implements; inhibits the growth or action of microorganisms

germicidal cabinet

box that uses ultraviolet light to provide a germ-free environment to store brushes, combs, and other implements used in spas

autoclave

device for heating substances above their boiling point, used to sterilize (spa) instruments

Therapeutic Day Spa
1234 Main Street
Any Town, NY 02101

SAFETY & SANITATION CHECKLIST

Keep this checklist, or one like it, in mind even if filling it out is not a part of your spa therapist's job description.

SPA EMPLOYEE INFORMATION

Name:	Date:

FACILITY SAFETY CHECKLIST

- ☐ Become familiar with all safety guidelines in Employee Manual.
- ☐ Report anything that appears unsafe to management immediately.
- ☐ Check that all exposed tile/ceramic/stone floors are dry and no areas remain for clients to slip on.
- ☐ Check that temperatures are set to correct levels in the sauna, steam, and whirlpool.
- ☐ Check that all non-skid floor mats are in place wherever needed.
- ☐ Know location and use of emergency medical kit.
- ☐ Direct clients' attention to safety signs and warnings wherever appropriate in spa.

FACILITY SANITATION CHECKLIST

- ☐ Become familiar with all sanitation guidelines in Employee Manual.
- ☐ Check stock of sanitary wipes, disinfectants and cleaning supplies available for use by spa therapists.
- ☐ Sanitize all surfaces that guests will come into contact with.
- ☐ Check for adequate supply of linens that have been sanitized by proper (hot water) washing.
- ☐ Assure all oils, lotions and body products are stored at appropriate temperature, off of floor in well-sealed containers.
- ☐ Wash all towels, sheets and other spa linens in hot water, not cold, in order to kill more microorganisms.

EQUIPMENT SAFETY CHECKLIST

- ☐ Become familiar with the safe operating procedure for all equipment in Employee Manual and Manufacturers' Manuals.
- ☐ Have grip bars, stepping stools and other aids available near all hydrotherapy equipment.
- ☐ Ensure that all electric plugs and connections for spa equipment are grounded and protected from water.
- ☐ Ensure that clients observe maximum usage of heat exposure

EQUIPMENT SANITATION CHECKLIST

- ☐ Wipe down hydrotherapy tub, wet table and other equipment with disinfectant after each use.
- ☐ Check for mold or build-up of product in drains, jets, crevices, beneath mats and other hard-to-reach areas.
- ☐ Assure that all instruments coming into contact with clients are sterilized (by autoclave, etc.).
- ☐ Refrigerate unused portions of open seaweeds, muds and other organic compounds (watch for mold).

MISCELLANEOUS ITEMS

- ☐ Therapists should keep clothing, jewelry, hair etc., clean and sanitary at all times while at work.
- ☐ Therapists should wash hands with antibacterial soap before each treatment and after eating, smoking and using washroom.
- ☐ Communicate with other spa therapists and employees regarding status of equipment and facilities (are repairs needed? potential sanitation problems noted?)
- ☐ When in doubt, therapists should stop and ask a superior before proceeding with a treatment they have any reason to believe may be harmful to a client or themselves.

FIGURE 3–28 To double-assure safety and sanitation in the spa, keep a checklist such as this in mind when you are on the job.

SPA PROFILE *Skip Williams, Resources and Development*

Spas, as you now see, are very complex businesses. Setting up and operating a spa can be so challenging that many spa developers seek the aid of experienced guides or consultants. One such guide is Skip Williams who, along with his partner Zahira J. Coll, runs Resources and Development, a company that focuses on the underlying financial and logistical realities of spa businesses and startups so that their owners can focus on the clients.

Williams began his career as a small business consultant who helped professionals from many industries improve their performance. It was while living in Sonoma, California, as a single parent that he happened upon the spa industry and saw the potential for making a big impact. "At first I had no clue what a spa was," says Williams, "but within two months after I started working with my first spa client in Calistoga, I fell in love with this industry. I found that I could help people discover the potential profits hidden in their spa businesses so they could afford to keep their doors open, serve their clients better and make a positive impact in the world."

Williams now has over 13 years of experience in the management, financial development, and operational fields, working as a spa director, controller, and business project consultant. He has been involved in the development of well over 300 spas throughout the U.S., Canada, and the Caribbean. He has seen over the years that many people who get into the spa industry are not fully prepared for all the complexities involved and the total immersion necessary to be successful. He wrote a book, *The Reluctant Spa Director and the Mission Dream*, which is a story about such a person. It is an educational tool as well as a captivating story. He has also developed some powerful tools, starting with his "Build-a-Spa" business model and culminating in the "Financial Blueprint" feasibility consulting package that gives spa owners and would-be spa owners the ability to accurately plan every aspect of their project, from budgets to square footage to equipment to staffing and beyond. See Figure 3–29 for a small example of some of the data generated by a Financial Blueprint analysis of a spa business plan.

"My mission in life," states Williams, "is to help those people who have the healer's heart, to keep their business sustainable and profitable in the real world so they can go forth, follow their dreams, and heal that many more people." He has a very practical point of view regarding this healing, one that some massage therapists may find hard to understand at first. "What the massage therapist is doing is an art, but it is not until the spa owner turns this art into a science that a real business has been created. Spa owners can no longer expect to have their service providers (i.e. massage therapists) be their business partners. Instead, spa owners need to take full responsibility for the risks and liabilities of running a business and pay their providers fair living wages and benefits."

Not surprisingly, one of Williams's main focuses now is on helping spa owners come up with appropriate compensation systems. In addition to creating Financial Blueprints for spas, Williams also spends time dealing with the controversial topics of how to pay spa staff, whether to pay commission versus straight wages and whether to hire them as employees versus contractors (see sidebar in Chapter 14, The Spa Hiring Paradox: A Lower Starting Wage Is Good for You). In all of this, he remains steadfastly dedicated to turning spas into viable and realistic businesses. Because, as he says with a smile, "You can't be altruistic if you're out of business."

(Continued)

SPA PROFILE

Skip Williams, Resources and Development *continued*

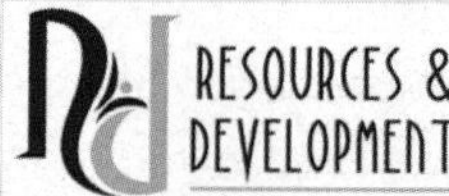

"Your Complete Resource for Spa and Hotel Development"

Is Your Dream Spa Viable?

- **How Large Will Your Spa Need to Be?**
- **How Much Money Will Your Spa Make?**
- **What Services Will Generate The Most Profit?**
- **How Will You Control Expenses?**
- **How Much Money Do You Need to Build Your Dream Spa?**
- **How Do You Create the Ultimate Spa Experience?**

Creating a feasibility analysis for a Day Spa, Resort Spa, Med Spa, or a Salon is far more complex than most businesses. Because each Spa has widely different variables such as:

- Menu Offering of Services
- Service Pricing
- Types of Locations
- Size
- Cost of Construction
- Rent Expense
- Ratio of Revenue Production Space vs. Amenity Space
- Types of Compensation Systems
- Types of Labor
- Labor Rates
- Hours of Operation
- Marketing Experience
- Marketing Budgets

The standard form of "Pro Forma" analysis is not adequate, nor can we ascertain much, if any, transferable information from other Spa businesses.

Even if you take the time to account for every little Revenue and Expense detail, a Pro Forma (also called a Projected Profit and Loss Statement) still will not allow you to:

- Compare the Profitability of Services Offered
- Calculate the Staffing Requirements
- Calculate Construction Costs
- Perform a Break-Even Analysis
- Analyze the Efficiency of Your Space
- Create a Master Purchase List
- Calculate other Setup and Equipment Costs

The standard Pro Forma simply does not give us a very good view of your "Vision" and is not a very efficient way to analyze your "Concepts". Many Spa Owners never have a clear understanding of where their profit is coming from and what expenses are draining potential from their business. Consequently, they take the risk of adding their Dream to the heap of Spa Failures Statistics.

www.ResourcesAndDevelopment.com – 702-436-0371

FIGURE 3–29 Financial Blueprint readout.

CONCLUSION

Spa facilities can be marble-studded palaces that feature stunning vistas of the world's most beautiful environments, or they can be humble windowless rooms in a corporate office park. Spa equipment can be high-tech and cost tens of thousands of dollars like computerized hydrotherapy tubs, or it can be simple and inexpensive like the small ice chests used to keep towels and products warm. Regardless of whether they cost millions or just a few dollars, spa facilities and the equipment in them are all dedicated to one main purpose: the health, well-being, and enjoyment of the clients. To ensure that clients have the best possible experience while at the spa, therapists need to place a strong emphasis on safety and sanitation, and they need to be sure of their ability to use every piece of equipment in its proper fashion. There is no substitute for training and ongoing practice to make therapists confident and efficient. Also, by knowing how a large array of spa equipment works, what goes into creating and installing it, and what its benefits are, spa therapists become more well-rounded and well-informed professionals, even if they do not end up using this equipment themselves on a daily basis.

REVIEW QUESTIONS

1. What are the main differences between a wet room and a dry room?
2. What are the advantages and disadvantages of a wet room versus a dry room?
3. What piece of equipment is the centerpiece for any successful spa dry room?
4. The equipment used in spa wet rooms or wet areas can be broken down into four main categories. What are they? Give examples of each type.
5. What are some general guidelines for dealing with all the laundry generated in a spa treatment area?
6. What risk factors do spas pose that are not found in such abundance in other environments where massage therapists work? What problems may arise because of them?
7. Therapists who perform spa treatments hold two key advantages regarding self-care, as compared to those who perform massage therapy alone. What are they?
8. Why is it a good idea to keep your spa treatment room (and your practical spa classroom) neat and organized?
9. What are the three main categories of risk management issues faced by spa businesses?
10. When should spa equipment, from the smallest brush to the largest hydrotherapy tub, be sanitized? What are some of the implements used for sanitizing in the spa?

through the application of water, which forms an integral part of most treatments. For example, an herbal wrap imparts much of its benefits through the hot water soaked into the sheets. The herbs in this case act as a catalyst, with the primary therapeutic agent being heated water. In other words, the herbs in this treatment contribute to and enhance the process which the heated water in the wrap instigates.

Other actions purportedly created by spa therapies include the detoxification, nourishment, or revitalization of bodily tissues. These effects will be discussed in detail in other chapters, along with the treatments that are most commonly reported to cause them. When reading these chapters, practicing these therapies, and especially when administering these therapies to paying clients in the spa setting, it is important that you not take any information for granted or parrot phrases you have heard secondhand. What are you really saying when you say, "This treatment will detoxify your body"? or "This treatment will help lower your blood pressure"? As a professional spa therapist, it will be up to you to know.

SPA TIP

Spa therapists need to be aware that, although "hydro" means water, the main therapeutic effects of hydrotherapy are caused by heat and cold, not the water itself. "Heat therapy" and "cold therapy" are also appropriate terms, though they are not commonly used in spas.

THE EFFECTS OF HYDROTHERAPY

As it applies to spa therapy, hydrotherapy can be defined as the application of water in its liquid, solid, or vapor forms, either externally or internally, to induce health benefits in the recipient. The primary physiological effects of hydrotherapy can be placed into three categories: thermal, mechanical, and chemical.

The thermal effects of hydrotherapy are caused by the application of water at temperatures above or below that of the body, with more pronounced effects created with greater differences in temperature. This differential in turn affects the internal heat-regulating mechanisms of the body, causing changes in circulation, digestion, perspiration, and other functions. Of the three primary physiological effects of hydrotherapy, the thermal effects are by far the most important. In fact, the term "hydrotherapy" may be misleading in a certain sense, because it leads people to believe that water (hydro) itself is the main therapeutic ingredient, while the most active agents in hydrotherapy are actually heat and cold themselves. Water is merely a vehicle for the transference of heat from or to the body. Other substances could be substituted, but none are so plentiful or so perfectly suited to the task.

When a large percentage of the body is immersed in heat, a widespread dilation of the blood vessels of the skin takes place, which helps the body eliminate heat from within. This process, which is accompanied by a shift of blood from the interior of the body to the surface, is known as the **hydrostatic effect** (Figure 4–1). This same effect is created in reverse when the entire body is immersed in cold.

Within the human body, the **hypothalamus** gland (Figure 4–2) regulates temperature and the transference of blood from one part of the body to another through the hydrostatic effect. Thus, the functioning of this gland, also known as the "master gland" because it has so many vital functions, is crucial to the effectiveness of hydrotherapy treatments.

When heat is transferred to or from an object, including the human body in spa therapies, it is through one of five methods: **conduction**, **convection**,

hydrostatic effect

a shifting of blood from the interior of the body to the surface

hypothalamus

also known as the "master gland," roughly the size of an almond and found in all mammalian brains, the hypothalamus links the nervous system to the endocrine system via the pituitary gland and regulates certain metabolic processes and other autonomic activities including the control of body temperature, crucial to the effects of hydrotherapy

conduction

heat transference via direct physical contact

convection

heat transference via moving currents of heated liquids or gases, as in a sauna or steam bath

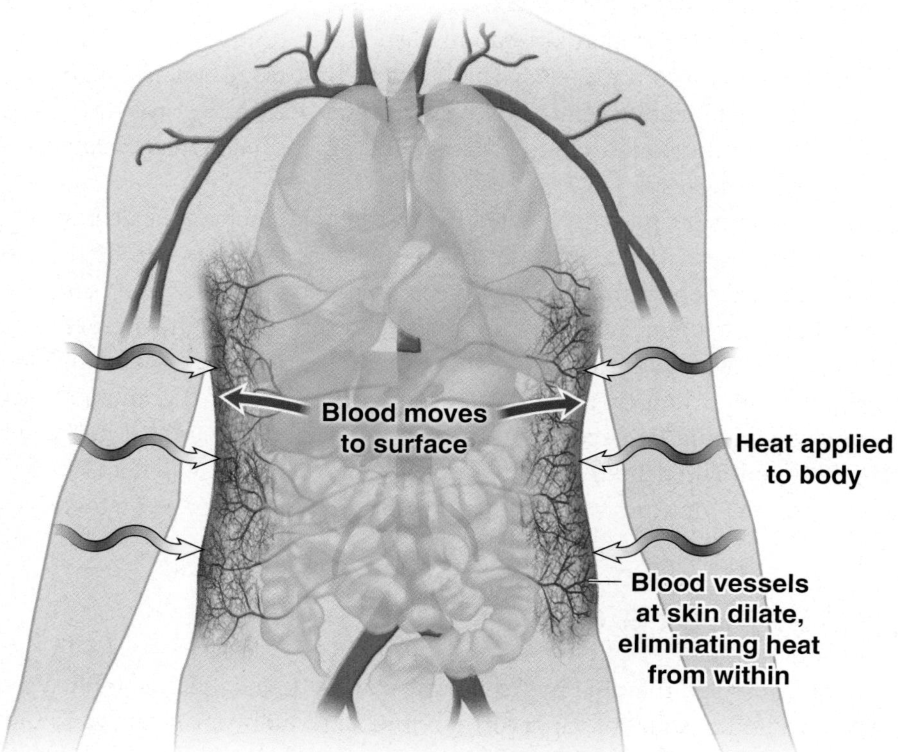

FIGURE 4–1 The hydrostatic effect is more pronounced the greater the temperature differential applied to the body in hydrotherapy.

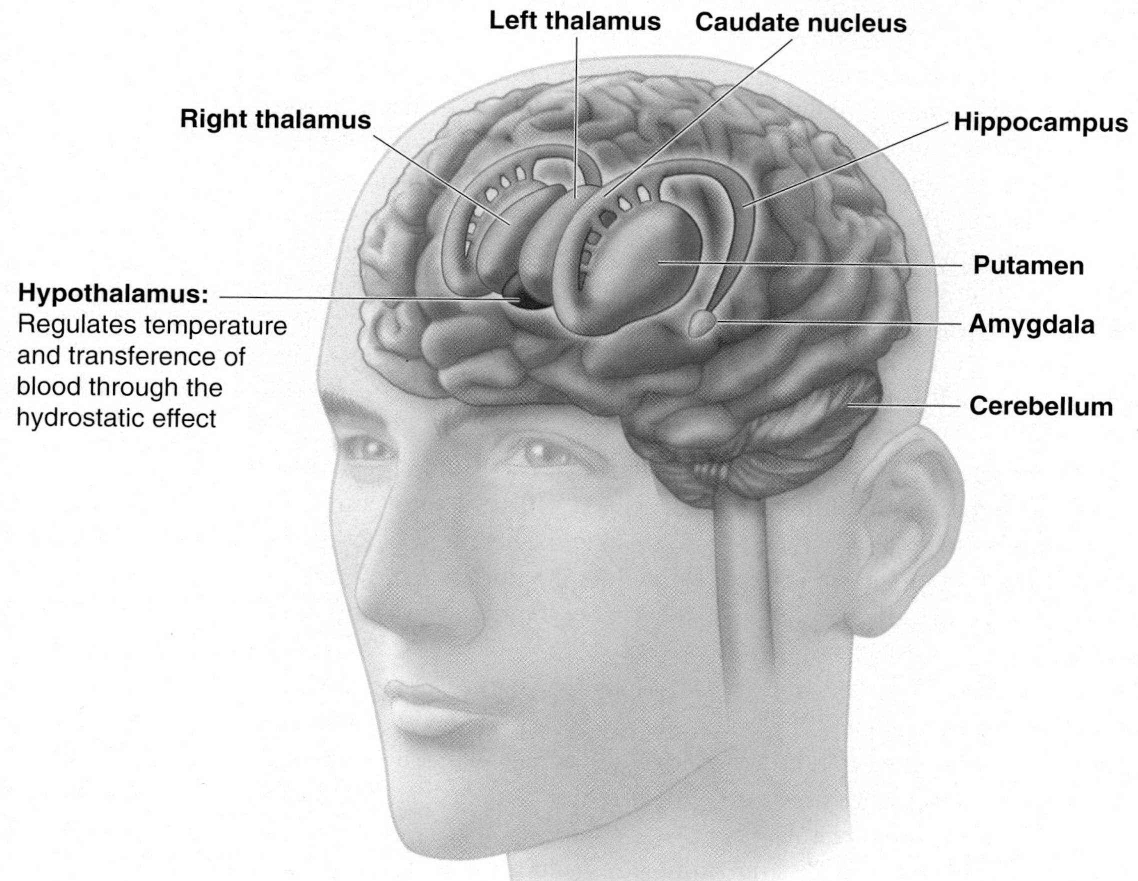

FIGURE 4–2 The hypothalamus gland is crucial to the effectiveness of hydrotherapy treatments.

conversion, **radiation**, and **evaporation**. Conduction takes place when one heated object is placed in direct physical contact with another object. One example of conduction with which many massage therapists are familiar is the hot pack or silicon gel pack. Most hydrotherapy treatments use conduction to transfer heat to or from the body. Convection takes place when heated liquids or gases are moved around a body, such as in the sauna or steam bath, which will be covered in the next chapter. In conversion, heat is created by passing energy, such as electricity or ultrasound waves, through a substance or body. Radiation heats the body through absorption of infrared rays, as from the sun and also in the infrared saunas which are used in some spas. Evaporation affects body temperature through the conversion of liquid into a vapor, removing heat in the process, which is how sweating cools the body.

conversion

heat transference via the passage of energy, such as electricity, through a substance or tissue

radiation

heat transfer to a body through direct exposure to infrared rays

evaporation

heat transfer through the change of substance from liquid to vapor form, as in sweating

The mechanical effects of hydrotherapy are caused by the impact of water on the surface of the body, as in hydrotherapy tubs, Jacuzzis and showers. These effects can be mild, as in a typical shower taken at home, or quite intense, as in a 104°F hydrotherapy bath with a high-pressure underwater massage hose. This impact stimulates local circulation and can help decrease muscle aches and pains, just as manual massage does (Figure 4–3).

The chemical effects of hydrotherapy are created when water is ingested or used for colonic irrigation. In most spas, external applications that produce thermal and mechanical effects are by far the most popular, but European spas in particular have made the internal use (through drinking) of mineral-laden spa waters an integral part of their health regimens.

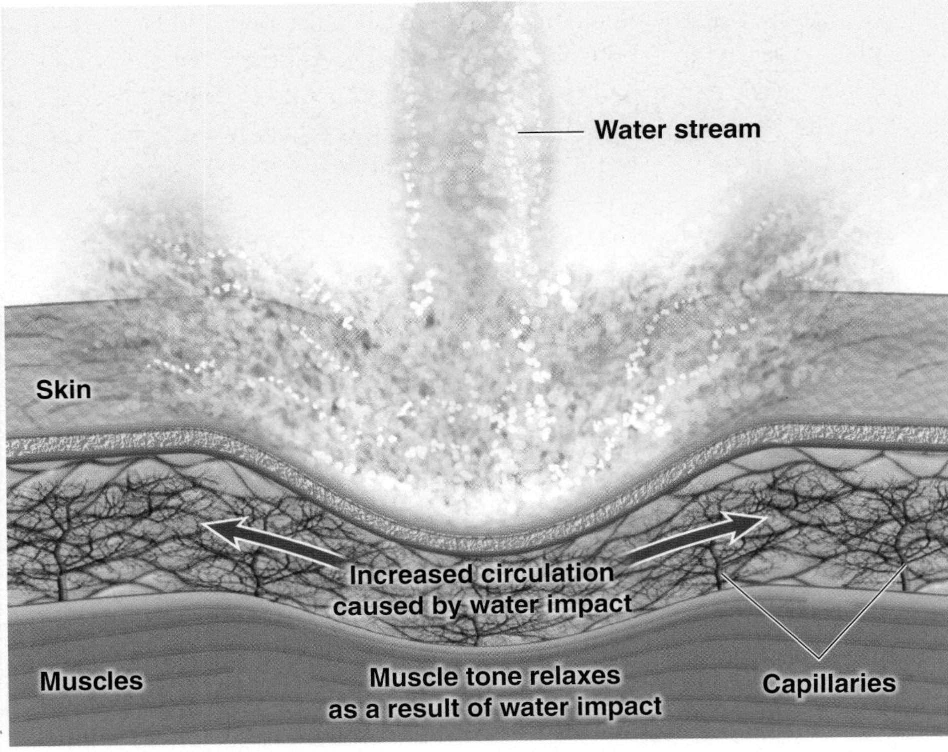

FIGURE 4–3 The mechanical effects of hydrotherapy can be quite pronounced.

DEFINITION	TEMPERATURE	USES
Extremely Hot	over 115°F	Hot showers (120°F), paraffin (128°F), hot packs (165°F)
Very Hot	104°F–114°F	Extra-hot soaks, hot mud
Hot	100°F–104°F	Jacuzzi, whirlpool, hot tub
Warm	92°F–99°F	Therapeutic baths
Tepid	80°F–91°F	Calming washes, neutral baths, showers and compresses
Cool	65°F–79°F	Cool compresses, cool showers
Cold	33°F–64°F	Cold gel packs, cold baths, cold showers, cold plunges
Very Cold/Ice	Below 32°F	Ice packs, ice cubes, cryotherapy
Contrast	Alternating 40°F/104°F	Contrast (heat/cold) baths and applications

TABLE 4–1 Water Temperature Definitions.

atonic effect

response produced by exposure to heat in hydrotherapy, in which the body exhibits a lack of muscle tone

tonic effect

response produced by initial exposure to cold in hydrotherapy, in which the body exhibits heightened muscle tone

thermalism

spa-specific term referring to the therapeutic use of naturally hot spring water (and sometimes cold seawater), specifically focusing on the temperature of the water

SPA CAUTION

After any type of therapeutic hot bath, it is always recommended that clients drink plenty of water. This may seem counterintuitive because the client is immersed in water throughout the treatment and ingesting more water will not seem necessary. However, the heat and increase in circulation created by these baths can stimulate fluid loss, and therefore fluid intake is recommended.

Water Temperature

When spa clients experience heat via a hydrotherapy treatment, the temperature of the water must be monitored closely using thermometers or the built-in thermostats found in some equipment. This is to assure the safety and comfort of the client. The definitions of what constitutes *cold water* versus *hot water, very cold* versus *very hot*, or *warm* versus *cool* vary from text to text and practitioner to practitioner. See Table 4–1 for temperatures that fall within the middle range of most commonly accepted definitions of these terms.

Hot water has a stimulating effect which then morphs gradually into a relaxing effect as the body recovers from the initial response to immersion in the heat. Cold water has a different kind of stimulating effect. It causes shivering, goose flesh, constricted blood vessels, higher pulse rate, and faster respiration, plus increased metabolism and muscle tone. Another way of saying this is that heat creates an **atonic effect** while cold creates a **tonic effect**, and these effects vary according to the duration of the heat or cold application. Cold can be stimulating when first applied, but over a longer period it begins to damage tissues.

Thermalism is a term that spa professionals use but that you will not find in most dictionaries. It can be defined as the use of thermal spring waters and sea waters at various temperatures for therapeutic purposes. Thermalism, in this sense, has been practiced for thousands of years. The use of this term by spa owners, directors, and therapists focuses attention on the most important therapeutic aspect of hydrotherapy, namely the heat (for spring water) and cold (for sea water) contained within the water. Its use, then, specifically refers to the thermal effects of hydrotherapy.

BATH TECHNIQUES

As long as they have existed, spas have been places where people bathe. Bathing has been, during many times and in many cultures, the essence of the spa experience. In much of the world, "taking the waters" is a term used interchangeably

The RICE Method

Did You Know?

Though most modern spa clients do not visit spas in order to receive remedial therapy for acute or chronic injuries, and are not seeking hydrotherapy for pain relief, it can sometimes happen. Therapists need to be aware of the spa's policy about treating injured clients, and they also need to be aware of the core therapeutic effects of heat and cold on the body in order to provide the most informed and beneficial treatment, if appropriate. If treatment of an injured client is not appropriate, therapists need to refer the case to another heath practitioner. Depending on the severity of the injury, the correct response may be to refer the client to a physician immediately.

If a spa client does happen to request treatment for an acute injury, spa therapists need to know that heat should normally not be applied for at least 72 hours following the injury, because increased blood flow caused by the heat application makes swelling and pain worse and may cause tissue damage to the injured area. This makes acute injuries a contraindication for many spa services.

The best protocol to follow in minor injuries is known by the acronym "**RICE**," which stands for Rest, Ice, Compression, and Elevation. The RICE method is definitely not a treatment commonly offered on the menus at luxurious modern spas, but it is a simple method spa therapists can use to help clients with many types of joint and muscle injuries. It helps ease pain and speed recovery, especially if it is used immediately after an injury.

REST: In most injuries, the area should remain at rest until pain sensations subside.

ICE: Apply ice as soon as possible after injury, even if the client is going to see a doctor. Ice reduces inflammation, pain, and swelling, and helps keep blood and fluid from building up in the injured area. Apply ice for 15 to 20 minutes every 2 or 3 hours. Crushed ice or small cubes can be placed in a plastic bag and wrapped with a moist towel. Ice should be used for the first 72 hours or until swelling lessens.

COMPRESSION: Between applications of ice, the injured area should be wrapped lightly with an elastic bandage or similar material to help control swelling and provide support. Start at the most distal point near the injury and wrap toward the heart.

ELEVATION: To speed recovery and ease pain, raise the injured area above the heart to allow gravity to drain excess fluids and help reduce swelling.

with "going to a spa." Modern spas have devised many versions of this ancient custom, and this chapter will familiarize you with their use and application. In addition to the myriad forms of bathing practiced in spas, several specialized spa showers will be explained in this chapter as well.

Spas sometimes use the term **balneotherapy** on their menus. The root of this term is the Latin word *balneum*, which means bath. However, the word has broader implications that spa therapists need to keep in mind. Specifically, *balneotherapy* refers to all the different types of water available for therapy, such as thermal spring waters, mineral laden waters, and silt-filled waters, plus such additives used in the waters as herbs, powders, oils, and gases. So, proper use of balneotherapy means that therapists need to be aware of the therapeutic effects created by the thermal, mechanical, and chemical properties of the waters used, plus the therapeutic properties of every product used in the waters.

RICE

an acronym that stands for Rest, Ice, Compression, and Elevation, the recommended preliminary treatment within the first 72 hours after an acute injury

balneotherapy

the use of baths to induce health benefits, often using thermal waters with specific therapeutic ingredients such as essential oils, herbs, and minerals

SPA CAUTION

As required by law in most areas, hot tubs, saunas, and other heat treatments in public areas should have signage indicating the risks involved posted clearly for all to see. Though this is often not required for hydrotherapy tubs in private treatment rooms, it is a good idea to remind clients of the potential risk either verbally or with a sign in the room.

SPA CAUTION

Therapists should monitor the pulse of clients in hot baths and hydrotherapy tubs, especially those clients who are old or weakened by sickness. Watch for signs of fatigue or dizziness, such as eyes floating upwards or skin blanching. Be prepared to support clients getting in or out of tubs, especially getting out when they may feel faint or light-headed.

We often overlook the health benefits of water. Professor Jonathan Paul De Vierville (see profile later in this chapter) states that "In America we look at what's pathological in water, not what's good." In other words, we spend a lot of time looking for impurities, pathogens, bacteria, and other matter that may cause harm, and then we spend a lot of money filtering and purifying water to eliminate these qualities. We spend relatively little if any time seeking out the positive qualities of certain waters and using them to our benefit. Balneotherapy, or "therapeutic bathing," takes the opposite approach and focuses instead on the positive, restorative properties of the waters being used. For those spas that use tap water that does not have any especially beneficial properties, therapeutic agents can be added. At times, the only therapeutic agent being added is heat itself, which is beneficial and qualifies the treatment as hydrotherapy. However, calling a hot bath in plain municipal tap water "balneotherapy" may be misleading.

There are many types of therapeutic baths, some more popular in spas than others. One type of extended, full-immersion, therapist-assisted bathing experience called Watsu™ is not covered here because it is described in Chapter 12. Study Table 4–2 to familiarize yourself with baths that are used therapeutically in many settings, including resorts, clinics, sports centers, convalescent centers, and, of course, spas. Then read the more detailed descriptions of therapeutic baths that follow the table and in subsequent chapters as well. A description of seaweed baths is offered in Chapter 7, herbal and mud baths in Chapter 8, aromatherapy baths in Chapter 11, and foot baths in Chapter 13. Detailed protocols are offered only for those baths that are popular in U.S. and Canadian spas. Certain treatments such as the sitz bath and **Hubbard tank**, which have proven therapeutic effects, will nevertheless not be covered in this book because they are not typically offered in modern spas.

Hubbard tank

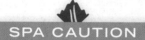

a large tank in which a patient can easily be assisted in exercises while in the water, developed by Leroy Watkins Hubbard (1857–1938), American orthopedic surgeon and physician to Franklin D. Roosevelt, who suffered from paralysis

Draping for Spa Bath Services

Draping is an issue when administering bath services, whether they be in a traditional bathtub or a high-tech hydrotherapy tub. It is difficult, if not impossible, to maintain full draping on a client who is stepping into a tub naked to receive bath therapy. For this reason, many spas have a same-sex policy when it comes to bath services. In these spas, only male therapists offer bath therapies for male clients and only female therapists offer bath therapies for female clients. In these cases, nudity is acceptable. In some localities, it is even common for therapists of the opposite sex to offer bath therapies, and the nudity is not an issue. Laws, regulations, and local traditions vary from state to state and region to region.

If it is preferable for any reason to maintain modest draping during bath therapies, three main alternatives present themselves:

1. Clients can wear bathing suits or shorts into the tub.
2. Clients can enter and exit the tub while alone in the room. This, however, presents serious risks of slip-and-fall accidents and increased liability for the spa.
3. Therapists can assist clients out of robes or towels in such a way as to preserve modesty to a large degree by using a bath entry draping protocol (Figures 4–4A through 4–4D).

BATH TREATMENT	DESCRIPTION	USES	CONTRAINDICATIONS	POPULARITY IN SPAS
Herbal Bath	client soaks in bath filled with warm or hot herbal solution	imparting qualities of herbs to clients for relaxation, invigoration and other effects	high blood pressure, heart disease, arteriosclerosis, allergies or reactions to certain herbs, pregnancy	medium
Essential Oil Bath	aromatherapy oils added to warm or hot bath	relaxation, invigoration, etc. imparting qualities of essential oils to clients	high blood pressure, heart disease, arteriosclerosis, allergies or reactions to certain essential oils, pregnancy	medium
Seaweed Bath	warm or hot bath with seaweed extracts added (see Chapter 7)	remineralizing of body	high blood pressure, heart disease, arteriosclerosis, allergies or reactions to iodine or shellfish, pregnancy	medium
Fango Bath/Mud Bath	either mud or fango powder is added to hot water to make a solution, or in some cases clients immerse in 100% mud	therapeutic for stiff joints and arthritis, relaxing and purifying through the use of **humic acid** (also see Chapter 8 for mud wraps)	high blood pressure, heart disease, arteriosclerosis, open sores or cuts, pregnancy	medium
Mineral Bath	warm or hot bath with added minerals such as calcium found in salts and other ingredients	to expose clients to desirable minerals that can be soaked in through the pores	high blood pressure, heart disease, arteriosclerosis, pregnancy	medium
Enzyme Bath	a treatment that uses active enzymes to produce heat and electrochemical reactions through a fermentation process	stimulates a natural cleansing processes in the skin, stimulates circulation and metabolism	high blood pressure, heart disease, arteriosclerosis, pregnancy	low in the West, very localized to specific spas, most in Japan
Whirlpool Bath	another name for a hot tub, with hot water agitated by high-pressure aerated jets	often in the common area of the spa, available for use by guests on their own at any time	recent injuries, open wounds, acute hematomas, varicosities, high blood pressure, heart disease, arteriosclerosis, pregnancy	high
Hydrotherapy Tub Bath	high-tech bath with multiple high-pressure water jets divided in therapist-controlled zones and often with underwater massage hose, used with a variety of additives	used in conjunction with therapeutic ingredients in stand-alone treatments for relaxation, remineralization, purification, etc. and also as part of larger services such as anti-cellulite therapy	recent injuries, open wounds, acute hematomas, varicosities, high blood pressure, heart disease, arteriosclerosis, pregnancy	high
Underwater Massage	therapist-held hose that directs stream of high-pressure water (usually hot) at client under the surface of a bath, usually found in hydrotherapy tubs	highly stimulating and deep-pressure massage can be given safely without excess force on sensitive tissues	recent injuries, open wounds, acute hematomas, varicosities, high blood pressure, heart disease, arteriosclerosis, pregnancy	high

TABLE 4–2 Types of Therapeutic Baths Offered in Spas. (*Continued*)

BATH TREATMENT	DESCRIPTION	USES	CONTRAINDICATIONS	POPULARITY IN SPAS
Cold Bath/Cold Plunge	cold water pool into which clients dip or plunge briefly, often adjacent to hot pool	quick immersion closes pores, improves circulation and stimulates skin and body after exposure to heat treatments (see Chapter 5)	infection, heart disease, chills, severe diabetes	medium
Carbon Dioxide Bath	warm bath with carbon dioxide (CO_2) either added or occurring naturally in spring water	usually an unintentional added effect of natural spring waters, sometimes used purposefully	high blood pressure, heart disease, arteriosclerosis, pregnancy	low
Hot Bath	hot water bath with no additional ingredients added	to wash off spa products, general relaxation, increase perspiration/elimination	high blood pressure, heart disease, arteriosclerosis, pregnancy	low
Contrast Bath	performed by going from one bath to another, such as a hydrotherapy tub to a cold plunge	alternating temperatures stimulates circulation and tones skin	infection, heart disease, chills, severe diabetes, high blood pressure, heart disease, arteriosclerosis, pregnancy	medium
Localized Bath	one body part at a time, such as the arm or leg, is submerged in water of a specific temperature to achieve desired results	used often for rehabilitation in case of injury to an extremity, localized soreness or sluggish circulation	abrasions, open sores, severe high blood pressure, lymph edema in the area, varicosities in the area	low
Foot Bath	the feet are placed in a receptacle of water, usually hot and often in combination with exfoliation, massage	often included in spa foot treatments, very luxurious	varicose veins on lower legs, severe hypertension, phlebitis	high
Sitz Bath	partial-immersion bath that covers the clientís pelvic area	used in cases of hypotonicity in the perineal region, after giving birth	infection, high blood pressure, heart disease, arteriosclerosis, pregnancy	low, used more often in rehabilitation centers

TABLE 4–2 Types of Therapeutic Baths Offered in Spas.

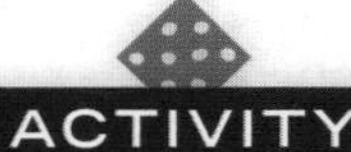

ACTIVITY

Practice Bath Entry Draping Protocol

Pair up with a classmate and practice the Bath Entry Draping Protocol while fully dressed. If your classroom is not outfitted with tubs, use a "virtual bathtub" for this activity by simply marking an area on the floor that will be used as the "tub." Or, to practice draping for the hydrotherapy tub, use the "virtual hydrotherapy tub" described in the Hydrotherapy Tub Safety Practice activity later in this chapter. This fully clothed and leisurely paced practice will make your movements more natural and fluid when you eventually use them in a real spa setting.

ADMINISTERING A THERAPEUTIC BATH

A therapeutic bath is one of the most simple and straightforward treatments offered in spas. During many baths, the client is left alone in the treatment area to soak, and no further assistance is needed from the therapist. In some spas, attendants or technicians prepare the baths, and therapists are not involved

humic acid

a substance found in muds used in spa treatments, it endows these muds with the ability to chelate (bind) positively charged ions, heavy metals, and free radicals so they become more available for elimination

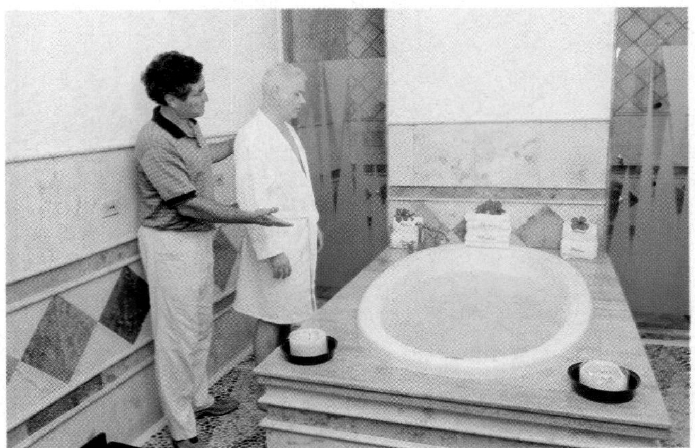

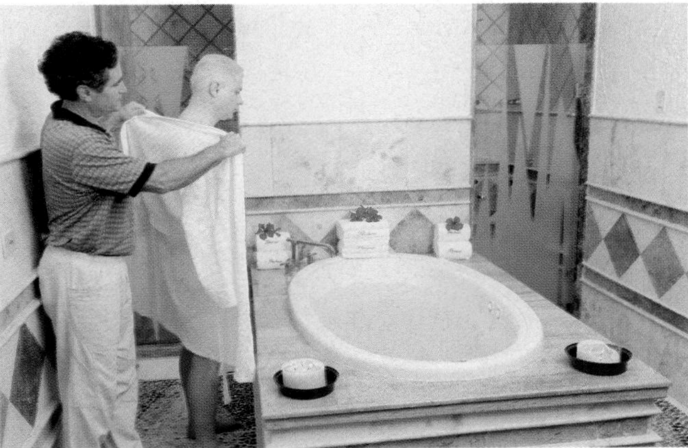

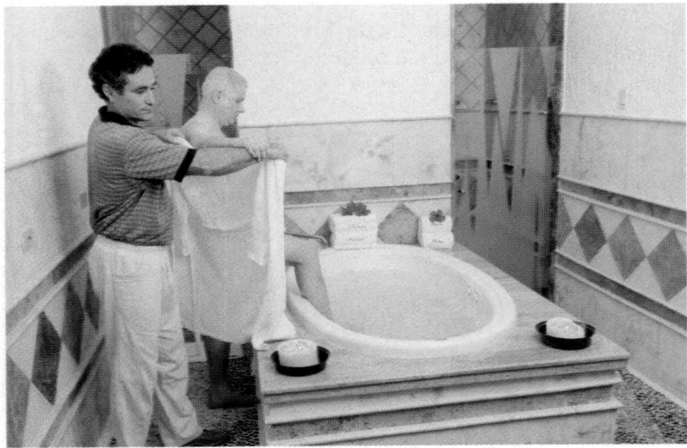

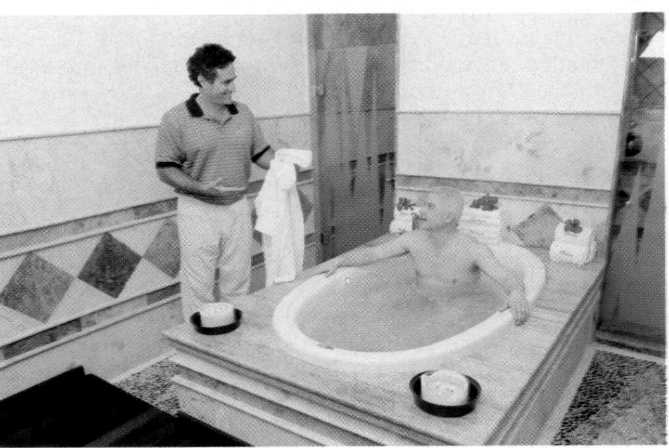

FIGURE 4–4 Use the bath entry draping protocol to preserve modesty. Instruct client to wear a bathrobe, large bath towel or bath sheet upon entering the bath area.

with the procedure at all. Practices vary depending upon the philosophy of the spa, the nature of the therapeutic additives, and local laws and regulations. During all therapeutic baths, the client's safety is the foremost concern. Care must be taken to assure that clients enter and exit the tub safely, that they remain for the recommended period of time, and that the water temperature and added ingredients are appropriate for the client's condition. Therapeutic baths can feature a wide range of added products with varied therapeutic intentions, as noted in Table 4–2, but the same protocol can be used for applying all of them.

Therapeutic Bath Protocol

TREATMENT: THERAPEUTIC BATH	
Wet Room/Dry Room	wet room
Tub Setup	bath tub filled with warm to hot water, therapeutic ingredients already added or nearby, bathmat at entrance, bowl of ice water
Treatment Duration	normally 20 minutes
Needed Supplies	bath mat, 2 bath towels, hand towel, bowl of ice water, wash cloth, therapeutic bath additives
Contraindications	high blood pressure, heart disease, arteriosclerosis, pregnancy, sensitivities or allergies to therapeutic bath additives
Draping	Depending on local laws, clients can be nude in tub when being treated by a therapist of the same sex, or they can wear bathing suits. Take extra care to maintain modesty while client is getting into and out of tub.
Treatment Order	usually given before massage/body treatments to soften and relax tissues
Safety, Sanitation Issues, & Clean-Up	The tub is sanitized after each use by wiping down entire interior surface with disinfectant. Clients need to be assisted into and out of tub and be warned about feeling weak after treatment.
Body Mechanics & Self-Care	Therapists need to protect lower back while bending over tub and be careful to avoid slipping on wet floors.
Product Cost	Costs vary with chosen bath additives but are generally $3 or less.
Treatment Price	Often free as an add-on to another spa treatment. *À la carte* price $20 to $50.
Physiological Effects	The primary action of the therapeutic bath is created by the heat in the water, relaxing muscle tone and softening connective tissues. Effects of the added therapeutic ingredients vary by type.
Pregnancy Issues (information provided by Elaine Stillerman, LMT, author and developer of MotherMassage®)	Therapeutic bath is contraindicated during each of the three trimesters of pregnancy. During postpartum recovery, the bath may be used once bleeding has stopped.

spa technician

a spa employee whose duties include preparing treatment rooms, stocking supplies and products, cleaning up after services, aiding clients to and from treatment areas, and other general tasks in support of therapists and management

Therapeutic Bath Preparation

1. The area is prepared by placing bath mats, non-slip surfaces, towels, ice water, wash cloth, and therapeutic ingredients within easy reach.
2. The bath is usually drawn by a therapist or **spa technician** before the client enters the room (Figure 4–5). Temperature is controlled for intended outcomes (see Table 4–1), the average temperature for a therapeutic bath being approximately 100°F.

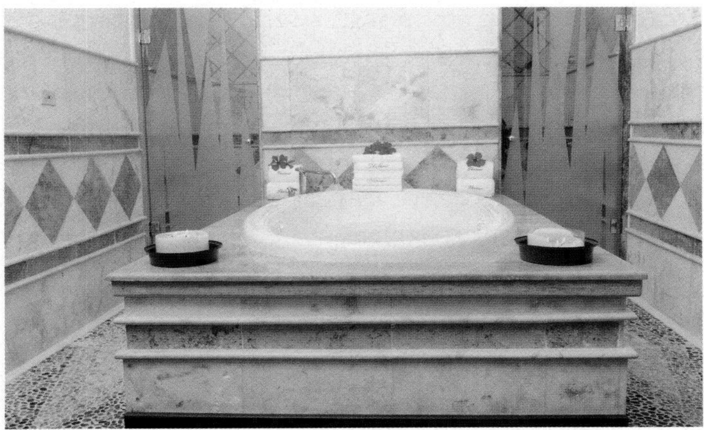

FIGURE 4–5 Therapeutic baths being drawn for client.

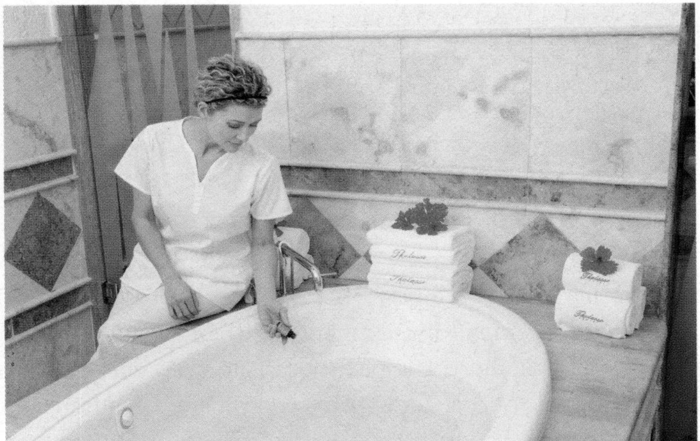

FIGURE 4–6 Therapeutic ingredients are added to bath.

3. Therapeutic ingredients are added to the bath while the tub is filling, or they are added after the client has entered the room so he or she can see the products (Figure 4–6).

Therapeutic Bath Procedure

1. The procedure, duration, and intended effects are explained to the client prior to the client's entering the tub.
2. The client is assisted into the tub (see Figures 4–4A through 4–4D, the Bath Entry Draping Protocol earlier in this chapter).
3. If the bathtub is jetted, the therapist will need to explain to the client how to turn the jets on and off.
4. Have cold compresses available to apply to the client's forehead if needed or desired.
5. Most therapeutic baths last 10 to 25 minutes, depending upon the client's age, health, tolerance for heat, and desired experience. The maximum time for hot baths (100°F or above) is usually 15 minutes, but therapeutic baths cool down over time, as compared

to Jacuzzis, hot tubs, hot springs, and whirlpools, which maintain a constant high temperature. Therefore, clients can remain in therapeutic baths longer.

6. Assist the client out of the tub. Offer a bathrobe, slippers, and a glass of water. Help the client into a nearby chair or lounger to relax afterward, or guide him or her to the next spa treatment.

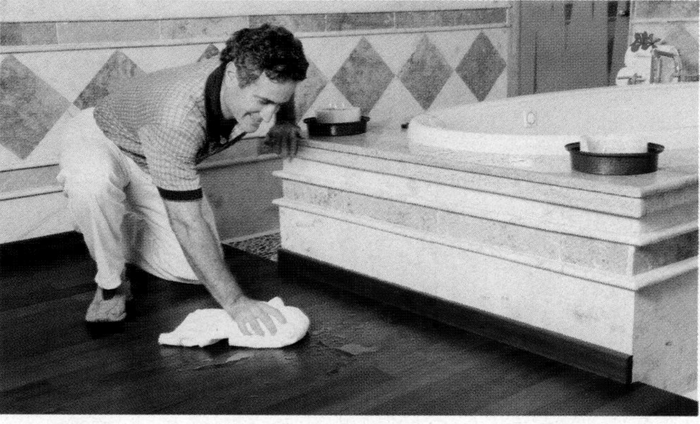

FIGURE 4–7 After therapeutic baths the floors are dried, the tub is sanitized and the room is prepared for the next treatment.

Therapeutic Bath Cleanup

1. The bathtub must be sanitized after every treatment with a disinfectant spray.
2. Floors must be dried between bath treatments to maintain a safe environment.
3. Towels and wash cloths are laundered, bowls cleaned, products stored, and the room tidied for the next treatment (Figure 4–7).

HYDROTHERAPY TUB BATH

The modern hydrotherapy tub is a powerful tool, and many of the top spas around the world feature hydrotherapy tub treatments on their menus. These tubs are not difficult to operate, but it is important for therapists to keep safety issues foremost in mind when administering services using this equipment, because clients generally need to climb up into the tub, which can have a slippery surface. Also, this exertion, combined with the effects of heat, can lead some clients to become light-headed and even faint. Therapists need to stay aware of their own body mechanics while administering treatments in these tubs as well, especially when bending over the edge to use underwater massage hoses. For safety purposes, the therapist generally stays in the treatment room while the client is in the tub.

Hydrotherapy tubs represent an evolutionary step up from the whirlpools and hot tubs that have been used in spas, fitness centers, and rehabilitation facilities for decades. Most hydrotherapy tubs have dozens of small jets that propel an aerated stream of water onto the client. These jets are separated into zones that are activated by the therapist or by computer, creating a customized treatment sequence. For example, the zone for jets aimed at muscles along the spine can be activated at full pressure for a client complaining of a tight back. For general relaxation, zones are activated in sequence for equal periods. In addition to the array of jets, many tubs feature an underwater massage hose that sprays a powerful stream of water at the client's body from a few inches away while submerged under the surface of the filled tub (Figure 4–8).

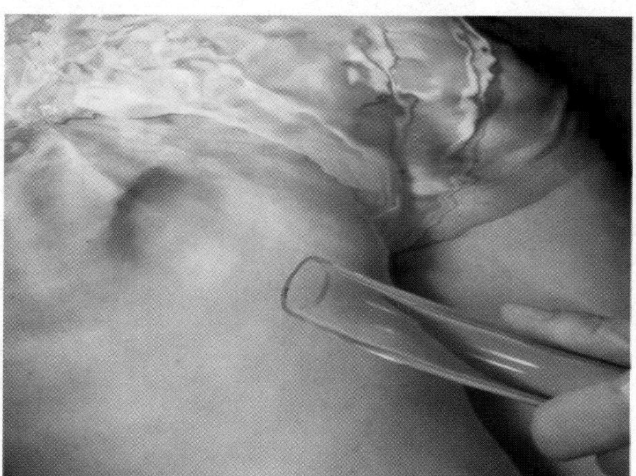

FIGURE 4–8 The underwater massage hose propels a powerful stream of water at clients' muscles.

ACTIVITY

Hydrotherapy Tub Safety Practice

If you eventually work in a large resort or destination spa, you will likely be trained on the use of hydrotherapy tubs while on the job. Though your classroom may not have an actual tub upon which to practice while you are in school, it is important to understand the basic safety procedures involved with their use. Practicing a couple basic tub safety procedures in the classroom, even without a tub, will reinforce them in your mind and make them second nature. This will make you a better prospective spa therapist. Practice the following "virtual" maneuvers to help you become accustomed to procedures used in hydrotherapy tub treatments. In place of a hydrotherapy tub, use a massage table set at the tallest height. Place a stepping stool to one side of the table and a bath mat in front of the stepping stool (Figure 4–9).

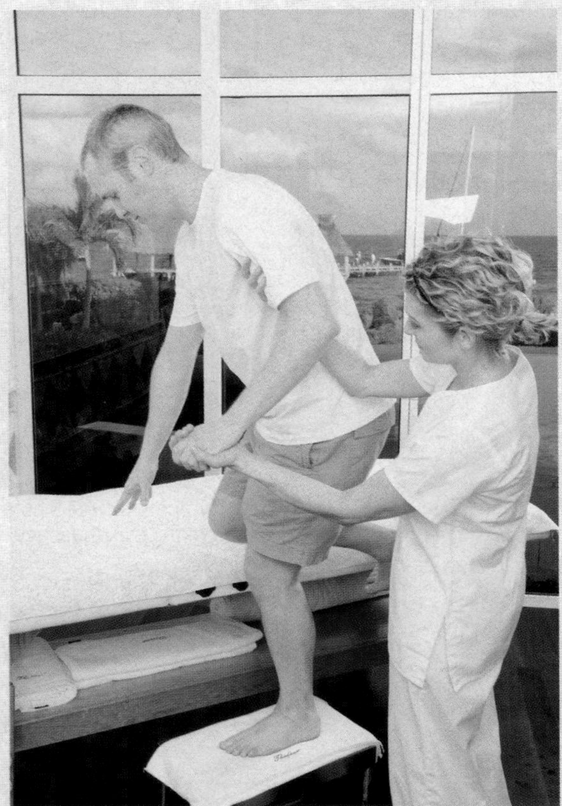

FIGURE 4–9 Create a makeshift hydrotherapy tub using a massage table and stool in order to practice safety issues.

1. Hydrotherapy tubs sit high off the floor and can be challenging for some clients to climb into. Therapists should always assist clients into and out of the tub. Practice assisting the "client" up onto a stepping stool and then onto the table, supporting the client's weight at the elbow with one hand and on the lower back with the other.
2. Water sometime spills over the top of the tub, making the floor slippery. Practice assisting the client by holding his or her forearm or elbow as the client steps from the bathmat directly into a pair of nearby sandals. Most spas furnish sandals for the guests for sanitary as well as safety reasons. Their use should be taken seriously.
3. The client should feign feeling weak or lightheaded while exiting the "tub" after a treatment. The therapist should support him or her, helping the client into a nearby chair.

Although the thermal and mechanical effects of water create the primary benefits of hydrotherapy tub treatments, the therapeutic ingredients that are often added to the water can also have an effect. Most commonly used therapeutic ingredients include essential oils, seaweed extracts, clay powders, and herbs.

Hydrotherapy Tub Protocol

TREATMENT: HYDROTHERAPY TUB BATH	
Wet Room/Dry Room	wet room
Tub Setup	filled tub with secure stepping stool for ease of access
Treatment Duration	usually 25 minutes, can be shorter if spot treatment as part of longer service such as cellulite
Needed Supplies	therapeutic agents, bowl of ice water, towels
Contraindications	recent injuries, open wounds, acute hematomas, varicosities, high blood pressure, heart disease, arteriosclerosis, pregnancy
Draping	Depending on local laws, clients can be nude in tub when being treated by a therapist of the same sex, or they can wear bathing suits. Take extra care to maintain modesty while client is getting into and out of tub.
Treatment Order	given before massage/body treatments or as part of cellulite protocols
Safety, Sanitation Issues, & Clean-Up	The tub is sanitized after each use by wiping down entire interior surface with disinfectant. Some tubs have self-cleaning modes. Also, clients need to be assisted into and out of tub and be warned about feeling weak after treatment.
Body Mechanics & Self-Care	Special care must be taken to avoid lower back strain while leaning over the tub to administer underwater massage with high-pressure hose. Brace yourself properly to support weight of client entering or exiting tub.
Product Cost	limited to cost of therapeutic ingredients added to bath plus water and electricity to fill and heat tub
Treatment Price	typically offered as a half-hour stand-alone treatment for $40 to $60 or as an add-on to cellulite or massage services
Physiological Effects	thermal effects of heat on body and mechanical effects of underwater massage hose and jets, relaxing muscles into an atonic state, combined with specific effects of therapeutic ingredients added to water
Pregnancy Issues (information provided by Elaine Stillerman, LMT, author and developer of MotherMassage®)	Hydrotherapy is contraindicated during each of the three trimesters of pregnancy. During postpartum recovery, hydrotherapy may be used after three months, once fibrinogenic activity normalizes to pre-pregnancy levels.

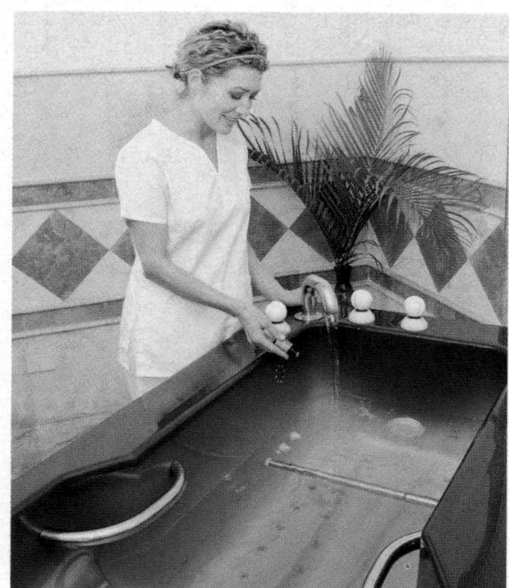

FIGURE 4–10 The therapist draws the bath and adds therapeutic ingredients to the hydrotherapy tub.

Hydrotherapy Tub Preparation

1. The area is prepared by placing bath mats, non-slip surfaces, towels, ice water, wash cloth, and therapeutic ingredients within easy reach.
2. The bath is usually drawn by the therapist before the client enters the room. Temperature is controlled for intended outcomes (see Table 4–1), the average temperature for a hydrotherapy tub bath being approxivmately 100°F.
3. Therapeutic ingredients are added to the bath while the tub is filling, or they are added after the client has entered the room so he or she can see the products (Figure 4–10).

Hydrotherapy Tub Procedure

1. The therapist assists the client as he or she enters the tub.
2. One by one, the therapist opens the valves to release water and air pressure onto specific parts of the client's body (Figure 4–11). Some hydrotherapy tubs feature computer-controlled valves (Figure 4–12). A typical routine will start with the extremities, then move to the core, for a total of 12 minutes, as in the following 7-step procedure:
   1. all zones turned on low: 1 minute
   2. arm zones: 2 minutes
   3. foot zones: 1 minute
   4. leg zones: 2 minutes
   5. shoulder zones: 2 minutes
   6. hip zones: 2 minutes
   7. pine zone: 2 minutes
3. The therapist turns off all jet valves, places the high-pressure underwater hose beneath the surface, and opens the valve for the hose.
4. The therapist uses the underwater hose to massage the client, maintaining the tip of the high-powered stream between 6 and 18 inches from the client's body, depending upon the sensitivity of the area being treated and the desired effects of the water massage (Figure 4–13). In order to test the strength of the hose, the therapist can direct the stream at his or her own hand from the same distance. The high-pressure water massage routine varies from spa to spa. One popular 10-minute sequence begins at the client's left foot and progresses up the left side of the body, then down the right, as follows:
   a. left foot top and bottom, avoiding tips of toes beneath nails: 1 minute
   b. left leg, inner and outer: 1 minute
   c. client turns slightly to right, massage left hip and back: 1.5 minutes
   d. left hand and arm: 1 minute

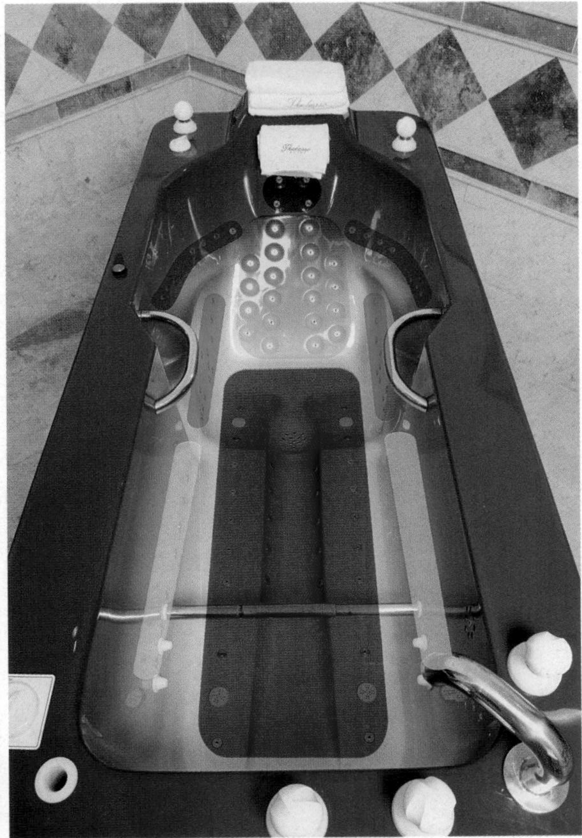

FIGURE 4–11 Hydrotherapy tubs feature multiple jets for specific body zones.

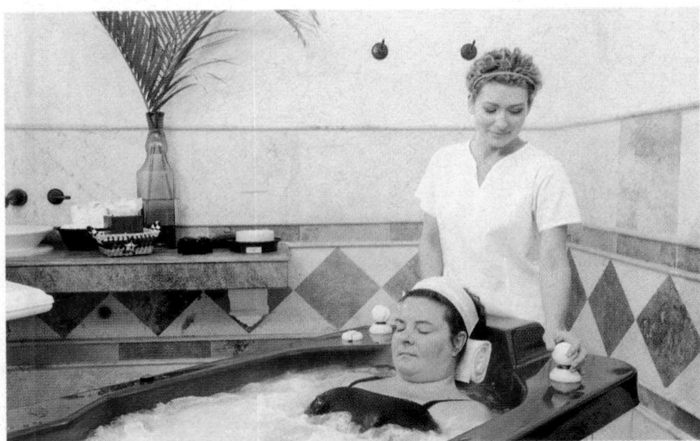

FIGURE 4–12 Selected valves for specific zones are operated by the therapist or by computer.

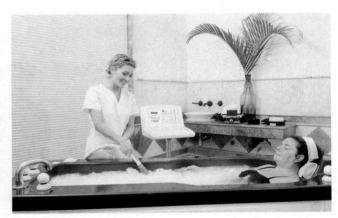

FIGURE 4–13 Care must be exercised when directing the high pressure water hose at the client's skin.

e. client slides further down into tub for shoulder massage, moving from left shoulder to right: 1 minute

f. right hand and arm: 1 minute

g. client turns slightly to left, massage right hip and back: 1.5 minutes

h. right leg, inner and outer: 1 minute

i. right foot top and bottom, avoiding tips of toes beneath nails: 1 minute

5. The therapist turns the high-pressure massage hose off and engages all jet zones at once for a short duration to create a final relaxation.
6. The therapist turns off all jets and pumps and assists the client from the tub, offering water to drink and a chair to rest in if needed.

SPA CAUTION

The high-pressure underwater massage hose in most hydrotherapy tubs is powerful and could cause pain or damage to delicate tissues. Avoid direct pressure over the same danger points that are contraindicated for manual massage, such as bony protuberances, axilla, inguinal crease, and others.

Hydrotherapy Tub Cleanup

1. The hydrotherapy tub must be sanitized after every treatment with a disinfectant spray. Some tubs feature a self-cleaning cycle.
2. Floors in the wet room must be dried between hydrotherapy treatments to maintain a safe environment.
3. Towels and wash cloths are laundered, bowls cleaned, products stored, and the room tidied for the next treatment.

THE COLD PLUNGE

The cold plunge (Figure 4–14) or cold bath is used extensively in spas, even though the amount of time spent in them can be measured in seconds. A quick way to close the pores and to refresh the body, the cold plunge is also said to improve immune functioning. As mentioned in Chapter 1, the Roman thermae featured cold plunges, with an entire room called the frigidarium dedicated to the cooling of spa goers' bodies, which was thought to be as important to the overall spa experience as warming the body. Centuries later, spa and natural

SPA CAUTION

Many clients report feeling weak for up to several hours after a hydrotherapy tub treatment. At the end of a treatment, therapists should suggest that clients rest and engage in only moderate exercise.

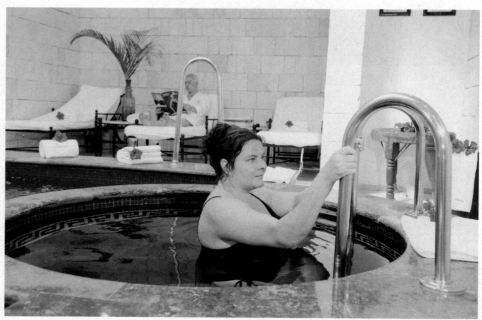

FIGURE 4–14 Often used with hot tubs, saunas and steam baths in contrast therapy, the cold plunge creates a systemic reaction to cold in the body.

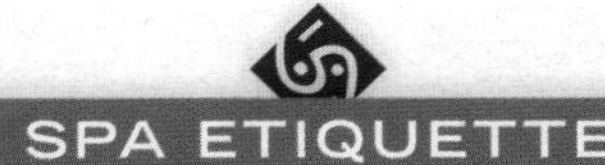

SPA ETIQUETTE

Modesty in the Spa

Although most spa clients appear comfortable wearing bathrobes in the public areas of the spa, therapists should not let the casual atmosphere of many spas lead them to the conclusion that clients do not care about personal boundaries and modesty. Even those therapists working in an all-male or all-female area of the spa need to pay attention to modesty issues. By adhering to the following suggestions regarding modesty, spa therapists will make clients feel secure and respected.

1. Make towels and robes easily accessible to clients wherever they might need them in the spa.
2. When it is safe, leave the hydrotherapy room when the client is disrobing and preparing to receive the treatment. When you need to assist the client, assure that he or she is modestly covered during transition phases before and after treatments, such as getting into a tub or climbing onto a wet table.
3. In co-ed areas where clients are wearing robes, be aware that some clients will want to avoid sitting close to members of the opposite sex. Help direct them to areas where they can feel comfortable.
4. In same-sex areas such as locker rooms and wet areas where nudity is common, therapists should respectfully maintain their attention away from the clients unless spoken to or asked for assistance.

health pioneer Sebastian Kneipp recommended cold baths as a core part of his health regime (see Chapter 1).

Some people like the cold plunge, but a majority of modern spa goers shy away from the shocking experience of immersion in the cold waters. Thus, many spas have cold plunges available, but they are underused. Spa clients therefore miss the benefits of contrast therapy and cold therapy. Spa therapists can help educate clients about the benefits of these therapies, which include decreased blood pressure, decreased heart rate, and increased circulation. Also, some spas post signage near the cold plunge to alert clients to the benefits and contraindications. See the section on Systemic Effects of Cold in Chapter 5 for more information.

Cold plunges are typically located in the female-only or male-only areas of the spa, such as the locker room or wet area, where clients enter them completely disrobed. Alternatively, cold plunges can be located in public areas where they are entered with bathing suits on. Some natural hot springs spas have cold plunges adjacent to the hot spring in an outdoor area.

SHOWER TECHNIQUES

Shower techniques in the spa can be defined as any directed spray of water for therapeutic purposes from one or more outlets, aimed at clients who are either standing or lying down. Though their roots are by no means as ancient as those of bathing, the various shower techniques applied in spas have been in use for many years. The three main types of therapeutic showers found in spa wet rooms are the Vichy shower, Swiss shower, and Scotch hose. A regular shower has some therapeutic effects as well, especially when applied hot, cold, or in contrast therapy. All shower therapies are percussive treatments that meld both mechanical and thermal therapeutic effects.

SHOWER TREATMENT	DESCRIPTION	USES	CONTRAINDICATIONS	POPULARITY IN SPAS
Swiss Shower	a walk-in shower with multiple jets on each wall that can alternate between high pressure/ low pressure, hot water/cold water	most popularly used to wash product from clients' skin after treatments, though originally meant as a means to fortify and tone the body and circulation	varicosities, blood pressure disorders, open skin ailments	medium; often installed but underused
Vichy Shower	a horizontal shower bar with several nozzles that spray water over clients lying on table below	used primarily to wash products from clients' skin and in combination with other spa services, such as massage, to add hydrotherapy benefits	open skin ailments, pregnancy, lymph edema	high (especially popular in high-end spas)
Handheld Shower	showerhead attached to a wall in a wet room that therapists use on clients receiving spa treatments on a wet table	used primarily to wash products from clients' skin on the wet table, such as exfoliants, seaweeds, and clay products	open skin ailments	high in spas with wet-table-equipped wet rooms
Scotch Hose	this treatment uses water sprayed at high pressure from a hose aimed at clients from a distance of approximately 10 feet	implemented in European-style spas with an extensive hydrotherapy program, often as a prelude to other spa treatments	varicose veins, inflammation, circulatory problems, open skin ailments, blood pressure disorders, pregnancy	low-medium, popular in some Europe-based or European-themed spas with elaborate hydrotherapy programs

TABLE 4–3 Types of Therapeutic Showers Offered in Spas.

SPA TIP

Clients can experience one of the main benefits of the shower—cleansing—without actually entering a shower or a wet room. This is accomplished in the dry room by using hot moist towels to perform the cleansing functions of a shower. Throughout the following chapters, you will find protocols that call for the use of towels in this fashion. When towels are used this way, they can effectively replace a shower.

Because spa showers feature multiple heads and/or high-pressure sprays, they entail the use of a large amount of water, much more than a typical home shower. This, in turn, necessitates an extra-wide drain for the water to escape the treatment area. Refer to the Plumbing and Electrical section in Chapter 17 for more installation concerns regarding showers. Table 4–3 offers brief descriptions of the main showers used in spas.

Showers are relatively new to spas because they are relatively new to mankind in general. Throughout most of history, a "shower" was reserved for royalty or the wealthy, and it consisted of a servant or slave pouring a container of (usually cold) water over his master's head. It was not until the mid-1800s that advances in plumbing led to modern showering capabilities. It was at this time that plumbers began constructing freestanding showers with hot and cold water. In the late 1800s, inventors developed showers that could be considered precursors to some used in spas to this day, such as the 1882 appearance of Ewart's Improved Spray Bath featuring 10 controls that manipulated various spouts. In 1889, J. L. Mott Iron Works began selling a device that could shower the bather from every angle, like today's Swiss shower, and other manufacturers offered a variety of options such as multiple heads, waterfall spouts, and body sprays. The anytime enjoyment of hot showers was made possible by Edwin Ruud, a Norwegian mechanical engineer who in 1889 invented the automatic storage water heater.

Vichy Shower

A Vichy shower (Figure 4–15) consists of a horizontal bar with multiple down-facing nozzles along its length, suspended above a wet table. Water from the nozzles showers the client lying on the table. Vichy showers are always located in a wet room. A typical Vichy shower room is 9' × 12' to 10' × 14', with an optimal space of 3 feet on all sides of the shower. Vichy showers represent a large investment on the part of the spa because they cost thousands of dollars to buy and install. In order to protect the spa's investment and assure the safety of clients, therapists need to know proper operation, safety, and sanitation procedures for this equipment.

The Vichy shower is named after Vichy, the famed spa town in France. First noted by the Romans for their curative powers in 52 BC, the thermal spring waters found at Vichy inspired early settlement of the area. A famed French writer in the seventeenth century, the Marquise de Sévigné, was a patient there and popularized Vichy's thermal baths through her work. After visits by the daughters of Louis XV, the bath facilities were greatly improved, and by the nineteenth century, Vichy was frequented by many celebrities, including Napoleon, who caused a profound transformation of the city, with landscaped gardens, newly laid out boulevards, and chalets and pavilions being built for the Emperor and his court. Many present-day spa clients who experience the Vichy shower report that the large quantity of water flowing over the body creates a luxurious sensation fit for an emperor.

Vichy showers are most typically incorporated into exfoliation and body wrap services, primarily to wash product from the body, though some spa menus

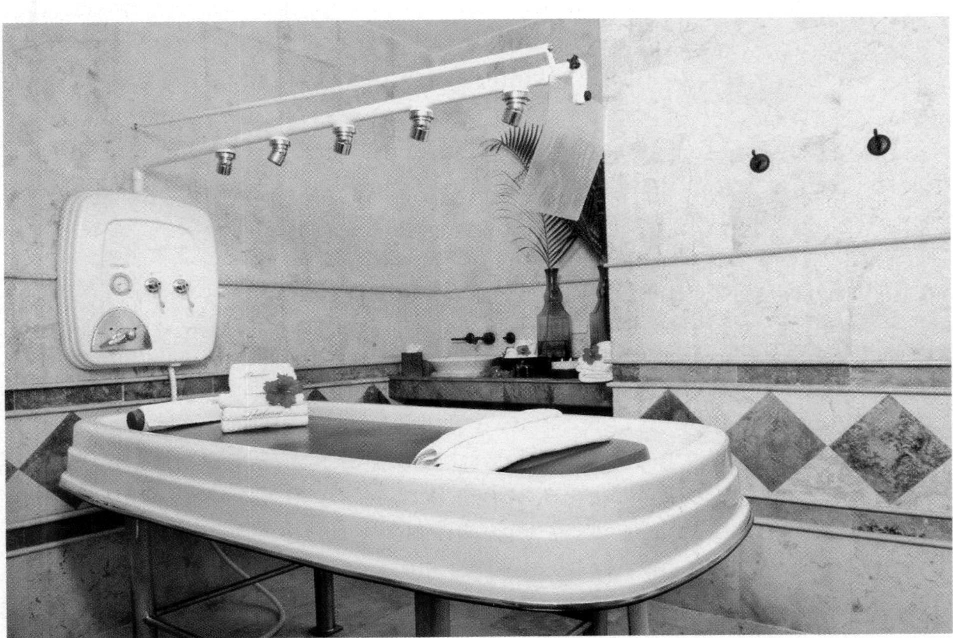

FIGURE 4–15 Vichy shower in a wet room.

offer a dedicated Vichy service that features an hour-long massage while under the flood of the multiple nozzles. The protocol for each of these services varies from spa to spa. The following chapters will contain a number of protocols for performing spa services using a Vichy shower and wet table. For all of these protocols, certain key points must be kept in mind:

1. The table can be layered with blankets, thermal blankets, and plastic wrap in order to administer a treatment. Afterwards, the layers are removed and the client can be washed with the Vichy shower without leaving the table.
2. For some treatments, the easiest way to clean products from the client's skin is to have the client step into a regular shower rather than stay on the wet table beneath the Vichy shower.
3. Sanitation of the table and all equipment after every treatment is especially important due to the abundance of water present, which can lead to bacteria growth and unsanitary conditions.
4. Proper modest draping must be maintained at all times (see "Draping on the Wet Table" section below).

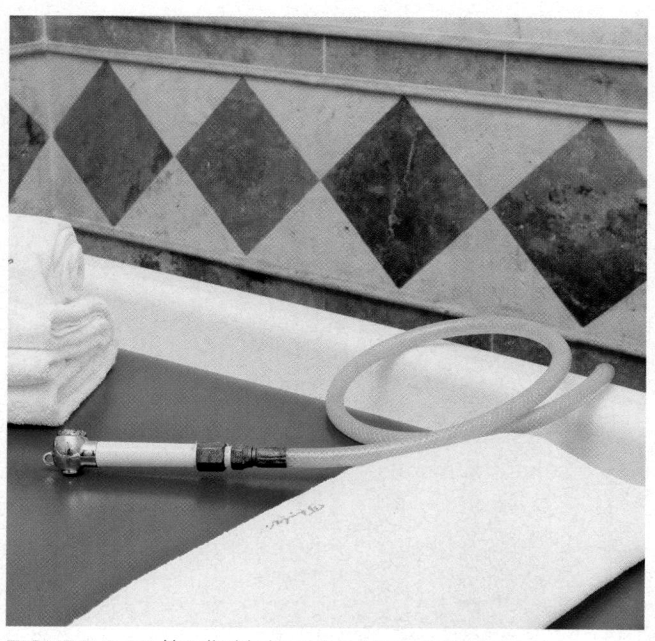

FIGURE 4–16 Handheld showerhead in wet room.

The Handheld Shower

Many wet rooms feature a handheld shower attached to the wall by an extra-long hose (Figure 4–16). This showerhead can be extended to all points over the wet table and is used to both moisten the skin prior to the application of certain exfoliants and also to wash all manner of spa products from the skin after application. In some wet rooms, this same showerhead is affixed to the wall and used by clients when showering off after a treatment. Therapists need to assure proper water temperature is attained prior to applying the shower spray to the client. The handheld shower, in effect, replaces the Vichy shower in many spas as it serves most of the same purposes.

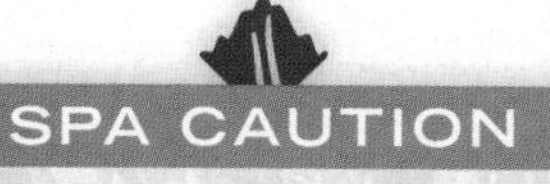

SPA CAUTION

If handheld showers are left on during treatment but a button on the showerhead is pushed to temporarily pause the flow, excess hot water can build up in the hose and can scald clients. Aim showerhead away from client when first releasing the flow during each phase of the treatment.

Draping on the Wet Table

Therapists are often curious about the most effective way to drape clients on the wet table during spa services that involve showers, specifically the handheld shower and Vichy shower. Draping is especially difficult on a wet table because of the amount of water used and the number of times the client must turn over. The drape, whether it be a sheet or towel, becomes waterlogged, unwieldy, and potentially uncomfortable for the client. Some spas opt to have their clients wear bathing suits or shorts for wet treatments, but many incorporate a modest Wet Table Draping Protocol that, with a little practice, can be mastered by therapists. See Figures 4–17A through 4–17J for an explanation of this draping procedure while using the handheld shower.

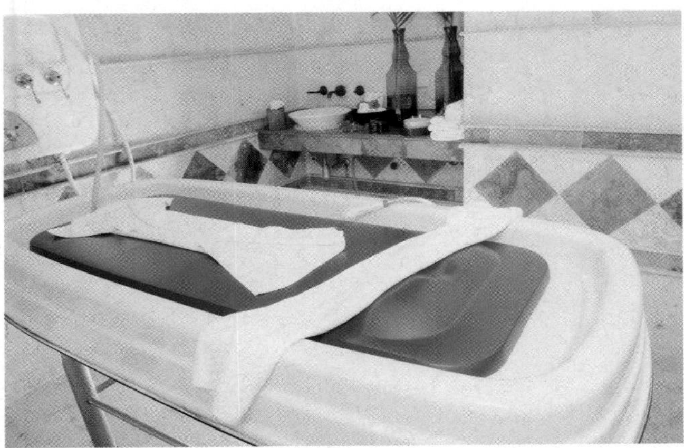
FIGURE 4–17A Before the client enters the room, a diaper drape using a large bath towel or a bath sheet is placed on the wet table.

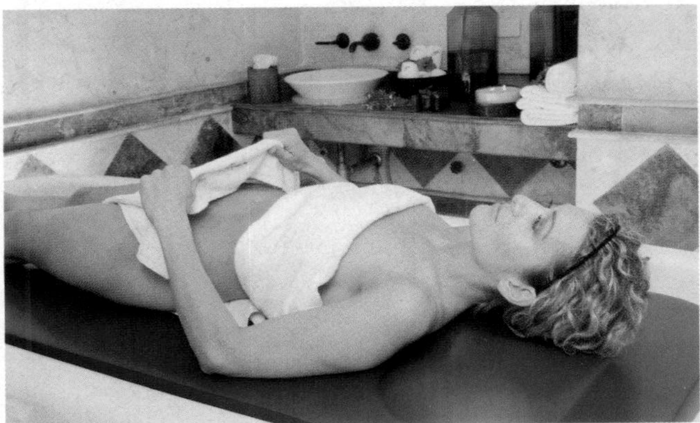
FIGURE 4–17B The client is left in the room alone to pull the diaper drape up and cover the front of the body.

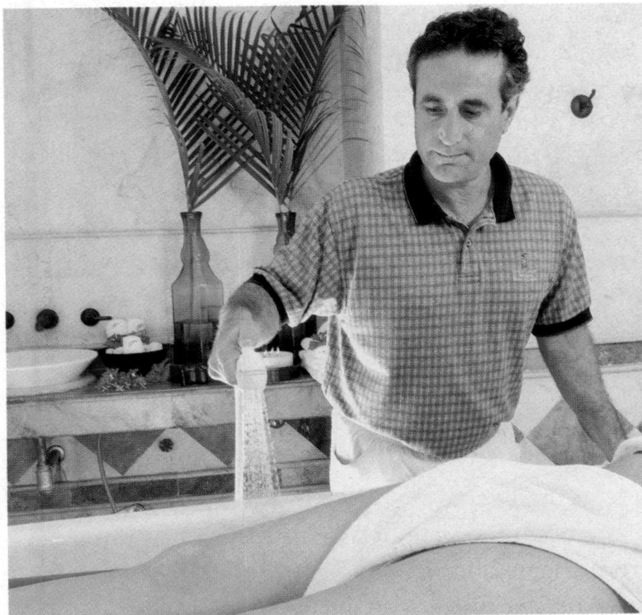
FIGURE 4–17C The therapist uses the handheld showerhead on the client's body when moistening the skin before product application or washing the product away after application. The drape is not sprayed directly but still becomes wet.

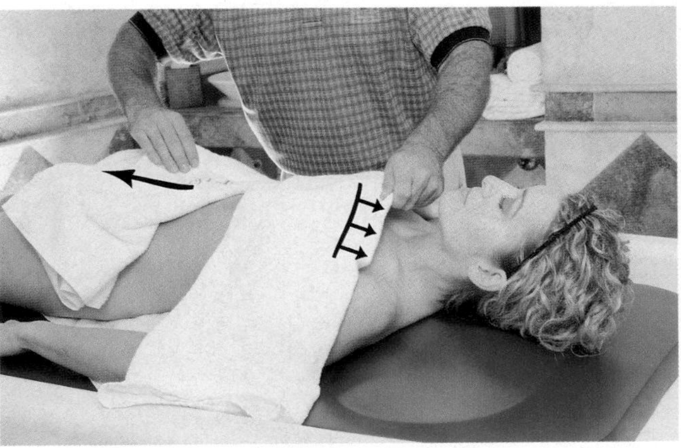
FIGURE 4–17D To shower the abdomen on female clients, a breast drape is placed over the top of the bath towel and held in place while the bath towel is pulled down to the hips.

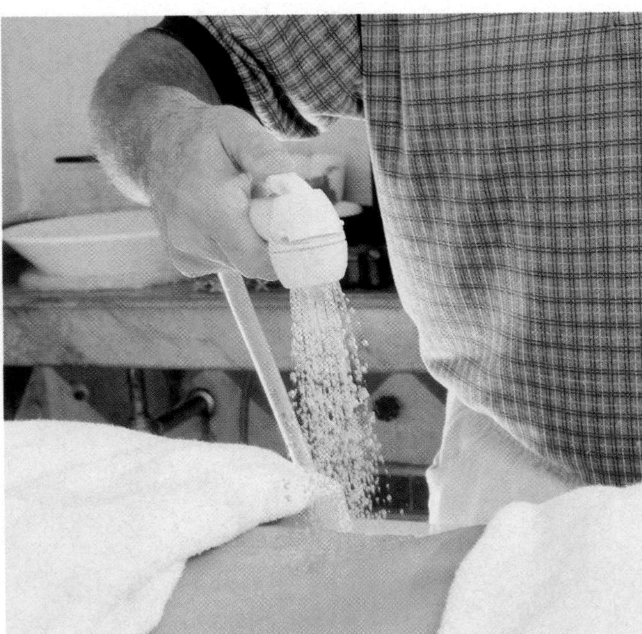
FIGURE 4–17E The abdomen is washed with the handheld shower.

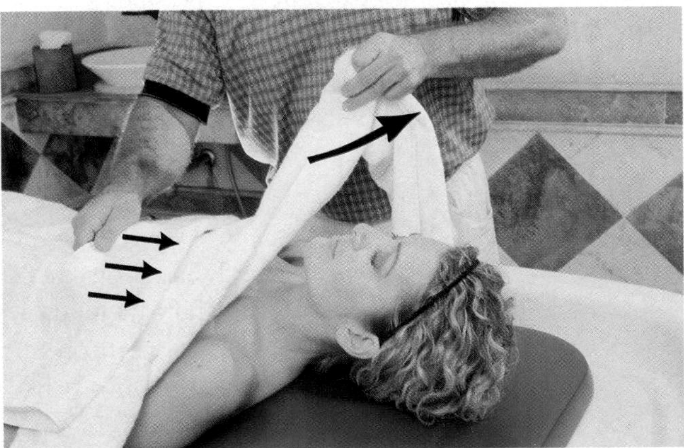
FIGURE 4–17F To turn the client over, first the diaper drape is pulled back up.

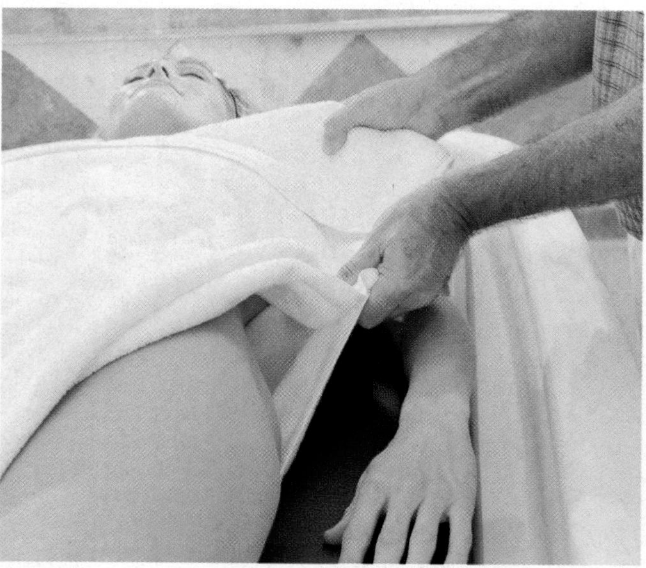

FIGURE 4–17G Then the therapist holds the top and bottom aspects of the drape together at the client's hip with one hand and the upper portion of the drape with the other hand.

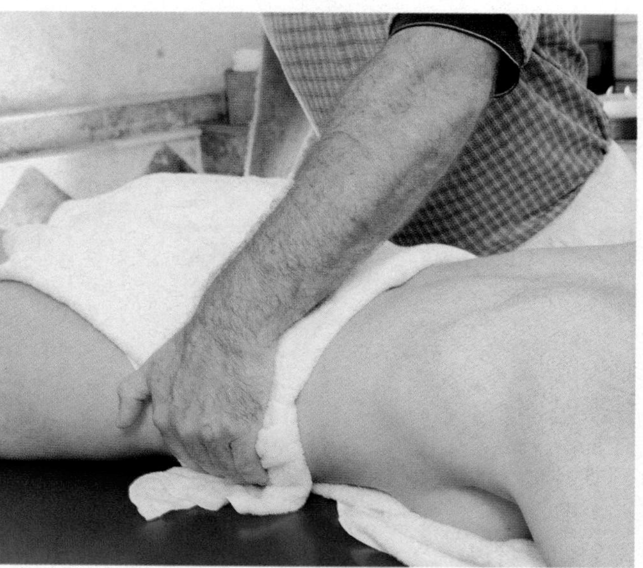

FIGURE 4–17I The diaper drape is pulled into place up over the buttocks.

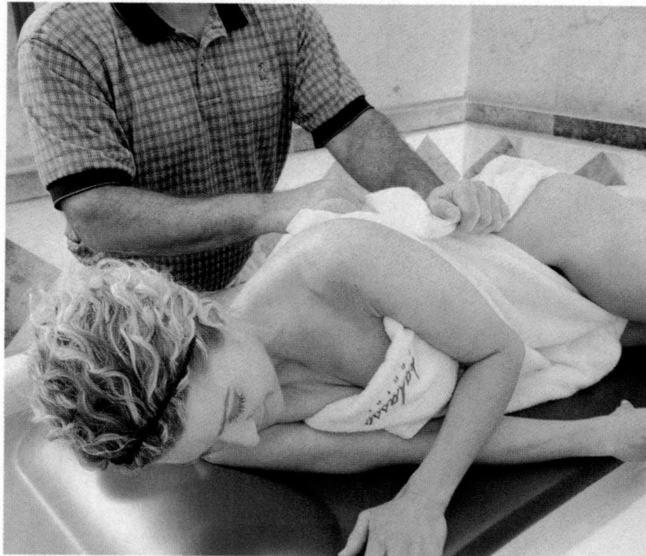

FIGURE 4–17H The client turns to the far side of the table while the therapist continues to hold the drape. This procedure can be reversed when client turns from face-down to face-up position.

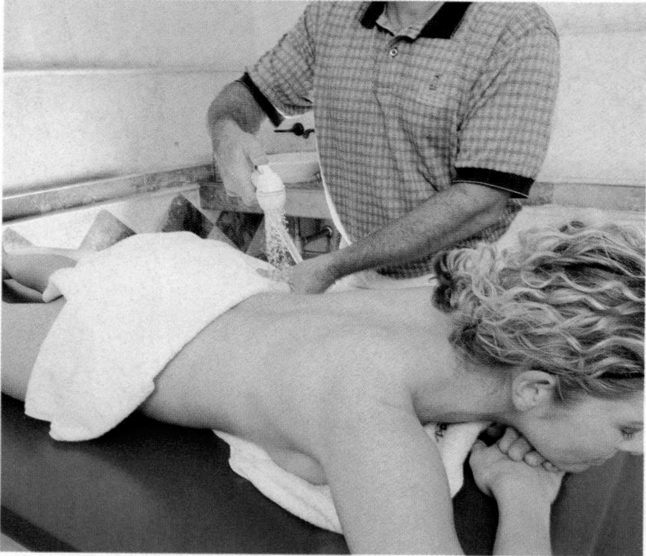

FIGURE 4–17J The therapist makes sure draping is secure and begins showering back of body.

Swiss Shower

The Swiss shower is a staple at many spas, yet paradoxically it is underused. Or, rather, its true therapeutic potential is underused because it is often used simply to wash products from clients after a mud, seaweed, or clay wrap. This underuse can occur because the spa staff is not aware of the intention of the spa designers. In order for the Swiss shower to be used as it was intended, therapists need to be aware of its therapeutic value. The Swiss shower is a highly stimulating treatment designed to benefit the circulation and provide relief from tension, insomnia, and stress. It is, in effect, a contrast-therapy hydro massage treatment that uses on average 10 sprays aimed at the body from multiple directions (Figure 4–18). A typical Swiss shower has three showerheads aimed horizontally at the client on each of three walls and one head directly above. This provides mechanical stimulation from all directions simultaneously and can be highly invigorating.

To perform a true Swiss shower treatment, the therapist must be on hand to control the temperature of the water throughout the duration. The temperature controls are usually found on a panel outside of the shower stall. The therapist works the panel to achieve the desired results. If clients simply enter the shower to rinse off, as happens at many spas, the results are not achieved.

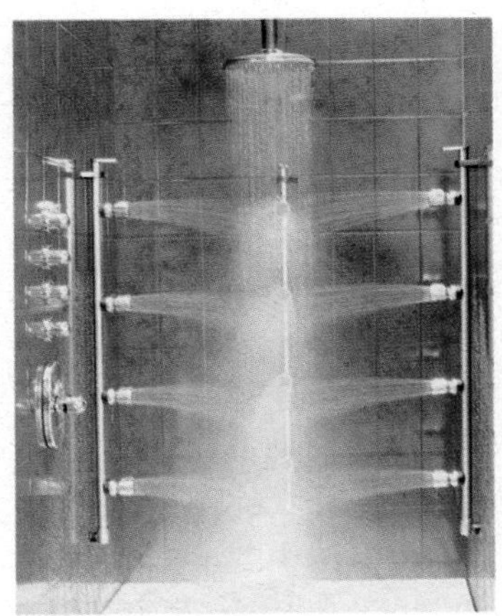

FIGURE 4–18 The Swiss shower utilizes 10 showerheads to administer a powerful dose of hydrotherapy.

Swiss Shower Protocol

TREATMENT: SWISS SHOWER	
Wet Room/Dry Room	wet room
Table Setup	no table
Treatment Duration	5 to 10 minutes
Needed Supplies	shower, towels, bath mat, body wash, soap, shampoo
Contraindications	varicosities, blood pressure disorders, thromboses, open skin ailments
Draping	Clients enter the Swiss shower completely undressed. If a therapist manipulates water pressure and temperature during treatment, it is always a therapist of the same sex.
Treatment Order	Swiss showers are often administered after body wraps to cleanse product from the skin, but they are also recommended before massage to relax tissues.
Safety, Sanitation Issues, & Clean-Up	The floor of the Swiss shower is kept sanitary through the use of bath mats or flooring that can be lifted and cleaned at the end of each day.
Body Mechanics & Self-Care	no ergonomic hazards for therapists
Product Cost	after installation of shower, only costs are soap/body wash, water, electricity to heat water, and cost of doing laundry associated with shower
Treatment Price	usually built into price of spa treatments given beforehand or afterwards, not charged for separately on most spa menus
Physiological Effects	strong mechanical effects due to multiple showerheads impacting body from various directions, highly stimulating to circulation, with added hydrostatic effect if administered as a contrast-application alternating hot and cold water flow
Pregnancy Issues (information provided by Elaine Stillerman, LMT, author and developer of MotherMassage)	As long as the pressure of the showerheads is not too strong on the abdomen or legs, and the temperature remains warm and not hot, a short Swiss shower can be very relaxing. Care must be given to support a pregnant client to prevent falls.

ACTIVITY

Practice Wet Table Draping Protocol

Pair up with a classmate and practice the Wet Table Draping Protocol while fully dressed, using regular massage tables instead of wet tables. Slowly and methodically perform the maneuvers shown in Figures 4–17A through 4–17J until they become natural.

SPA ETIQUETTE

When towels used as drapes become soaked during treatments on wet tables, proceed as normal with the treatment. As long as the water and the room remain warm, the client will not feel uncomfortable.

SPA ETIQUETTE

The temperature in wet rooms should be turned up to 80°F or higher during wet table treatments, even if this makes the therapist uncomfortably warm. Clients easily become chilled during wet table treatments, even when draped.

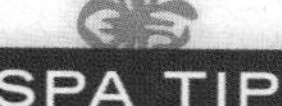

SPA TIP

In order for clients to understand that the Swiss shower is more than just a souped-up shower, they need to be educated, and this job often falls to the therapist who is there with them and can explain the proper use and benefits of the equipment. Therapists should always be prepared to offer this kind of educational assistance, even if the spa's brochure and menu do not cover it or if spa management does not seem especially concerned about explaining the proper use of the Swiss shower to clients.

Swiss Shower Preparation

1. Test equipment to make sure water temperature controls are working properly and calibrated for therapist use.
2. Turn on the shower and set the temperature and pressure to desired levels.
3. Explain the treatment to the client, including therapeutic benefits that go beyond a typical shower.

Swiss Shower Procedure

1. Instruct the client to enter the shower and stand in the spray. Observe and monitor the client's response to temperature and pressure to gauge appropriate settings. Adjust if necessary. Also, ask the client for verbal feedback about temperature and pressure. Some clients may feel overwhelmed at first in a Swiss shower.
2. Start with a temperate shower between 90°F and 100°F, increasing to 120°F within 30 seconds. Maintain this temperature for a full minute, then switch to cold (55°F to 70°F) for 30 seconds, then back again 3 times. The temperature differential can be larger and times extended as clients become accustomed to the treatment.
3. Turn off the showers. Escort the client from the shower area, and offer towels, a robe, a glass of water, and a comfortable area to sit in. Make sure the client is warm and dry before proceeding to his or her next treatment.

Swiss Shower Cleanup

1. Bath mats and towels are restocked.
2. The entire area should be sanitized at the end of each work day.

Scotch Hose

Also called an "affusion under pressure," "percussion douche," "Scotch douche," or "Scotch shower," the Scotch hose treatment was developed for use in those European spas which had a strong emphasis on hydrotherapy and in many cases thalassotherapy (see Chapter 7). Today, it is used in many spas around the world but is most prevalent in those spas that maintain a strong connection to their European therapeutic traditions. The Scotch hose is often applied as a form of contrast therapy, with the water temperature set between 55°F and 70°F for the cold application and 100°F to 120°F for the hot application. A temperate spray of approximately 90°F is used at the beginning and end of the cold application. The therapist stands 9 to 10 feet from the client and controls the water temperature and pressure while simultaneously aiming the spray at the client's body. Traditionally, the Scotch hose treatment had been administered for those clients who seek to increase mental alertness or to generally tone the body and nervous system. As part of a more extensive hydrotherapy "cure" at some European spas, the Scotch hose was given to all clients as part of their course of treatments. More recently it has been offered as an *à la carte* service which spa clients can choose to add to their other treatments.

Scotch Hose Protocol

TREATMENT: SCOTCH HOSE	
Wet Room/Dry Room	wet room
Table Setup	no table
Treatment Duration	2 to 3 minutes, slightly longer for contrast application
Needed Supplies	temperature and pressure-controlled water hose in a spa wet room area, towels, bath mat
Contraindications	varicose veins, inflammation, circulatory problems, open skin ailments, thromboses, blood pressure disorders, pregnancy
Draping	Clients wear bathing suits or shorts, or they enter the Scotch hose treatment area nude if the service is given in an all-male or all-female area of the spa and the therapist is the same sex as the client. Note: if clients are nude, they should be instructed to cover breasts (for women) or genitals (for men) to protect against strong spray.
Treatment Order	hot or contrast Scotch hose prior to massage or spa treatments, cold Scotch hose after exertion or heat treatments
Safety, Sanitation Issues, & Clean-Up	Safety bars are often fastened to walls for clients to grasp while experiencing high-pressure spray, and non-skid surfaces are used on floor. Entire area is sanitized at end of each day the same way a shower stall is cleaned and disinfected.
Body Mechanics & Self-Care	Scotch hose poses no ergonomic hazards for therapists, but caution should be taken to control water temperature and avoid scalding self or client.
Product Cost	after installation of equipment, only costs are water, electricity to heat water, and cost of doing laundry associated with treatment
Treatment Price	often built into price of spa treatments or overall hydrotherapy offerings at spa, but *à la carte* prices range from $20 to $30
Physiological Effects	strong mechanical effects due to high-pressure impact of water, highly stimulating to circulation
Pregnancy Issues (information provided by Elaine Stillerman, LMT, author and developer of MotherMassage)	The Scotch hose is contraindicated during the three trimesters of pregnancy. It may be used after three months postpartum, once fibrinogenic activity returns to pre-pregnancy levels.

Scotch Hose Preparation

1. Test equipment to make sure water temperature and pressure controls are working properly and calibrated for therapist use.
2. Turn on the shower and set the temperature and pressure to desired levels.
3. Explain the treatment to the client, including safety measures such as firmly grasping handrails when present, and then guide the client into the treatment area.

Scotch Hose Procedure

1. Treatments are usually begun at the feet so as to gradually introduce the spray to the client, as it can sometimes be shocking (Figure 4–19).
2. The spray is directed up the client's leg and torso, then down the arm, then switched to the opposite side of the body, with the column of water constantly moving over the client's body (Figure 4–20). The therapist can

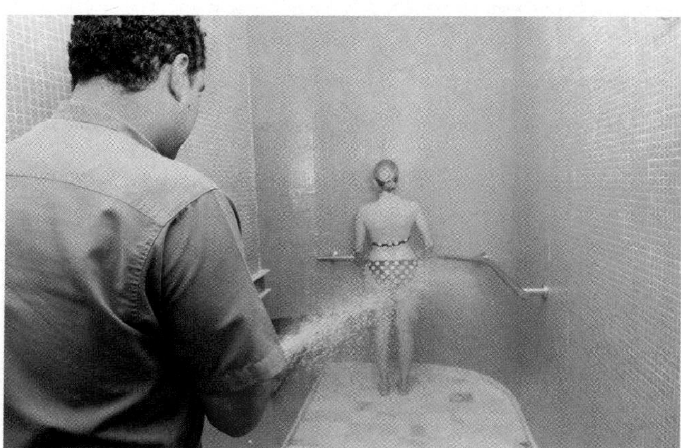

FIGURE 4–19 The Scotch hose treatment is usually begun at the client's feet and moves up the legs.

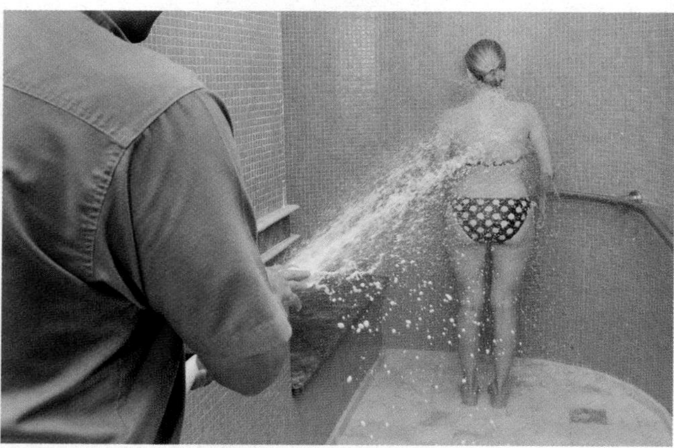

FIGURE 4–20 The Scotch hose is administered by moving the water stream over the client's body, "fanning" the spray over delicate areas.

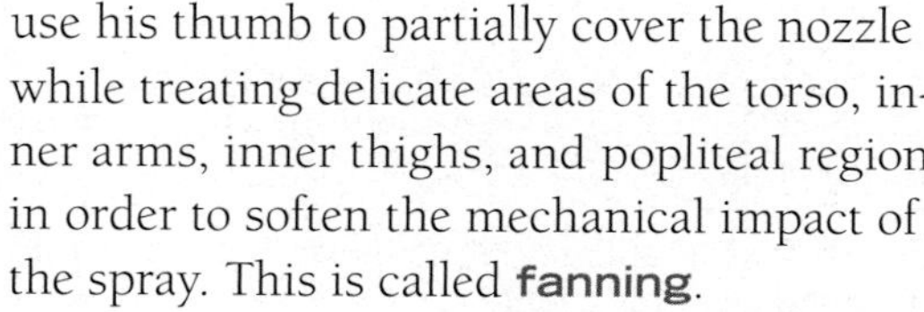

use his thumb to partially cover the nozzle while treating delicate areas of the torso, inner arms, inner thighs, and popliteal region in order to soften the mechanical impact of the spray. This is called **fanning**.

3. Constantly monitor water temperature and pressure, adjusting for desired treatment. The exact temperature should be dictated by the client's observed reactions and intention for the treatment. More extreme temperature differences create a more stimulating treatment.

    a. In a contrast treatment, start with heat for one minute, then cold for 30 seconds, switching three times between the two temperatures.

    b. Hot treatments start with slightly cooler water, then work up within 30 seconds to the desired maximum for the duration of the 2 to 3 minutes, finishing with a brief cold application (15 seconds).

    c. Cold Scotch hose treatments start with slightly more temperate water, which is then cooled for the duration of the 2 to 3 minutes at the cold temperature and finished with a brief temperate application (15 seconds).

4. Escort the client from the shower area, and offer towels, a robe, a glass of water, and a comfortable area to sit in. Make sure the client is warm and dry before proceeding to his or her next treatment.

fanning

technique used by therapists and spa technicians of partially covering nozzle with the thumb to soften impact of water spray in certain hydrotherapy treatments such as the Scotch hose

Scotch Hose Cleanup

1. The floor in the treatment area should be dried if clients walk directly on tiles, which can become slippery.
2. Bath mats and towels are restocked.
3. The entire area should be sanitized at the end of each work day.

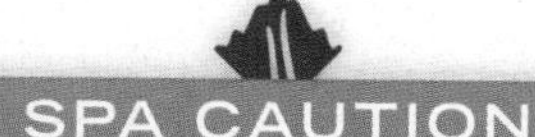

SPA CAUTION

Clients need to be thoroughly prepared prior to the start of a Scotch hose treatment, because the pressure of the spray and can be quite shocking. Therapists should talk to clients about the intensity of the treatment before it begins. Always begin the treatment gently, usually on the feet, with a moderate temperature to gauge the client's reaction. This reaction needs to be constantly monitored throughout the treatment. Stop the treatment immediately if the client appears to be weak or distressed.

SPA PROFILE

Spa = Water × (Time + Temperature)

This is the equation that Professor Jonathan Paul De Vierville, Ph.D., uses to distill the true meaning of spa therapy and **spa culture**. He is director and founder of the Alamo Plaza Spa in San Antonio, Texas. He is also a well-known expert on hydrotherapy and leads a group of spa professionals and enthusiasts on tours of European spa facilities each year. If there is anyone in the modern spa industry who can provide deep insights into the meaning and importance of spas, spa culture, water, and hydrotherapy, Dr. De Vierville is the man.

"Water is a mystery within us," he states. "It is the universal agent for transition, transformation, healing and balance. Water is soft, sensuous and musical, directly associated with the world of the unconscious and dreams. We are the waters and dreams and the waters and dreams are us."

While some look to water as the root of spa therapy, Professor De Vierville tends to look at it more as the entire tree. "It is true that the historical origins of spa are in water," he says, "and also the true life of spa lies in the essential miracle of water. Many therapists today are learning 'dry massage,' but the ideal should be to expand that to a 'wet massage.' Therapists can honor both our internal aqueous environment and the external hydrotherapy environment through spa treatments, as in skin affusions and the ingesting of spa waters for example. The massage therapist should become the spa master, the bath master, and be able to do both the dry and the wet treatments."

This is why it is important for spa therapists to become familiar with spa services as well as massage therapy. When therapists know about and believe in the power of water-based spa therapies, their work can complete the overall mission of the spa, rather than stand alongside it as something separate. "Massage is the steak of spa," admits Dr. De Vierville, "but it needs to be complemented with all the traditional spa side dishes in order to be truly satisfying."

Dr. De Vierville believes that, "We all need to work together to provide the ultimate experience for our clients. It is no longer the time of the lone wolf. It is the time of community. A good spa will allow therapists to maintain uniqueness but within a context of that community, and to make this possible requires enlightened spa management. There are some greedy managers out there, but only the fair ones can help usher in the full potential of the spa vision. To be on that kind of team is one of the great joys and privileges spa therapists can have today.

"I do not believe there will ever be a glut of spa therapists or massage therapists in the world," he says. "There will always be a need to develop more spas as cultural institutions for social regeneration. And we will need many 'spa social workers,' also known as massage therapists, to help with this regeneration.

"These highly evolved spa therapists will need to understand the full scope of what a spa can be, not just techniques but philosophy too. What really makes spas helpful to people is as much ethereal as it is empirical and practical. As much invisible as visible. Spa needs to have that sense of spirit and soul and not just get lost in protocols. The key to creating a true spa experience for clients is the integration of water into the entire process. People are asking for more authenticity now, more evidence-based, results-based services. We need to ask ourselves, 'What's the outcome?' Spas are no longer just an escape, a place to get away from other things. Now they are places to engage in life. There is a sense of sanctuary, but spas are now trying to turn clients around to face life. Individuals can escape to a spa, but once there they then encounter the social aspect, the community, once again. Therapists are an integral part of that new social support system of the spa.

"Going to a spa is like going on a pilgrimage," he says. "On a pilgrimage, you go away, but that's only half the journey. To me, the more important thing is

(Continued)

SPA PROFILE

Spa = Water × (Time + Temperature) continued

the return. It's the full cycle. If the spa industry is to sustain itself, it has to honor that full cycle. It can't just be a self-indulgent, luxurious escape. Spas are the very epitome of getting back in touch with the Self, and with nature. The blood of nature is water. Nature's blood is water. We in the spa industry have to realize that."

For those who want to delve deeply into the world of water therapy and the true meaning of spa, information about hydrotherapy and experiential spa pilgrimages to Europe is available at http://www.alamoplazaspa.com or by phone at (210) 822-7238.

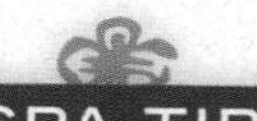

SPA TIP

While hot showers definitely create the sensation of warmth for clients who take them, they are nonetheless not immersive heat treatments and therefore do not raise the core body temperature significantly. Showers, then, are not used to warm clients prior to heat treatments such as the herbal wrap (see Chapter 8). For this, hot baths, whirlpools, steam, or sauna are recommended.

RESEARCH

Using the Internet or searching at local spas in your area, find a spa that offers either a hydrotherapy tub bath, Vichy shower, Scotch hose, or other hydrotherapy treatment. At the top of a sheet of paper, write down verbatim the description of this treatment given by the spa. Lower on the page, rewrite this description using some of the therapeutic know-how you have gained in this chapter. At the bottom of the page, discuss your rationale for changing the wording.

spa culture

the entire lifestyle and worldview inspired by a close focus on hydrotherapy, natural healing techniques, products such as herbs, connection with nature, and healthful well-rounded living, as promoted and adhered to in spas

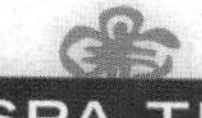

SPA TIP

"In order for you to get a really get a big perspective, look at the Earth as just a big drop of mineral water. It's a garden in space. The origins of spa are in that garden."

—Professor Jonathan Paul De Vierville

CONCLUSION

Bathing has been a central part of the spa experience for hundreds of years, and it still plays a key role in modern spas. The grandest of spa resorts feature lavish bathing facilities that rival the ancient baths of Rome, and even small massage-therapist-owned spas without extensive bathing facilities can offer the power of hydrotherapy to clients through the application of water in foot baths, hot towels, and other inexpensive supplies. Special tubs and showers have been developed to enhance the age-old effectiveness of water therapies, and massage therapists are most often in charge of administering them. It is important, then, for spa therapists to remember that their therapeutic roots lie in the rich history of bathing, and that it is not just massage alone that produces the results that spa clients seek. Rather, it is a combination of massage skills and the inherently healing properties of water that leads to the full expression and impact of spa therapy.

REVIEW QUESTIONS

1. Name and explain the three main types of effects produced by hydrotherapy.
2. Explain the workings of the hypothalamus. How does it relate to spa therapies?
3. What are the five methods of heat transference in the body, and which one is most important to the majority of spa therapies?
4. Explain the basic effects of hot water versus cold water.
5. What is the RICE technique, and when is it appropriate to use in spas?
6. Why can clients remain in therapeutic baths longer than Jacuzzis, hot tubs, hot springs, and whirlpools?
7. Describe a typical high-tech hydrotherapy tub used in top spas.
8. What are the benefits of a cold plunge?
9. Name and describe the three main types of therapeutic showers used in spas.

CHAPTER

5

Heat and Cold Applications

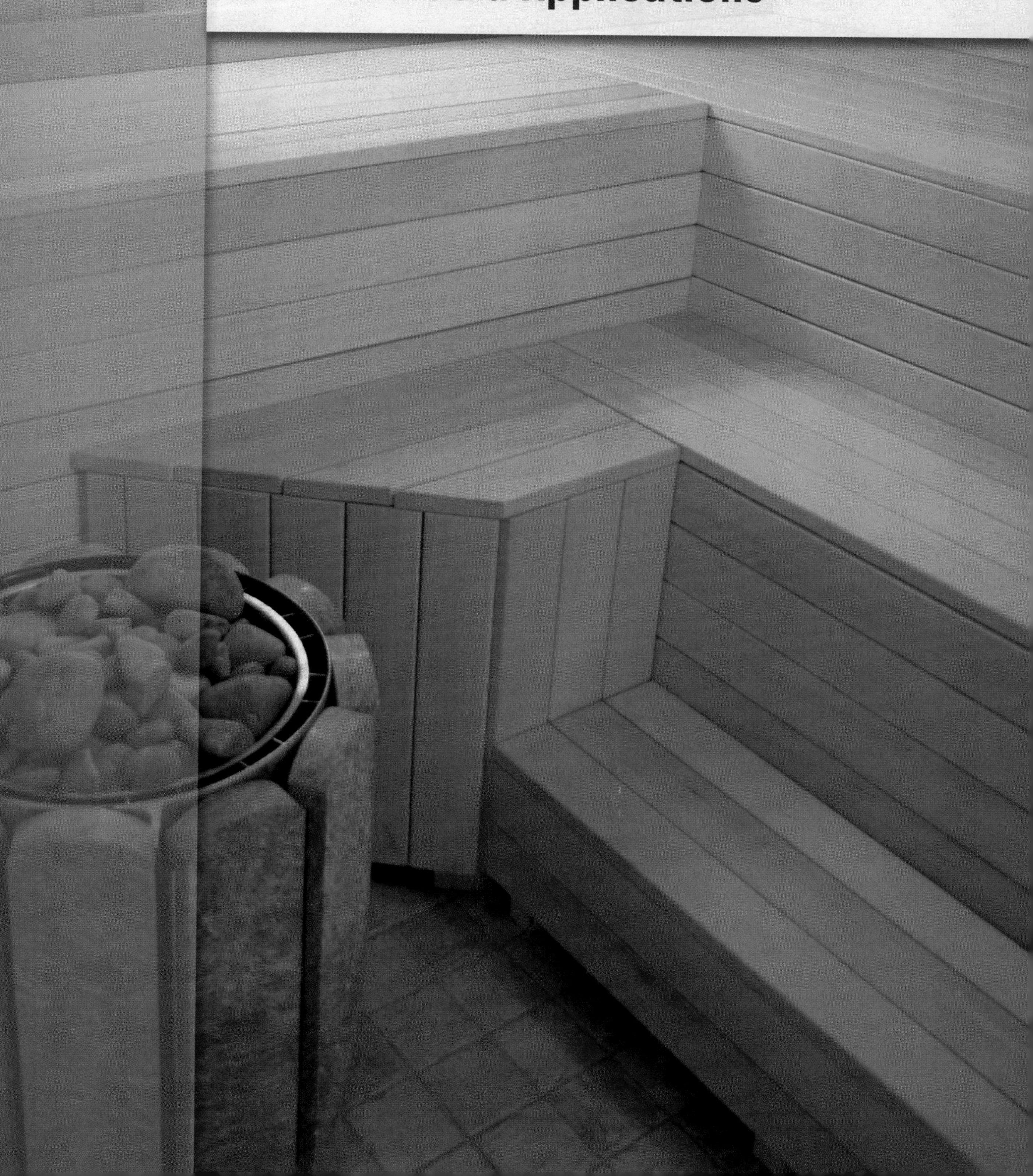

LEARNING OBJECTIVES

1. **Explain how the body regulates temperature in reaction to spa treatments.**
2. **Describe the primary effects of heat and cold therapy as produced in popular spa treatments.**
3. **List and explain the major contraindications for spa treatments involving heat.**
4. **List and describe major spa hot and cold applications.**
5. **Describe and demonstrate ability to perform affusion treatments.**
6. **Describe and demonstrate ability to perform ablution treatments.**
7. **Describe the histories and uses of saunas and steam baths around the world.**
8. **Describe and demonstrate ability to perform paraffin treatments.**
9. **Explain the use of cooling treatments in spa therapy.**
10. **Demonstrate ability to perform cold spa treatments.**

INTRODUCTION

As you learned in the last chapter, many of the major benefits of spa treatments are created through the effects of hydrotherapy. You also learned that these effects are actually created by the heat within the water used in the treatments. This chapter is specifically about those spa treatments and amenities that are designed to transmit heat to or from the body, whether water is involved or not. These include hot and cold compresses, ice packs, fomentations, ablutions, affusions, steam baths, saunas, paraffin wax applications, and cooling anti-sunburn procedures. Many spa body products, such as muds, clays, herbs, and seaweed can also be applied hot and transfer heat to the body. They will not be discussed here, however, because they are covered in Chapters 7 and 8. Also, hot stones definitely transfer heat to the body and are quite popular in spas. Chapter 10 is devoted to this modality.

While the transfer of heat to and from the body certainly represents one of the main therapeutic benefits of spa treatments, it is interesting to note that some traditional hydrotherapy treatments that accomplish this objective have fallen into disfavor in most modern spas. These treatments include the wet sheet wrap and cold mitten friction, for example. This disfavor is perhaps due to the discomfort some spa clients report experiencing during application of these treatments. Spas today need to offer treatments with the benefits of heat and cold application but without the discomfort. Certainly, Sebastian Kneipp (see Chapter 1) would have frowned upon such an attitude, and certain spas, especially those in Europe, still have a focus on traditional, effective heat and cold treatments, regardless of how uncomfortable some clients might find them. See Table 5–1 for a list of heat and cold treatments and their relative popularity in modern spas.

TREATMENT	DESCRIPTION	USES	CONTRAINDICATIONS	POPULARITY IN SPAS
Ablutions	washing down the entire body or certain parts with a coarse wet linen cloth, usually with cold water	produces heat in the body as a reaction to the cold cloth application, stimulates circulation and digestion	oversensitivity to cold, bladder or kidney infection	low
Affusions	the regulated streaming of (usually cold) water onto the surface of the entire body or specific areas of the body	stimulates and improves circulation, improves immune function, tone muscles	depending on area of body treated: kidney or bladder infections, blood pressure disorders, menstruation, sciatic pain	low
Cold Compresses	cloth which has been wrung out in ice water is held in place on a specific area	used to supply local moist cold therapy to an area, often used on head during hot body wraps	none	high
Cold Mitten Friction	application of cold water with loofah mitts or similar exfoliating device	helps cool the body after fevers, exfoliates skin, stimulates circulation and builds resistance to cold	acute skin conditions, delicate skin, open cuts and abrasions, lesions, oversensitivity to cold	low
Cold Wraps	cold moist sheets and dry blankets are wrapped around the client	depending upon duration of wrap; absorbs body heat at first, increases circulation, then induces perspiration	oversensitivity to cold, claustrophobia, blood pressure irregularities	low
Fomentations	substance or material used as a warm, moist compress to ease pain and/or relax tissues	most common use is hydrocollator pack prior to massage or spa treatment	inflammation in treatment area	high
Ice Packs	application of ice or frozen gel pack to local area	reduces swelling and pain	oversensitivity to cold, diabetes (if applied to extremities)	low, more common in rehabilitation facilities

TABLE 5–1 Popularity of Heat and Cold Treatments in Modern Spas. *(Continued)*

TREATMENT	DESCRIPTION	USES	CONTRAINDICATIONS	POPULARITY IN SPAS
Paraffin Treatments	extremities are dipped in 128°F paraffin wax or larger body areas covered with gauze with paraffin brush-applied	used by both therapists and estheticians to warm, moisten, and relax tissues, penetrates to soothe joints	skin conditions for localized applications, heat contraindications for full-body wrap application	high
Rasul Chamber	chamber inlaid with mosaic tiles in which clients self-apply muds that are later steamed and washed off	creates an exotic environment to apply therapeutic muds and the benefits of steam	all heat contraindications, sensitivities to specific muds and clays	medium, limited to exclusive facilities because of high cost
Sauna	systemic dry heat application in a room or cabinet with heating elements such as stones, electric coils, and ceramic infrared emitters	warms and relaxes clients prior to massage or other spa services, especially heat applications such as the herbal wrap, raises core temperature	all heat contraindications	high
Steam Bath	steam can be applied in a canopy, a small cabinet and other manners as well as in a full traditional steam room	moisturizes skin, warms and relaxes clients prior to massage or other spa services, especially heat applications such as the herbal wrap, raises core temperature	all heat contraindications, acute respiratory infections	high
Sunburn-Relief Cooling Treatments	soothing and cooling preparations such as aloe applied to skin, may also include wraps and baths	in spas where clients present sunburned skin, these services offer pain relief and skin protection	sensitivities or allergies to products used in soothing applications	high in tropical settings, lower in others
Turkish Bath	a form of large steam chamber in which body washing, massage and exfoliation are applied	creates an exotic atmosphere, adds benefits of heat to application massage and exfoliation	all heat contraindications	medium, gaining popularity

TABLE 5–1 Popularity of Heat and Cold Treatments in Modern Spas.

Before exploring the details of specific modalities and their applications, this chapter first explains how the heat and cold in these treatments affects the body. Understanding these basic physiological mechanisms is an important part of becoming a knowledgeable and professional spa therapist.

THE EFFECTS OF HEAT AND COLD THERAPY

The overwhelming majority of spa treatments involve the application of heat to the client's body, as compared to cold. In some spas, however, the cold plunge serves as a tool for creating contrast therapy, and many spas offer cooling compresses and applications, especially in hot, dry climates or where sun damage to clients' skin is prevalent. It is therefore important to understand the basic effects of both heat and cold on the body. The three main types of effects created by both heat and cold are local, systemic, and reflex. These three types of effects are markedly different for heat and cold. Local effects manifest themselves only in the area where the heat or cold is applied, which includes the skin and superficial tissues directly below the skin. Systemic effects occur throughout the body. Reflex effects occur in specific body parts other than the site of application, through actions of the nervous system. The physiological changes that occur in the body during these applications is due in large measure to the temperature change, length of application, and total body surface area where the heat or cold is applied (Figure 5–1).

Temperature Regulation

Many factors combine to make water such a powerful therapeutic medium, and foremost among these is its unparalleled ability to transfer heat to and from the body (see the section entitled "The Effects of Hydrotherapy" in Chapter 4). The reason water is so conducive to heat transfer is that it has the highest specific heat of any substance. This is another way of saying that it takes a large amount of energy to raise its temperature. As it heats up, water absorbs more heat per unit of weight than other compounds, and as it cools down, water releases more heat. When it melts or boils, water releases an incredible amount of **latent heat,** which can then be put to therapeutic use in spa treatments (Figure 5–2). Because the specific heat of water is 1, it takes 1 calorie of heat loss per gram to lower the temperature 1 degree Celsius. A gram of water at 40°C would require a 40 calorie heat loss to reach 0°C. Then, the magic of latent heat takes over, requiring a further loss of 40 more calories in order to change the water into ice. The ice then needs to absorb those 40 extra calories once again in order to turn back into water. This is what makes ice such a powerful therapeutic tool; it absorbs massive amounts of heat. On the other end of the temperature spectrum, water requires an even greater amount of energy to transform itself into steam. That same gram of 40°C water would require 60 calories of heat to achieve 100°C and then another 540 calories to transform into steam. The water does not get hotter while it is absorbing this energy; it remains at 100°C. The heat building within it at this point is

latent heat

the quantity of heat absorbed or released by a substance undergoing a change of state, such as ice changing to water or water to steam, at constant temperature and pressure

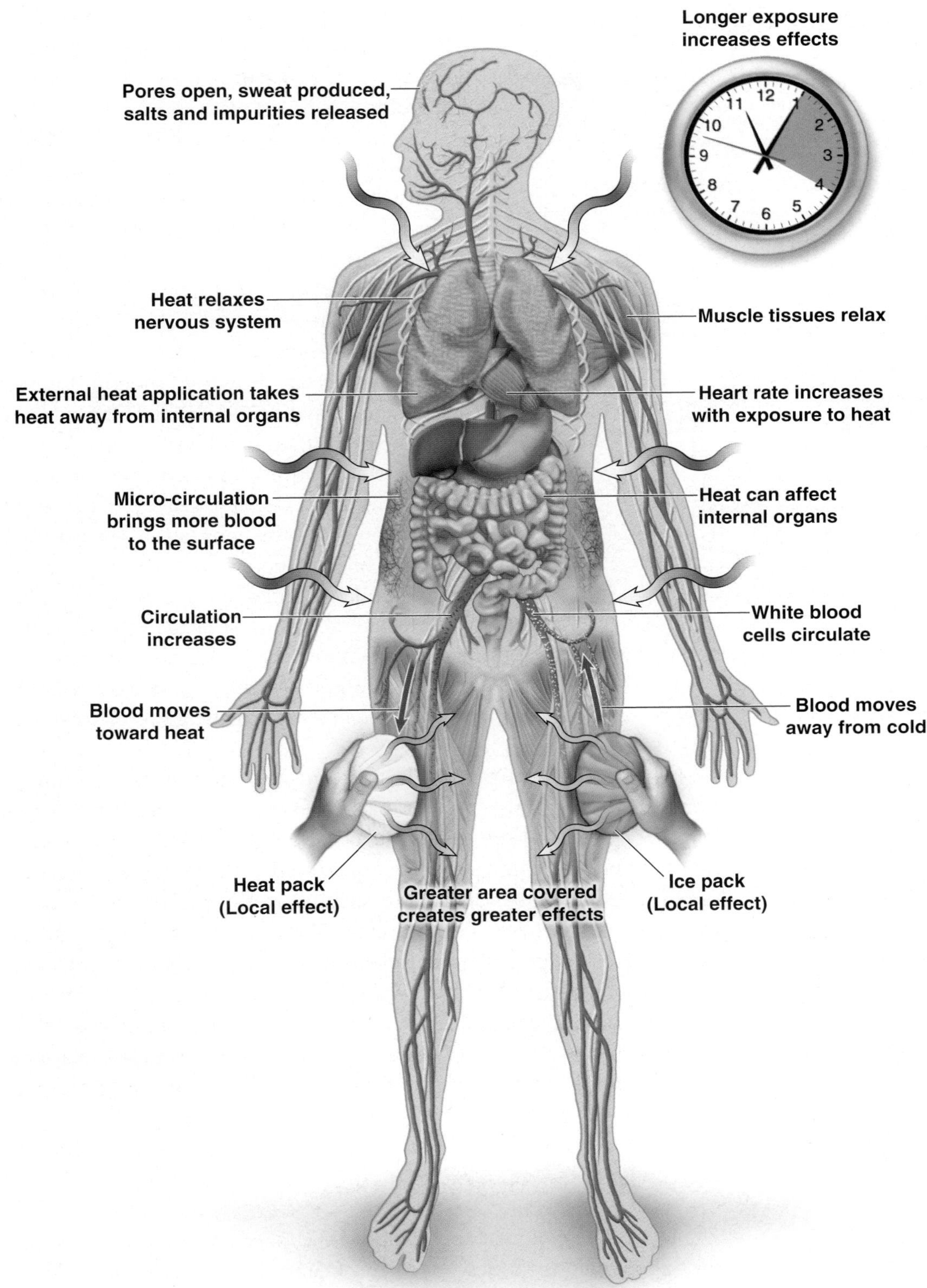
Longer exposure
increases effects
Pores open, sweat produced,
salts and impurities released
Heat relaxes
nervous system
Muscle tissues relax
External heat application takes
heat away from internal organs
Heart rate increases
with exposure to heat
Micro-circulation
brings more blood
to the surface
Heat can affect
internal organs
Circulation
increases
White blood
cells circulate
Blood moves
toward heat
Blood moves
away from cold
Heat pack
(Local effect)
Greater area covered
creates greater effects
Ice pack
(Local effect)

FIGURE 5–1 Heat has a profound effect on the human body.

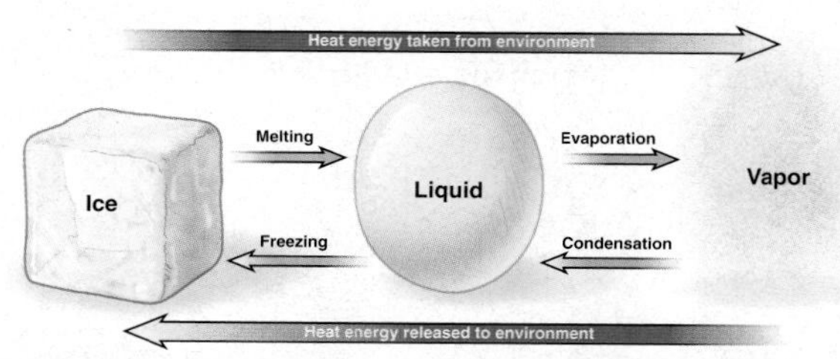

FIGURE 5–2 Latent heat is stored in water in its various forms and released during spa treatments.

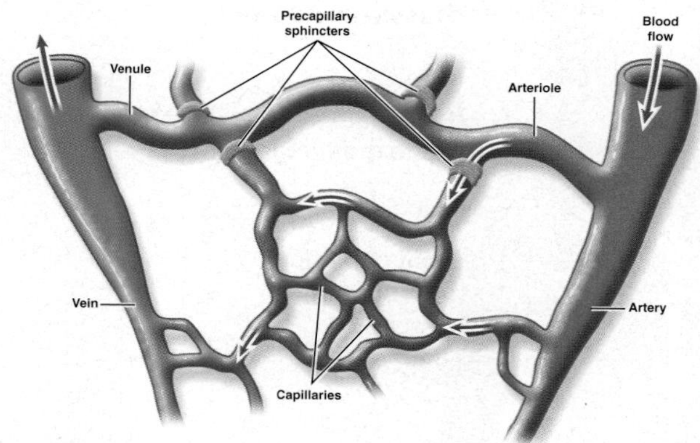

FIGURE 5–3 Precapillary sphincters control blood flow to the skin surface.

latent heat, which is then trapped in the steam when the water vaporizes. When the steam condenses to water again, it releases all that energy. That is why steam can scald the skin so easily.

When the body is heated up or cooled down through the application of spa treatments, blood flow is powerfully manipulated, which creates correspondingly powerful physiological effects. When blood or lymph is drawn away from one part of the body by increasing the amount sent flowing to another area, this is known as the principle of **derivation**. For example, in order to relieve congestive headaches, heat can be applied to the feet, drawing blood and lymph toward the feet and away from the head. Conversely, when cold is used to drive blood and lymph away from a particular area, this is known as **retrostasis**. Ice applied to the head in the case of a headache drives blood and lymph away from the congestion toward the lower extremities. Both principles of derivation and retrostasis can be applied simultaneously, as when heat is applied to the feet and cold to the head at the same time to treat headaches. When the entire body is immersed in heat or cold, blood is moved from the interior to the exterior or vice versa according to the temperature, creating the hydrostatic effect, as discussed in Chapter 4.

derivation

the drawing of blood and lymph away from an area of the body by applying heat to another area

retrostasis

the driving of blood and lymph away from an area of the body by applying cold to that area

precapillary sphincter

a band of smooth muscle that adjusts the blood flow into each capillary

One of the most important anatomical structures involved in the movement of blood during spa therapies is known as the **precapillary sphincter** (Figure 5–3). These sphincters are located in the muscular walls of the arteriole just before the capillaries. They are strongly affected by temperature change, opening when heat is applied to specific areas or to the entire body surface, and tightening when cold is applied. Massage and other mechanical stimulation, such as a high-pressure underwater jet, affects them as well. Thus, a combination of massage and spa hydrotherapy treatments can create an amplified effect on these structures. The entire process of blood and lymph manipulation through spa treatments creates an intricate internal ballet as anatomical structures respond precisely to the range of temperatures and pressures applied (Figure 5–4).

Local Effects of Heat

The local effects of heat applications take place primarily in the skin itself and the subcutaneous tissues up to 3 or 4 centimeters below the surface. The heat increases circulation and metabolic processes on the cellular level within the tissues directly affected. This can facilitate tissue repair and healing as interstitial tissues are more efficiently rid of inflammatory by-products and excess fluids. Heat also helps bring extra white blood cells into circulation in the affected area, which also aids in healing of tissues and expulsion of unwanted materials.

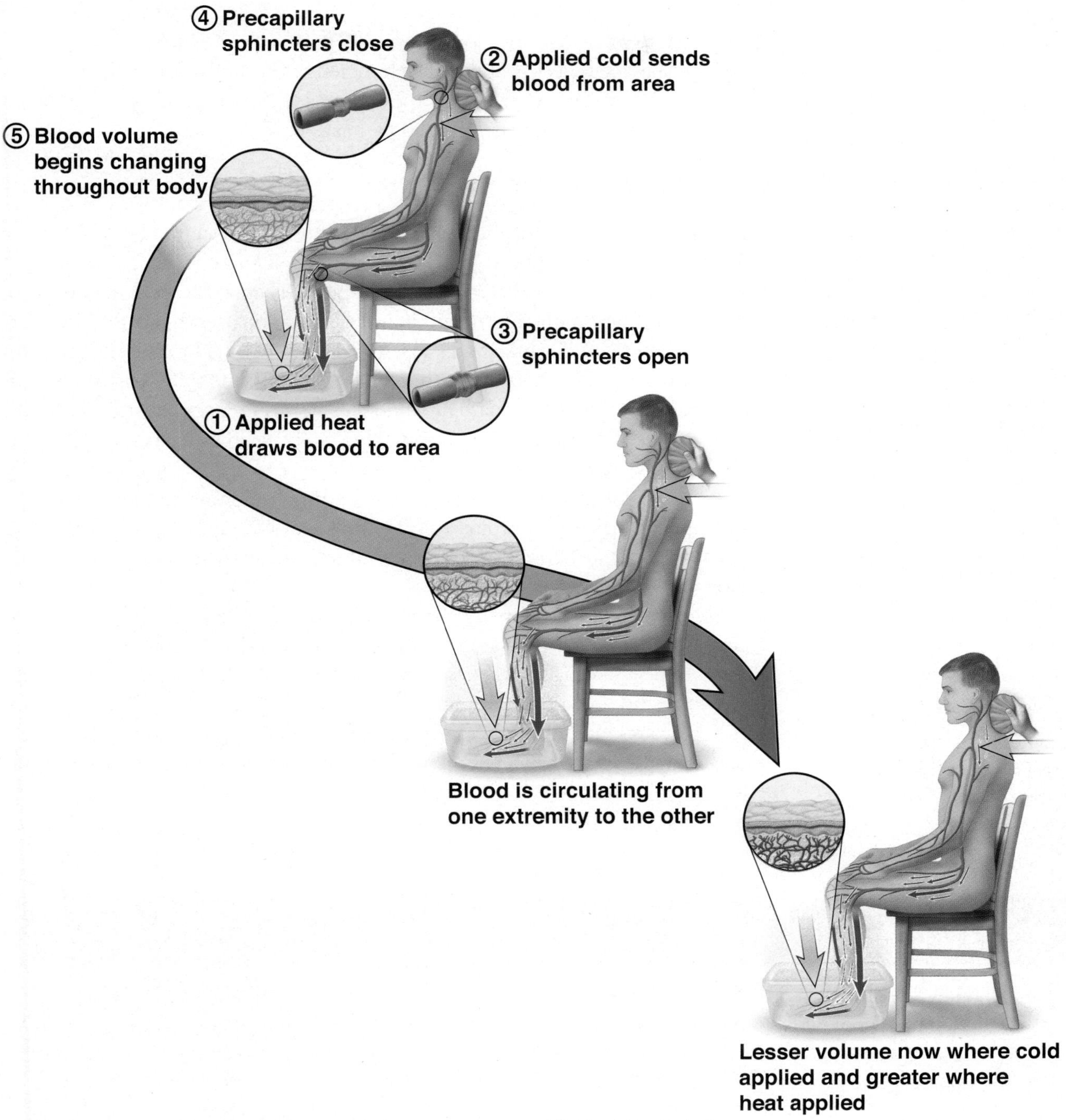
④ Precapillary sphincters close
② Applied cold sends blood from area
⑤ Blood volume begins changing throughout body
③ Precapillary sphincters open
① Applied heat draws blood to area
Blood is circulating from one extremity to the other
Lesser volume now where cold applied and greater where heat applied

FIGURE 5–4 A, B, C Spa treatments create an intricate movement of fluids within the body.

Another major effect of local heat is **vasodilation**. Because local heat application sends more blood to the skin, the vessels there, including the precapillary sphincters as previously noted, dilate. This extra blood then naturally carries away some of the excess heat, protecting the delicate skin. Also, the heat helps diminish pain and muscle spasms. Because the vessels are dilated, the blood

vasodilation

dilation of blood vessels

pressure in the immediate area is lowered. This can help relieve pain from conditions such as arthritis.

In the spa, local heat is applied with fomentations and hydrocollator packs. Also, many site-specific applications such as back treatments and foot treatments involve localized areas that are affected by heat.

diaphoresis

the process of sweating; *diaphoretic* substances or procedures induce sweating

diuresis

increased secretion of urine, often brought about during whole-body applications of heat such as hot tubs, saunas, and steam baths

eccrine sweat glands

the approximately 2,500,000 coiled tubular glands in the adult human's skin that secrete sweat

apocrine sweat glands

scent glands that develop in puberty, responsible for sweat's odor

Systemic Effects of Heat

Spa treatments such as full-body heat wraps produce systemic heating effects in the body, as do all immersive heat applications such as saunas, steam baths, and whirlpools. These system-wide, whole-body reactions to heat include generalized vasodilation of superficial blood vessels, increased heart rate, accelerated pulse, and a quick spike and subsequent drop in blood pressure. The drop in blood pressure surprises many therapists, who assume that because general heat immersion raises the heart rate and can be so intense and stimulating, it must raise the blood pressure as well. This drop in pressure is counterintuitive, but it is very real, and it accounts for the fact that during or immediately after general heat treatments, clients may be prone to fainting due to reduced blood supply to the brain brought on by the lower blood pressure. See the Did You Know? sidebar about contraindications for heat treatments later in this chapter.

Other systemic effects include increased **diaphoresis** as the body strives to dissipate excess heat through evaporation. Muscles and soft tissues soften when exposed to heat, aiding in relaxation and reduction of muscle pain. This also facilitates stretching and therefore physical activity such as exercise. The joints are more supple and move more freely during general heat application. And **diuresis** increases as the kidneys excrete more fluid, helping the body rid itself of metabolic by-products.

Spa Treatments and Sweat

Did You Know?

Sweating is the body's most efficient way of cooling itself down. When body temperature rises through exertion, an increase in ambient temperature, or exposure to an external heat source such as a spa treatment, sweating occurs. Heat is removed from the body when the sweat evaporates on the skin. This heat dissipates in the surrounding air through the process of convection.

Sweat glands are coiled tubular glands that extend from the skin surface down into the hypodermis (Figure 5–5). **Eccrine sweat glands** cover the entire body, but a higher concentration is found in certain areas, such as the palms, soles of the feet, and armpits. These are the glands primarily involved in temperature regulation, overseen by the hypothalamus, as discussed in Chapter 4. **Apocrine sweat glands** develop in puberty. They are located wherever there is body hair, but are more plentiful in the armpits and in the genital area. Essentially serving as scent glands, they produce sweat that contains fatty materials which are the main culprit in sweat's odor, due to the bacteria that break down these fatty materials. Emotional stress can increase extra sweat production from these glands.

(Continued)

Spa Treatments and Sweat *continued*

Did You Know?

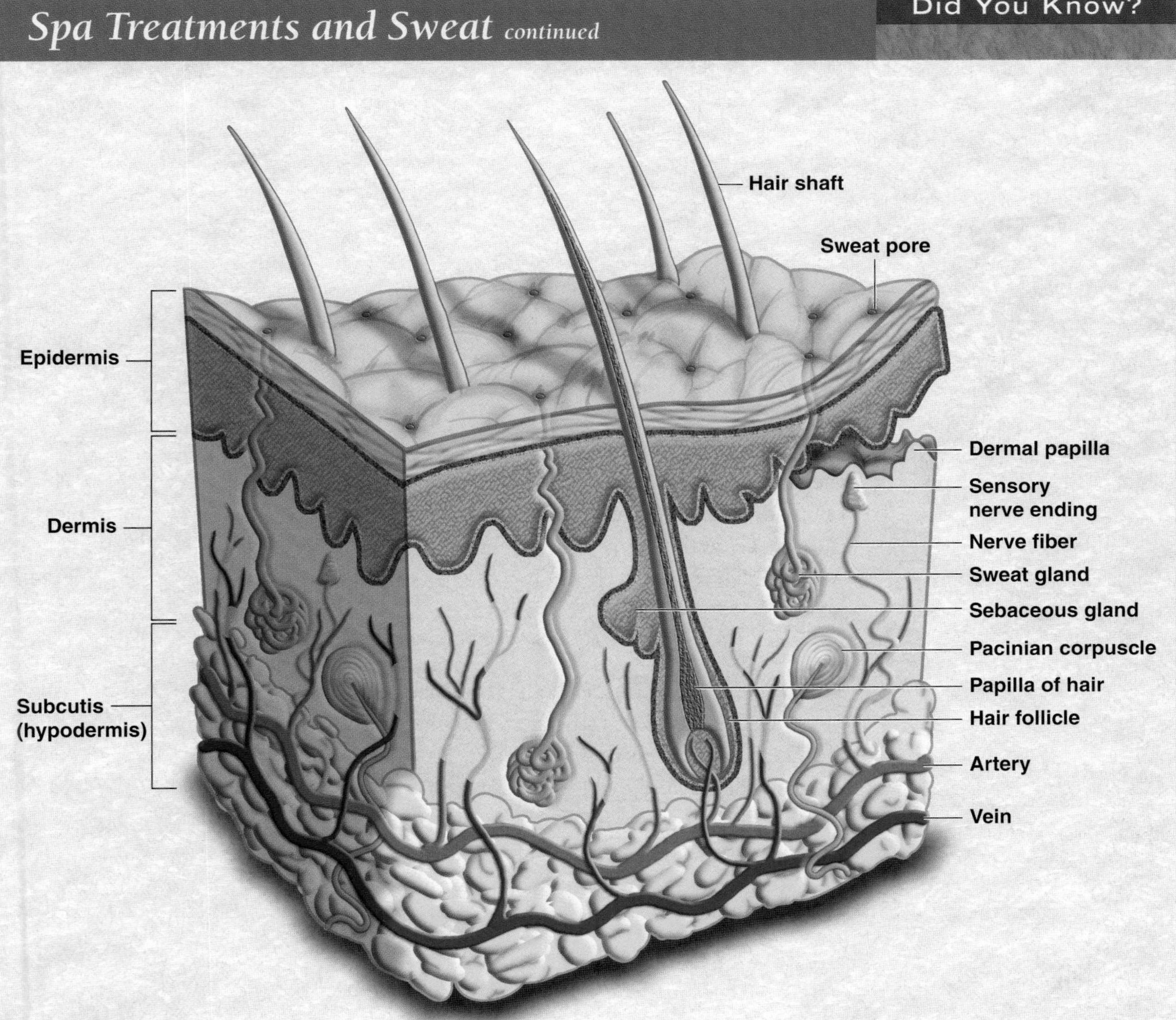

FIGURE 5-5 Sweat glands embedded in the hypodermis.

As massage therapists are aware, the skin is the largest organ in the body. Approximately 30 percent of body wastes are passed through the skin, and sweating enhances this process by opening pores and increasing the amount of waste expelled. The main reason that certain people sweat more than others is because they have a higher number of sweat glands in their bodies. This number can vary widely, depending upon the number of sweat glands with which a person is born. The average adult male has approximately 2,500,000. Women actually have more sweat glands than men, but their glands are less active than men's, and so women tend to sweat less. These facts explain why different clients have such varied reactions to the same heat treatments in the spa. While some sweat profusely, others seem to be hardly affected at all. This is due to no fault of the therapist or the technique, but rather just the natural response of the particular client's body to heat.

SPA TIP

Sweat consists almost entirely of water, with only trace amounts of salts, fatty materials, urea, and other wastes. Spa clients primarily lose water when they sweat during heat treatments, and water is what they need to drink in order to replenish their bodies. Teas, juices, and soft drinks do not help replenish the body with the same efficiency as water. Alcoholic and caffeinated drinks actually deplete the body of water. Besides pure water—spring water is best, but purified water is acceptable as well—the only other viable choice to offer clients after sweat-inducing spa treatments is vitamin or mineral water. Some spas give clients a glass of such fortified water after treatments and then offer larger bottles for sale.

vasoconstriction

decrease in the diameter of blood vessels, caused by the application of cold in certain spa therapies

analgesic

a technique or substance capable of relieving pain, such as application of ice

cryotherapy

the therapeutic use of cold

hypertension

high blood pressure

hypotension

low blood pressure

arteriosclerosis

hardening of the arteries

thrombosis

a clot of coagulated blood attached at the site of its formation in a blood vessel

phlebitis

inflammation of a vein, most commonly in the legs

diabetic peripheral neuropathy

nerve damage in the toes, feet, and sometimes hands caused by diabetes, often causing lack of sensation in the affected area

Reflex Effects of Heat

When local heat is applied to an area of the body, nerve fibers carry the stimulation up into the spinal cord, through synapses, and out to an organ supplied by the same nerve. An application of heat to one area can result in an increase in circulation and heat in corresponding organs. Thus, when spa treatments include the heating of the skin surface, they are also having an effect on internal organs as well, though these effects are not usually specified for any particular spa modality.

Local Effects of Cold

The immediate response to cold is the opposite of that to heat—**vasoconstriction**. Blood flow is restricted, the skin blanches, circulation in the area is slowed, and local tissue temperature is lowered. Prolonged cold exposure (more than 10 to 20 minutes) lowers local temperature further and results in a lessening of normal metabolic processes. Brief applications of cold are considered stimulating, while prolonged applications are sedative.

Cold lessens sensibility to pain and other sensations in the area, and diminishes the responsiveness to stimulation. It is therefore considered **analgesic**. Muscle tone in the area is increased through cold application, and cold also makes connective tissues denser and less malleable.

Very few spa treatments involve the application of cold, unless it is used in contrast to a heat application or when a cooling effect is desired to combat burns or overheating due to sun exposure. **Cryotherapy** is another term for the therapeutic use of cold, though some therapists mistakenly think it involves the use of ice exclusively. Cold baths and plunges are also cryotherapy, as is the use of cold compresses.

Systemic and Reflex Effects of Cold

When the entire body is exposed to cold, the sensations experienced, in sequential order, include cold, painful cold, less cold, painful burning, and eventual numbness. Respiration increases, while heart rate and metabolic processes decrease. Blood pressure initially increases, but then lowers during continued exposure. The effects of cold water or ice application are more pronounced and dramatic than the systemic effects of warm or hot water because there is a greater temperature difference between the body and the water. If the cold application is too long or intense, tissues can be damaged, but in healthy

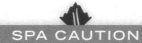

SPA CAUTION

Spa Therapies' Major Contraindications

The most common contraindications for spa treatments involve the effects produced in the human body by the application of heat. Rather than restating why these conditions are contraindicated in every protocol throughout the following chapters, the reasons are listed here. In the event any of these contraindications are present for a particular client, heat treatments should not be administered. In some cases, it is possible to obtain written permission from a physician that will allow treatment. If written medical permission is impossible to obtain, some spas allow clients to sign a release form excusing the spa from liability. Spas should use release forms with caution, however. Should injury result from a heat treatment, a signed release form may not be enough to shield a spa from legal responsibility.

Heat Contraindication 1: High or Low Blood Pressure

People with **hypertension** are usually counseled to avoid heat treatments. Heat raises blood pressure upon initial application, which may overly stimulate a client and lead to cardiac problems, perhaps even a heart attack. A physician's permission must always be obtained prior to administering a heat treatment to a hypertensive client. If the client is taking medication to treat the hypertension, his or her blood pressure may be abnormally low. Because the overall effect of prolonged exposure to heat is a lowering of blood pressure, the effects of the medication could combine with the effects of the heat, lowering blood pressure dramatically, resulting in the client's fainting. For the same reason, clients with **hypotension** need to be cautious about receiving heat treatments as well.

Heat Contraindication 2: Cardiovascular Conditions

A number of cardiovascular conditions could potentially be negatively impacted by the heat in spa treatments, including **arteriosclerosis**, **thrombosis**, and **phlebitis**. Clients with a weak heart or heart valve problems may also experience excessive stress during heat treatments that could put them at risk.

Heat Contraindication 3: Diabetes

Up to 50 percent of clients with diabetes may experience a condition known as **diabetic peripheral neuropathy**. People with this condition sometimes have no feeling in their extremities, most commonly in their feet. This makes it dangerous to apply heat treatments to these clients, who may be unaware of tissue damage being inflicted by the heat because they are insensitive to the pain it would otherwise cause.

Heat Contraindication 4: Fever

Clients experiencing fever and related symptoms caused by flu, inflammatory diseases, and acute infections should not undergo heat treatments, which may aggravate or further inflame the condition, weakening the client.

Heat Contraindication 5: Pregnancy

Pregnant clients should avoid heat treatments, especially in the earlier stages of the pregnancy, because a significantly raised body temperature at this stage could have an adverse impact on the developing fetus. Spot heat treatments that do not affect core temperature are not contraindicated during pregnancy.

In addition to the main contraindications listed above, clients should be informed that taking recreational drugs, alcohol, or some prescription medications prior to or during heat treatments may put them at risk. Any medical conditions should also be checked by a physician prior to heat application. It must be remembered that cold, not heat, is recommended for acute injuries. And finally, varicose veins can be affected negatively by certain impact heat treatments, such as the high-pressure water hose or Scotch hose.

SPA CAUTION

In general, the colder the application, the greater the risk for potential tissue damage. Therefore, caution is advised when using any kind of cold application, especially those involving ice.

hunting response

the body's response to prolonged exposure to cold (as while hunting), which includes intermittent supply of warm blood to cold-exposed extremities

hypothermia

a condition in which more heat escapes from the body than the body can produce, symptoms of which may include gradual loss of mental and physical abilities

blood pump

action created by contrast therapy whereby alternating heat and cold bring in fresh blood to an area and help flush out wastes

individuals reacting to normal cold application, the body will defend itself by increasing blood flow to cold areas. If the body is exposed to extreme cold for an extended period, it will attempt to re-warm itself by initiating a cycle of blood vessel dilation and contraction known as the **hunting response**. This response could occur, for example, in clients who remain in the cold plunge for too long. This exposure would eventually result in **hypothermia** and could even be life-threatening. See Chapter 4 for more information about the cold plunge.

During the application of cold, spa clients may experience several reflex responses in regions of the body generally underlying the application site. For example, when cold is applied to the abdominal area, the intestines beneath will experience an increase in blood flow and acid secretion. And when cold is applied to the scalp, the blood vessels in the brain will contract.

Effects of Hot and Cold Contrast Therapy

The general effect of heat and cold contrast therapy is stimulating, resulting in an increase of local circulation. Contrast therapy produces a significant flow of blood from one part of the body to another. For example, during contrast immersion baths of the upper extremities, clients experience first a large increase—as much as 100 percent—in blood flow to the area during immersion in hot water, followed by a large flow of blood away from the area during cold immersion. This creates a **blood pump** within the body that removes wastes from the area while bringing in new blood with its oxygen and nutrients (Figure 5–6). Cold application can help stimulate the production of white blood cells, which are responsible for fighting infection.

The timing of contrast therapy treatments involves longer applications of heat interspersed with shorter cold applications. Typically, heat will be applied four or five times as long as the cold applications, which should not extend past one minute. The cold plunge is often used to create contrast treatments in the spa, with clients immersing first in a whirlpool, steam bath, or sauna for several minutes before plunging into the cold water for 30 to 60 seconds. This process is repeated for a total duration of 20 to 30 minutes.

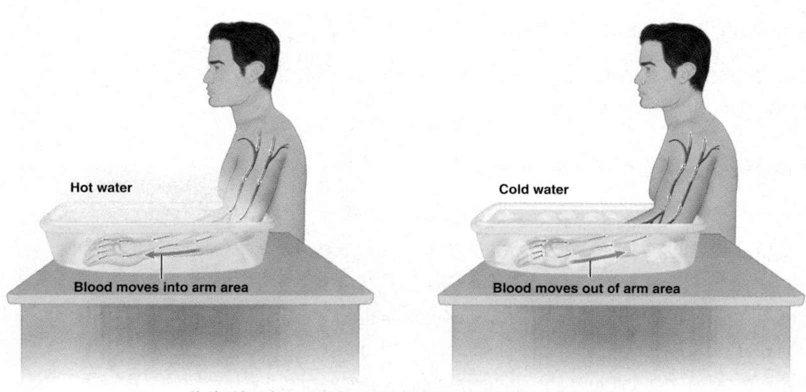
Hot water
Blood moves into arm area
Cold water
Blood moves out of arm area
Hot/cold cycle repeated several times to create blood pump action

FIGURE 5–6 Contrast therapy induces a "blood pump" in the affected area.

Pregnancy and Spa Therapies

Elaine Stillerman, LMT, has been a licensed therapist since 1978, and began her pioneering work with pregnant women in 1980. She is the developer and instructor of the professional certification seminar "MotherMassage: Massage during Pregnancy" and the author of numerous articles and several books on the subject, including *MotherMassage* and *Prenatal Massage: A Textbook of Pregnancy, Labor,*

1,001 High-Risk Pharmaceuticals for Heat Therapies

Did You Know?

The following list is excerpted from The Essential Massage Companion: Everything You Need to Know to Navigate Safely through Today's Drugs and Diseases, by Dr. Bryan A. Born. This is only a partial list of commonly prescribed medicines that alter the body's ability to maintain proper core temperature, either by altering circulatory system control or neurological control. The list should be used only as a general reference and not as the ultimate source of information.

Barbiturates

phenobarbital (Luminal), pentobarbital (Nembutal), amobarbital (Amytal), secobarbital (Seconal), thiopental (Pentothal), methohexital (Brevital), and butalbital (component of Fiorinal and Fioricet).

Diuretics

Thiazide diuretics (hydrochlorothiazide), Loop diuretics (furosemide), Potassium sparing diuretics (spironolactone)

Alpha Blockers

alfuzosin (UroXatral) doxazosin (Cardura), prazosin (Minipress, Minizide), tamsulosin (Flomax), and terazosin (Hytrin).

Beta blockers

acebutolol (Sectral), atenolol (Tenormin), bisoprolol (Zebeta), metoprolol (Lopressor), nadolol (Corgard), and timolol (Blocadren), nebivolol (Bystolic).

Tricyclic Antidepressants (TCAs)

amitriptyline (Elavil, Endep), clomipramine (Anafranil), desipramine (Norpramin), doxepin (Sinequan, Adapin), imipramine (Tofranil), nortriptyline (Pamelor, Aventyl), protriptyline (Vivactil), trimipramine (Surmontil)

Antipsychotic Medications

chlorpromazine (Thorazine), fluphenazine (Permitil, Prolixin), haloperidol (Haldol), loxapine (Loxitane), mesoridazine (Serentil), molindone (Moban), perphenazine (Trilafon), thiothixene (Navane), and trifluoperazine (Stelazine).

Atypical Antipsychotics

aripiprazole (Abilify), clozapine (Clozaril), olanzapine (Zyprexa, Zydis), quetiapine (Seroquel), risperidone (Risperdal) and ziprasi-done (Geodon).

Antihistamines and cold remedies

(too many to list common names)

Hormone Replacement Medications

thyroglobulin (Proloid), and thyroid (Armour Thyroid, Desiccated thyroid, S-P-T, Thyrar, Thyroid Strong, Westhroid).

Antiemetic Medications

Promethazine (Phenergan, Mepergan) Prochlorperazine (compazine), serotonin receptor antagonists including granisetron (kytril), dolasetron (anzemet), ondansetron (zofran), Aprepitant (Emend), Dronabinol (marinol)

Courtesy of Dr. Bryan A. Born, B.S., D.C., Concepts Born, LLC, www.TheEssentialMassageCompanion.com

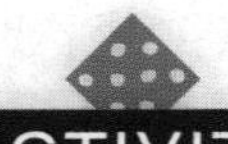

ACTIVITY

The Temperature Test

In order to speak knowledgeably about the physiological effects of heat treatments on the body, all spa therapists should experience and monitor these effects in their own bodies. For this research project, you will record your own or a fellow student's heart rate, blood pressure, and body temperature at four distinct times—before, during, and after the application of heat—and make a chart to graph the results. See the example in Figure 5–7. Choose an immersive therapy such as a hot bath, whirlpool, sauna, steam chamber, or herbal wrap (see Chapter 8) to apply the heat.

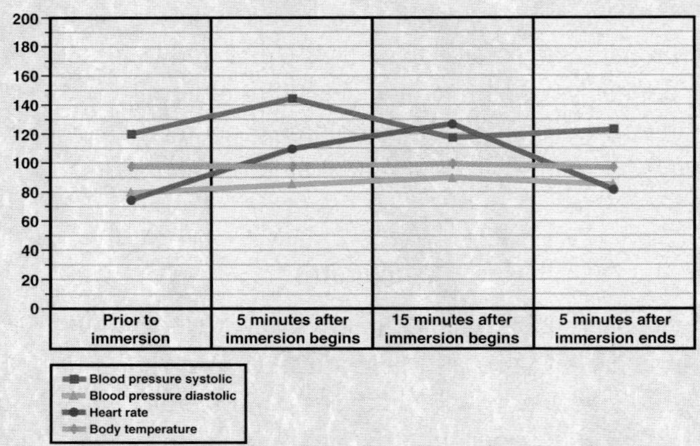

FIGURE 5–7 Monitor the physiological effects of heat treatments within your own body to form a full understanding of spa therapies.

and Postpartum Bodywork. She is also the award-winning writer for the PBS-TV show *Real Moms, Real Stories, Real Savvy*. Thus, Stillerman speaks with authority when it comes to pregnancy as a contraindication for certain spa therapies.

deep vein thrombosis

the formation of a blood clot, "thrombus," in a deep vein, commonly affecting the leg veins, especially during pregnancy, and thus any spa treatment that delivers deep strokes or heat to this area must be avoided during pregnancy

"Heat application to the legs should be avoided during pregnancy," she states. "Starting in the early second trimester, women develop more clotting factor, with higher fibrinogenic activity. Their risk of developing **deep vein thrombosis** is heightened five or six fold. Therefore, all deep treatments, deep strokes, and penetrating heat must be avoided during pregnancy and up to three months postpartum in order to protect against dislodging a blood clot.

"It is strongly recommended that before any massage or spa treatments are administered, therapists should perform pretreatment evaluations for pitting edema and blood clots, which I teach to students in my workshops. Also, it is important that these tests continue three months postpartum."

Stillerman suggests that only massage or spa professionals certified in prenatal/postpartum massage should be working with pregnant women in the spa setting, because so much of this hands-on work requires an intimate knowledge of anatomy and physiology during the childbearing year.

affusion

spa treatment popularized by Kneipp featuring a stream of water of specific temperatures over the entire body or certain areas; an affusion under pressure is the same, but with water directed at high pressure at the body to produce more pronounced mechanical effects

AFFUSIONS

Simply defined, an **affusion** is the pouring of a liquid onto the body (Figure 5–8). In spas, this liquid is water, and it is applied through a hose. The word *affusion*, which is used when describing baptisms, comes from the Latin *affsus*, past participle of *affundere*, "to pour on." The use of affusions in spas is limited primarily to Kneipp-inspired facilities that specialize in treating people with specific ailments. However, therapists who perform these simple therapies in their own private spa practices can achieve positive benefits for their clients with a minimum investment. In order to achieve this, care must be taken to follow protocols and see treatment series through to their full completion.

Three important factors to consider when applying an affusion are (1) direction of the water flow, (2) temperature of the water, and (3) particular body part affected. Affusions are typically applied cold, with a water temperature of approximately 60°F, although alternate-temperature and increasing-temperature affusions are also used. See Table 5–2 for a description of various affusion procedures. Using a hose, the therapist surrounds the area of the body being treated with a coat of water until the client begins to have a visible reddening of the skin. Separate treatment areas include the arms, legs, knees, chest, back, neck, and face. Several potential affusion treatments are possible for each body area, such as a cold knee affusion, an increasing-temperature knee affusion, and an alternate-temperature knee affusion. Affusions can be further categorized as either *simple affusions* or *affusions under pressure*, such as the Scotch hose discussed in Chapter 4, thus offering mechanical effects as well as therapeutic.

Affusion treatments are low in popularity in modern U.S. spas, but they are quite effective and provide an important therapeutic tool for use by spa therapists. According to hydrotherapy expert Dr. Reinhard Bergel, it takes time for the cumulative effects of affusion treatments to be

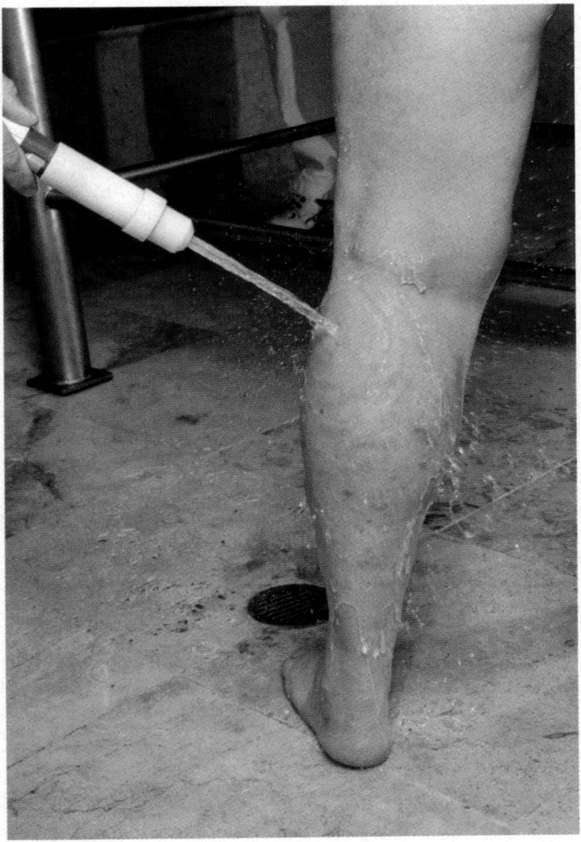

FIGURE 5–8 Affusions involve pouring water of varied temperatures onto the body.

SPA AFFUSION TREATMENTS				
AREA	**TEMPERATURE**	**EFFECTS**	**TECHNIQUES**	**CONTRAINDICATIONS**
Arm	cold: 55°F to 65°F	refreshing and stimulating, indicated for fatigue	move up outside of arm to shoulder then down inside on each arm, 4 repetitions	heart problems, asthma, oversensitivity to cold
	alternate: 60°F/100°F	refreshing and stimulating, indicated for fatigue and poor circulation to hands	move up outside of arm to shoulder then down inside on each arm, first with cold water, then hot, 4 repetitions	heart problems, asthma
Leg	cold: 55°F to 65°F	toning effect on varicose veins, stimulates circulation in legs, reduces blood pressure	start at foot, move up ITB, hold at gluteal then down back of leg to heel, repeat on other leg, then up front of leg to inguinal and down inside, repeat on other leg, repeat whole process 3 times	low blood pressure, oversensitivity to cold, menstrual cramps, kidney infections
	alternate: 60°F/100°F	stimulates circulation, reduces blood pressure, relaxes	same as one repetition of cold leg affusion, then repeat with warm water, repeat whole process two times	oversensitivity to cold, menstrual cramps, kidney infections

TABLE 5–2 Affusion Treatments. *(Continued)*

SPA AFFUSION TREATMENTS				
AREA	**TEMPERATURE**	**EFFECTS**	**TECHNIQUES**	**CONTRAINDICATIONS**
Body	cold: 55°F to 65°F	stimulates immune system and nervous system, increases metabolism and circulation	warm body first in sauna, whirlpool, etc., start at foot, move up ITB then down back of leg, up other leg, switch to hand, up arm to shoulder, down body, other hand up to shoulder then down body and down leg, repeat on front, focusing circular movements on abdomen, then down leg to finish with both feet	menstrual cramps, bladder infections, heat contraindications, oversensitivity to cold
Knee	cold: 55°F to 65°F	reduces blood pressure, stimulates circulation	up outside of calf from foot, hold above back of knee until skin reddens then down back of calf to heel, repeat on other knee, then switch to front, running water up above kneecap until reddening, then back down, repeat on other leg and finish with both feet	low blood pressure, oversensitivity to cold
	alternate: 60°F/ 100°F	relieves headache, increases blood flow, reduces blood pressure	perform knee protocol above, alternating with warm water first then cold, two times each	varicose veins, low blood pressure
Chest	cold: 55°F to 65°F	reduces fatigue, increases metabolic rate, stimulates circulation	start at hand, move up outside of arm and stay at shoulder until skin reddens, down inside arm, repeat on other arm, then move up arm again and crisscross over chest several times, then down one arm to hand	asthma, oversensitivity to cold
	alternate: 60°F/ 100°F	increases metabolic rate, stimulates circulation	repeat procedure for cold chest affusion, starting with warm application, then cold, two times each	asthma, heart conditions
Back	increasing: 93°F to 110°F	relieves back soreness and tension, increases blood flow, reduces spasm	start with lower temperature and gradually warm up while running water over back until skin reddens	acute back pain, blood pressure disorders
Neck	increasing: 93°F to 110°F	relieves neck strain and tension increases blood flow, reduces spasm	start with lower temperature and gradually warm up while running water over back of neck and over shoulders until skin reddens	acute neck pain, blood pressure disorders
Face	cold: 55°F to 65°F	refreshes, relieves fatigue and headache, stimulates circulation	start on one side of face near chin, go up over cheek, temple, and forehead, then down left side of face, being careful so client can breathe freely; repeat 3 times	eye infections, sinus infections, oversensitivity to cold

TABLE 5–2 Affusion Treatments.

fully felt. As he says, "True hydrotherapy conditioning takes three weeks of daily application." The following is a protocol for just one spa affusion therapy application. Use Table 5–2 to adjust the procedure for various treatment sites and temperatures.

Alternate-Temperature Leg Affusion Protocol

TREATMENT: ALTERNATE-TEMPERATURE LEG AFFUSION	
Wet Room/Dry Room	wet room
Table Setup	No treatment table is needed; client is standing or seated over floor drain or bathtub.
Treatment Duration	10 to 20 minutes, depending on client's tolerance and resistance
Needed Supplies	hose or pail to pour water, bath towel, hand towel, a bathtub, shower or drain in floor
Contraindications	oversensitivity to cold, blood pressure disorders, infections or abrasions in treatment areas
Draping	A bathing suit can be worn, leaving skin over treatment area as exposed as possible.
Treatment Order	Affusions are administered as a separate treatment with a rest or exercise period afterward, or before massage or other spa treatments.
Safety, Sanitation Issues, & Clean-Up	Therapists need to be aware of potential dangers from slipping due to moisture present in treatment area. All water needs to be drained or wiped from area to avoid mold buildup.
Body Mechanics & Self-Care	To protect lower back, therapist should take care not to stoop while applying water with hose or bucket.
Product Cost	none
Treatment Price	\$30 to \$50 or included in hydrotherapy package
Physiological Effects	relaxes body, lowers blood pressure, stimulates circulation, tones area treated, refreshes, reduces headaches and fatigue
Pregnancy Issues (information provided by Elaine Stillerman, LMT, author and developer of MotherMassage)	Leg affusion treatments are not recommended during pregnancy. Pressure on the legs during pregnancy must be 10 to 30 gm of pressure, rendering this treatment unsafe. Application of any heat to the legs must be avoided to prevent dislodging potential blood clots often found in the deeper femoral, iliac, and saphenous veins.

Alternate-Temperature Leg Affusion Preparation

1. Test the water source with a thermometer for accurate temperature reading.
2. Fill the pails with water if no hose is available near the client.
3. Assure that the room is warm and without drafts.
4. Have a hand towel available to wipe up excess water or spills.

Alternate-Temperature Leg Affusion Procedure

1. With the client standing over a drain or in a bathtub, begin the affusion with 100°F water on the left foot, hosing up the outside of the leg to the gluteal muscles.

SPA TIP

Spa therapists should lengthen clients' exposure to cold temperatures gradually to build tolerance. Cold affusions can be applied with cool water at first. Then, the temperature can be lowered a few degrees each day, until reaching a true cold therapy application level at 60°F or lower. Water temperatures of 55°F to 65°F are ideal for affusion treatments.

SPA TIP

When a hose is not available to perform an affusion, the therapist can pour water from a pail on a client who is seated or standing in an empty bathtub.

2. Keep the water pouring on the gluteals until the skin begins to turn red.
3. Move the water flow down the back of the leg.
4. Repeat on the right leg.
5. Move to the front of body and, starting at the foot, hose up the front of the left leg.
6. Keep the water pouring on the inguinal space until the skin begins to turn red.
7. Hose down the inside front of the leg.
8. Repeat on the other leg.
9. Repeat the entire procedure with 55°F to 65°F water.
10. Repeat the warm-water affusion and cold-water affusion one more time each, finishing with cold water on the feet.
11. Wipe away excess water from the client's body with your hands rather than a towel.
12. Have the client rest, wrapped up in a blanket if he or she is chilled.

ablution

a treatment that involves washing the skin of a spa client, usually with a coarse linen cloth or sponge and cold water, either over the entire body or a certain area, such as the legs or abdomen

Alternate-Temperature Leg Affusion Cleanup

1. If a bathtub is used, disinfect areas where clients stand.
2. Wipe down areas where clients sit or stand to avoid slippery surfaces.
3. Place used towels in the laundry.

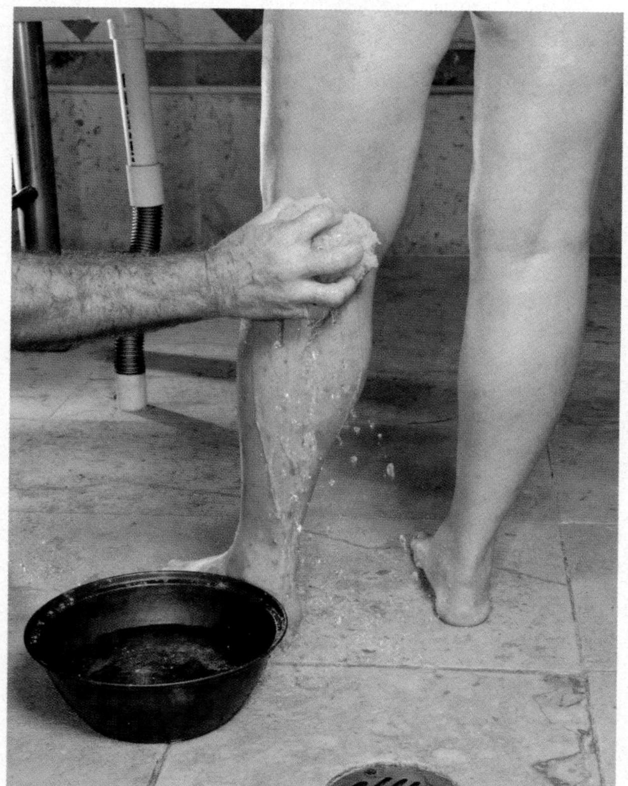

FIGURE 5–9 Ablutions consist of cold water applied with a sponge or towel.

ABLUTIONS

An **ablution**, also known as *wet brushing*, is a sponge or towel bath with cold water ranging from 55°F to 70°F (Figure 5–9). This is another Kneipp therapy used primarily in European spas. The ablution is extremely simple, though effective, and has proven therapeutic value as demonstrated in German studies. In order to gradually acclimate the client to cold water, ablutions are sometimes started with slightly warmer water, above 70°F, and then cooled incrementally during successive treatments until the client is experiencing the true benefits of the therapy with water at 55°F to 65°F. Ablutions can be applied to the upper body, lower body, abdomen, or entire body, and help to stimulate circulation and generate heat in the body, aiding in elimination of metabolic by-products and waste. Though not generally popular in most modern U.S. spas, when used correctly, ablutions can have true health benefits, especially when implemented over several weeks as traditionally prescribed.

TREATMENT: FULL-BODY ABLUTION	
Wet Room/Dry Room	wet or dry room
Table Setup	protective waterproof covering, sheet, draping materials
Treatment Duration	5 minutes for partial-body ablution, 10 minutes for whole-body ablution; does not include body-warming in blankets afterward if needed
Needed Supplies	basin to hold water, hand towel/wash cloth/sponge for bathing, bath towels, thermometer to check water temperature
Contraindications	oversensitivity to cold
Draping	bathing suit or wet table exfoliation draping (see Chapter 6)
Treatment Order	Clients are often counseled to rest after ablutions, as it is a rehabilitative therapy. If given in conjunction with other therapies, apply ablutions first before body treatments or massage.
Safety, Sanitation Issues, & Clean-Up	Ablutions are safe and mild. Take care not to chill client with cold water application and to dry all surfaces thoroughly after treatment. If client shivers uncontrollably, cease treatment immediately and wrap in blankets.
Body Mechanics & Self-Care	Therapist should not stoop over treatment table while applying wet sponge or cloth. Also, assure hands are warmed after treatment, especially when administering more than one successively.
Product Cost	none
Treatment Price	usually included in cost of overall hydrotherapy program or treatment package
Physiological Effects	cools body in case of fever, stimulates circulation, "hardens" body with repeated cold water application to strengthen immune response, promotes digestion, and stimulates circulation
Pregnancy Issues (information provided by Elaine Stillerman, LMT, author and developer of MotherMassage)	This short ablution may be welcomed by many pregnant women, who often feel overheated. Care must be taken to position the client comfortably during the full-body ablution, limit exposure to body-warming blankets after the treatment, and regulate a cooler temperature.

Full-Body Affusion Preparation

1. Protect the treatment table with a waterproof covering.
2. Fill a basin with water: 70°F for clients unaccustomed to cold therapies, and progressively cooler as they become accustomed to an ideal of 55°F to 65°F.

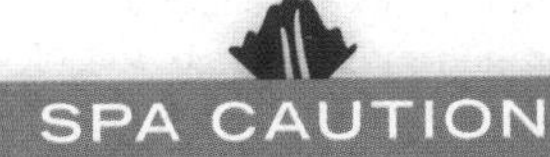

SPA CAUTION

Clients need to be kept warm after a cold-water affusion, either by staying active with light exercise, by wearing warm clothes, or being wrapped in blankets and resting.

Full-Body Affusion Procedure

1. Begin with the client lying supine.
2. Dip a coarse wash cloth or sponge in the water and only squeeze out enough to stop the water from dripping.
3. Wash up the outside of the left arm and down the inside of the arm.
4. Move up the arm again, then across the shoulder, neck, and chest.
5. Repeat on the right arm, moving up to the shoulder, neck, and chest.
6. Move down to wash the abdomen, making clockwise circular motions over the colon.

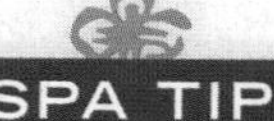

SPA TIP

During ablutions, dip the sponge or wash cloth in the basin repeatedly to keep it filled with water, but not dripping.

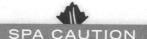

7. Move to the right foot and wash up the front of the leg, then back down.
8. Repeat on the left leg.
9. Ask the client to turn over onto her abdomen, and wash down the back from the neck to the sacrum and on both sides of the back, three or four times.
10. Starting at the foot, wash up the left leg and back down.
11. Repeat on the other leg.
12. Do not dry skin, but let water evaporate naturally.
13. Assure that the client is warm after treatment.

SPA CAUTION

Always be sure that clients are sufficiently warm during and after ablution treatments, especially if they are unaccustomed to cold therapies. Wrap them in blankets or warm clothing and socks after an ablution. In case of intense shivering or discomfort during treatment, discontinue immediately.

Full-Body Affusion Cleanup

1. Launder the wash cloth and towels.
2. If a sponge was used, disinfect.
3. Empty and clean the basin.
4. Wipe down and disinfect the waterproof covering on the treatment table.

SAUNAS

Spas use a wide variety of heated chambers, cabinets, rooms, and enclosures for the purpose of raising clients' body temperatures and effecting all the benefits of systemic heat application (Figure 5–10). These heating chambers, as you will see in this chapter, take many forms, but the most popular traditional forms are the sauna and the steam room, which date back all the way to spas in the days of the Roman Empire as explained in Chapter 1. The main benefits of these heat chambers include:

- stimulation of circulation
- deep cleansing of the pores and skin through sweat
- flushing wastes and impurities from the body

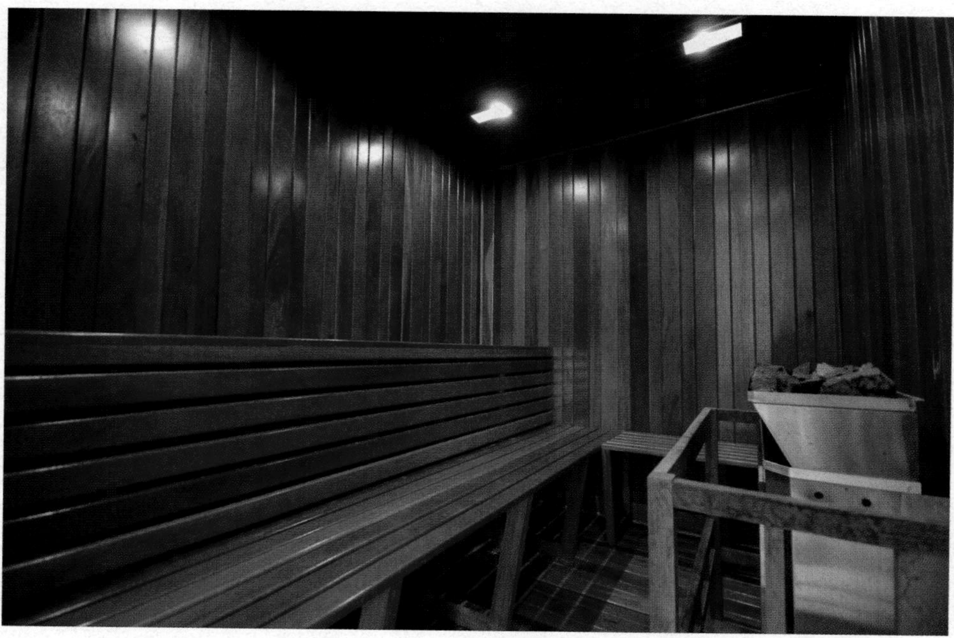

FIGURE 5–10 Spas today incorporate a wide range of beautiful sauna designs.

STEAM BATHS

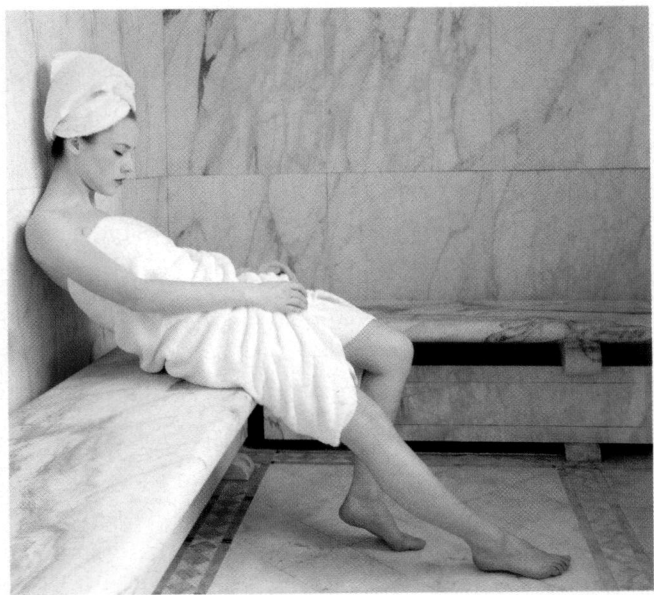
FIGURE 5–14 Steam room.

Several different types of steam applications are used in the spa setting, including the aromatherapy steam tube, the Russian steam cabinet, and the tabletop steam canopy, yet the most commonly seen in spas remains the traditional steam room. This is a room with tiles on all four walls, floor, and ceiling, with a steam generator embedded in one wall or in an adjacent room (Figure 5–14). A thermostat or timer triggers the generator, which pipes in new steam periodically, keeping the room hot and humid, providing a substantially different experience than the Finnish sauna. Even when water is poured on the rocks in a sauna, the steam generated is not nearly as dense. The temperature in steam rooms is lower than saunas, but the air often feels hotter because of the moisture present. Many spa clients have a distinct preference for this moist heat.

Steam baths, as compared to dry saunas, offer spa clients more benefits for respiratory conditions. The steam can help relieve throat irritation and stimulate mucous discharge from the lungs, offering relief to bronchitis sufferers. It can also relieve congestion in the upper respiratory mucous membranes, which helps clients suffering from sinus inflammation. Many spas install a bottle of eucalyptus essence in their steam rooms so that clients can spray it into the steam and breathe it in, further enhancing these positive effects.

The aromatherapy steam tube is a mini-steam room that is portable and much less expensive than installing a traditional steam room. A small reservoir of water at the base of the unit is heated until it produces steam. Drops of essential oil placed on top of the heating unit evaporate and mingle with the steam, creating a pleasant and therapeutic heat treatment for one client at a time. For clients who report feeling claustrophobic inside of the steam chamber, a good option is the Russian steam cabinet, which has a similar steam generator at the base but a cabinet that leaves the head exposed to fresh air. The Russian steam cabinet should not be confused with the traditional Russian steam bath known as the **banya** (see Did You Know? sidebar).

banya
traditional Russian communal steam bath

Some spas offer men and women separate sauna and steam facilities in their wet areas, adjacent to the locker rooms, but in smaller spas, the sauna and steam facilities are often co-ed, which brings up modesty issues. While clients often enter single-sex saunas and steam baths nude, with nudity actually being strictly enforced in some European countries, in co-ed U.S. spa facilities, bathing suits are usually worn. Even when using the facilities while nude, clients are encouraged to sit on towels for sanitary reasons and because the wood or tile can become uncomfortably hot.

Steam baths have the same heat contraindications as saunas, and one extra precaution must be taken with clients who have a compromised respiratory system, for example in the case of the flu or a chest cold. Though it is rare, such an infection could occasionally be spread as mucous is loosened and moves throughout the lungs.

The Russian Banya

Did You Know?

The banya is the traditional Russian steam bath. It is a popular and pervasive part of Russian life, much as the sauna is for the Finns. The temperature in a banya is not as hot as in a sauna, but a large amount of water is poured on the heated rocks, creating copious amounts of steam that prompts many banya users to don a special felt hat called a **chapka** to protect their heads from the searing air.

Traditional banyas have three rooms: an entry room, a washing room, and the steam room. Bathers remove clothing and wash before entering the steam chamber. When everyone is inside, seated on wooden benches, the door is closed. Warmed water is poured on the heated rocks only after bathers have already begun to sweat. Sometimes, aromatherapy oils are added to the water as well.

After the first round of heat, bathers leave the banya to cool off in cold air, or in lakes or rivers if available. In wintertime, some bathers roll in the snow. When they enter for the second time, more water is added to the rocks. During this session, bathers use bunches of dried branches and leaves, usually birch, to hit themselves and fellow bathers in order to further stimulate circulation. The Russians call this a **venik**, and it is also used to fan hot air over the body, thus increasing heat through convection and intensifying the sweat.

Several cycles of heat and cold are enjoyed, between which many bathers relax with a drink or a game. Just as in Finland's sauna, the Russian banya experience is part of the fabric of daily life for many people. A wide range of banya facilities are available for people from all walks of life, and some Russians build banyas on their own property, which they share with friends or rent for a fee.

chapka

felt hat worn to protect the head from heat in a Russian banya

venik

similar to the Finnish *vasta*, a bunch of branches and leaves used in the Russian banya to stimulate circulation

Tabletop Steam Canopies

Popularly known by the brand name Steamy Wonder, steam canopies that fit over the top of massage tables simplify the process of immersing spa clients in heat (Figure 5–15). The units generate steam in a small crock pot placed on the floor beneath the table. The steam is propelled by a fan through a vent into the canopy which fits snugly over the table. Clients rest supine on the table with their heads outside the canopy while the steam envelopes them, creating all the beneficial systemic effects of heat without the need of a full sauna, whirlpool, or steam bath. This is an economical choice for many spas, and even award-winning spas choose to use a steam canopy rather than build an expensive heating chamber.

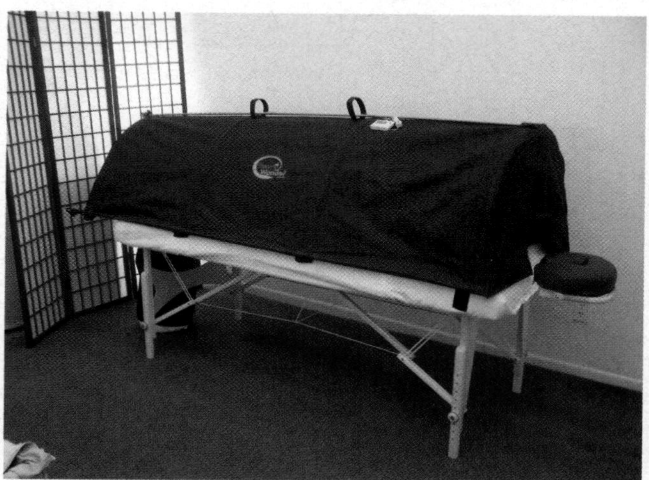

FIGURE 5–15 The Steamy Wonder™.

Steam canopies are used for the same duration and the same purpose as any other full-body heat immersion process. Their most typical application is immediately before a body wrap service, particularly an herbal wrap, for which the core body temperature must be raised slightly. The canopies can also be used as a stand-alone service, simply to provide the benefits of heat. They can be hung from the ceiling in a massage or spa room, eliminating the need for a storage space. A cover is placed over the massage table to protect it from heat and moisture while using the canopy. After an application of heat, the canopy can be lifted

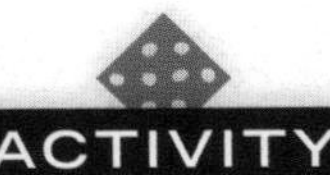

ACTIVITY

Contrast Immersions

Many U.S. spa goers have not felt the therapeutic power of full-immersion contrast therapies, such as those in the Finnish sauna tradition and the Russian banya tradition. Even when the facilities are available at a spa, they are often underused. This is unfortunate, because full-immersion contrast hydrotherapy provides some of the most pervasive overall health benefits of any therapy offered in the spa setting. In order for spa therapists to confidently recommend this type of therapy, they must first experience its effects and benefits themselves.

Even if you are reluctant to immerse yourself in heat and cold contrast therapies, you owe it to your future clients to discover this ancient technique for yourself so you can speak knowledgeably about it and encourage clients to fully avail themselves of the spa's facilities, which were, after all, patterned after age-old, time-tested traditions. This activity can be experienced while at school or afterward at a spa, health club, resort, private home, or other facility that is equipped with a steam canopy, whirlpool, sauna, or other heating unit. In addition, a cold plunge, cold bath, lake, river, snow, or—at a minimum—a cold shower is needed for the contrast. Finnish saunas are often built on sites that offer natural contrast therapy, and some North American spas, such as Spa Scandinave in Quebec, are located in natural settings as well, but many spas are not. Although the experience is esthetically more appealing in nature and some people claim they receive extra benefits from the negative ions found near moving water and burning wood flames, the essential effects of heat and cold can be achieved in the plainest of rooms in any location, given the proper equipment and timing of the immersions.

Note: Be sure to check for any contraindications prior to engaging in this activity.

Full-body heat immersion: 10 to 15 minutes
- Recommended water temperature = 100°F to 104°F
- Recommended sauna temperature = 180°F
- Recommended steam chamber temperature = 115°F

Full-body cold immersion: 1 to 3 minutes
- Recommended water temperature = 50°F to 65°F

Repeat the heat–cold cycle three times. Intense contrast therapy such as this should be experienced with at least one other partner. Do not attempt alone. After the immersions, wrap yourself in a blanket and rest for 20 minutes, observing your reactions to the immersion. Was it stimulating? Relaxing? Exhausting? If steam was used, notice its effects on respiratory mucosa. Over the following several hours, periodically focus attention on your body and any residual sensations you may be feeling as a result of the immersions. Note anything of interest. Then, write one page describing your experience and an assessment of the value of full-immersion contrast therapy.

and the client can receive a massage or spa treatment while still on the table, or the therapist can direct the client to another table. All the benefits of and contraindications for heat apply when using a steam canopy.

SPA CAUTION

Only attempt immersing in near-freezing water or rolling in snow if you are accustomed to it or have received approval from a physician for this activity.

Turkish Baths and Rasul Chambers

The Turkish bath, as it is incorporated into North American spas, consists of a large steam chamber kept at a low enough temperature that the therapist can work in the steamy room, applying bath, exfoliation, and massage modalities. This modern application is of course based on the ancient hammam tradition as described in Chapter 1. The Westernized version sometimes remains true to this tradition, but many spas omit the contrast therapy and the vigorous massage and exfoliation treatments that are such an integral part of the original hammam experience.

Spa therapists who work in spas featuring Turkish baths need to be prepared to perform massage in a steam-filled room at over 100°F. Not all therapists are capable of this, and it is reasonable to refuse such an assignment if you believe it would be injurious to your health. Those therapists who do feel capable of working inside the Turkish bath need to take more frequent breaks than usual and remember to stay hydrated. Therapists working in a Turkish bath are essentially performing the traditional role of a tellak in a hammam.

Found in many of the most luxurious spas, Rasul chambers are a variation on the Turkish bath. Inspired by Moorish design, these small chambers are elaborately decorated with mosaic tiles, and their ceilings feature little sparkling lights meant to represent the heavens at night. Clients enter the Rasul chamber either alone or with one or more partners, and are given a supply of muds, which they spread on their faces, bodies, and through their hair. Once covered in the mud, they rest on benches inside the chamber while the lights become progressively dimmer, simulating nightfall in the desert, and fragrant steam begins to fill the space. The moisture helps the mud penetrate the pores for approximately half an hour, until shower jets overhead begin a gentle spray to rinse the body clean. The experience is often followed by a massage. Rasul chambers are increasingly popular in North American and European spas. They offer clients an exotic and therapeutic treatment that is more private than most, as a therapist need not be present in the chamber.

PARAFFIN APPLICATIONS

For many years, the application of hot therapeutic paraffin wax products to the skin in spa settings has primarily been the province of estheticians and cosmetologists, who use the wax in a number of procedures, including facials, manicures, pedicures, and cellulite treatments. Some aspects of these treatments can now be legally performed by massage therapists in spas, and the use of paraffin by therapists is rising. The application of paraffin can be defined as a heat treatment, as well as an esthetic one, and massage therapists are well-prepared to administer this type of heat therapy. Chapter 13, Esthetic Modalities for Spa Therapists, will include protocols for a face treatment which incorporates paraffin wax.

Paraffin wax is a petroleum-based hydrocarbon that was discovered by German scientist Carl Reichenbach in 1830. Paraffin is important for spa therapy because of its ability to store heat and its power as an **emollient**. Emollients are useful in spa services because of their three main properties: **occlusion**, lubrication, and **humectation**.

- *Occlusion*: Paraffin creates an occlusive barrier on the surface of the skin that retards water loss, thus increasing the moisture content of the skin.
- *Lubrication*: Paraffin softens the skin, making it feel suppler and smoother, in addition to making it easier for therapists' hands to glide across the skin surface during spa treatments after the wax is removed.
- *Humectation*: As an efficient **humectant**, paraffin increases the water-retaining capacity of the **stratum corneum**.

emollient
a substance which softens and soothes the skin

occlusion
closure or blockage, used when describing paraffin wax, which creates an occlusive barrier that retains moisture in the skin

humectation
the action or process of moistening

humectant
a substance that promotes retention of moisture

stratum corneum
the outermost layer of the epidermis consisting of dead cells that slough off

Paraffin is used primarily as an adjunct to other treatments, not as a main treatment in its own right, although a full-body paraffin wrap can be administered apart from other services. Some types of paraffin are pre-blended with therapeutic agents such as herbs and essential oils to enhance the effects and make treatments more attractive to clients. The optimal temperature for paraffin wax used in spa applications is approximately 128°F. The wax is just warm enough to be kept in a liquid state at this temperature, and it is just cool enough for application to the skin. The wax is maintained at the proper temperature in thermostatically controlled basins (Figure 5–16), which come in various sizes and shapes according to intended use.

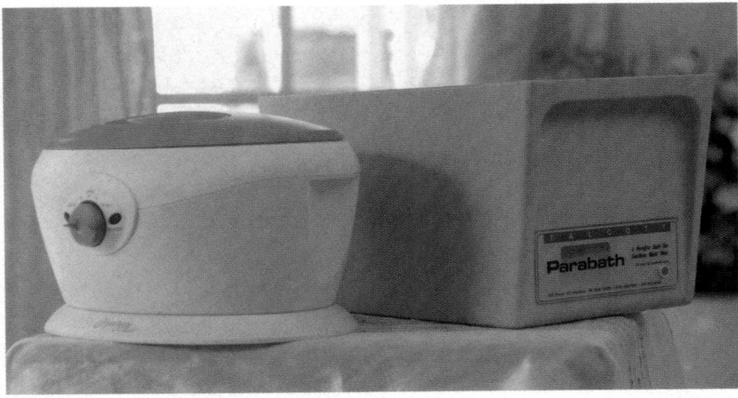

FIGURE 5–16 Various Paraffin heating basins.

In spas, paraffin wax is applied using two main techniques: dipping and brushing. For dipping, clients immerse a part of the body, most popularly the hand or foot, into the basin for a moment, then lift it out, allowing the paraffin to cool and harden slightly on the skin before dipping again. The process is repeated three to five times, and the area is then usually wrapped in plastic or some other insulating material. Some spas offer boots or mittens custom-made for this purpose (Figure 5–17). The paraffin is left on the skin for 10 to 20 minutes and is then pulled off *en masse*, leaving the skin supple and the underlying tissues relaxed. When a brush is used for application, the paraffin is spread over the skin of the targeted area. Sometimes gauze is used to help set the wax in place (Figure 5–18). After the paraffin has been allowed to cool for 10 to 20 minutes, it is peeled away.

Paraffin application is especially beneficial for people with stiff joints, sore muscles, fibromyalgia, and inflammatory conditions such as arthritis, bursitis, and tendonitis. It also provides relief for eczema, psoriasis, and dehydrated skin. Because the occlusive barrier it creates seals out impurities as well as sealing

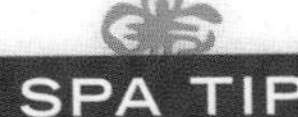

SPA TIP

Some spa therapists mistakenly use the noun "emollient" when referring to a face or body cream, as in, "Try this emollient. It's good for your skin." This is incorrect. You can correctly use the word as an adjective, referring to a product as an "emollient cream or lotion," but only specific single substances, such as paraffin wax, can be correctly referred to by the noun "emollient." Paraffin is an emollient. Creams and lotions are moisturizers.

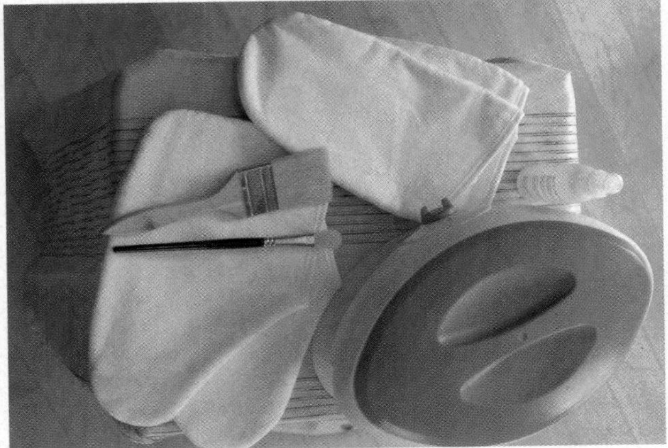

FIGURE 5–17 Insulating boots and mittens worn over paraffin applications.

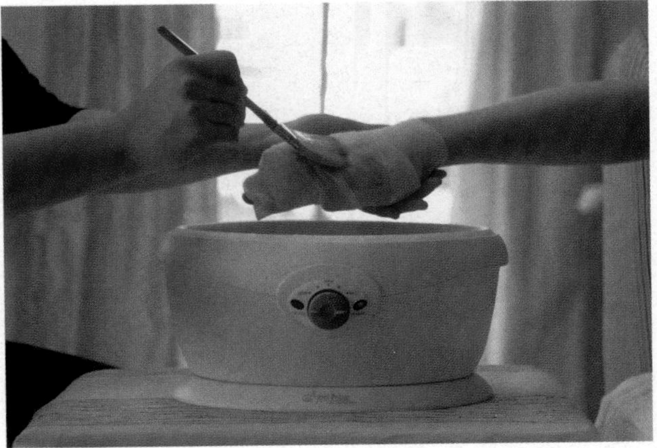

FIGURE 5–18 For brush-on paraffin applications, gauze is often used.

in moisture, some people have used it to aid the healing process of minor cuts and abrasions. Overall, the paraffinic medium is excellent at providing deep-penetrating heat that stimulates circulation while also rejuvenating, hydrating, and nourishing the skin.

Paraffin Hand Dip Procedure

The paraffin hand dip is used by spa therapists during a number of spa services, such as scalp treatments and foot treatments. The client's hands are first dipped in the paraffin and wrapped using the following procedure, and the therapist then carries on with the treatment. Having the hands surrounded by the warm paraffin during the treatment aids relaxation and creates a comforting sense of warmth. Also, the application of heat to the hands draws blood away from other areas of the body through the principle of derivation. Clients report increased enjoyment and value when such a hand dip is added to treatments.

Paraffin Dip Preparation

1. Preheat the basin to the proper temperature.
2. Position the basin near the treatment table.
3. Have mittens or plastic wrap nearby.
4. Have the client wash her hands.

TREATMENT: PARAFFIN DIP	
Wet Room/Dry Room	dry room
Table Setup	no special setup for paraffin dip
Treatment Duration	10 to 20 minutes
Needed Supplies	brush, gauze, dipping basin, mittens, plastic wrap, hand towels
Contraindications	diabetic peripheral neuropathy
Draping	not needed for hand treatment
Treatment Order	applied simultaneously with other spa treatments
Safety, Sanitation Issues, & Clean-Up	Paraffin is kept at 128°F, which can damage tissues over periods of immersion more than a few seconds. Discard all paraffin that has come into contact with client. Multiple clients can dip in basin, as bacteria do not spread in hot paraffin, though hands should be cleansed prior to dipping.
Body Mechanics & Self-Care	Paraffin aids therapist self-care. See SPA TIP, Paraffin Self-Care for Therapists.
Product Cost	under $1 per treatment's worth of paraffin for dipping
Treatment Price	usually included in overall cost of main treatment of which the paraffin dip is part
Physiological Effects	Heat stimulates local circulation, and occlusive barrier promotes moisture retention in skin tissues.
Pregnancy Issues (information provided by Elaine Stillerman, LMT, author and developer of MotherMassage)	Hand paraffin dip is safe during pregnancy. Therapists should keep the client's wrists neutral and work gently if the client experiences carpal tunnel or deQuervains syndromes. Stroking should always be toward the heart. If her hands are swollen, elevate her arms to encourage lymphatic drainage. Avoid stimulating large intestine 4, found in the webbing of both hands.

Paraffin Dip Procedure

1. Dip the client's hand into the basin for 1 to 3 seconds until fully coated with wax (Figure 5–19). Remove the hand and let any excess drip into the basin (Figure 5–20). Ask the client if the sensation was comfortable. If not, make subsequent dipping times shorter.
2. Wait 5 to 10 seconds before dipping the hand once again. Then, repeat for a total of 3 to 5 times, building up a thick layer of wax. The thicker the layer, the greater the sensation of heat.
3. As each hand is finished dipping, wrap it in plastic wrap and cover it with a hand towel (Figures 5–21A and 5–21B) or insert it into a mitten (Figure 5–22).
4. Repeat on the other hand.

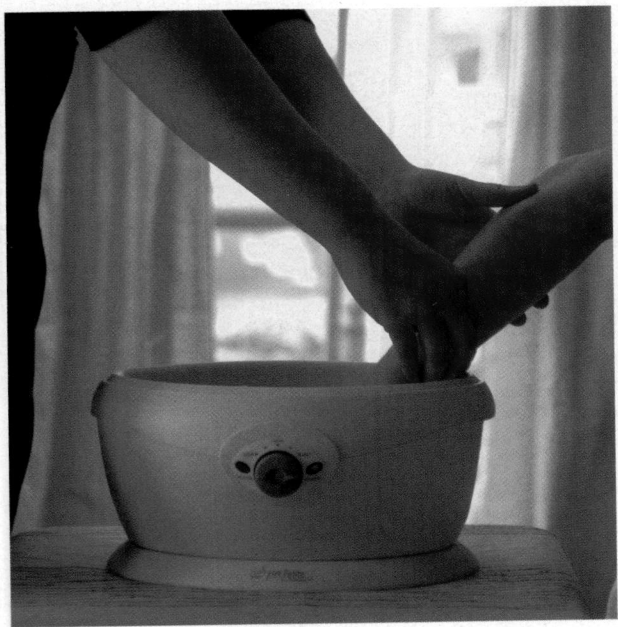

FIGURE 5–19 Dip hand into basin.

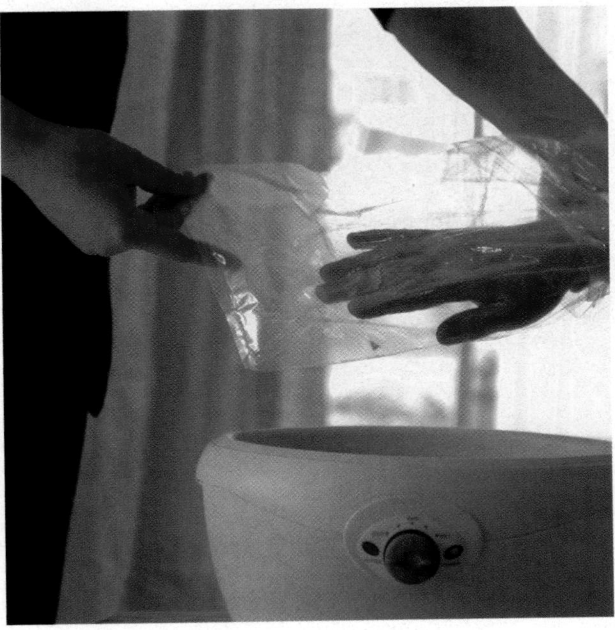

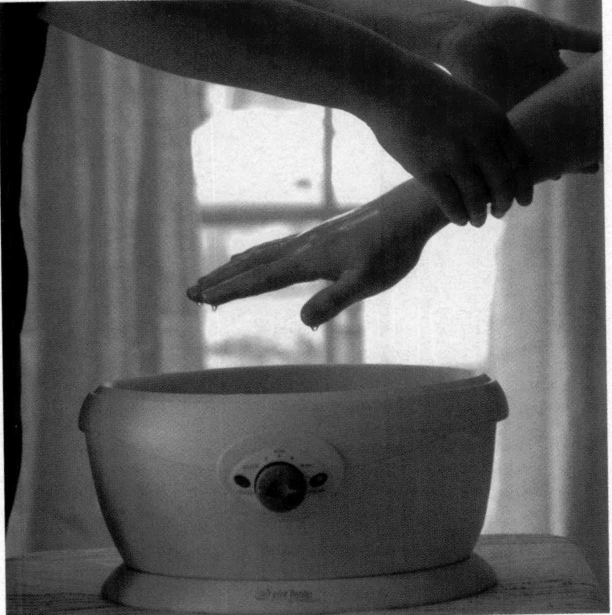

FIGURE 5–20 Remove hand and let wax drip off.

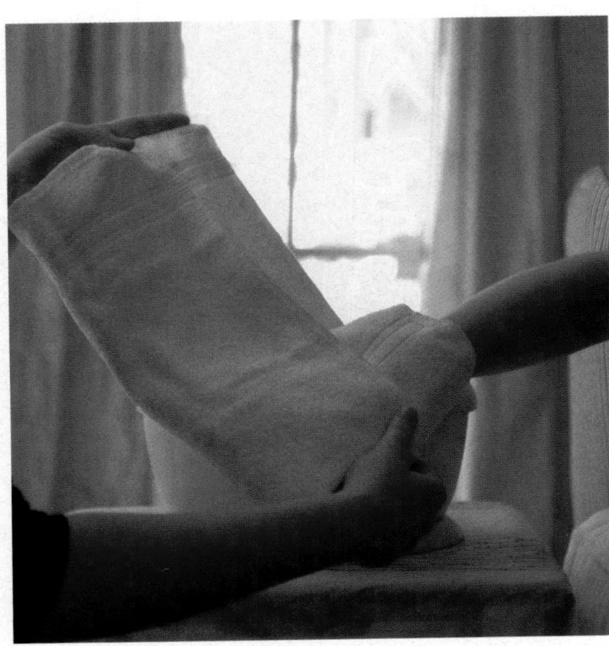

FIGURE 5–21A and B Wrapping hand in plastic and towel.

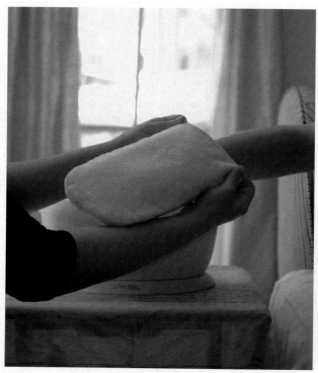

FIGURE 5–22 Wrapping hand in mitt.

5. Apply scalp massage while the paraffin remains on wrapped hands for 10 to 20 minutes (Figure 5–23).

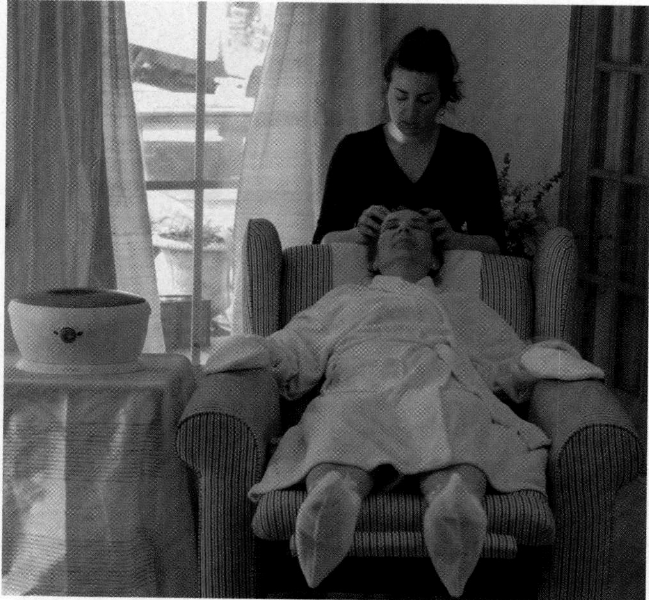

FIGURE 5–23 Apply scalp massage.

Paraffin Dip Cleanup

1. Remove the mittens/wrap and paraffin all together, starting at the wrists and wiping down toward the fingers (Figure 5–24). Most if not all of the paraffin should slip away.
2. Remove excess paraffin from the skin using a moist wash cloth or hand towel (Figure 5–25).

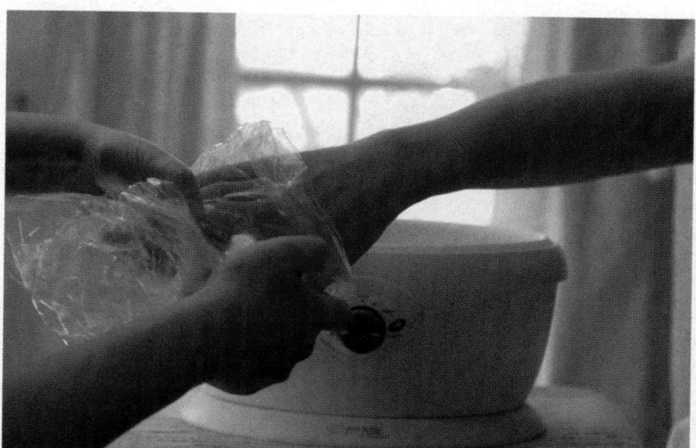

FIGURE 5–24 Removing paraffin.

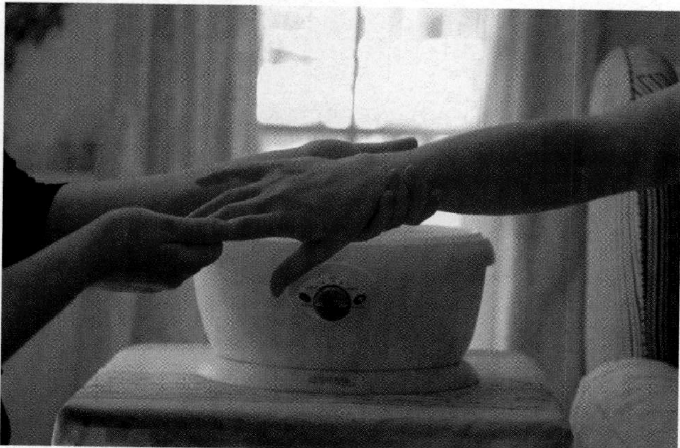

FIGURE 5–25 Cleaning excess paraffin from skin.

3. Massage lotion or cream into the hands for 5 minutes (Figure 5–26).

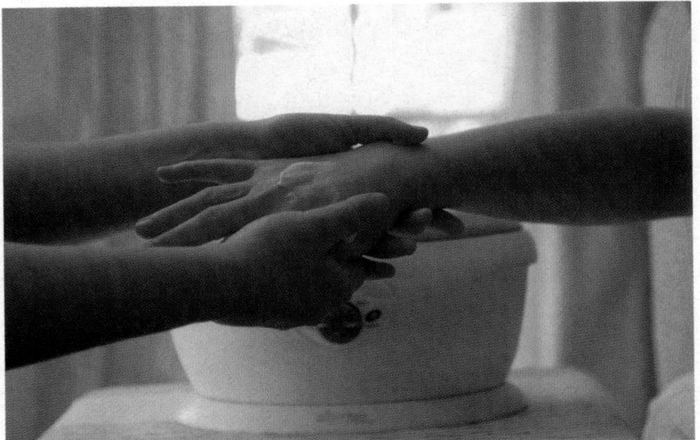

FIGURE 5–26 Massaging lotion or cream into hands after paraffin application.

SPA TIP

An alternative to the dipping basin is the paraffin pouch. The pouches are activated chemically to warm and melt the wax inside before the client slips her hand in. No heating unit is needed. The pouches are for one-time use and are disposed of after each treatment.

SPA COLD TREATMENTS

Though not as popular as heat treatments, cold treatments still have a place in the spa. The most popular cold application is the cold plunge, as mentioned in Chapter 4. Other therapies include wet sheet wraps, sunburn-relief cooling treatments, cold mitten friction, and localized applications such as the ice pack and cold compress. It must be remembered that, when it comes to cryotherapy, the main effects are created through the removal of heat from the body. These treatments are recommended, then, for reducing fever and inflammation, soothing minor sunburn, and cooling the body during and after heat applications.

These spa cold treatments also exert effects on the body through the process of retrostasis, as heat is removed from one area and sent to another. This can help relieve headaches and congestion. The intensity of the effects created through spa cold therapies depends upon several factors:

- The water temperature used in the application, which ranges from ice to 60°F.
- The duration of the cold application.

SPA TIP

In order to generate heat with cold, the wet sheet must be wrapped closely against the skin in all areas during this procedure.

fomentation

the application of hot, moist substances to the body to ease pain; also refers to the actual material applied

Did You Know?

Fomentation Use in Spas

Direct, localized moist heat applications are sometimes used when spa clients present chronic minor aches or pains, or in order to relax tissues prior to or during a massage or spa treatment. These hot applications are called **fomentations.** A fomentation describes any hot, moist substance that is applied to the body to ease pain. So, in that sense, paraffin wax could be considered a fomentation, as could an herbal wrap. However, as it is commonly used, the word almost always refers to a hot compress of some kind, such as a Thermophore® heating pad, a hydrocollator pack, a Fomentek™ bag, or simply a hot, wrung-out wash cloth. These devices, though sometimes found in spas, are more often used in therapeutic massage practices.

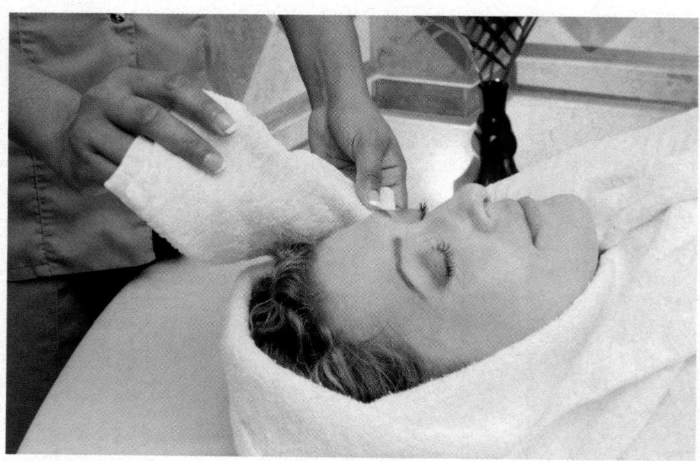

FIGURE 5–27 Cold compress being applied during spa heat treatment.

- The frequency with which the application material—wash cloth, loofah, towel, etc.—is dipped in cold water.
- In the case of cold mitten friction, the vigor of the friction applied.

Ice packs are not on most spas' treatment menus and are normally used only in case of an acute injury suffered while on the premises. They reduce swelling and pain. Cold compresses are used much more frequently by spa therapists, primarily on the forehead during heat treatments such as the herbal wrap (Figure 5–27). They are also sometimes applied to the back of the neck and chest. The compresses soothe clients and help them feel less claustrophobic during the heat application. They are also used to wipe away excess perspiration. Spas most often use wash cloths for cold compresses, but at times, small hand towels or strips of linen are used. These are kept in a bowl of ice water near the treatment table.

SPA TIP

Paraffin Self-Care for Therapists

Busy spa therapists often perform five, six, or even more hours of hard work every day, and their hands can begin to feel the strain of overuse. One trick that many therapists have found effective is to dip their hands in the paraffin bath at the end of a shift and let them soak in the penetrating warmth, soothing sore joints and muscles. This custom, combined with proper body mechanics and self-care, can improve health, quality of life, and career longevity. Always receive permission from management prior to personal use of the spa's paraffin dip.

Wet Sheet Wrap

The wet sheet wrap surprises people. The technique consists of being wrapped in a cold wet sheet, which sends shivers up most potential spa clients' spines, but once they are in the wrap they find themselves, in a surprisingly short period of time, warming up to the point of sweating. In this sense, the wet sheet wrap is both a cold and a heat treatment. Being wrapped in a cold sheet stimulates the body's heat-producing mechanisms so that, after an initial few minutes of cold, the interior of the wrap goes through a warming period until it eventually becomes hot. The wet sheet wrap, then, can be defined as having three distinct stages—cooling, neutral, and heating. Each stage has its own benefits.

During the cooling stage of the wrap, clients with fever, hot flashes, or inflammation are soothed. During the neutral stage, while the wrap is neither cold nor hot, clients relax as their bodies no longer have to produce so much heat to combat the cold temperature. This physiological relaxation leads to mental relaxation as well. Finally, the wrap heats up enough to causing sweating, which helps to purge impurities through the skin in a manner similar to, but not as intense as, the herbal wrap, which is explained in Chapter 8.

TREATMENT: WET SHEET WRAP	
Wet Room/Dry Room	dry room
Table Setup	blanket, thermal blanket, wet sheet, bath towels to tuck around head and feet
Treatment Duration	30 minutes
Needed Supplies	blanket, sheet, bolster, basin or sink for cold water, optional hot foot bath
Contraindications	oversensitivity to cold, claustrophobia, blood pressure irregularities

(Continued)

TREATMENT: WET SHEET WRAP	
Draping	special wet sheet wrapping technique shown in procedure
Treatment Order	The wet sheet wrap can be performed as a stand-alone treatment or as part of a contrast heat–cold hydrotherapy regime. Massage and other spa treatments can be administered afterward as well.
Safety, Sanitation Issues, & Clean-Up	Be sure the water for dipping sheets is not much colder than 60°F to avoid over-chilling of client. Use small amount of soap to launder sheets.
Body Mechanics & Self-Care	To protect lower back, take care not to bend too far over client when wrapping sheet. Avoid prolonged exposure of hands to extremely cold water. Warm hands intermittently during wringing if necessary.
Product Cost	none
Treatment Price	usually included as part of overall hydrotherapy program
Physiological Effects	three-tiered, with cold effects at first stimulating circulation and lowering skin temperature; then, neutral temperature relaxing mind and body; finally, heat inducing sweating and purging of impurities
Pregnancy Issues (information provided by Elaine Stillerman, LMT, author and developer of MotherMassage)	Avoid during the first trimester. Wet sheet wrapping should be kept to cooler temperatures and the sheets should fit loosely and be more of a cover than a wrap, especially on the lower extremities. At all times, the pregnant client must be positioned safely and comfortably—with her upper torso (from her hips) at an angle between 45° and 70° and her legs and feet elevated. Pillows should be placed under her neck. Heat applications are not appropriate during pregnancy.

Wet Sheet Wrap Preparation

1. Prepare a table with a blanket overlapping the head of the table by 1 foot, with a thermal blanket 3 inches from the top.
2. Optionally, have the client place his feet in a hot foot bath for 10 minutes.
3. Fill the basin with cold water and wring out the sheet.

Wet Sheet Wrap Procedure

1. Lay the wrung-out sheet atop thermal blanket.
2. Instruct the client to lie supine on the sheet, and then wrap closely against the skin in all areas for this procedure (Figures 5–28 through 5–33).
3. Place a bolster under his or her knees and allow the client to rest for 20 to 25 minutes, applying a cold compress to the forehead near the end of the wrap if the client begins perspiring. For additional heat, add more blankets atop the wrap.
4. Unwrap and assist the client off the table.
5. Offer water and help the client to a chair to relax after the treatment.

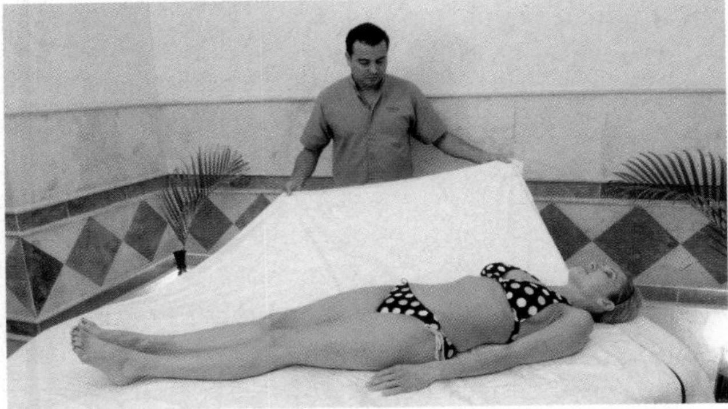

FIGURE 5–28 Lay the sheet atop the thermal blanket and have client lie upon it supine. Note shoulder position 3 inches below top of sheet.

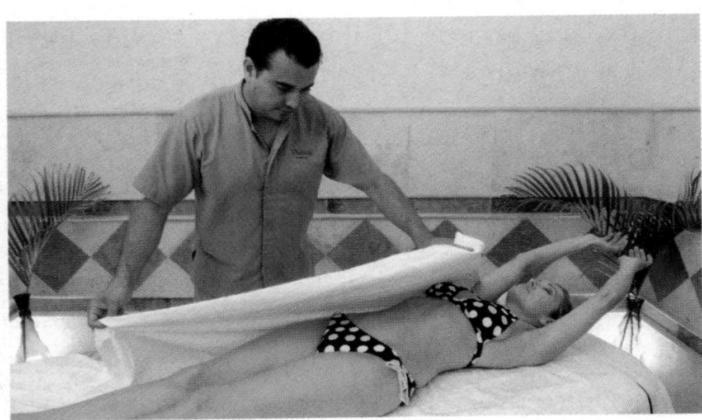

FIGURE 5–29 Client raises both hands while sheet is wrapped around the body from one side and tucked under the opposite side.

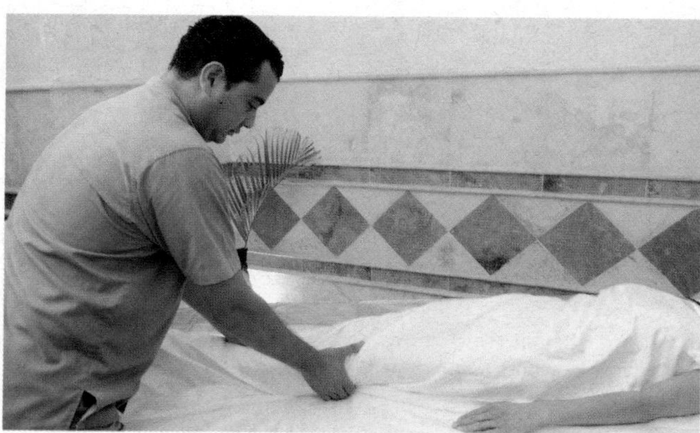

FIGURE 5–30 Client lowers hands while sheet is tucked under opposite leg.

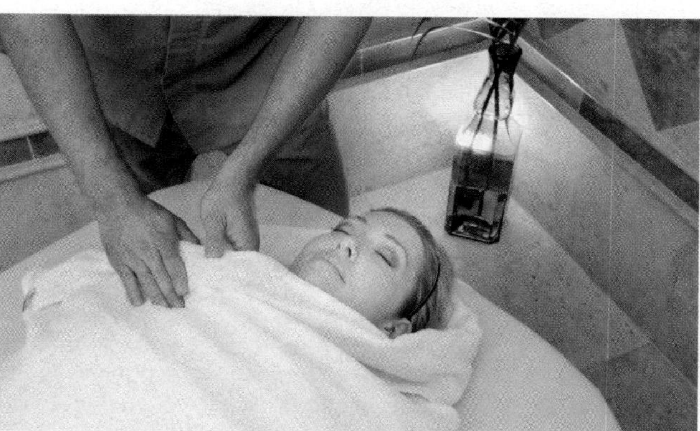

FIGURE 5–32 The blanket is then pulled up, one side at a time, over the entire body, being careful to cover the tops of the shoulders.

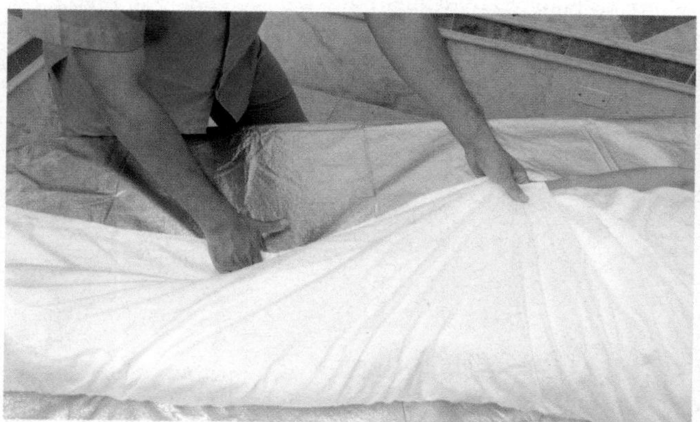

FIGURE 5–31 Pull the untucked side of the sheet up over the entire body and tuck on opposite side.

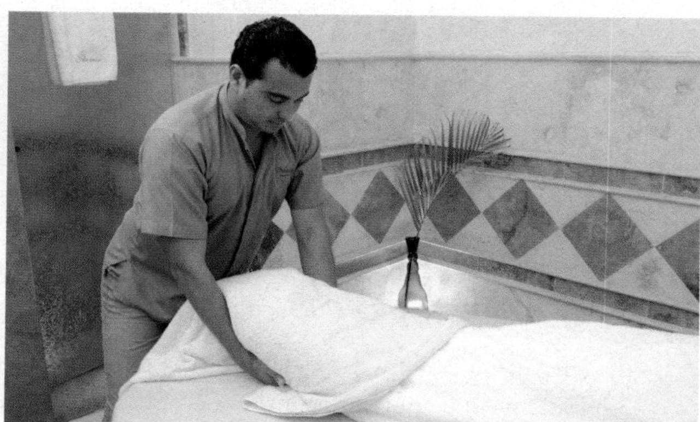

FIGURE 5–33 Bath towels can be used around neck and feet to exclude air.

Wet Sheet Wrap Cleanup

1. Launder the sheet and towels.
2. Use antiseptic spray to clean the thermal blanket.

Cold Mitten Friction

Cold mitten friction is a traditional hydrotherapy treatment used for building immune resistance and helping clients recover from fevers. It stimulates circulation and white blood cell activity and enhances tone in the neuromuscular system. Used as part of an overall hydrotherapy program in customary European style, cold mitten friction is applied in a successive program over several weeks, with colder water being applied in each consecutive treatment, starting at or above 60°F and gradually lowering in one- or two-degree increments to 50°F or below, depending on the health and strength of the client.

Cold mitten friction is extremely intense. Most U.S. spa clients would not sign up for such a treatment unless it was part of a health-improvement regime that included diet, exercise, and internal cleansing practices such as the ingesting of herbs and colonic irrigation. That being said, some individuals welcome such invigorating treatments for their toning and strengthening effects.

SPA CAUTION

As with all cold spa treatments, the wet sheet wrap has the potential to overly chill clients and make them uncomfortable. This is especially true if the client feels cold before the treatment even begins. Therefore, it is important to be sure that clients are sufficiently warm before the wet sheet wrap. Clients can immerse their feet in a hot foot bath for 10 minutes prior to the treatment in order to avoid feeling excessively chilled once it commences.

TREATMENT: COLD MITTEN FRICTION	
Wet Room/Dry Room	wet room or dry room
Table Setup	protective layer of a rubber sheet, thermal blanket or other waterproof covering, with sheets and draping towels on top
Treatment Duration	5 minutes
Needed Supplies	a basin of cold water and two loofah mitts; loofah pads or exfoliating gloves may also be substituted for loofah mitts
Contraindications	acute skin conditions, delicate skin, open cuts and abrasions, lesions, oversensitivity to cold
Draping	Use wet table draping protocol or normal massage draping.
Treatment Order	Cold mitten friction is applied as a stand-alone treatment or prior to spa heat treatments or massage.
Safety, Sanitation Issues, & Clean-Up	Do not expose more than one part of the body at a time. Make sure client does not get overly chilled. Warm client in blankets after treatment. Keep feet warm at all times.
Body Mechanics & Self-Care	Cold water and abrasive mitts can aggravate therapists' hands. Be sure to warm hands after treatments and apply emollient lotion.
Product Cost	none
Treatment Price	usually included as part of overall hydrotherapy program
Physiological Effects	stimulates circulation, stimulates metabolism, increases immune response and white blood cell activity, neuromuscular tonic
Pregnancy Issues (information provided by Elaine Stillerman, LMT, author and developer of MotherMassage)	This rigorous rubbing is not recommended on the lower extremities or anterior torso, or during the first trimester. During the second and third trimesters, arms and back may be treated carefully with the client sitting upright and draped appropriately. Prone positioning on the body support system is also appropriate.

Cold Mitten Friciton Preparation

1. Fill a basin with cold water at 40°F to 60°F, lower for each subsequent treatment.
2. Place loofah mitts in cold water.
3. Prepare the table with protective covering, sheet, and drapes.

Cold Mitten Friction Procedure

1. Ask the client to lie supine on the table, draped as for a massage or Wet Table Draping Protocol as described in Chapter 4.
2. Wring the mitts out in the cold water and put them on.
3. Uncover one area at a time and rub vigorously for 5 to 10 seconds, starting with the left leg, then the right leg, right arm, left arm, and torso (Figure 5–34). Apply a breast drape for female clients. After each area, rub vigorously with a dry towel for 3 seconds

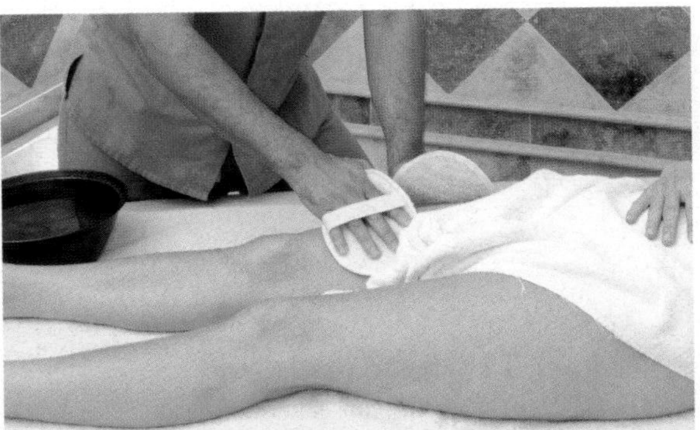

FIGURE 5–34 The therapist uses two loofah mittens dipped in cold water to apply vigorous friction for 5 to 10 seconds.

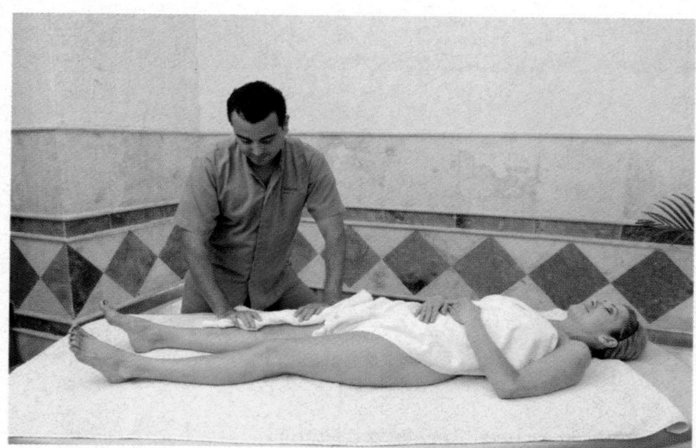

FIGURE 5–35 After cold mittens, apply a towel and use friction to dry the area.

(Figure 5–35), then re-cover, dip mitts in water again, and proceed to the next area.

4. Ask the client to turn over, and repeat the application on the backs of the legs and the back, one area at a time.
5. Have the client relax, wrapped in a blanket or warm robe, after the treatment. Offer a cup of warm herbal tea. Be sure the client is not chilled (Figure 5–36).

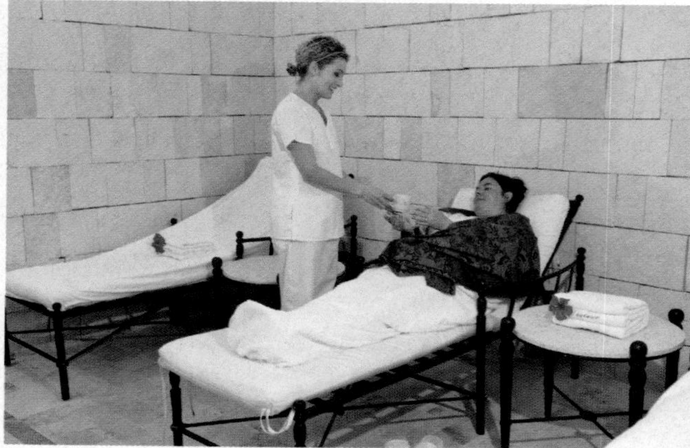

FIGURE 5–36 After cold treatments, make sure client is not chilled.

Cold Mitten Friction Cleanup

1. Empty and clean the basin.
2. Remove sheets from the table and launder them with the towels.
3. Clean the waterproof table covering with antiseptic.

Sunburn-Relief Cooling Treatments

Many spas that offer swimming pool or beach amenities also offer sunburn-relief cooling treatments. These treatments serve three main purposes: to repair damaged skin cells, to hydrate dried-out tissues, and to soothe discomfort. The products applied to the skin in such treatments are often all-natural, such as fresh aloe vera, yogurt, milk, or tea. Aloe has been used on cuts, sores, abrasions, and sunburns for many years. Its thick, soothing gel provides relief and can aid the skin in repairing sun damage. The fat and lactic acid in milk and yogurt are thought to be soothing for red, inflamed skin. Tea, in the form of brewed liquid or fresh leaves if available, is applied for its tannin content, which also helps soothe the skin. All of these natural products need to be rinsed from the skin with water after application. Often, this is followed by an application of cool compresses or even a wrap with moist, chilled sheets.

SPA TIP

St. John's wort, a popular herb said to have anti-depressant properties, has also been used as a balm for burns and to soothe nerve pain. These properties can help relieve some of the discomfort of sunburn. A tea is prepared from the plant. After the tea cools, it is used to dip compresses, which are then applied to the affected areas.

hydrosphere

the combined mass of water found on, under, and over the surface of a planet

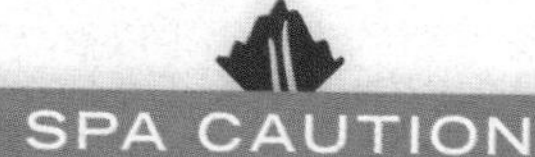

SPA CAUTION

Exfoliation is contraindicated for clients with sunburns, because sunburned skin is too sensitive to receive these treatments. If a client becomes sunburned after scheduling an exfoliation treatment, the spa should offer to change the service to a cooling treatment instead. Severe sunburns or blistering should be referred to a physician for treatment.

SPA PROFILE

100 Trillion Cells of Hydrotherapeutic Power

Richard Eidson—author, therapist, inventor, and hydrotherapy expert—is a firm believer in the power of hydrotherapy to touch people's lives on many levels. When he begins speaking about his favorite topic, his voice brightens and he launches into a well-thought-out explanation of exactly how and why spa treatments can be so effective.

"I've been able to travel a lot, fortunately," remarks Eidson, "visiting many of the great hydrotherapy centers around the world: Baden Baden. Vichy, Japan, Greece where Hippocrates lived, and Turkey, among others, and through this I've been able to develop an historical perspective on the subject. It seems to me that over time we have been gradually developing a new paradigm, a new understanding of human physiology. Finally, just now, we are starting to move away from the gross anatomy paradigm and beginning to look at the body as it truly is— this miraculous system made up of 100 trillion cells that live in an extremely dynamic fluid matrix, which is mainly water. The system is maintained by the heart pumping 3,600 gallons of blood per day out to 10 billion capillary beds where nutrients are exchanged. It's amazing when you consider the average body contains approximately 10 gallons of water. That's 84 pounds! This water creates a huge capacity for transferring heat, for movement, for buoyancy, all of which we can work with through hydrotherapy. This is the new paradigm I am most excited about, the connection between our bodies, the outer world in which our bodies exist, and the treatments we can perform to directly affect our bodies in relation to the world."

Eidson has turned his passion and his understanding of hydrotherapy into something concrete that many massage therapists use every day in their practices. As the inventor of the Steamy Wonder system, he has made it possible for countless therapists to offer hydrotherapy in a dry room setting. The Steamy Wonder is popular in spas and is mentioned several times in this book because it is such a valuable tool.

Eidson has recently developed a more advanced all-in-one hydrotherapeutic tool called the Integrated Spa System, which includes a wet table, Vichy shower, steam canopy, and massage platform. Using this new system, spa clients never get cold, therapists never get wet, and clients can stay on the same table for two or three hours at a time. He markets these to therapists and to spas all around the world, seeking to spread the benefits of hydrotherapy far and wide. "Hydrotherapeutic tools like the ones I invent for use by therapists can alter our metabolic rate 7 percent for every degree of increased temperature," he states. "So, if we can raise the core temperature from 98.6 degrees to 101.6 degrees, we're creating a 21 percent increase in circulation! This can offer outstanding benefits. As soon as you increase the temperature of the white blood cells, they become much more effective, while at the same time heat makes viruses less effective, stimulating the immune system. It is no wonder that these treatments have been a fundamental part of worldwide healing traditions for centuries. It's all based on increasing the core temperature. This is fundamental science—we're not talking about esoteric concepts here."

Eidson's book, *Hydrotherapy for Health and Wellness*, outlines a number of hands-on treatments, and in addition it offers the reader some philosophical insights into what he calls the **hydrosphere** (Figure 5–37). "We exist within and are an integral part of the Earth's self-contained watery environment," he says. "Every 20 days we naturally lose 100 pounds of water, and we have to bring that back in somehow from the outside world in the form of plain water, beverages, and food. In a way, we are large, walking, talking water filters. Students in massage school need to learn about this symbiotic relationship between our bodies and the planet, and, in my opinion, they need to do that within a well-structured hydrotherapy program."

(Continued)

SPA PROFILE

100 Trillion Cells of Hydrotherapeutic Power *continued*

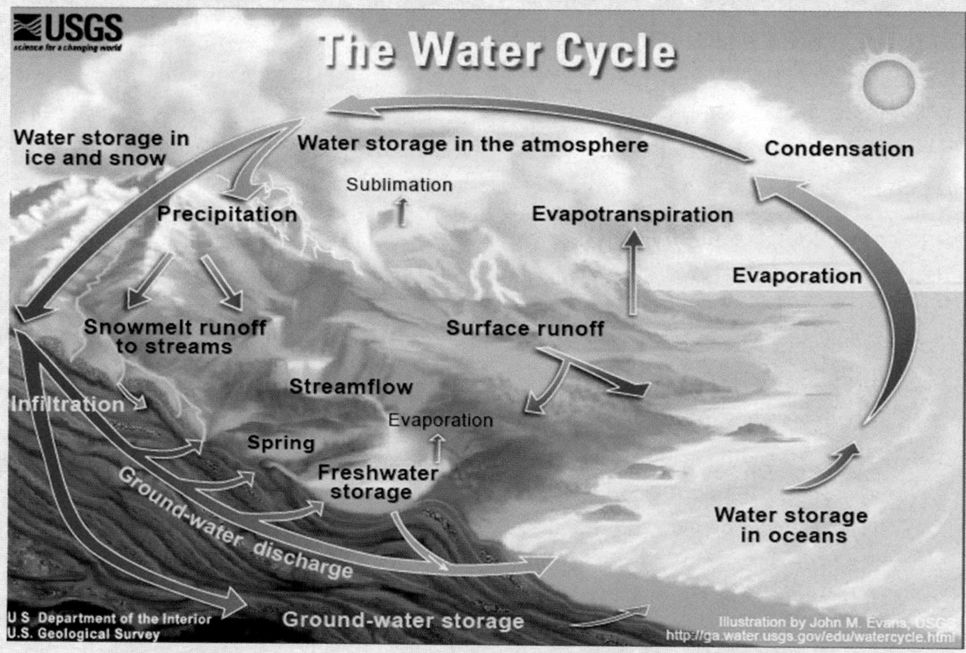

FIGURE 5–37 The hydrosphere consists of Earth's static water supply, constantly changing, of which our bodies form a part.

Being the inventor of a famous steam unit, it is no surprise that Eidson's favorite spa treatments should feature moist heat. "I believe steam treatments are very therapeutic," he says, "especially when the treatment is brought to the client on a massage table. Hydrotherapy tub treatments also have great potential benefits, and they can even be offered in a deep bathtub. As therapists become more highly trained, hydrotherapy protocols such as steam, shower, and bath treatments will become even more therapeutic. Also, they could be better combined with other spa treatments, for example massage and skincare treatments, in ways that enhance the overall wellness transformation."

After all of his spa travels, his writings on hydrotherapy and his invention of much-used spa equipment, Eidson has some very specific advice for therapists just getting into the field. "Go to Germany," he says. "They have more than 100 amazing high-tech facilities with natural mineral water, hydrotherapy treatments, and full wellness programs." (See the "Exotic Modalities" sidebar in Chapter 12 for one example.) "There, and elsewhere, we are learning more every day about the marvels of heat and cold therapies. Cryotherapy, for example, has been shown to decrease the amount of secondary hypoxic damage that takes place during heart attacks. I predict huge developments in the future use of hydrotherapy, not just in spas but in medicine as well, and all walks of life. When we increase or decrease the core temperature just a few degrees with these techniques, we can make a huge difference in peoples' lives."

As a man whose inventions and words have already literally touched the lives of thousands of people around the world, we can safely assume that Eidson's predictions may indeed come true.

RESEARCH

Exfoliation in History

Choose one of the exfoliation techniques listed in this chapter or another one of your own liking, and research its use in history. Any exfoliation technique from any culture and any time up through the first half of the twentieth century can be chosen. Write one page explaining the development, rationale, usage, and popularity of this technique.

will sink through the pores more quickly. Herbs will be able to penetrate and detoxify that much better. Essential oils will reach the blood stream with less to impede them. For this reason, exfoliation is always applied before other spa treatments, not afterwards. The skin is already in a state of natural and continuous exfoliation. Spa services simply aid and enhance this process, which is sometimes atrophied in modern people, especially those who do not engage in physical exertion or spend much time outdoors. As a secondary benefit to exfoliation, superficial circulation is stimulated. Afterwards, clients are left with skin that can literally glow. This is why these treatments are often referred to as a "salt glow" or "body glow." Not only does skin glow afterwards, it is also softer and smoother to the touch. Removing excess dead skin cells can reveal the younger and healthier-looking skin underneath.

micronized

pulverized into particles a few micrometers (millionths of a meter) in diameter

salicylic acid

the only beta hydroxy acid, common in many plants and willow bark, causes dead cells to slough off and the top layer of skin to be removed, unclogging pores

glycolic acid

translucent crystalline compound found in sugar cane, sugar beets, and unripe grapes; one of the alpha hydroxy acids

citric acid

a weak, water-soluble acid found in many fruits, especially citrus fruits; one of the alpha hydroxy acids used in chemical exfoliation products

malic acid

a colorless, crystalline solid acid found in fruits such as apples; used in some chemical exfoliants; one of the alpha hydroxy acids

trichloroacetic acid

a strong acid made by chlorinating acetic acid, used by physicians in chemical peels of the skin

Exfoliant Types

Two main categories of exfoliation treatments are used in the spa setting: mechanical and chemical. Mechanical exfoliants include **micronized** buffing beads, crushed nut shells or seed pits, sugar or salt crystals, pumice stones, abrasive cloths, and loofahs. Chemical exfoliants are comprised of compounds containing **salicylic acid**, **glycolic acid**, fruit enzymes, **citric acid**, or **malic acid**. In spas, these chemical exfoliants are typically applied by estheticians, while dermatologists and other physicians are the only ones licensed to apply powerful chemical peels using compounds such as **trichloroacetic acid**. In general, massage therapists do not receive the training needed to perform chemical exfoliation services, with the exception of small amounts of certain fruit enzymes such as papaya. This chapter, then, will cover applications of mechanical exfoliation techniques, which are the type performed by massage therapists in spas. These treatments, though similar in effect, are called by a wide variety of names, depending on the products and techniques used. See Table 6–1 for a list of common exfoliation treatment names found on spa menus. See Table 6–2 for a list of the products used in these treatments.

Salts and Sugars

Salt is the single most popular exfoliating product in use in modern spas, and the most widely used type of salt is sourced from the Dead Sea in Israel (Figure 6–3). This salt is prized for the size of its granules, which range from fine to semi-coarse (Figure 6–4). They contain high concentrations of magnesium chloride, potassium chloride, and calcium, three vitally important minerals, which soak into the pores when the salts are applied to the skin. Other types of salt can be used as well, especially sea salts, but average table salt is not

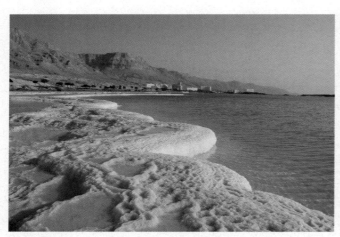

FIGURE 6–3 The Dead Sea.

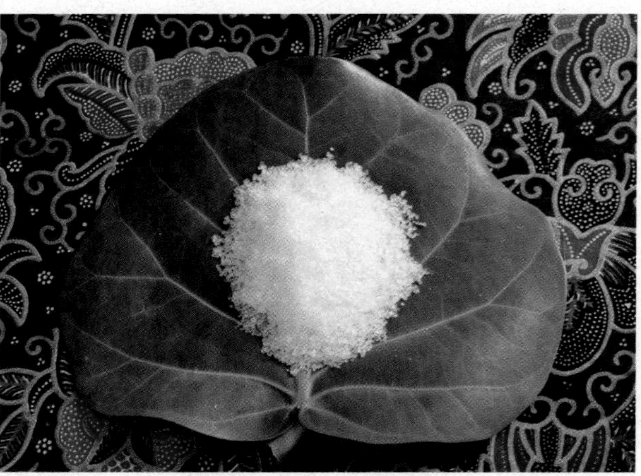

FIGURE 6–4 Dead Sea Salts are the most popular kind for spa exfoliation services.

EXFOLIATION TYPE	DESCRIPTION
Exfoliation	generic term used to describe all mechanical and chemical processes which slough away topmost layer of dead skin cells of the stratum corneum
Body Scrub	a generic term for all mechanical exfoliation services with the exception of salt
Salt Scrub	used to describe all mechanical exfoliation procedures involving the use of salt
Body Glow	used to describe all mechanical exfoliation procedures except for those involving the use of salt
Salt Glow	another term used to describe all mechanical exfoliation procedures involving the use of salt
Body Polish	used to describe all non-salt exfoliation services but particularly those applied with fine-grain exfoliants that create a gentle experience for clients
Sugar Scrub	use of sugar granules to exfoliate the skin, combining the mechanical action of granules with the chemical action of glycolic acid
Peel	used by estheticians for chemical exfoliation procedures, often incorporating alpha or beta hydroxy acids
"Ingredient" Scrub	examples include "almond scrub," "ginger scrub," "peppermint scrub," and others which cite a specific ingredient which is either the primary exfoliating agent or key component in a spa service
Dry Brushing	use of a dry bristle brush, with no water or moisturizer of any kind, to exfoliate the skin, often prior to cellulite services or body wraps, especially noted for its beneficial effects on the lymphatic system
Loofah Scrub	use of loofah mitts or pads to exfoliate, often in combination with other exfoliating agents and/or body baths
Herbal Scrub	the use of dried herbs to exfoliate the skin, often Ayurvedic in origin, sometimes applied dry, sometimes moistened
Body Gommage	a French term literally meaning "scouring" that refers to an exfoliation service incorporating a cream application that dries on the skin and is scrubbed away

TABLE 6–1 Common Spa Exfoliation Terms.

hyperemia

increased blood in an organ or other body part; can refer to reddening of the skin surface caused by spa services such as exfoliation and vigorous massage

recommended because it is too finely ground and would not provide enough friction to adequately exfoliate the skin.

Many spa clients find salt too abrasive, especially those with fair complexions and delicate skin. In this type of client, salt can cause **hyperemia** and possible discomfort. To perform exfoliation, salt must be mixed with other ingredients, typically water, massage oil, and essential oils, in order to make the

EXFOLIANT	DESCRIPTION	EFFECTS/BENEFITS	CONTRAINDICATIONS	POPULARITY
Buffing Beads	perfectly round particles of micronized polyethylene	because of their true spherical nature, these man-made beads roll more smoothly than other products over the skin, offering a gentle exfoliation	sunburn, cuts, abrasions, sores, eczema, some clients prefer not to have a synthetic exfoliant on their skin	low
Dry Bristle Brush	dry brush made of boar bristle, Tampico fiber, etc., used directly on skin to exfoliate without moisture	especially stimulating to the lymph system, helping lymph flow, improving elimination, often recommended during purification/detoxification spa programs, cellulite services, and fasting	sunburn, cuts, abrasions, sores, eczema, thin/delicate skin	low-medium
Fruit & Milk Sugars	primarily glycolic acid and lactic, commonly known as *alpha hydroxy acids* (AHAs)	used in peels, masks and creams, AHAs cause the cells of the epidermis to become "unglued," allowing the dead skin cells to slough off, making room for regrowth of new skin	sunburn, cuts, abrasions, sores, recent shaving, eczema, application makes skin extremely photosensitive so sunscreen must be used extensively	high but only among estheticians
Gloves	gloves fabricated from nylon and worn when applying exfoliation maneuvers	a gentle and simple way to exfoliate, especially over dry skin	sunburn, cuts, abrasions, sores, eczema, thin/delicate skin	low
Herbal Scrubs	powdered herbs used dry or blended with water to form a paste, popular in Ayurvedic applications	the herbs soak into the skin, providing internal benefits while exfoliating the surface	sunburn, cuts, abrasions, sores, eczema, allergies to the herbs used	medium
Jojoba Beads	tiny rounded particles of jojoba wax	softer than polyethylene buffing beads, but with similar properties of roundness for a smooth buffing experience	sunburn, cuts, abrasions, sores, eczema	medium
Loofah Granule Powder	ground powder of a dried loofah	added to cream-based exfoliants for delicate scrubbing action	sunburn, cuts, abrasions, sores, eczema	medium

TABLE 6–2 List of Typical Mechanical Exfoliant Products Used in Spa Treatments. *(Continued)*

EXFOLIANT	DESCRIPTION	EFFECTS/BENEFITS	CONTRAINDICATIONS	POPULARITY
Loofah Sponges, Mitts, & Pads	the dried, fibrous part of the gourd-like fruit of a plant of the genus *Luffa*	the naturally abrasive honeycomb-like structure of this dried fruit makes an efficient exfoliating tool when used whole or fashioned into mitts and pads	sunburn, cuts, abrasions, sores, eczema, thin/delicate skin	high
Nut Meal	the finely ground shells of certain nuts, commonly almond and walnut	when added to a moisturizing exfoliant, the tiny shell particles add friction to scrub dead skin cells from the surface	sunburn, cuts, abrasions, sores, eczema, allergies to nuts used	high
Pumice	a volcanic glass full of cavities and very light in weight formed on the surface of some lavas; used as an abrasive	pumice stones often used in salons during the pedicure process to remove dry and excess skin from the bottom of the foot and also calluses	sunburn, cuts, abrasions, sores, eczema, thin/delicate skin	high with manicurists and cosmetologists but lower with massage therapists
Salt	often from the Dead Sea, but also from other areas, salts prized for their buffing properties, sometimes combined with oils and other therapeutic ingredients	use of salt crystals of various sizes and consistencies for mechanical exfoliation combined with penetration of beneficial minerals into the skin	sunburn, cuts, abrasions, sores, eczema, allergies, recent shaving, thin/delicate skin	high
Seed Meal	the finely ground shells of certain fruit seeds, commonly apricot and peach	when added to a moisturizing exfoliant, the tiny seed particles add friction to scrub dead skin cells from the surface	sunburn, cuts, abrasions, sores, eczema, allergies to fruits used	high
Silica Particles	finely ground sand-like compound used in microdermabrasion machines which shoot them out under high-pressure to remove dead skin cells; aluminum oxide, zinc oxide, and other particles are also used	effectively scours the skin of dead cells, usually used by estheticians on the face only, a treatment that can be powerful enough to cause scarring if used improperly	sunburn, cuts, abrasions, sores, eczema, allergies, thin/delicate skin	high with estheticians but not used by therapists
Sugar Granules	large-grain sugar often used in combination with oils and other therapeutic ingredients	combines mechanical exfoliating effects of sugar crystals with chemical effects of glycolic acid	sunburn, cuts, abrasions, sores, eczema	high

TABLE 6–2 List of Typical Mechanical Exfoliant Products Used in Spa Treatments.

salt easier to work with on the skin. Dry salts are overly abrasive. Salts are typically mixed with these additives prior to application to the skin. However, in some cases, especially in wet rooms where a large supply of water is available, the skin is thoroughly wet first and then dry salts are applied, mixing with the moisture already on the body.

Occasionally salts are combined with other exfoliants, such as corn meal or jojoba buffing beads, for example, to create a dual-layered effect, the salt acting as the more abrasive product and the other ingredient adding a softer feel that still scrubs the skin. Some products contain two or three sizes of salt grains in the same scrub, claiming that the larger grains slough away the majority of dead skin cells and then the smaller grains polish and refine the skin further. In general, the larger the salt grain, the more intense the exfoliating action will be.

Sugar

Sugar is used as an exfoliant in many spas. It is not as abrasive as salt, except for those cases in which extra-large sugar granules are used. The sugar crystals have the same exfoliating action as salt crystals, with two notable differences: (1) They do not contain the minerals that salts do and therefore do not offer the mineralizing benefits of salt, but (2) they do contain naturally occurring glycolic acid, one of the **alpha hydroxy acids** (AHAs), which helps to eat away dead skin cells as well as scrub them away. Sugar is often blended with aromatic essential oils and ingredients such as honey to create a luxurious exfoliation experience for spa clients.

alpha hydroxy acids

a wide range of exfoliants, such as glycolic acid and malic acid derived from fruit and milk sugars; they unglue dead skin cells from the surface, allowing them to slough off; best used on thickened, sun-damaged skin without oily buildup

Nut and Seed Meals

Almond, walnut, and other nut shells, as well as fruit seeds such as apricot and peach—ground down to a size smaller than a grain of sand—are often added to a moisturizing base to form gentle exfoliants. Sometimes they are used as the sole scrubbing agent, and in other products they are blended with a number of exfoliants. The tiny, irregularly shaped particles rub against the skin, pulling dead cells along with them during the exfoliation process. In some products, soaps or body baths are included to add a cleansing effect to the exfoliation process.

Herbal Scrubs

Herb powders, when moistened and applied to the skin in paste form, eventually dry and form a hard flaky layer that can be rubbed away with the hands and fingers, creating a gentle exfoliation with the added health benefits afforded by the herbs soaking into the pores. **Ayurvedic** herbs are often used in this process. Thought not as popular as wet herbal pastes, some exfoliation procedures use dry powdered herbs directly on the skin.

Ayurvedic

referring to the holistic alternative medicine that is the traditional system of medicine of India

Body Gommage

A process more typically employed by estheticians on the face, the gommage process involves the use of cream-like products that dry on the skin and are then buffed away with the palms and fingers, exfoliating the skin in the process. These body products are typically offered by European spa or cosmetic companies that have a strong emphasis on beauty.

Loofah

The loofah (also spelled l-u-f-f-a) is a multipurpose exfoliation tool (Figure 6–5). It is used in its natural state or manufactured into a number of shapes such as

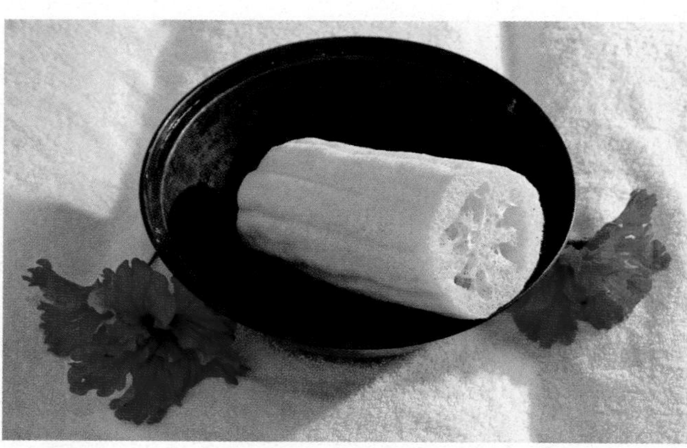

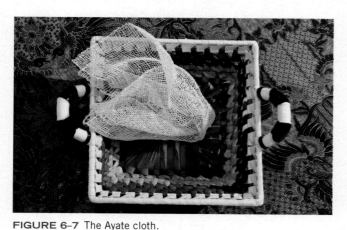

FIGURE 6–5 Loofah, fruit of an annual tropical vine, genus Luffa.

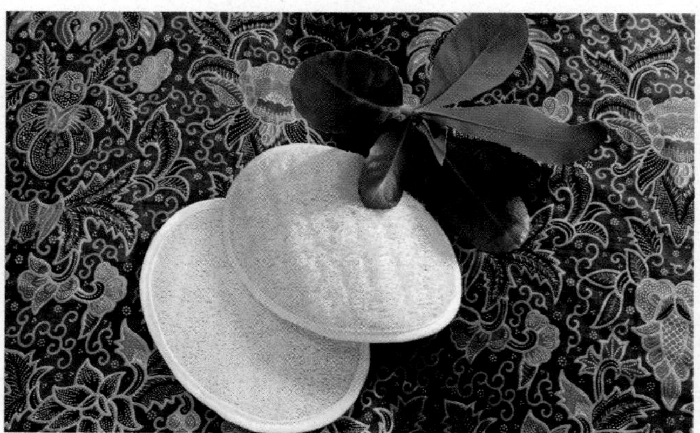

FIGURE 6–6 Loofah is made into several exfoliating tools.

SPA CAUTION

Loofahs can harbor bacteria and must be thoroughly sanitized after each use if they are to be used on multiple clients. Loofah mitts and pads are often meant for one-time use and given to clients afterwards, which avoids the sanitation issue.

pads and mitts (Figure 6–6). It is also ground into a fine powder and added to other ingredients to form exfoliating creams. The term "loofah sponge" is often used, but the loofah is actually a fruit. It grows on a vine in the tropics. When dried out, the "skeleton" of fibrous tissue left behind inside the fruit is what we sometimes call a loofah sponge or shower sponge. Loofahs can be quite abrasive and should be used with caution at first until spa clients' tolerance is ascertained. They are more abrasive when used dry, as they are in many pre-wrap procedures. When used wet, they can provide a more gentle exfoliation.

Ayate Cloths

Ayate cloth is made from the agave cactus in Mexico (Figure 6–7). When used dry, the cloth exfoliates and stimulates circulation. When soaked in water, it turns smooth and can be used to wash the body after exfoliation. The use of these cloths is popular at Southwestern U.S. spas. They are similar to **sisal** cloths, also made from agave cacti.

FIGURE 6–7 The Ayate cloth.

Exfoliating Gloves

One of the simplest ways to exfoliate the skin is to don a pair of exfoliating gloves and to run them over the skin using the exfoliation maneuvers described in this chapter (Figure 6–8). These gloves can be easily incorporated into a regular massage service, as they do not require any water to work. They are also inexpensive and can be offered to clients after each treatment.

A special type of exfoliating glove, **garshana gloves** are used in an Ayurvedic spa service called *garshan massage*. This consists of a dry lymphatic brushing with the gloves, which are made of raw silk. The procedure is often incorporated into a full regime of Ayurvedic practices as part of a lifestyle program. See Chapter 12 for more information about Ayurvedic spa services.

Ayate

fiber from the agave cactus used to make exfoliating cloths for spa services; also see *sisal*

sisal

fiber from the agave cactus used to make exfoliating cloths for spa services; also see *ayate*

Pumice Stone

Whole pumice stones are not generally used by massage therapists for full-body exfoliation services. They are more popular with manicure and pedicure specialists for use on the hands and feet. However, ground pumice is often used as a key

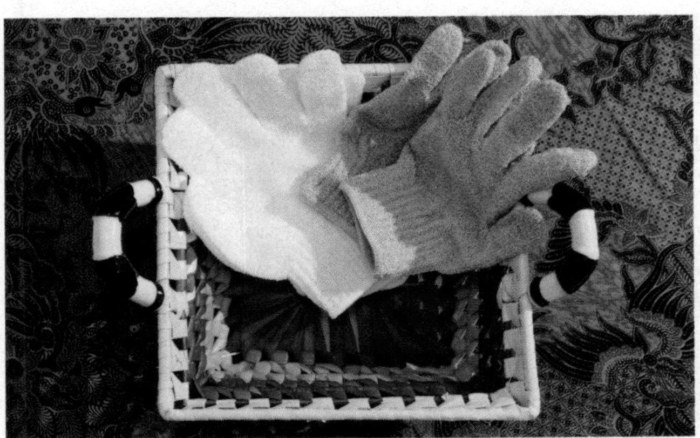

FIGURE 6–8 Exfoliation gloves.

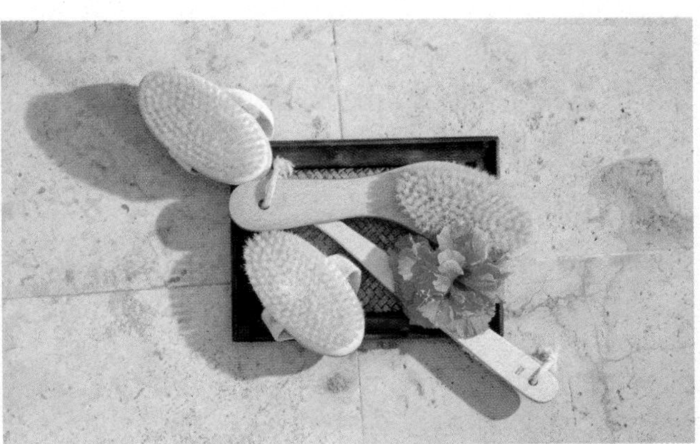

FIGURE 6–9 The dry bristle brush exfoliates the skin and stimulates lymph flow.

ingredient in body exfoliating mixtures. Pumice is an extremely lightweight and fine buffing material. Its source is a kind of solidified foam formed from volcanic eruptions and magma flow. Once formed, pumice is so light that it floats on water.

garshana gloves

silk gloves used for exfoliation in Ayurvedic healing tradition

Dry Bristle Brush

The dry bristle brush (Figure 6–9) is often used for short, full-body exfoliations, with a duration of only 5 to 10 minutes, immediately preceding product applications and spa body wraps. When used this way, the brushing is incorporated into the treatment, with no additional fee charged to the spa client. Also, some spas offer stand-alone dry bristle brush exfoliation services, which usually last half an hour. These are charged separately. Dry bristle brushing has two main benefits for the spa client: exfoliation and stimulation of lymph flow. Bristle brushes are made from a variety of sources, including goat hair, boar bristle, **Tampico fiber**, and coconut fiber. Some brushes are more abrasive than others, so care has to be taken when using them with spa clients. Bristle brushing is always applied dry—see the protocol later in this chapter.

Tampico fiber

made from the agave lechugilla plant found in Mexico, fiber used in exfoliating brushes with a high liquid absorption rate and a rough texture created by calcium oxalate crystals embedded in the surface

Buffing Beads

Many exfoliating spa products incorporate buffing beads. These tiny spheres can be synthetic, as in the case of polyethylene buffing beads which are made from plastic, or organic, as with jojoba buffing beads, which are fashioned from jojoba wax. They roll over the surface of the skin, as opposed to abrading it, as do most rough-ground nut and seed meals, as well as sugar and salt granules. This makes buffing beads one of the gentlest of all exfoliants, and as such the beads are incorporated into many products.

beta hydroxy acid

salicylic acid, a lipid-soluble exfoliant able to penetrate into pores which contain sebum in order to dislodge the dead skin cells there; best used on oily skin with blackheads and whiteheads

Alpha Hydroxy Acids

Though not generally applied by massage therapists, low concentrations of AHAs are sometimes included in the formulas for widely used cream-based exfoliants. Therapists, therefore, should be familiar with their properties and effects. Alpha hydroxy acids are derived from fruit and milk sugars. The five main types of AHAs found in spa exfoliation products and their sources are listed in Table 6–3. The only **beta hydroxy acid** is salicylic acid. It is oil-soluble

ALPHA HYDROXY ACID	SOURCE
glycolic acid	sugar cane
lactic acid	milk
malic acid	apples and pears
citric acid	oranges and lemons
tartaric acid	grapes

TABLE 6–3 Five Main Alpha Hydroxy Acids.

Extreme Exfoliation

Did You Know?

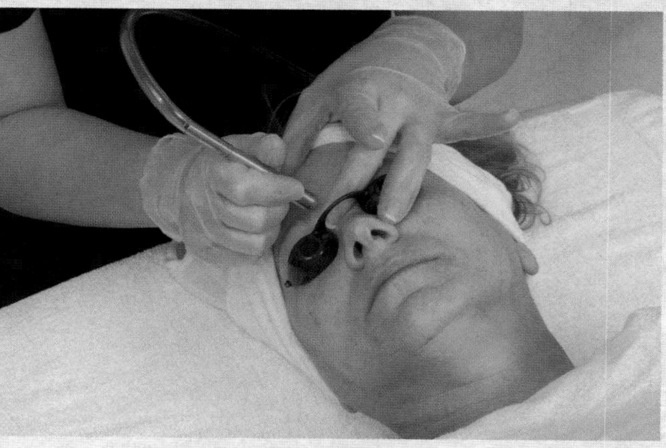

FIGURE 6–10 Microdermabrasion is an extreme form of exfoliation used in some spas.

Microdermabrasion (Figure 6–10) and **laser skin resurfacing** are extreme cases of exfoliation that are offered in some spas, usually medical day spas. In microdermabrasion, the stratum corneum is partially or completely removed by light abrasion created by a pressurized stream of zinc oxide, aluminum oxide crystals, silica, or other fine particles, or sometimes with a roughened surface. These particles and the removed skin cells are suctioned away. The procedure is used to remove sun-damaged skin and to improve the appearance of scars and dark spots. It is not very painful, requires no anesthetic, and can be performed by a trained technician. **Dermabrasion** refers to a more extreme medical procedure carried out under anesthesia to remove tattoos or scars. A physician must, of course, be present to perform this procedure, which is also the case for laser skin resurfacing, sometimes called a *laser peel*. In this procedure, a carbon dioxide (CO_2) laser is used to remove, layer by layer, areas of damaged skin, scarring, uneven pigmentation, wrinkles, and fine lines.

ACTIVITY

Comparing Exfoliants

Different exfoliants offer spa clients a wide array of sensations and results from which to choose. Knowledgeable spa therapists should be able to inform clients about the nuances of these sensations and results, aiding them in choosing a product or procedure. While the spa's menu should offer an adequate description, nothing beats a first-person recommendation. A spa therapist, in this regard, can be like a sommelier in a fine restaurant, guiding patrons to the most rewarding experience. In order for you to be able to adequately describe various exfoliation products, you must, of course, experience them for yourself. In this activity, you will choose just two products to start with and compare them on your skin. Later, expand your horizons by trying a wide range of exfoliation procedures. Any two products will do, as long as they are substantially different from each other. You would not, for instance, choose an almond body scrub and a walnut body scrub. Good choices for contrast and comparison include:

loofah mitt vs. dry bristle brush
seed meal vs. sugar
nut meal vs. sea salt
herbal scrub vs. gloves

Once you have chosen your two exfoliants, either apply them yourself, one to each arm, or work with a partner and apply one to each leg, using the exfoliation strokes described in this chapter. Spend several minutes on each extremity in order to fully experience the sensations created by each. Note the difference between the two. Afterwards, write a paragraph describing these differences and how you would explain them to spa guests.

and thus able to penetrate into pores, which contain sebum, and release the dead skin cells there, making it especially effective at treating oily skin with pimples. AHAs, in comparison, are water-soluble.

AHAs cause dead skin cells on the skin's surface to become "unglued," allowing them to slough off. Some practitioners claim that AHAs can, over time, improve the appearance of wrinkles as well as rough, sun-damaged skin. According to FDA guidelines, spa clients can purchase retail products containing small amounts of alpha hydroxy acids at concentrations of 10% or less. Estheticians can use AHAs with concentrations of 20% to 30%, and physicians can use alpha hydroxy acid products that have concentrations of 50% to 70%. The higher the concentration, the longer-lasting the effects, but more irritation, redness, itching, and pain can occur as well. Another major side effect is sun sensitivity. All spa clients who receive exfoliation with AHA products need to have a good sunscreen with UVA and UVB protection applied as well, either within the exfoliant mixture itself or in addition to it. This also applies to retail AHAs sold to the client for use at home.

microdermabrasion

an exfoliation procedure usually performed on the face, in which the stratum corneum is partially or completely removed by light abrasion created by a pressurized stream of zinc oxide, aluminum oxide crystals, or other fine particles, or sometimes with a roughened surface

laser skin resurfacing

procedure in which a laser is used to remove areas of damaged skin, scarring, uneven pigmentation, wrinkles, and fine lines

THE SKIN AND HOW EXFOLIATION AFFECTS IT

Human skin consists of two distinct layers (Figure 6–11). The deeper layer, called the **dermis**, is filled with nerve endings, capillaries, sweat glands, sebaceous glands, and hair follicles. The superficial layer, called the **epidermis**, comprises only a small fraction of the skin's total thickness, less than 1/200th of an inch thick in most places. Yet, of course, it is this thinnest of layers that most of us think about when we think about the skin. It is the visible part, the part we touch when we reach out to make contact with another person. It is also the part on which spa therapists work during exfoliation services.

The entire epidermis is regenerated every two weeks. It consists of four or five layers—one layer exists only in the palms and soles. These are, from deepest

dermabrasion

medical procedure that involves anesthetizing the skin surface, then sanding or wire brushing an area to remove tattoos or scars; carried out under anesthesia

dermis

the deep, vascular, inner layer of the skin

epidermis

thin, outermost layer of the skin, above the dermis, itself consisting of four or five layers

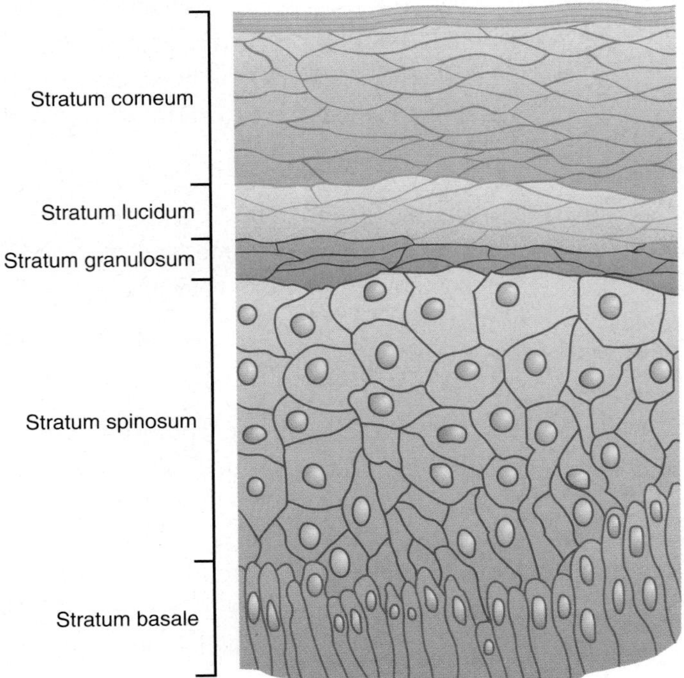

FIGURE 6–11 Cross section of the skin. The stratum basal layer is where keratinocytes are formed, which gradually move up and die, to be shed in desquamation to stratum corneum.

SPA PROFILE

Susan Wheeler, Spa Director, The Spa at the Equinox

"Exfoliation is a key part of the spa experience here for our guests, our therapists, and for me, too," states Susan Wheeler, spa director at the Equinox Resort and Spa in Manchester Village, Vermont. "In fact, my personal philosophy is that when you go away to a spa for retreat or renewal, the first thing you should do is cleanse. This tradition goes back to the ancient rituals of Japan and other great bathing cultures. So, when people ask me or my therapists our advice regarding which treatment to receive first, we always recommend exfoliation, especially if the guest is going to be here for a period of time and have a variety of therapies. Literally and figuratively, exfoliation prepares you to receive everything else the spa has to offer—the creams, oils and natural products—plus it prepares you to receive the spiritual benefits of rest and renewal found at a spa such as ours. We do not have a specific program to induce a sense of spiritual renewal. Here, it just happens. We give you the tools—but you make the discoveries. Exfoliation can play a part in that."

The therapists on staff at the Equinox find that performing exfoliation services offers a certain degree of renewal for their own bodies as well. "Most therapists love performing these treatments because they are relatively easy on your body and they offer a break between back-to-back massages," says Wheeler. "I think that taking care of therapists' health like this is extremely important. With exfoliation, you don't have to grind the scrubbing particles hard into the skin. You have to be gentle. Certain areas like bottoms of feet have calluses that need to be treated more vigorously, but in general, as far as exfoliation goes, gentle is best."

Wheeler has created a long-lasting career at the Equinox. "I've been here for 20 years," she says, "during which I've helped develop amenities, treatment menus, and product mixes. But more than anything, it is the heart and soul of the place that matter. The elusive quality of 'spirit' is the most important thing for spas today. A spa director can buy anything—fancy showers, expensive products, high-tech equipment, you name it—but you can't buy spirit, and that's what this spa has. A lot of it has to do with the beautiful environment we have in Vermont. Most spas have to work very hard to achieve what we already have naturally. We are a green environment, every hue of green that's in the world."

The products that Wheeler has chosen for the exfoliation treatments at the Equinox reflect that naturally beautiful environment. "We use the B. Kamins line, which is based on maple, which of course is indigenous to the area," she notes. "When people think of Vermont they think of maple, but they may not know that maple sugar has lots of wonderful influences on the skin, and it's also one of those products that very few people are allergic to. It's gentle but not too gentle. It's our signature scrub. We also carry other exfoliating products, such as salt, because people have varied preferences. We try to have many scrubs available at all times. Every once in a while we have to make a quick trip to the health food store to get a certain ingredient!

"Our clients choose which scrub they want every single time they sign up for exfoliation. Not everyone's skin is the same, so it would be very presumptuous for me to have just one product.

(Continued)

keratinocytes

skin cells found in the epidermis, generated in the stratum basale and eventually moving up to the stratum corneum, where they are shed through natural means or through exfoliation services

to most superficial: the stratum basale, the stratum spinosum, the stratum granulosum, the stratum lucidum—only present in thick skin such as palms of hand and soles of feet—and the stratum corneum. Cells called **keratinocytes** are generated in the stratum basale and gradually move outward to die and form the waterproof, resistant protein called *keratin*. Eventually, this substance flakes off naturally in a process called **desquamation**. Spa exfoliation procedures, then, are a type of therapist-aided desquamation in which keratinocytes are purposefully swept away from the stratum corneum.

SPA PROFILE *Susan Wheeler, Spa Director, The Spa at the Equinox* continued

Depending on your skin type and what you're looking for, we have something for everyone. Scrubs actually take off your dead skin cells, after all! This is important. Our therapists analyze what's needed for each guest and recommend the appropriate product. I try to empower the therapists to use their analytical skills in that way and to take charge of the situation. Just because someone booked a certain treatment, that's not what they always get. We try to guide them. Guests going in to estheticians for facial treatments are analyzed so much, but not when they go to massage therapists for body treatments. That's not proper. Our team is good at analyzing people. To use salt on someone who's fair and has delicate skin would probably not be what they need, for example."

Wheeler has found that most therapists enjoy being part of the spa body treatment staff and have no problem performing exfoliation services. Occasionally, though, therapists have requested to opt out for specific reasons. Some, for example, prefer not to get wet. Wheeler will still hire a therapist who does not do exfoliation services, as long as the therapist's massage and teamwork skills are strong enough, but she has had to make that choice only rarely. "Therapists in general are great," she says, "and the most important quality I look for in them is the ability to work as part of our whole spa team. The clientele that comes here can go anywhere they want, and our mission is to give them a truly meaningful experience. They'll forget other things—but they're not going to let go of the memories, of the experience they've had. Our therapists are a big part of that, whether they're performing massage or any other service. They have the power to turn a simple exfoliation treatment into an unforgettable experience of cleansing, renewal and awakening."

Menu of Exfoliation Services at the Spa at the Equinox

- **Body Exfoliation:** A pure sea salt, maple, or citrus scrub. Brings your skin to a radiant glow; the warm rain of the Vichy shower relaxes the mind and body; and a rich body cream is massaged into the skin for a smooth touch.
- **Skin Rejuvenation:** A gentle exfoliation followed by a soothing massage with warm blended essential oils.
- **The Autumnal Ritual:** Inspired by the Egyptian rituals, this full-body treatment is a delicate combination of pure gold mineral and Egyptian chamomile. Allow yourself to be transformed from head to toe as you are exfoliated, enveloped, and massaged in a golden hue that will leave you relaxed and rejuvenated.
- **Equinox Legend:** Reconnect to nature by discovering the essences that speak most profoundly to your own spirit. In this very special treatment, designed exclusively for The Spa, your therapist will assist you in choosing from an exotic selection of fragrance infused sugars, salts, and crushed nuts. You'll then choose a mask from an array of mud, seaweed, and oils to enhance your wrap. And finally, you will select your own finishing moisturizer of essential blended oils or fine hydrating lotions. The Legend is ever-changing, ever-renewing, uniquely personal, and awakens your spirit.

Spa clients frequently ask how often they should receive an exfoliation service. They wonder if too many exfoliations will be bad for their skin. It should be remembered that the body has its own innate wisdom; if nature did not intend for dead skin cells to remain on its surface, they would fall off by themselves—which, in fact, they do. In that regard, exfoliation is natural and should be encouraged, and even aided, by our efforts in the spa. However, a certain amount of dead skin cells need to remain on the body to act as a barrier against light and heat energy and to protect against water loss, microorganisms, and many chemicals. As you can see,

desquamation

peeling off in scales; from the Latin *desquamare,* which means "to scrape the scales off a fish;" used when referring to the natural process of shedding dead skin cells, as compared to the mechanical or chemical process of exfoliation

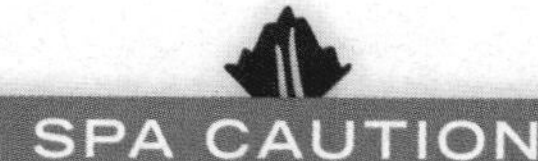

SPA CAUTION

Exfoliation Major Contraindications

Exfoliation treatments are safe under almost all circumstances for almost all clients. However, the following conditions are contraindicated and should be noted on spa intake forms. If no intake form is used, spa therapists should ask clients about these conditions prior to performing an exfoliation.

Exfoliation Contraindication 1: Sunburn

Sunburned skin is much too sensitive to receive exfoliation services.

Exfoliation Contraindication 2: Cuts, Abrasions, or Sores

Exfoliants, especially salt, can seep into openings in the skin and produce painful reactions. In addition, the abrasive action used in exfoliation can pull injured tissues, further damaging them.

Exfoliation Contraindication 3: Eczema

Eczema and all inflammatory conditions of the skin, including rashes, should be avoided.

Exfoliation Contraindication 4: Recent Shaving

Never perform exfoliation on an area of the body that has been recently shaved. This is true for the use of all exfoliants, which may irritate the area, but it is especially important regarding salt, which can cause severe discomfort and burning sensations. Allow 12 to 24 hours to pass after shaving or depilation before applying salt.

Exfoliation Contraindication 5: Allergies

Some clients may have an allergy to certain products used in exfoliation preparations, especially those containing nut meals such as almond or walnut. Allergies and sensitivities to any products used in exfoliants need to be ascertained prior to beginning the treatment during the intake process. See the intake form in Chapter 3, Figure 3–25. If this allergy was not discovered prior to treatment and an allergic response such as a rash, redness, itching, or pain occurs, stop the treatment, cleanse the product from the area and have a nurse or physician check the reaction as soon as possible.

Exfoliation Contraindication 6: Delicate Skin

Older skin or skin damaged by overexposure or weakened by disease should not be aggressively exfoliated. However, gentle exfoliation with mild products or soft exfoliation devices can usually be tolerated.

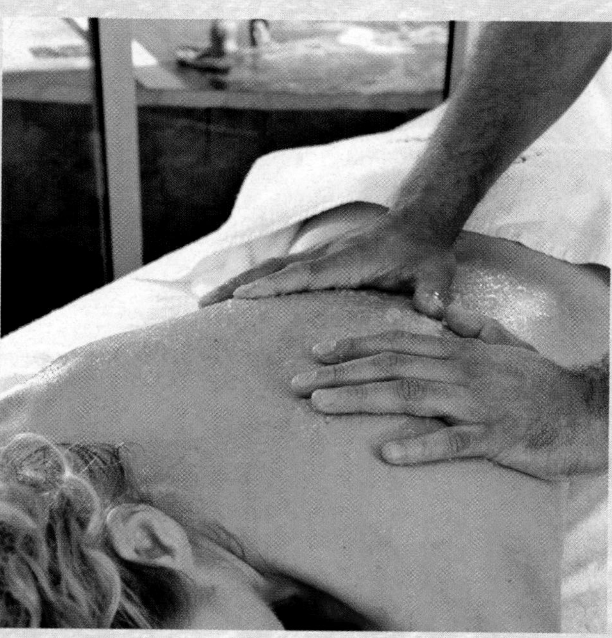

FIGURE 6–12

SPA TIP

If you see the skin start to redden a bit during an exfoliation treatment, do not be alarmed. This hyperemia is completely natural, especially for those people with fair complexions, and it is nothing to worry about. If someone is extremely sensitive, though, a gentler exfoliant should be applied. In rare cases, when using nut meal exfoliants and certain essential oils, an allergy or sensitivity may be to blame. If so, the treatment should be stopped, the exfoliant should be washed from the skin, and a nurse or physician should be called to check the reaction if it does not disappear immediately.

SPA ETIQUETTE

Treatment Room Temperature for Exfoliation Services

The water applied to clients' skin during exfoliation services creates a chilling effect that far exceeds mere temperature alone. Thus, a treatment room at 77°F could feel perfectly comfortable for a client receiving a massage, while the same temperature would feel extremely cold for a client experiencing exfoliation with wet towels or a shower. Clients receiving exfoliation services may begin shivering in rooms that feel comfortable or even warm to the therapists working in them. Good technique and high-quality exfoliation ingredients cannot compensate for the discomfort caused by low temperatures. To avoid this problem, therapists need to make sure that showers used in exfoliation rooms are kept at skin temperature (91°F) or above, depending on the temperature of the room. The hotter the room, the cooler the water can be while still maintaining client comfort, but the water should never drop below 91°F. Wrung-out towels need to be hot to the touch. Also, exfoliants themselves should be kept warm, especially if the treatment room is cool. Spa clients do not want to pay to have cold salt slathered on their skin. Exfoliants can be warmed in the same manner as massage oils, either placed beneath a stream of hot water, heated in a bottle warmer, nestled among hot towels in a roaster or towel cabbie, or floated atop hot water in a hydrocollator or other heating device. The air temperature in the exfoliation room should be a minimum of 82°F. Even though this will cause some therapists to sweat somewhat while administering a treatment, the client's comfort and health are paramount and should be respected.

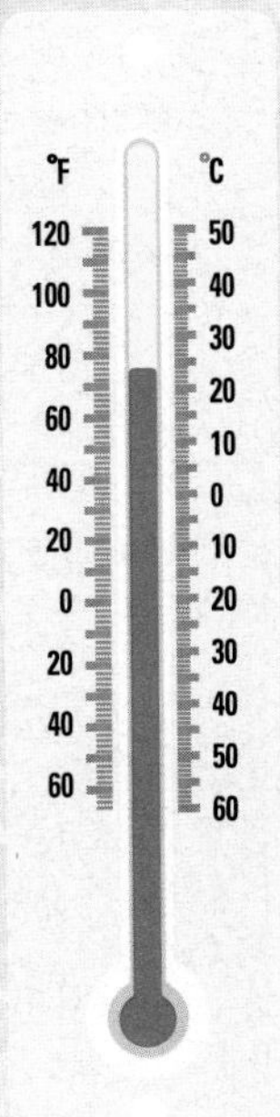

FIGURE 6-13

it would not be beneficial to constantly scrape dead skin cells off. An occasional sloughing, though, especially when combined with other nourishing, replenishing treatments, can actually help the skin in its constant process of renewal. Most spa visitors receive exfoliation once a week, perhaps two or three times if the exfoliation is included within a larger service such as a body wrap or cellulite treatment. Any more than this may be overdoing it for full-body exfoliations. The exception to this is the application of a daily exfoliator, usually meant for the face.

WET ROOM AND DRY ROOM EXFOLIATION TECHNIQUES

This section offers three distinct protocols, one for performing exfoliation services in a dry room, one for performing exfoliation services in a wet room, and one for a dry brushing procedure. An exfoliating procedure using Ayurvedic

The Exfoliation Stroke

Did You Know?

The actual manipulation you will perform during exfoliation services is not like any of the massage strokes you typically learn in school. In fact, it is sometimes more difficult to train experienced massage therapists in the art of exfoliation than it is to teach beginning therapists or non-therapists. This is due to the fact that experienced therapists have become accustomed to applying massage strokes to the body, strokes that aim to affect the tissues beneath the skin, not the skin itself. It is sometimes difficult for therapists to "think surface" because they are so used to "thinking depth." When it comes time to perform an exfoliation service, often their tendency is to palpate the underlying tissues rather than focus on the maneuvers required to skillfully remove the uppermost layers of dead skin cells in the stratum corneum (Figures 6–14 and 6–15).

In order to perfect the exfoliation stroke, therapists need to become comfortable working on the surface, at least temporarily. There are three primary components of successful exfoliation strokes:

1. They are applied in a circular motion so as not to pull delicate skin fibers too far in one direction or another.
2. They are applied with the palms and fingers open and flat.
3. They are applied with "gentle but firm" pressure in order to create a pleasurable scrubbing sensation and to effectively scour dead skin cells from the surface. This type of stroke also helps stimulate circulation of blood and lymph.

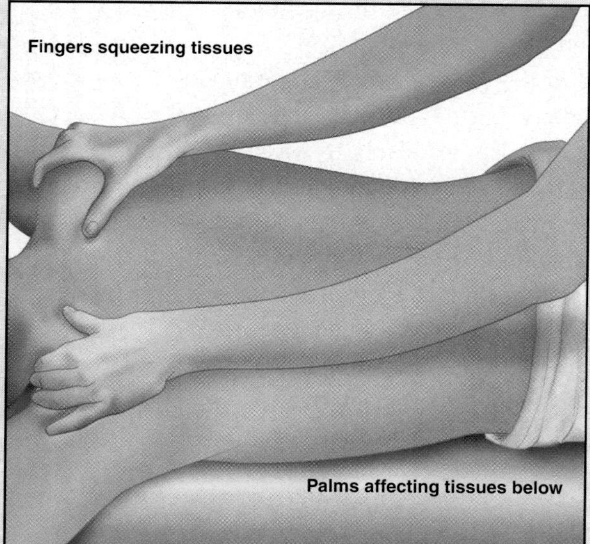

FIGURE 6–14 INCORRECT EXFOLIATION STROKE: Massage strokes penetrate beneath the skin to affect the tissues below.

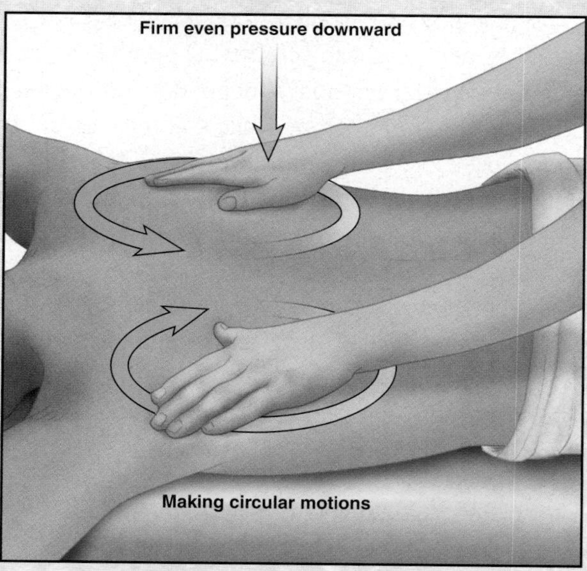

FIGURE 6–15 CORRECT EXFOLIATION STROKE: Exfoliation strokes are meant to affect the skin surface.

herbs will be featured in Chapter 12. In each of the procedures, the product used will be referred to simply as "the exfoliant" rather than any specific brand or product type. All components and products used in these treatments are interchangeable. Some treatments use one product alone. Others feature several exfoliants working in concert to create a specific effect. Some include a bathing component using body washes in addition to exfoliants. Others do not. For example, the dry room exfoliation procedure given here features an extra

SPA TIP

When applying exfoliation to smaller surface areas such as around the ankles, knees, or elbows, use all of your fingertips held together to form a small flat surface (Figure 6–16).

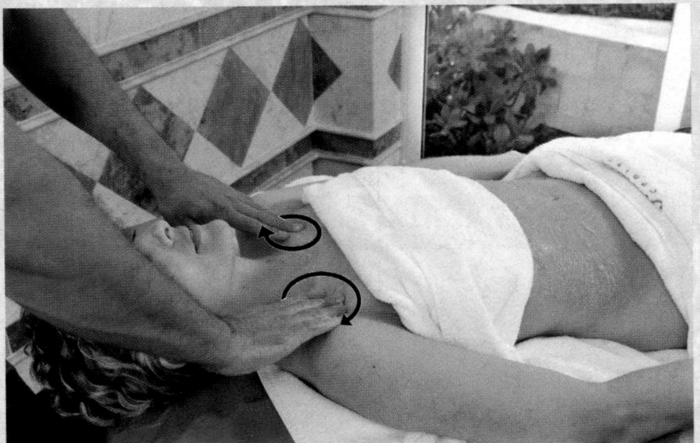

FIGURE 6–16 Hold your fingertips together to exfoliate hard-to-reach areas.

Hydrocollator Use in Spas

Did You Know?

One of the most popular options therapists choose to heat their towels, exfoliants, and other spa products is the hydrocollator, which can serve a pivotal role in the spa treatment room. In addition to its intended use as a heating basin for therapeutic silicon gel packs, the hydrocollator is also a good choice for immersing the towels used in so many dry room spa treatments. At the same time, rubberized spa bowls filled with spa products can be floated on the water's surface in the hydrocollator, heating them prior to application.

step using loofah mitts and a body bath. This step could be left out, and the procedure would still be an effective exfoliation. On the other hand, this step could be added to the wet room exfoliation protocol. Many variations on these treatments are practiced at spas around the world. In the end, any of these procedures can be effective as long as they achieve the goals of removing dead skin cells, stimulating circulation, and leaving clients' skin texture and appearance improved.

Applying exfoliation treatments in a wet room versus a dry room involves one main distinction between protocols. In wet rooms, a shower is used to apply water and prepare the skin before exfoliant application, and to wash the exfoliant off after application. In a dry room, wash cloths, towels, loofah mitts, and sponges are used instead of a shower. These differences will be reflected in the following protocols. If you do not have access to a wet room during your training, this will not impede your learning. In spite of their obvious differences, wet room and dry room exfoliation procedures are extremely similar. If you have learned the procedures in a dry room and later find work at a spa with a wet room, it will be a simple process to adjust to the new environment.

SPA TIP

In order to avoid pulling body hair, make sure enough moisture is present when applying exfoliation strokes. A slightly moist exfoliant layer will make the scrubbing smoother, while completely dry exfoliants can be overly abrasive. Remoisten the skin at any point during exfoliation treatments if you feel a dry, grainy sensation or a dragging of the exfoliant over the skin.

Exfoliation services have their own subset of problems related to draping. As a general guideline, the Wet Table Draping Protocol explained in Chapter 4 can be used effectively during exfoliation services, but when the water used in these treatments is combined with the exfoliants themselves, the treatment surface can become messy and potentially uncomfortable for clients. Care must be taken to keep the surface of the treatment table and the draping as clean as possible, as will be discussed in the following protocols.

Wet Room Exfoliation Protocol

TREATMENT: WET ROOM EXFOLIATION	
Wet Room/Dry Room	wet room
Table Setup	wet table cushion with towel or bath sheet atop it and towels for draping
Treatment Duration	30 minutes
Needed Supplies	bath towel, bath sheet, ¼ cup exfoliant in small bowl, emollient lotion
Contraindications	sunburn, cuts, abrasions, sores, eczema, thin/delicate skin, allergies to exfoliants, recent shaving when using salt
Draping	Wet Table Draping Protocol—see Chapter 4
Treatment Order	Exfoliation services are always first, before other spa services or massage.
Safety, Sanitation Issues, & Clean-Up	Exfoliants, especially oil-based ones, can be slippery on smooth surfaces and floor. Water for heating products needs to be maintained at proper temperature to avoid overheating.
Body Mechanics & Self-Care	Continual use of shower can and slick exfoliants on tiles can cause potential slip and fall dangers. While working over high, wide wet tables, care must be taken not to strain lower back.
Product Cost	depending upon chosen exfoliant, 50¢ to $3, extra cost of disposable loofah or similar exfoliating tool built into treatment if used
Treatment Price	$30 to $80
Physiological Effects	Provides the three main benefits of exfoliation: to cleanse the pores and prepare skin for absorption of products, help the skin perform its natural processes, and leave client's skin texture and appearance improved. Also, some exfoliants add benefits such as minerals in salts.
Pregnancy Issues (information provided by Elaine Stillerman, LMT, author and developer of MotherMassage)	Exfoliation must be avoided on the lower extremities and anterior torso and during the first trimester. During the second and third trimesters, the arms and back may carefully be treated with the client sitting upright and draped appropriately or prone on the body support system.

Wet Room Exfoliation Preparation

1. Prepare the table for the wet table draping protocol.
2. Have exfoliant and emollient lotion at hand. Warm the exfoliant and body bath, especially if the treatment room is cool.
3. Assure that water temperature in the shower heads is set to an appropriate level so the first contact will not shock the client.

Wet Room Exfoliation Procedure

1. The client starts prone on the wet table. With the handheld shower—or Vichy shower, if available—wet the client's skin (Figure 6–17). Ask for client feedback about water temperature.

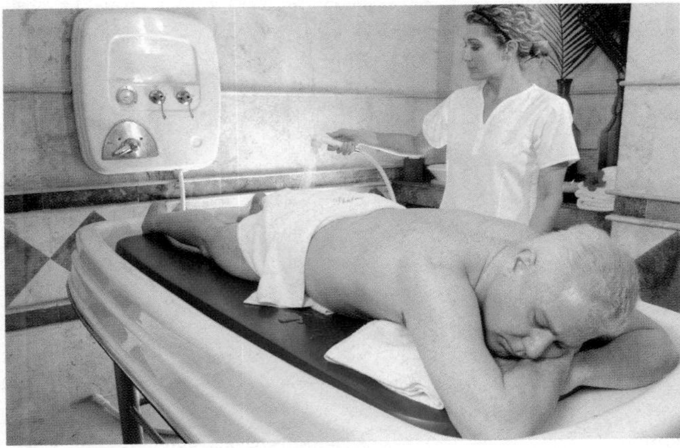

FIGURE 6–17

2. Place a tablespoon of exfoliant into one hand, rubbing your palms together to warm it if necessary. Using both hands, apply it first to the back of the left leg, then the back of the right leg, and finally the back itself (Figure 6–18). The sides of the body along the ribcage, the shoulders, and the triceps region can be exfoliated as well. Replenish exfoliant in your hands as you begin each new area, or as needed.

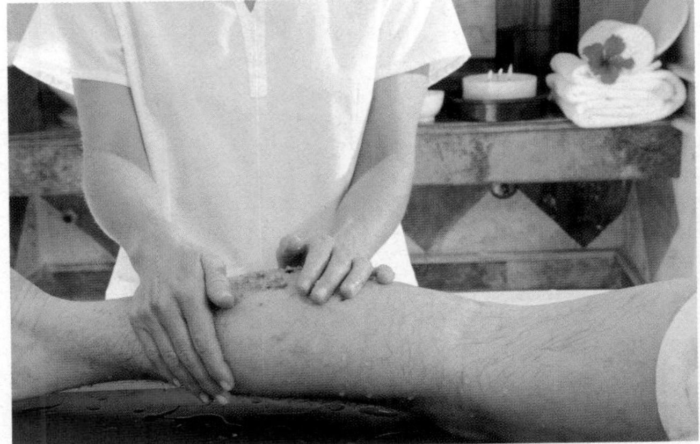

FIGURE 6–18

3. With the handheld shower or Vichy shower, wash exfoliant from the client's skin (Figure 6–19).

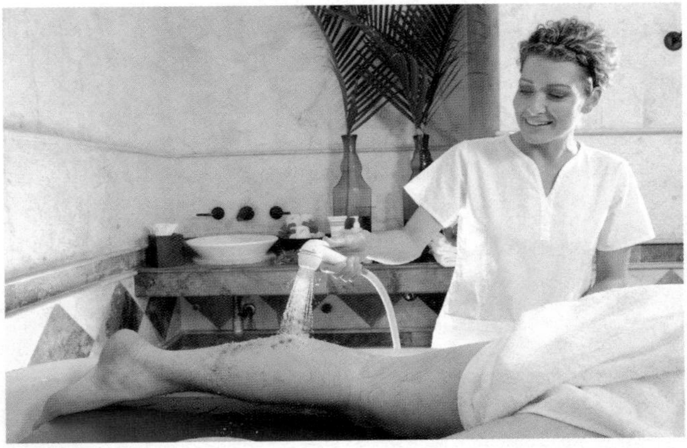

FIGURE 6–19

4. Maintain the drape in place while the client rolls over into a supine position.
5. With the handheld shower—or Vichy shower if available—wet the client's skin (Figure 6–20).

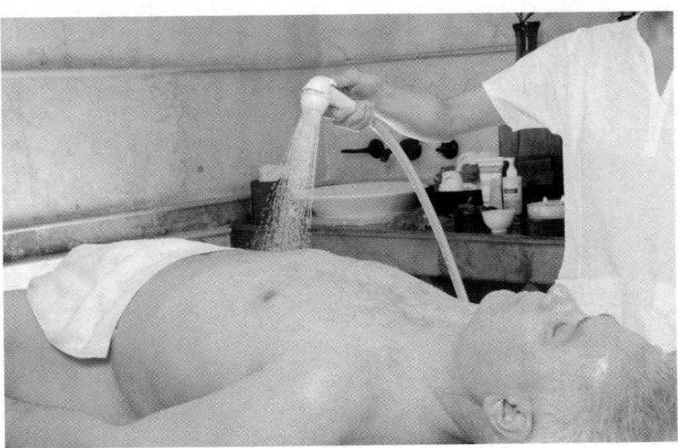

FIGURE 6–20

6. Use a tablespoon of exfoliant, beginning on the right foot and moving up the right leg (Figure 6–21). Then repeat on the left leg.

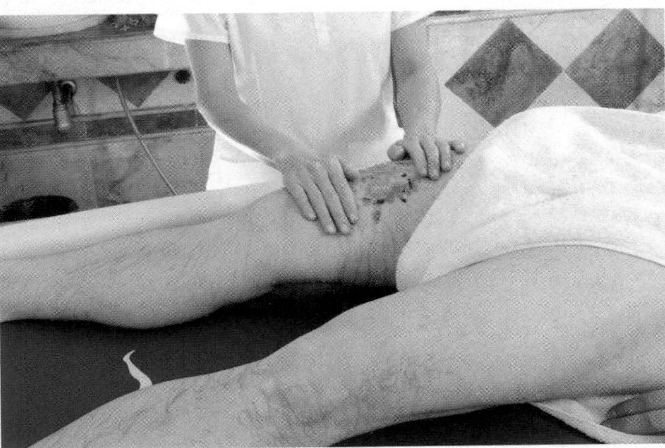

FIGURE 6–21

Move to the abdomen, using gentle, large, circular exfoliation movements, because this is a sensitive area (Figure 6–22). Use a breast drape for female clients. Exfoliate the left hand and arm (Figure 6–23), then move across the upper chest to the right hand and arm. Do not apply body exfoliant to the neck or face.

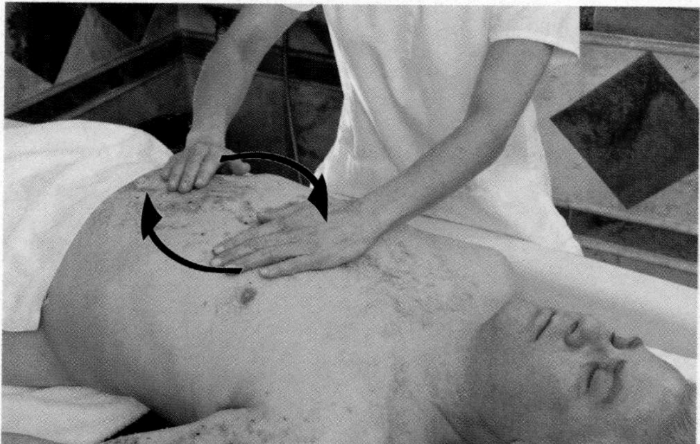

FIGURE 6–22

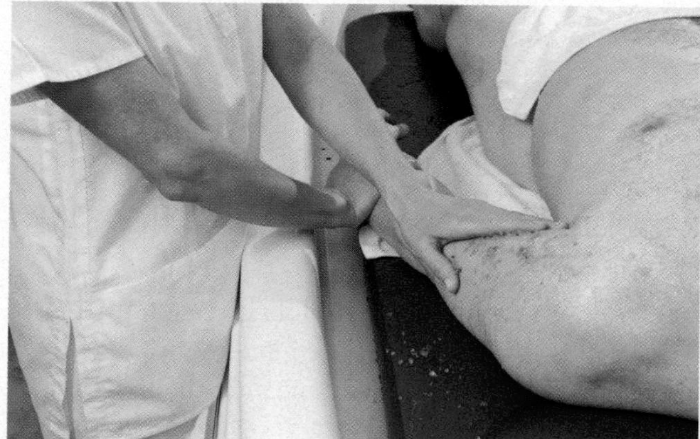

FIGURE 6–23

7. With the handheld shower or Vichy shower, wash exfoliant from the client's skin (Figure 6–24). Pat the client dry with a clean bath towel (Figure 6–25).
8. Apply emollient cream or lotion to the front of the body, starting with the right leg (Figure 6–26). After two minutes, ask the client to turn over. On the final turn, quickly slide a bath sheet under the client to provide a dry surface to lie on (Figure 6–27). The client will end lying face-down on the bath sheet for the final two-minute application of cream or lotion to the back of the legs, shoulders, triceps area, and back (Figure 6–28).

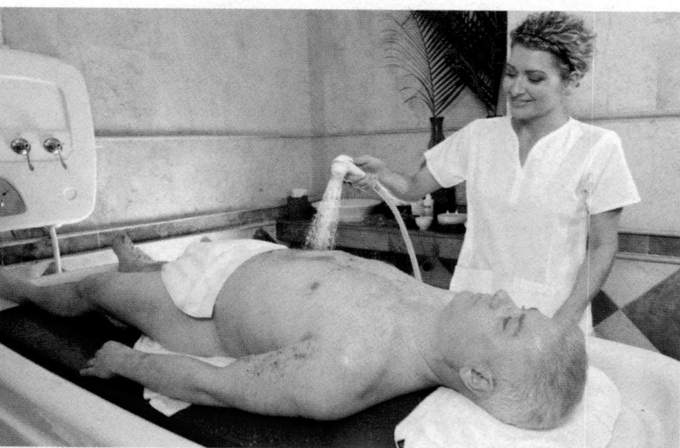

FIGURE 6–24

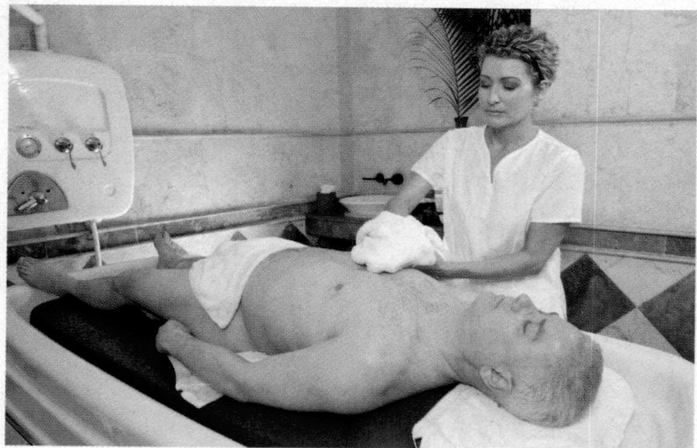

FIGURE 6–25

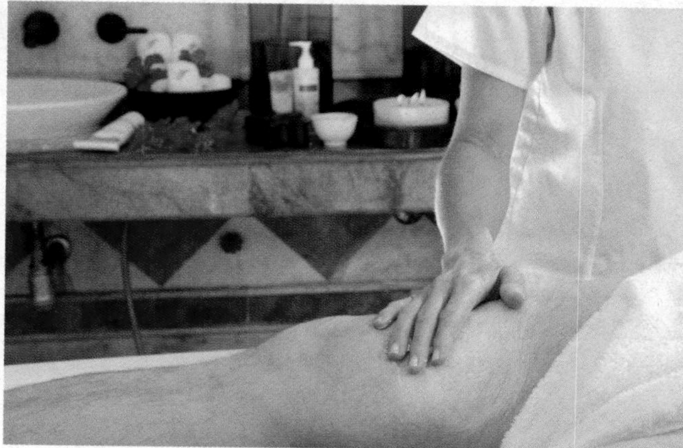

FIGURE 6–26

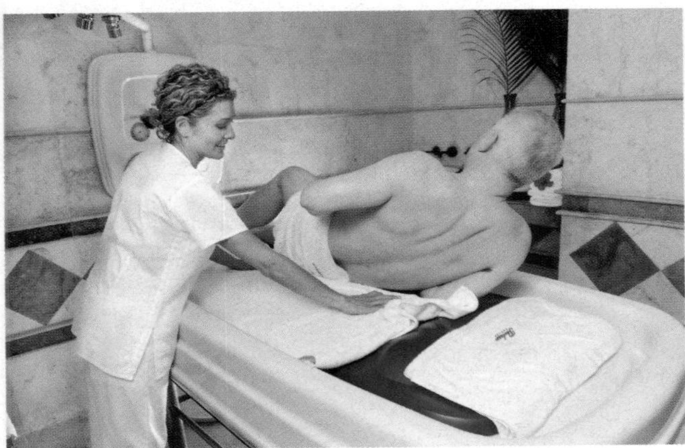
FIGURE 6–27

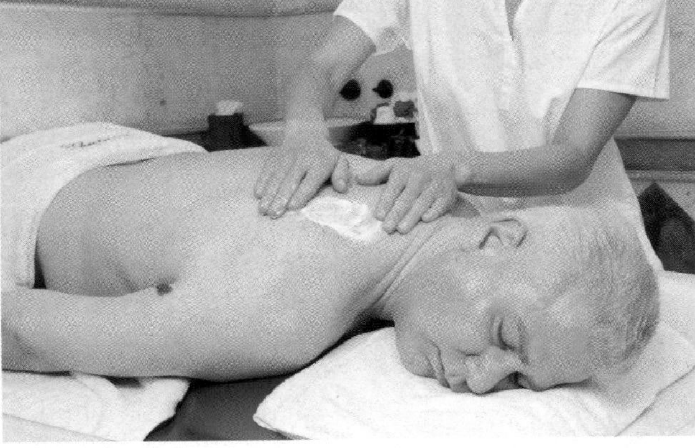
FIGURE 6–28

Wet Room Exfoliation Cleanup

1. Clean and dry the top of the wet table.
2. Launder the sheets and towels.
3. Clean the bowls and utensils.
4. Wipe up any water or product on the floor to avoid slipping.

SPA TIP

If you are moving from an exfoliation procedure directly to a body wrap with seaweed, mud, clay, or herbs, do not apply moisturizing cream to the skin, as it will block the freshly cleaned pores, slowing absorption of therapeutic products. Alternatively, the application of a moisturizing cream or oil can be extended into an hour-long procedure, creating a combination exfoliation/massage treatment.

Dry Room Exfoliation Protocol

TREATMENT: DRY ROOM EXFOLIATION	
Wet Room/Dry Room	dry room
Table Setup	protective covering such as a thermal blanket or rubberized sheet, bed sheet, bath sheet, draping towels
Treatment Duration	30 minutes
Needed Supplies	3 bath towels, 4 hand towels, wash cloth, plastic bowl, loofah pad, ¼ cup exfoliant in small bowl, 2 tablespoons body wash, insulated container, heating unit (hydrocollator or crock pot), emollient lotion
Contraindications	sunburn, cuts, abrasions, sores, eczema, thin/delicate skin, allergies to exfoliants, recent shaving when using salt
Draping	massage draping technique with towel or sheet, and hand towel for breast drape for female clients
Treatment Order	Exfoliation services are always first, before other spa services or massage.

(Continued)

TREATMENT: DRY ROOM EXFOLIATION	
Safety, Sanitation Issues, & Clean-Up	Exfoliants, especially oil-based ones, can be slippery on smooth surfaces and floor. Water for heating towels and products needs to be maintained at proper temperature to avoid overheating. Hot towels need to be thoroughly wrung out to avoid scalding. Loofahs and similar tools need to be sterilized, disposed of, or given to client after use.
Body Mechanics & Self-Care	Maintain same body mechanics for dry room exfoliation as those used for massage, taking care to use legs muscles to avoid straining lower back. Exfoliants and water keep therapists' hands supple, but salt can irritate.
Product Cost	depending upon chosen exfoliant, 50¢ to $3, extra cost of disposable loofah or similar exfoliating tool built into treatment if used
Treatment Price	$40 to $70
Physiological Effects	Provides the three main benefits of exfoliation: to cleanse the pores and prepare skin for absorption of products, help the skin perform its natural processes, and leave client's skin texture and appearance improved. Also, some exfoliants add benefits, such as minerals in salts.
Pregnancy Issues (information provided by Elaine Stillerman, LMT, author and developer of MotherMassage)	Exfoliation and heat must be avoided on the lower extremities and anterior torso and the first trimester. During the second and third trimesters, the arms and back may carefully be treated with the client sitting upright and draped appropriately or prone on the body support system.

SPA TIP

For the sake of ease and modesty in the group setting, students in the classroom may choose to wear bathing suits when practicing the dry room exfoliation procedure.

Dry Room Exfoliation Preparation

1. Prepare the massage table with a protective covering such as a thermal blanket or rubberized sheet. Place a bottom sheet atop this, then a large towel or bath sheet, and finally draping towels.
2. Take four hand towels, fold them into quarters, roll them up lengthwise, and dip them in very hot, but not boiling, water. Wearing rubber gloves to protect your hands, wring out the towels and place them in an insulated container. Alternatively, you can dip towels in room temperature water, wring them out, and warm them in a crock pot, roaster or hot towel cabbie. See the sections on insulated containers and heating units in Chapter 3.
3. Have exfoliant, body bath, and lotion at hand. If available, place these products on a wheeled cart for easy accessibility in all areas of the treatment room. Warm the exfoliant and body bath, especially if the treatment room is cool.
4. Fill the bowl with hot water and soak the loofah pad in the bowl.

Dry Room Exfoliation Procedure

1. With the client face-down on top of the bath sheet, dip the wash cloth in the bowl of hot water, wring it out, and moisten the client's back and back of the legs. The backs of some loofah pads are made of cloth and can be used for this step instead, making the wash cloth unnecessary (Figure 6–29). This step is performed in the place of the initial spraying with shower head or Vichy shower at the beginning of the previous protocol.
2. Place a tablespoon of exfoliant into one hand, rubbing your palms together to warm it if necessary. Using both hands, apply it first to the back of the left leg, then the back of the right leg, and finally the back itself (Figure 6–30). The sides of the body along

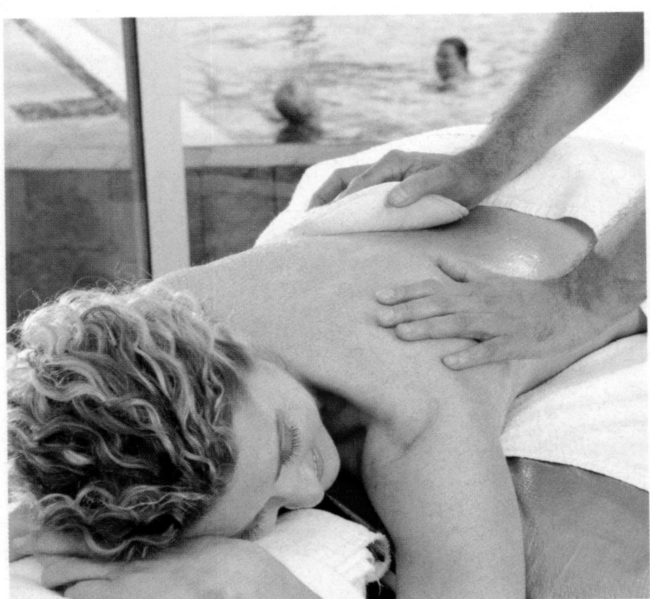

FIGURE 6–29

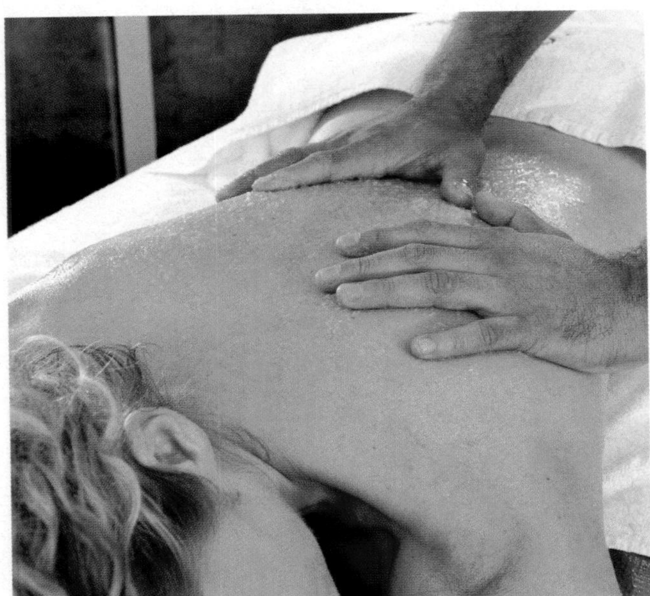

FIGURE 6–30

the ribcage, the shoulders, and the triceps region can be exfoliated as well. Replenish exfoliant in your hands as you begin each new area. If the client feels chilled, you can cover each area of the body with a drape after exfoliating it.

3. Take the first preheated towel out of the heating unit or insulated container, unfold it, and wave it in the air for a few seconds if it is still too hot to apply (Figure 6–31). Under normal conditions, the towel can be placed on the

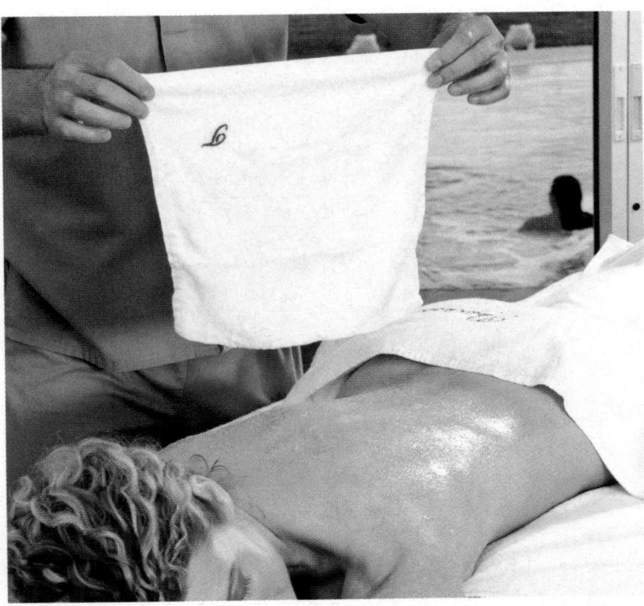

FIGURE 6–31

client's back even if it still feels quite hot to your hands, which are more sensitive. Press the hot, moist towel into the client's back for a moment, and then use it first to wipe off the exfoliant from the back (Figure 6–32). Then, fold the towel in half and use the clean side to remove exfoliant from the left leg (Figure 6–33). Turn the towel over and remove exfoliant from the right leg (Figure 6–34). It is not necessary to wipe off every last grain of exfoliant in this step.

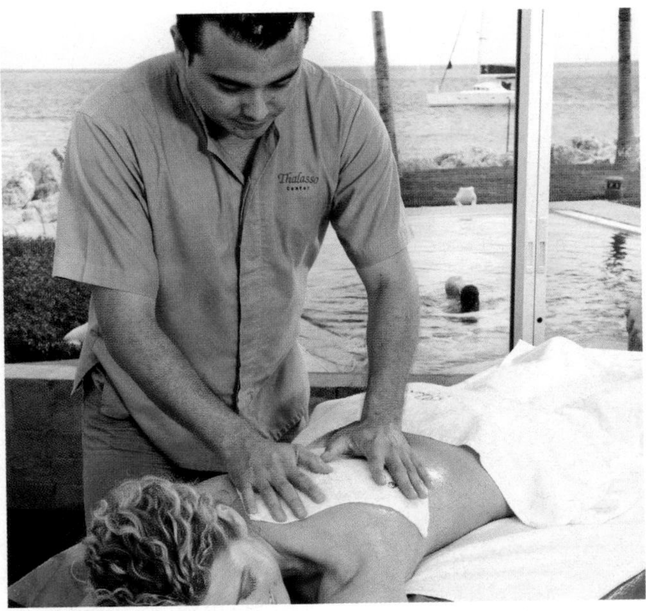

FIGURE 6–32

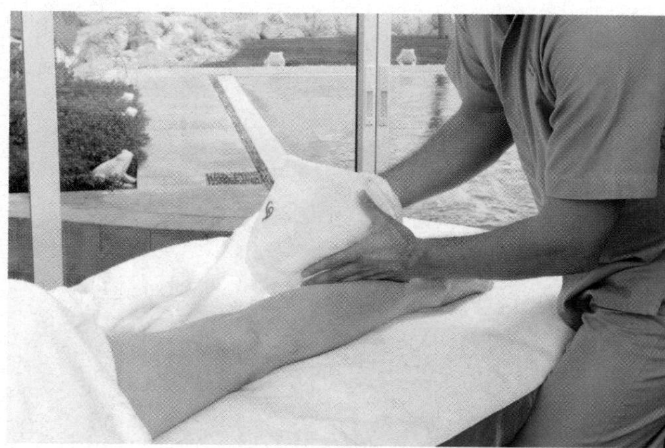

FIGURE 6–33

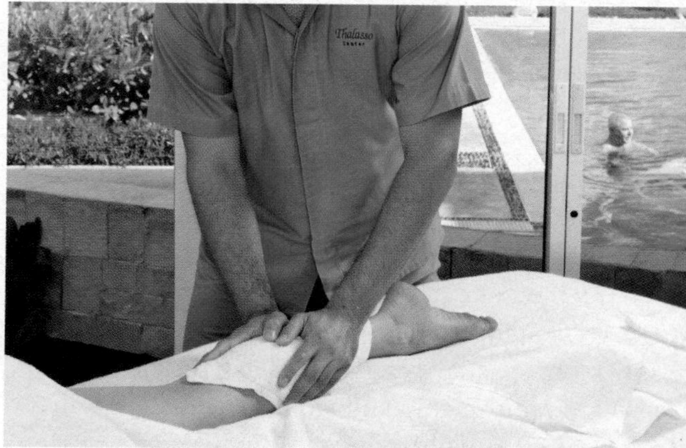

FIGURE 6–34

4. Dip the loofah pad in the bowl of hot water, apply one tablespoon of body bath to the scrubbing surface, and use it to wash the skin of the left leg, right leg, and back (Figure 6–35). This, in effect, is a second exfoliation combined with a cleansing.

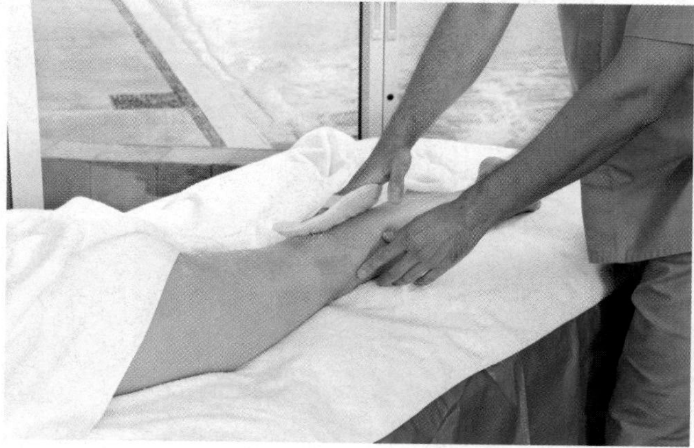

FIGURE 6–35

5. Using the second towel, repeat Step 3, this time wiping away the body bath and any left-over exfoliant (Figure 6–36).

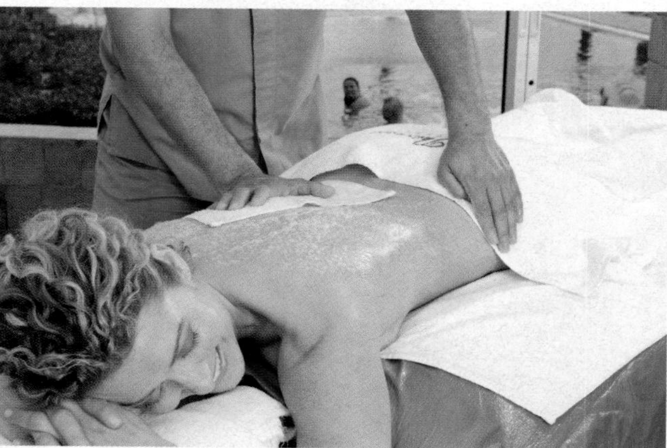

FIGURE 6–36

6. The client turns supine. Moisten the front of the body with the wash cloth or loofah pad (Figure 6–37).

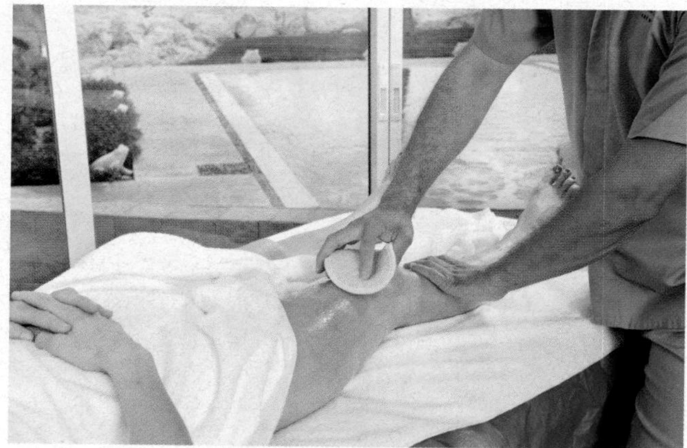

FIGURE 6–37

7. Use a tablespoon of exfoliant, beginning on the right foot and moving up the right leg. Then repeat on the left leg (Figure 6–38).

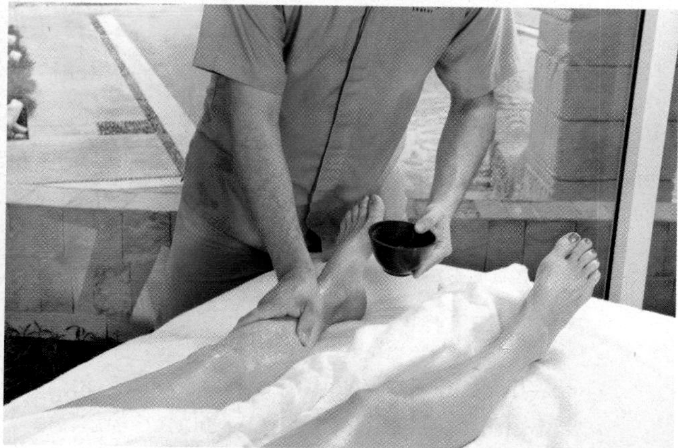

FIGURE 6–38

Move to the abdomen, using gentle, large, circular exfoliation movements, because this is a sensitive area (Figure 6–39). Use a breast drape for female clients. Exfoliate the left hand and arm, then move across the upper chest to the right hand and arm (Figure 6–40). Do not apply body exfoliant to the neck or face.

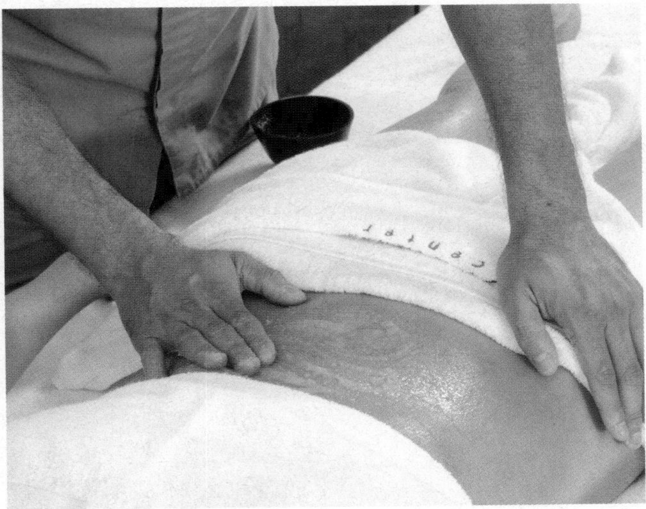

FIGURE 6–39

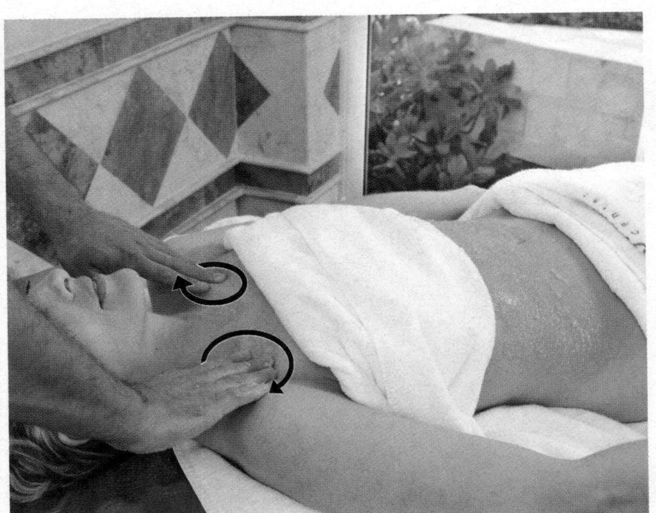

FIGURE 6–40

8. With the third hot towel, wipe away the exfoliant, starting with the abdomen (Figure 6–41). Move from the abdomen to the shoulders, arms, and hands. Then, fold the towel in half and use the clean side to remove exfoliant from the right leg. Turn the towel over and remove exfoliant from the left leg.

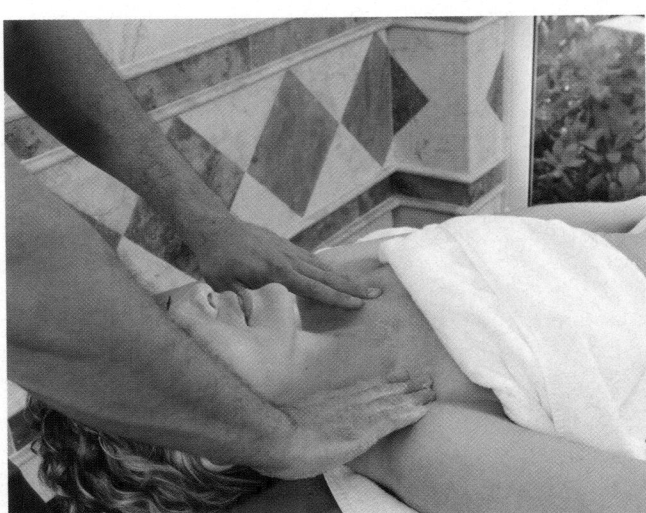

FIGURE 6–41

9. Dip the loofah pad in the water once again, add a tablespoon of body bath, and use it to wash the skin of the right leg, left leg, abdomen, and arms. Dip the loofah into the water whenever necessary to keep the pad moist. Spend extra time on those areas of calluses and toughened skin, such as the elbows and heels (Figure 6–42).

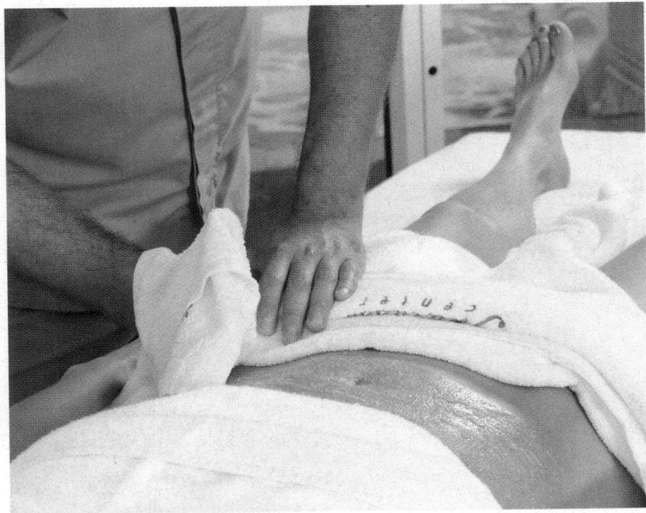

FIGURE 6–42

10. With the last hot towel, remove the soap and any excess exfoliant from the abdomen, arms, and legs (Figure 6–43). Pat the client dry with a clean bath towel (Figure 6–44).

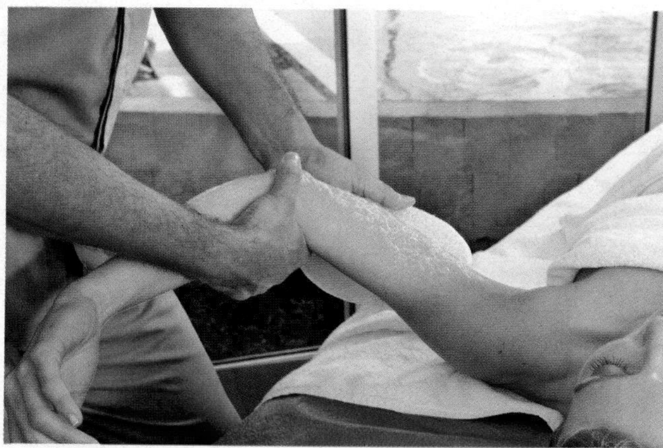

FIGURES 6–43

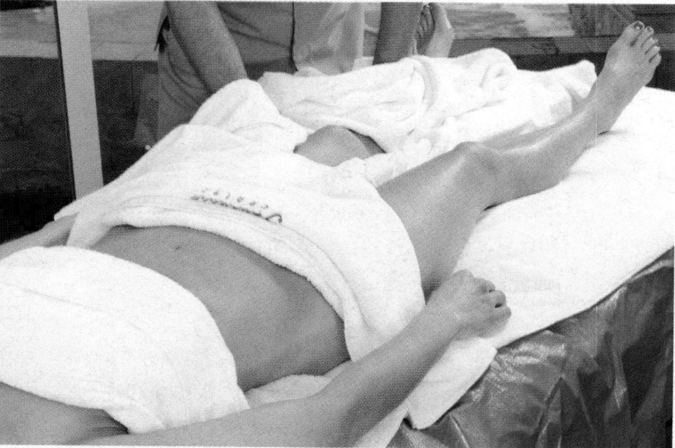

FIGURES 6–44

11. Apply emollient cream or lotion to the front of the body, starting with the right foot. After two minutes, ask the client to turn over. On the final turn, quickly roll the bath sheet the client was lying on out from underneath. The client will end lying face-down on the clean sheet for the final two-minute application of cream or lotion to the back of the legs, shoulders, triceps area, and back (Figures 6–45 through 6–47).

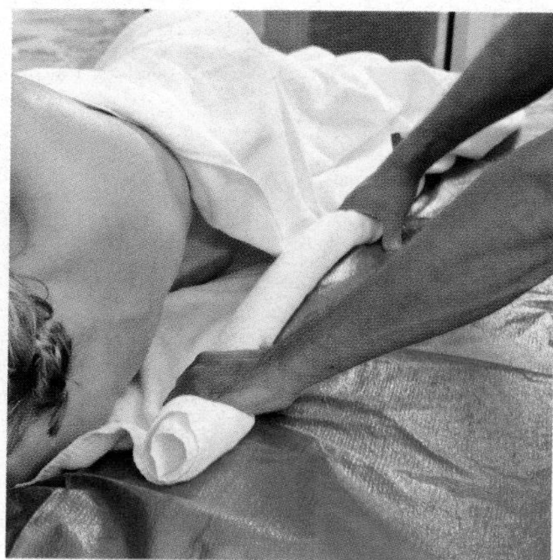

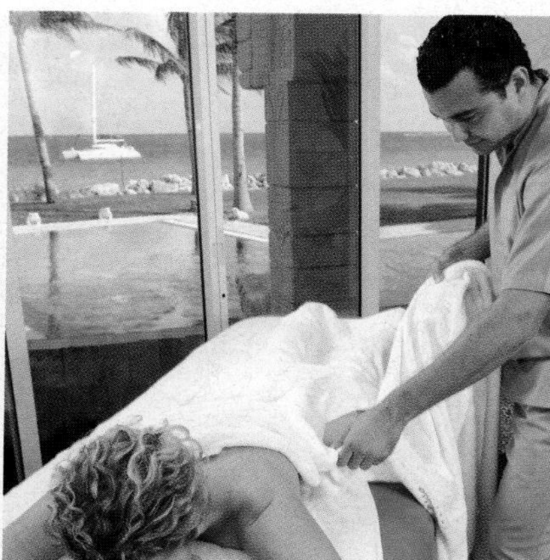

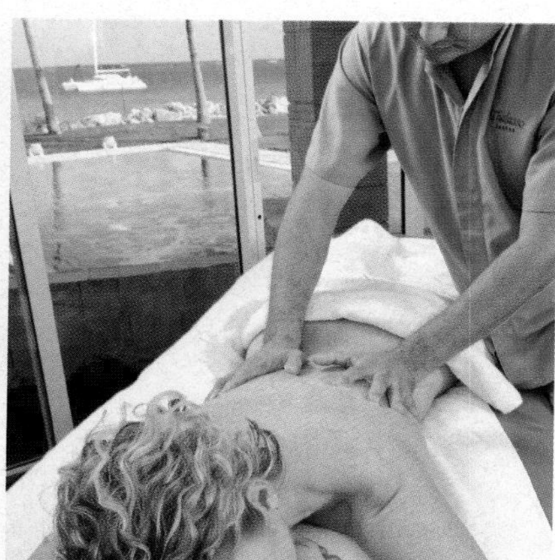

FIGURES 6–45, 6–46, 6–47 Client rolls over as bath sheet is removed from under body.

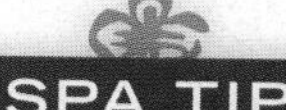

SPA TIP

Timing is important for exfoliation services. The steps in this dry room protocol take approximately five minutes each. Applying the exfoliant to the back of the body and wiping it off takes five minutes. Using the loofah and body bath on the back of the body, then wiping it off, takes five minutes as well. The same timing is repeated on the front of the body, making 20 minutes of total exfoliation. Five minutes are then spent applying emollient lotion to the entire body and five more minutes to clean the room and prepare for the next client, making a total of 30 minutes. For the wet room exfoliation protocol explained above, the scrubbing step takes 10 minutes on each side instead of five.

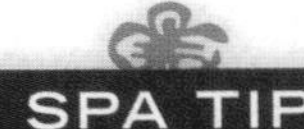

SPA TIP

More than four towels can be used in this protocol, as long as they are available in the treatment room and the extra laundry is not a problem. In general, the more hot towels used, the more luxurious dry room exfoliation feels.

Dry Room Exfoliation Cleanup

1. Launder the sheets and towels and disinfect the waterproof table covering.
2. Wash the bowl and utensils with soap and hot water.
3. Dispose of the loofah pad or place it inside a plastic bag and offer it to the client, included in the price of treatment (Figure 6–48).
4. Wipe or sweep up any excess exfoliant that has fallen to the floor to avoid slippery surfaces.

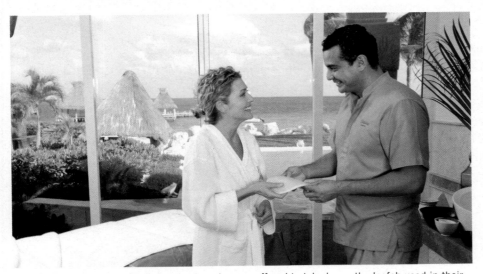

FIGURE 6–48 Clients appreciate it when they are offered to take home the loofah used in their exfoliation treatments.

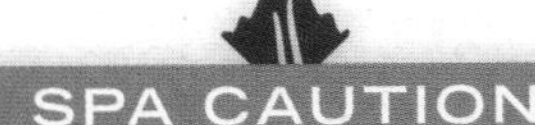

SPA CAUTION

Do not waste exfoliating products. Some therapists have a tendency to apply excess exfoliant, which does not provide increased benefits to the client. It is not necessary to create a thick paste of exfoliant on the skin. A thin layer that completely covers the epidermis is sufficient. If therapists exceed this amount, money is being wasted in each service. Some spa directors have had to ration product because of overuse by therapists. Use the amounts of product recommended in the protocols. After you have gauged the effectiveness of the amount applied, you may even find that you can lower it and still give an effective treatment.

SPA TIP

You can easily omit the loofah scrub portion of the dry room exfoliation protocol. Simply skip Steps 4 and 9 and spend an extra 5 minutes on Steps 2 and 7. You will use two hot towels per side of the body, one on the hips and legs, and one on the torso and arms. In brief, this treatment sequence would be:

1. Exfoliate the backs of legs and hips.
2. Use a hot towel to clean the area.
3. Exfoliate the back, shoulders, and triceps area.
4. Use a hot towel to clean the area. (the client turns over)
5. Exfoliate feet and fronts of legs.
6. Use a hot towel to clean the area.
7. Exfoliate the torso and arms.
8. Use a hot towel to clean the area.
9. Apply lotion to the front of the body. (the client turns and the bath sheet is removed from beneath the body)
10. Apply lotion to the back of the body.

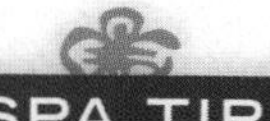

SPA TIP

Using a hot, moist towel to wipe off exfoliating products does not create a second-rate experience for the client. In fact, many clients find the sensation more pleasurable and luxurious than stepping into a shower or lying beneath a Vichy shower to have the product washed off. Showers are a common occurrence for most spa goers. Being gently and caringly hand-cleansed with hot towels by an attentive spa therapist is an out-of-the-ordinary experience. When done properly, it adds enjoyment to a spa treatment.

For treatments in a dry room, practice getting the towels as hot as possible and then storing them in such a way that their heat is maintained for as long as possible. An insulated container or Spa Thermal Unit, as described in Chapter 3, can be used, as long as the towels are sufficiently hot to begin with. Once you have the system down, you'll have a setup that allows you to simulate a hot shower treatment room with amazing accuracy, and perhaps even improve upon it.

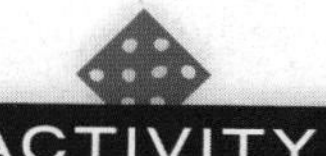

ACTIVITY

Create an Exfoliant

Exfoliants are available everywhere, it seems. In addition to spas, many beauty supply stores, salons, and even well-stocked drug stores carry dozens of options in the realm of scrubbing agents. Most spas use exfoliation products produced by other companies, though some, such as the Green Valley Spa in Utah and Charlie's Spa at the San Souci resort in Jamaica, formulate their own blends on-site. Try making your own version of Charlie's Spa's sea salt and cornmeal blend, and test it in comparison to commercially available scrubs. Do you think it is just as good? Better? Experiment with changing the essential oils or the ratio of salt to cornmeal. Use less water, or a little bit more. Or substitute massage oil for the water. If you like, you can use this self-created blend for the protocols and activities in this chapter.

Cornmeal and Sea Salt Exfoliant

Mix the following ingredients thoroughly into a grainy paste:

- ½ cup of sea salts
- ½ cup organic corn meal
- 2 tablespoons spring water
- 3 drops each lavender, chamomile, and rosemary essential oils

DRY BRISTLE BRUSHING

Dry bristle brushing is a technique primarily used in spas that have a focus on natural health. It is not considered luxurious by most standards, and clients who receive this treatment need to be educated about its benefits, which include a powerful stimulation of lymph flow in addition to the more obvious effects of exfoliation (Figure 6–49). Often incorporated into the first 5 or 10 minutes of a more involved procedure such as body wrapping or cellulite services, dry brushing can also be performed as an invigorating stand-alone treatment. Spas with high-intensity detoxification programs often offer dry bristle brushing in conjunction with fasting, colon-cleansing, herbal purification diets, and colonic irrigation procedures because it stimulates the elimination of the toxins that can be circulated through these procedures.

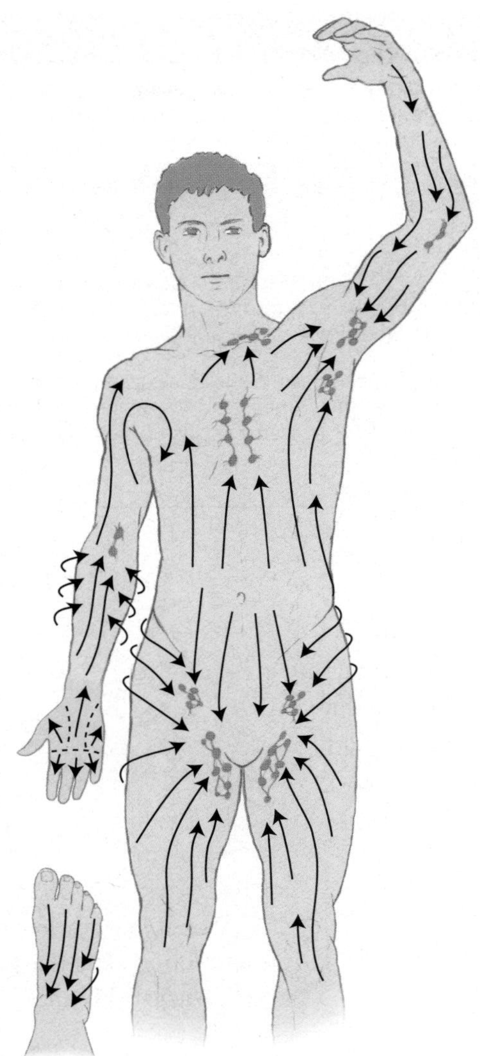

FIGURE 6–49 Dry brushing movements are always toward primary lymph nodes and the heart.

Dry Bristle Brush Protocol

TREATMENT: DRY BRISTLE BRUSH	
Wet Room/Dry Room	dry room
Table Setup	sheet to cover table, draping towels or sheet
Treatment Duration	20 to 30 minutes
Needed Supplies	dry bristle body brush, emollient lotion
Contraindications	sunburn, cuts, abrasions, sores, eczema, thin/delicate skin
Draping	massage draping techniques apply
Treatment Order	As an exfoliation service, dry brushing is scheduled before other spa treatments and massage.
Safety, Sanitation Issues, & Clean-Up	Brushes must be sanitized after use. Even though they are for the most part invisible, sloughed-off dead skin cells still gather on sheets, towels, and treatment surfaces after dry brushing, and these must be cleaned as after any other spa service. Some brushes can be too abrasive on clients with sensitive skin.

(Continued)

TREATMENT: DRY BRISTLE BRUSH	
Body Mechanics & Self-Care	Take care not to grip brush too tightly to avoid stressing wrists and hands. Apply same body mechanics as massage, bending legs and avoiding strain to lower back while bending over table to perform exfoliation.
Product Cost	only cost of emollient lotion applied at end of treatment
Treatment Price	$30 to $60
Physiological Effects	Provides the three main benefits of exfoliation: to cleanse the pores and prepare it for absorption of products, help the skin perform its natural processes, and leave client's skin texture and appearance improved. Particularly stimulating for lymph flow.
Pregnancy Issues (information provided by Elaine Stillerman, LMT, author and developer of MotherMassage)	Dry bristle brushing is contraindicated on the lower extremities, anterior torso, and during the first trimester. During the second trimester, dry brushing may carefully be administered to the arms and back with the client in a sitting position and appropriately draped or prone on the body support system.

Dry Bristle Brush Preparation

1. Cover the table with a sheet and draping materials.
2. The client should not enter a steam room or other heating area prior to service, because the skin should be dry for this exfoliation.
3. Confirm that the brush has been sanitized and is ready for use.

Dry Bristle Brush Procedure

1. Start with the client prone. Begin on the foot and lower left leg. Where appropriate, such as around the ankles, knees, and other joints, apply circular exfoliation movements as described in this chapter (Figure 6–50). On larger surfaces, such as the calves, hamstrings, back, and other areas, use longer, straight strokes, always in the direction of circulation toward the primary lymph nodes and the heart (Figure 6–51).

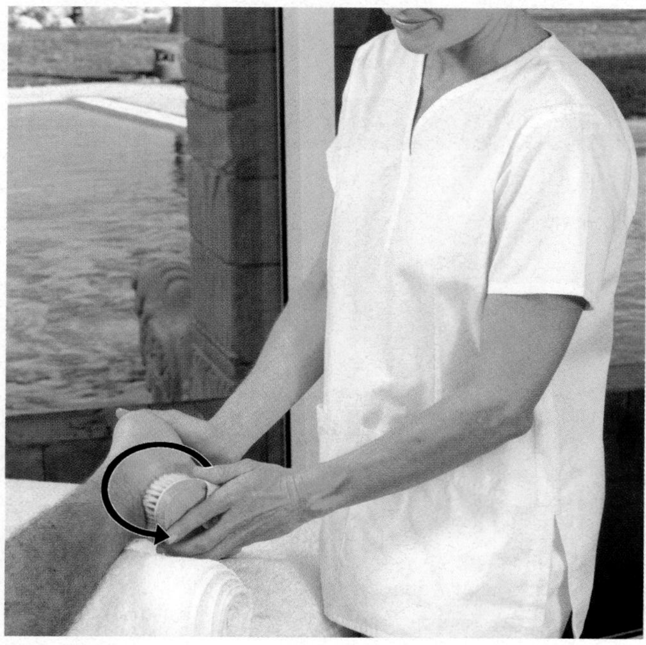

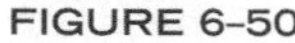
FIGURE 6–50

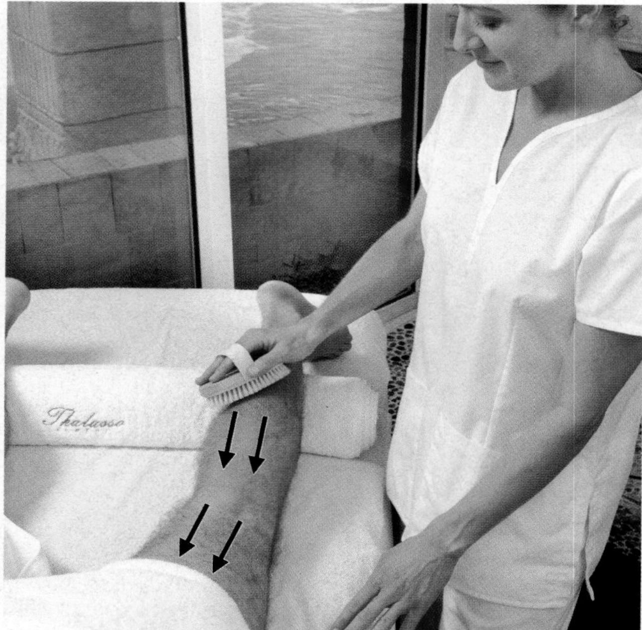
FIGURE 6–51

2. Repeat on the back of the right leg.
3. Dry brush the back, shoulders, and upper arms (Figure 6–52).

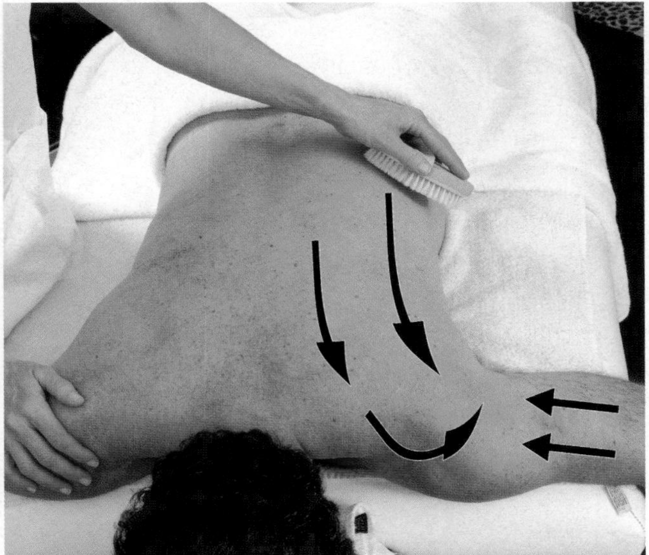

FIGURE 6–52

4. The client turns supine. Apply dry brush exfoliation to the left foot and leg (Figure 6–53).

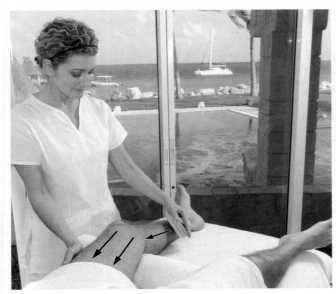

FIGURE 6–53

5. Repeat on the right foot and front of leg.
6. Apply circular dry brushing around the belly in a clockwise direction using a gentle, rhythmic stroke (Figure 6–54).
7. Dry brush the right arm first (Figure 6–55).
8. Repeat on the left arm.

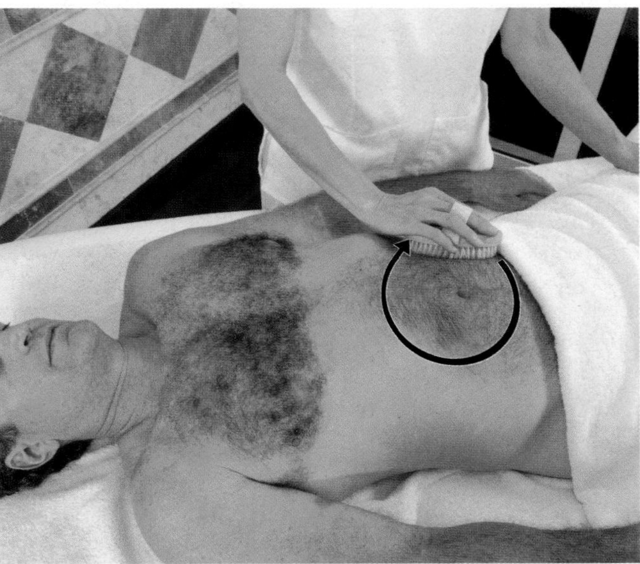

FIGURE 6–54

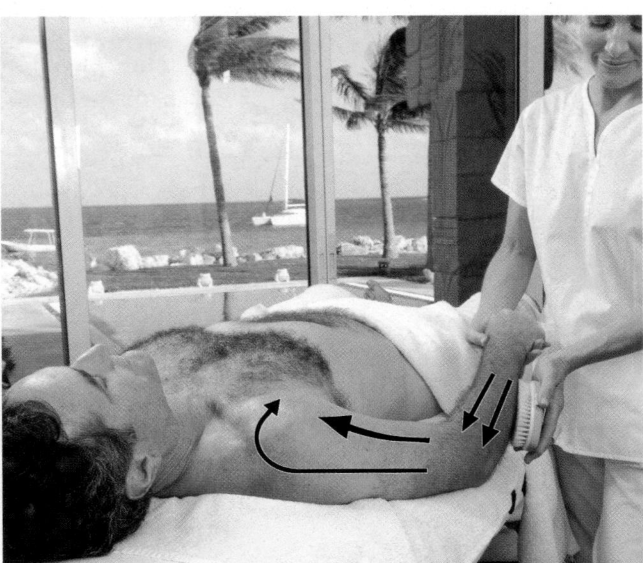

FIGURE 6–55

9. Dry brush the chest, using a breast drape for female clients. Avoid the neck and face, because these areas are too delicate for dry brushing.
10. Apply an emollient lotion when finished, starting at the chest and moving over the body in reverse order from the dry brushing. If desired, place a clean sheet underneath when the client turns into prone position again, although this is not necessary as it is in the dry room exfoliation procedure above. Apply lotion to the backs of the legs and the back.

ACTIVITY

Self-Exfoliation

You can perform many of the steps outlined in the protocols above on yourself. One popular way to exfoliate your own skin is to use a combination bath/body scrub product in the shower. Although it is difficult to exfoliate your own back, it can be accomplished with a long-handled brush. Why, then, is it worth the time and expense to pay for spa exfoliation services when self-exfoliation is such a viable option?

As an experiment, contrast and compare the sensations of exfoliating yourself with the sensations of receiving a full exfoliation service from a classmate or at a spa. Use a dry bristle body brush, or self-exfoliate in the shower with a loofah mitt, sisal mitt, or exfoliating gel. Afterwards, write down at least three differences that you found between the two experiences, describing them in your own words. This will help you to speak with authority to spa clients who ask about the benefits of spa exfoliation services.

Dry Bristle Brush Cleanup

1. Launder the sheets and towels.
2. Sanitize the dry brush. See Spa Room Sanitation section in Chapter 3.

CONCLUSION

Exfoliation services lay the foundation for all other spa treatments that follow. Without clean pores through which to enter the body, even the best spa products will be less than optimally effective. Although simple to perform, exfoliation is often misapplied by therapists who do not have a full appreciation for the differences between massage techniques and exfoliation techniques. Some therapists, in fact, feel that exfoliation services are not worthy of their skill level, and they are therefore reluctant to perform them. However, when applied by knowledgeable therapists using proper technique and exhibiting sensitivity to the client, exfoliation treatments can be not only pleasurable but profoundly therapeutic as well. These services are a mainstay on spa service menus, and therapists should know as much as possible about their background and efficacy. Therapists with their own private practices can offer exfoliation services to their clients with very little investment in new supplies or equipment. It is one of the quickest ways to expand offerings while at the same time creating an excellent opportunity for retail sales—see Chapter 16. Performing exfoliations and recommending appropriate products to spa clients is a way for therapists to take more responsibility for their clients' overall health and well-being. Who else, after all, is better qualified to recommend procedures and products to be applied to the skin than the therapist whose career is based on touching that skin every day?

SPA TIP

Dry brushing is intrinsically stimulating. Some people find it too abrasive. It is a good idea to remind clients of this when they choose dry brushing from a spa menu, to make sure they are prepared for the sensation and give them an opportunity to choose another exfoliation service if they are especially sensitive.

opened what many consider the first modern thalassotherapy center. These facilities have proliferated ever since, and today France has dozens of such centers. Many others dot the globe in resort areas, especially in the tropics, including the Seychelles, Mauritius, Mexico, and others. In the U.S., only a couple of spas located on the coast are known for using fresh seawater in their treatments and thus can be considered thalassotherapy centers, most notably Gurney's Inn in Montauk, on the far eastern tip of Long Island.

In true thalassotherapy, the living organisms in fresh seawater, loaded with minerals and trace elements, are absorbed through the skin through the process of **osmosis**. This can only happen if three important criteria are met:

1. In order to be effective and keep the microorganisms in it alive, seawater should be warmed to approximately 98°F before coming into contact with the skin.
2. The water itself is pumped directly from the sea at a certain depth and a certain distance from the coast in order to maintain its purity.
3. Because the living organisms in seawater die within hours of being pumped from the ocean, thalassotherapy centers must be located on the shore or very near it in order to ensure effective treatments.

Additionally, in order to be considered a true thalassotherapy center, the facility must be supervised by a physician and use seawater and sea product treatments exclusively. Often, thalassotherapy centers will have a spa featuring other treatments, including massage, adjacent to or incorporated within them. This is not necessary in order to be considered a bona fide thalassotherapy center, however.

osmosis

diffusion of molecules through a membrane from a place of higher concentration to a place of lower concentration until the concentration on both sides is equal, a process that can take place through the skin when substances such as seaweed are applied to it

RESEARCH

Pick a thalassotherapy center anywhere in the world and research the treatments offered there, the history of the facility, the clientele, results obtained, and any outstanding features that make the center unique. Write a one-page report about your findings.

Algae: The Foundation of Thalassotherapy

We can, quite literally, thank algae for making our lives on this planet possible. Without algae, which transform sunlight into oxygen through the process of **photosynthesis**, there would not be sufficient oxygen to support terrestrial life. We would all die. Or rather, we would have never come to be here in the first place. Seaweeds, specifically, are a type of multicellular algae. There are several types, or phyla, of algae, used in spa applications: red, green, blue-green (now classified as *cyanobacteria*), and brown (Table 7–1). In addition to providing 70 to 80 percent of the world's oxygen, algae also display a number of other benefits for mankind. Many cultures, notably the Japanese, use algae as a major source of nutrition, eating it in great quantities. Sea plants consumed in this manner provide crucial elements such as iodine, which supports thyroid function and prevents **goiter**, a serious health problem, especially in landlocked areas, far from the sea, with iodine-poor soils.

Thousands of types of algae thrive in the oceans, in inland waterways, on land, and even in ice-bound regions near the poles. They range in size from microscopic single-cell entities to the colossal strands of kelp trailing almost 200 feet from the seabed. Because it needs sunlight to survive, algae grow in only a

photosynthesis

the conversion of light energy into chemical energy by certain living organisms such as algae

goiter

an enlargement of the thyroid gland visible as a swelling of the front of the neck, sometimes caused by insufficient iodine intake; seaweed provided in spa treatment applications or through ingestion provides this iodine

ALGAE	PHYLUM	DESCRIPTION	EXAMPLES USED IN SPAS	BENEFITS
Green Algae	Chlorophyta	approximately 7,000 species, cells contain plantlike chlorophyll pigments that give algae their grass-green color, found in lakes and oceans, and on land in soil and on tree trunks	ulva lactuca, a type of sea lettuce	a concentrated source of vitamin C, chlorophyll and antioxidants, used in spa treatments to nourish and tone the skin
Red Algae	Rhodophyta	approximately 6,000 species, deepest-dwelling algae, high in amino acids and polysaccharides, may contain red pigment to capture light, source of **carrageenan**, a thickener used in ice cream, medicines, cosmetics, and spa products	Irish moss, dulse, porphyra	common ingredient in many thalassotherapy products, gently stimulates sensitive skin, storehouse of calcium magnesium
Brown Algae	Phaeophyta	approximately 1,500 species, including some of the largest algae used in spas	fucus, bladderwrack and the most popular—laminaria digitata—known as *kelp*	highly remineralizing, used for body wraps, cellulite services and slimming programs as a diuretic
Cyanobacteria (also known as blue-green algae)	Cyanophyta	cells lack nucleus, common in fresh water, also found in the ocean and on land habitats in soil, tree trunks, desert rocks, etc.	aphanizomenon flos-aquae, spirulina	high in amino acids, stimulates cellular metabolism

TABLE 7–1 Seaweed Phyla.

carrageenan

a colloid extracted from various red algae (as Irish moss) used as a thickener or stabilizer in ice cream, medicines, cosmetics, and spa products

carbon cycle

the cycle of carbon in the Earth's ecosystems in which carbon dioxide is transformed through photosynthesis into organic nutrients, like oxygen, then ultimately turned back into an inorganic state, as through human respiration

limited depth range, typically from the surface down to not more than 879 feet deep, with the vast majority above 200 feet. Of all these algae, only a dozen or so commonly find their way into spa treatment rooms.

In order to create the benefits enjoyed by spa clients during thalassotherapy applications, algae must undergo photosynthesis, in which absorbed sunlight goes through a chemical transformation, converting it into potential energy which the algae store for later use. In addition to algae, two other types of living things can perform photosynthesis: plants and certain bacteria. Almost every living organism is dependent upon photosynthesis for food. Photosynthesis is also the process by which algae free oxygen from carbon dioxide. Chlorophyll is the green pigment used by most plants to absorb energy from the sun, but in algae, a wide variety of other pigments may be used to perform photosynthesis. This is the reason algae come in so many hues. The endless cycle of plants and algae converting carbon dioxide into oxygen through photosynthesis, only to have this oxygen inhaled by animals who then exhale carbon dioxide yet again, is part of a key process in nature known as the **carbon cycle** (Figure 7–2).

All in all, algae are much more interesting, and vital to life as we know it, than most people expect. An entire branch of science, known as **phycology** or **algology**, is devoted to the study of algae.

Most of the seaweeds used in the spa industry are sourced from the northwest coast of France, off the shores of Brittany and Normandy. The seaweed is not typically applied in its fresh state, but rather processed for ease of transportation and application. After kelp is harvested, for example, its nutrient-dense material is separated from the fibrous cell walls, and the concentrated portion is then made suitable for packing and shipment, either through freeze-drying, micronization, or other processes. Spas and spa product companies then reconstitute this powder and mix it with other ingredients such as essential oils to create the finished products used on clients' skin.

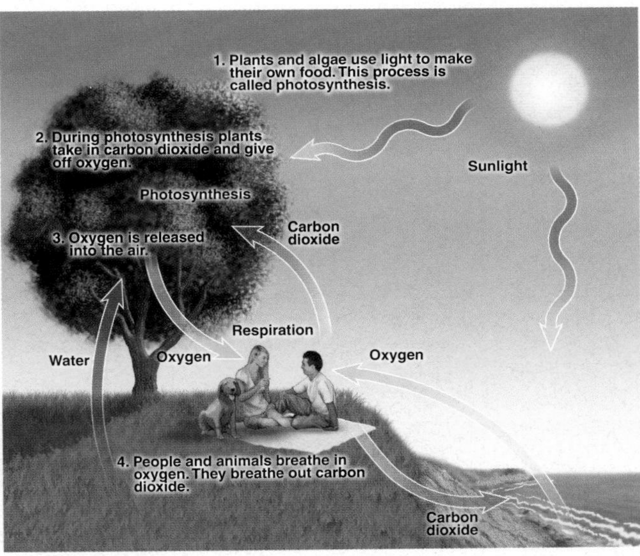
1. Plants and algae use light to make their own food. This process is called photosynthesis.
2. During photosynthesis plants take in carbon dioxide and give off oxygen.
Photosynthesis
3. Oxygen is released into the air.
Carbon dioxide
Sunlight
Respiration
Water
Oxygen
Oxygen
4. People and animals breathe in oxygen. They breathe out carbon dioxide.
Carbon dioxide

FIGURE 7–2 Algae form a crucial part of the carbon cycle.

SPA TIP

Speaking Properly of Algae

Only larger, multicelled algae are considered seaweed. Thus, in a classic rectangles-versus-squares scenario, all seaweeds are a type of algae, but not all algae are seaweed. Also, the word *algae* is the plural form of the less common singular "**alga**."

EFFECTS AND BENEFITS OF THALASSOTHERAPY

Perhaps the most important and certainly the most talked-about benefit of all thalassotherapy treatments is **remineralization**. The microscopic life packed into every drop of seawater and algae carries with it a high density of minerals such as magnesium, potassium, calcium, and sodium. Table 7–2 lists the primary elements in seawater, while Table 7–3 shows them all, including trace elements present in minute amounts. See the profile in this chapter of Dan Fryda, president of Spa Technologies, for more information about the importance of minerals found in seaweed products.

Because our soil and environment have been depleted of minerals, we cannot rely on food to supply these vital elements in our diet. Unless farmers remineralize the soil, our food lacks many of these elements, making it necessary to supplement our diets with sea salt or mineral supplements. Refined table salt is

SPA TIP

Ancient Algae

Until recently, the classification *cyanobacteria* used to be called *blue-green algae*. Scientists found, though, that these organisms are more like bacteria than plants. They are still used in spa treatments, and they are really, really old. In fact, they comprise the absolute oldest known fossil of any type on Earth. Fossils consisting of cyanobacteria discovered in western Australia were dated at 3.5 billion years old, just slightly younger than the oldest known rocks on the Earth, which are 3.8 billion years old. So, when this type of "seaweed" is used in the spa, clients are literally having the oldest, most elemental form of life applied to their skin and absorbed into their pores.

alga
singular form of *algae*; refers to aquatic plants or plantlike chlorophyll-containing nonvascular organisms

phycology
the science and study of algae; see also *algology*

algology
the science and study of algae; see also *phycology*

remineralization
the process of supplying the body with minerals that have been depleted through lifestyle and/or environmental factors; the main benefit of thalassotherapy treatments

ELEMENT	PERCENT	ELEMENT	PERCENT
Oxygen	85.84	Sulfur	0.091
Hydrogen	10.82	Calcium	0.04
Chlorine	1.94	Potassium	0.04
Sodium	1.08	Bromine	0.0067
Magnesium	0.1292	Carbon	0.0028

TABLE 7–2 Seawater Composition by Percentage of Mass.

ELEMENT NAME	CHEMICAL SYMBOL	ELEMENT NAME	CHEMICAL SYMBOL
Aluminum	AL	Gold	AU
Antimony	SB	Hafnium	HF
Arsenic	AS	Holmium	HO
Barium	BA	Indium	IN
Beryllium	BE	Iodine	I
Bismuth	BI	Iridium	IR
Boron	B	Iron	FE
Bromine	BR	Lanthanum	LA
Cadmium	CD	Lead	PB
Calcium	CA	Lithium	LI
Carbon	C	Lutetium	LU
Cerium	CE	Magnesium	MG
Cesium	CS	Manganese	MN
Chloride	CL	Mercury	HG
Chromium	CR	Molybdenum	MO
Cobalt	CO	Neodymium	ND
Copper	CU	Nickel	NI
Dysprosium	DY	Niobium	NB
Erbium	ER	Osmium	OS
Europium	EU	Palladium	PD
Fluoride	F	Phosphorus	P
Gadolinium	GD	Platinum	PT
Gallium	GA	Potassium	K
Germanium	GE	Praseodymium	PR

TABLE 7–3 Complete List of Elements in Seawater. *(Continued)*

ELEMENT NAME	CHEMICAL SYMBOL	ELEMENT NAME	CHEMICAL SYMBOL
Rhenium	RE	Terbium	TB
Rhodium	RH	Thallium	TL
Rubidium	RB	Thorium	TH
Ruthenium	RU	Thulium	TM
Samarium	SM	Tin	SN
Scandium	SC	Titanium	TI
Selenium	SE	Tungsten	W
Silicon	SI	Vanadium	V
Silver	AG	Ytterbium	YB
Sodium	NA	Yttrium	Y
Strontium	SR	Zinc	ZN
Sulfur (sulfate)	S	Zirconium	ZR
Tantalum	TA	Oxygen	O
Tellurium	TE	Hydrogen	H

TABLE 7–3 Complete List of Elements in Seawater.

a poor substitute, as it increases appetite and lacks trace minerals, and the excess iodine added to it may increase hypothyroidism. The sea, on the other hand, is replete with every mineral and element imaginable.

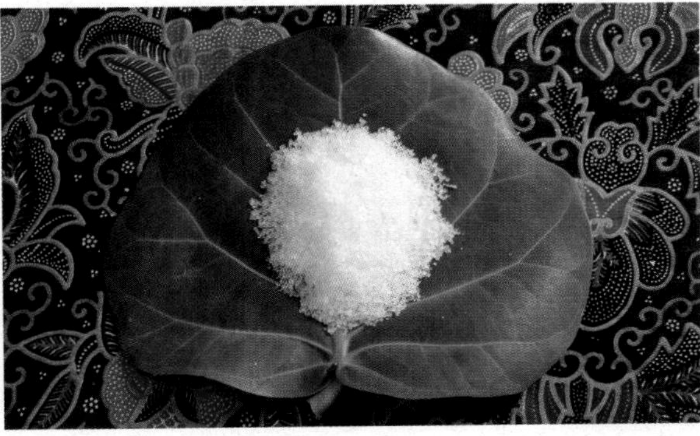

FIGURE 7–3 Crystals of sea salt.

Seawater, of course, contains plentiful concentrations of salt (Figure 7–3), averaging 3.5 percent or 35 parts per thousand. Salt is vital to the healthy functioning of the human body, helping to balance and replenish the body's **electrolytes**. In parts of the world where no land-based salt deposits have been available, humans have gone to great lengths to procure their salt from the sea. The Japanese, for example, relied upon the sea for centuries to provide their necessary salt because they had no terrestrial salt sources. The many minerals found in sea salt, seaweeds, and seawater can be broken down into two main categories: major minerals and trace minerals. Trace minerals are defined as those substances of which the body needs less than 100 milligrams per day, while major minerals include those of which we require more than 100 milligrams. Minerals help support normal metabolism in a number of ways (Table 7–4). In fact, without minerals, your body would not be able to absorb vitamins, and many biological processes including muscle movement and the sending of nerve impulses would be impossible.

Seawater also contains other important therapeutic components in addition to minerals. Some of those most often cited by seaweed suppliers include **phytoplankton** and **zooplankton**. Phytoplankton is the plant constituent of plankton, mainly consisting of unicellular algae, and zooplankton is the animal constituent of plankton, consisting primarily of minuscule crustaceans and fish

electrolyte

any of the ions, such as sodium or calcium, that in biological fluid regulate or affect most metabolic processes, e.g. the flow of nutrients into and waste products out of cells

phytoplankton

plant constituent of plankton; mainly unicellular algae

zooplankton

animal constituent of plankton; mainly small crustaceans and fish larvae

MAJOR MINERALS IN SEA SALTS	
Calcium	needed for building and repairing many tissues in the body, particularly bone, neutralizes acidity
Chlorine	controls the flow of body fluids, maintains proper electrolyte balance, helps reduce excess acid levels, aids digestion inside stomach in the form of hydrochloric acid
Magnesium	promotes assimilation of carbohydrates, assures metabolism of vitamin C and calcium, helps prevent calcium deposits and kidney stones
Phosphorus	essential for biochemical synthesis and nerve cell functions related to the brain, important for bone mineralization
Potassium	maintains healthy nervous system and regular heart rhythm, aids muscle contraction, works with sodium to control the body's water balance, helps maintain stable blood pressure
Sodium	essential to digestion and metabolism, regulates body fluids, nerve and muscular functions
SOME OF THE TRACE MINERALS IN THE SEA SALTS	
Bromine	regulates nervous system, vital for pituitary hormonal function
Chromium	required in trace amounts for sugar metabolism
Cobalt	required for biosynthesis of vitamin B_{12}
Copper	required component of many enzymes
Iodine	production of thyroid hormones, needed for immune defense
Iron	required for many proteins and enzymes, especially hemoglobin
Manganese	needed for oxygen processing
Selenium	required for certain enzymes, has antioxidant properties
Silicon	needed for skin and hair balance, bone and cartilage formation
Sulfur	required for three essential amino acids and many proteins
Zinc	required for several enzymes

TABLE 7–4 Minerals in Sea Salt.

larvae. Plankton, of course, are loaded with nutrients, as they are at the absolute bottom of the planet's food chain and thus contain energy converted directly from sunlight. They have been said to contain antibiotic, bacteria-inhibiting, and anti-viral substances. Algae contain **polysaccharides**, complex chains of carbohydrates that promote the absorption of moisture on the surface of the skin, giving it an improved, healthier, more hydrated appearance. Algae also contain proteins, amino acids, vitamins, and **phytohormones**, which seaweed suppliers claim help to moisturize and nourish the skin, as well as defend it against UV radiation.

polysaccharides
complex carbohydrates found in seaweeds that help skin absorb moisture

phytohormones
plant hormones that regulate physiological process; found in seaweeds

In addition to remineralization and the therapeutic benefits that it implies, thalassotherapy treatments are also recommended to spa clients to treat a number of specific conditions. Over the past several decades, therapists and physicians at thalassotherapy centers have administered seawater and seaweed treatments as part of programs such as weight loss, anti-cellulite, and stress reduction programs, as well as beautifying treatments. Some of the particular conditions for

That "Sea Smell"

Did You Know?

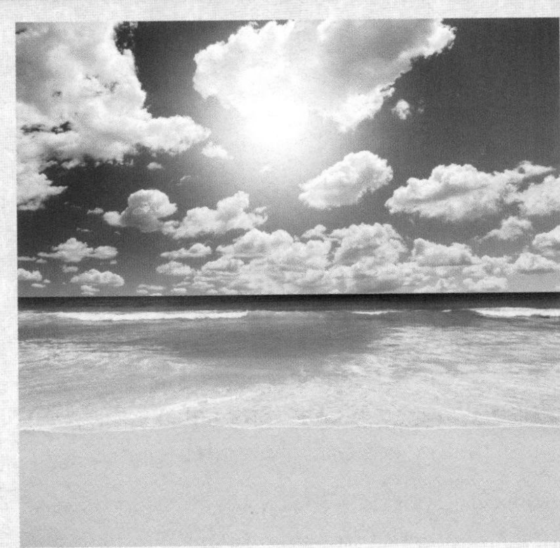

If you have ever had the experience of walking along the sea shore and breathing in a deep, pungent lungful of ocean air, you have experienced the effects of **dimethyl sulfide (DMS)**. This compound is the ingredient in the ocean responsible for its unique smell. Across the ocean and along the coasts all around the world, millions of tons of DMS are released by microbes that live in seaweed and plankton, giving off this unmistakable, living odor. The gas also has an effect on the formation of clouds over the ocean, thus impacting the climate of the whole planet.

DMS has been known to scientists for years, and recently, researchers at the University of East Anglia in the United Kingdom were able to extract a single gene responsible for its emission. In a kind of old wives' tale passed down for years, many people have referred to the sea's smell as being caused by "ozone," which was often credited with healing or rehabilitative powers. But in fact, as pointed out by the scientists, it is DMS that causes the smell, which is simply a gas released by a microbe. No particular curative properties have as yet been ascribed to it.

For more information about the "spa smell"—the pleasant commingling of aromas in many spas which usually includes a seaweed component—and how to create it in your own spa environment, see Chapter 17 in the "Spa Aromas for the Massage Room" section.

which thalassotherapy has been recommended in traditional thalassotherapy centers include:

- Depression
- Obesity
- Cellulite
- Rheumatism
- Peripheral circulatory problems
- Recovery from surgery or illness

SPA TIP

"The main benefit of seaweeds used in spa services is to provide intense nourishment to the skin."

—Dan Fryda

Thalassotherapy Contraindications

There are few contraindications for thalassotherapy treatments, which make them particularly safe for a majority of spa clients. In fact, the most commonly cited contraindication, allergy to shellfish, is actually unnecessary. See the Did You Know? sidebar, The Iodine Allergy Fallacy. However, it is important to keep the following two points in mind and, if one or more of them presents itself, to possibly advise clients against receiving these services.

Thalassotherapy Contraindication 1: Claustrophobia

Clients receiving a seaweed body wrap can sometimes experience claustrophobia, especially if the wrap is wound too tightly around the body, pinning the arms.

dimethyl sulfide (DMS)

gas released by microbes that live in seaweed and plankton; responsible for the sea's particular smell

The Iodine Allergy Fallacy

Did You Know?

For years, many spa therapists and managers have unintentionally misled clients by claiming "allergies to shellfish" as a contraindication for thalassotherapy treatments. Their line of reasoning was as follows: The ingredient to which people are allergic in shellfish is iodine, and seaweed also contains iodine. Therefore, if people are allergic to shellfish, they will be allergic to seaweed and it should not be applied. This reasoning is wrong.

It is not actually iodine that people are allergic to in shellfish. Scientists have proven that what causes allergic reactions to shellfish are certain shellfish proteins, such as the muscle protein tropomyosin. Tulane University Health Sciences Center researcher Dr. Samuel B. Lehrer, who has published articles on the topic in the journal *Marine Biotechnology*, states, "This misconception of iodine and seafood allergy has persisted in spite of the fact that there is little or no evidence to support it and data over the past 20 years has identified the protein allergens which cause seafood allergy." He also notes that the proteins responsible for these allergic reactions are animal proteins, which means that they do not exist in the kelp and other algae that spa therapists apply to their clients' skin.

While it is possible that a client could have a reaction or sensitivity to some ingredient in a thalassotherapy application, that ingredient is likely not iodine. Verifiable cases of iodine allergy, in fact, have not been scientifically documented.

The bottom line? Being allergic to shellfish does not mean clients should not receive seaweed wraps or other sea-based product applications. Do not perpetuate this error yourself and keep clients from receiving perfectly safe spa treatments.

This, however, is not a contraindication specific to thalassotherapy. Rather, the act of wrapping itself is what causes the reaction, which would occur even if no spa product were applied to the body. Because seaweed body wraps are not heat treatments, insulation is not as important as it is for an herbal wrap, for example, during which as much heat as possible must be retained within the wrapping layers in order for the treatment to be effective. During seaweed wraps, then, the blanket and sheets can surround the body in a looser and more comfortable manner if so desired, avoiding almost all concerns regarding claustrophobia. See the Did You Know sidebar, Fear of Being Wrapped, in Chapter 8.

Thalassotherapy Contraindication 2: Sensitivities to Essential Oils and Additives

Often, pre-blended seaweed products contain essential oils or fragrances that may trigger sensitivities in certain clients. Whenever a pre-blended product is used, each ingredient should be disclosed to the client prior to application in order to avoid a reaction. Before adding an essential oil to reconstituted seaweed, always check with clients for sensitivities.

SEAWEED APPLICATIONS

A wide array of thalassotherapy applications are offered in spas, including many focused on the face, applied primarily by estheticians. The majority of seaweed and seawater treatments performed by massage therapists are body wraps, baths, and

FORM USED	DESCRIPTION	ADVANTAGES	DISADVANTAGES
Seawater	water pumped directly from the ocean and warmed for use in the spa	the purest and most direct use of seawater	restricted to specialized coastal facilities
Mud/Clay	mud sourced from the sea shore or sea bed; also, seaweed is sometimes combined with clay and mud to add drawing/purifying properties	spreads evenly on clients' skin and purifies the body effectively	can be messy during cleanup
Spray Mist	seaweed extracts mixed with other liquid components to create a spray-on application often used at the end of seaweed wraps	quick and easy to apply	can sometimes be overly cooling on skin
Powder	the micronized or freeze-dried nutrient-dense core of sea plants	allows for on-site reconstitution	possible unpleasant odor, difficult to mix
Lotion	seaweed extracts blended with body lotion	ease of application	some products have unknown amounts of seaweed
Extracts	a concentrated form of seawater or seaweed, usually added to other substances such as bath water, body creams, or lotions	powerful even in small amounts; softens, hydrate and smooth skin, improves product texture	can be expensive
Oil	massage oil infused with seaweed extracts	adds benefits of thalassotherapy to massage	some products have unknown amounts of seaweed

TABLE 7–5 Sea Products Used in Spas.

cellulite services, which will be covered in this section. Sea salt exfoliation services can also be considered a type of sea-based treatment because their primary ingredient, sea salt, comes from the ocean, though typically these treatments are not classified under thalassotherapy on spa menus. See Chapter 6 for more information about sea salt exfoliation. The ingredients used in the many manifestations of thalassotherapy in the spa range from straight seawater to highly processed body creams. See Table 7–5 for more information on these products.

Although it is not as fashionable as it once was, drinking seawater for its therapeutic benefits is still practiced by some diehard believers. For instance,

SPA TIP

Powdered versus Pre-Packaged Seaweeds

While some therapists have a strong preference for using pure micronized seaweed, which is reconstituted right in the treatment room, others swear by pre-packaged seaweed products that come from manufacturers ready to be applied to the body. Each has its advantages. Pure seaweed powder is unadulterated and free of any additives, and therapists can feel assured that what they are applying to their clients' skin is whole and natural. What's more, therapists can control the addition of any other ingredients to the seaweed, including water, oils, and scents. On the other hand, this process takes time, and some clients are not interested in the pedigree of particular products. Packaged seaweed brands are simpler to prepare and apply, and some clients have an affinity to certain suppliers, but therapists have no control over the ingredients. In the end, the choice is a matter of personal preference. Both types of seaweed product work. It is up to the therapist to represent the most positive aspect of each to the client.

Nick Monte, founder of Gurney's Inn and the International Health & Beauty Sea Water Spa on the tip of Long Island, had his daily drink of seawater shipped fresh from the Atlantic to his home in Las Vegas until he passed away in 2007 at the age of 90. He credited much of his health and longevity to this internal thalassotherapy. Scientists and physicians warn that drinking seawater is harmful and potentially fatal, as has been proven by countless castaways dying of thirst who were tempted to drink the water all around them, only to have the excess salts in the seawater hasten dehydration, wreak havoc with cell metabolism, create delirium, and ultimately result in death. However, small amounts of seawater diluted to the proper 0.9 percent salinity and ingested over long periods of time apparently have no such side effects and may even be beneficial, as proven by long-lived thalassotherapy proponents such as Mr. Monte.

Seaweed has also been shown to be an effective tool in weight-loss programs. Kazuo Miyashita, a professor at Hokkaido University in Japan, has studied the effects of seaweed on weight loss, with some positive results. In research funded by the Japanese government, he focused on **fucoxanthin**, a pigment found in brown algae but not in green or red. He found that this pigment promotes fat burning within fat cells in white adipose tissue by increasing the action of the protein thermogenin. In laboratory experiments, he and his team supplemented the diet of obese rodents with fucoxanthin, resulting in weight losses of up to 10 percent. The seaweed ingredient has been formulated into products for human use to help fight the growing obesity epidemic, but research on its effectiveness has so far been inconclusive. Soon, though, spas might be able to boast that thalassotherapy's benefits include weight loss in addition to wellness and remineralization—a trifecta for health-conscious spa clients.

fucoxanthin

brown pigment occurring in the chloroplasts of brown algae, found in scientific studies to help reduce fat

ACTIVITY

If Our Bodies Come from the Sea, Why Is the Sea Saltier than We Are?

When the first living organisms evolved in the oceans, seawater had a salt content much lower than it is today. Over the eons, the seas became saltier as fresh water captured salts in the soils and rocks it flows through on the way to the ocean. At the same time, water has continually evaporated from the oceans, leaving the salts behind. This has created today's 3.5 percent salinity level, compared to the 0.9 percent level found in the oceans when life first evolved. The fluids in our bodies still have this lower salinity level, which helps explain why drinking straight seawater today is ill-advised.

As an experiment, create two salt solutions, one with a salinity level equal to the ocean's and one equal to that in our bodies. To accomplish this, place 9 grams of salt in 1 liter of water to simulate our bodies' salinity, and place 35 grams of salt in another liter of water to simulate the salinity of the sea. Note: 9 grams of salt is approximately 1.5 teaspoons and 35 grams is approximately 6 teaspoons. Now, taste a few drops of each solution. Can you discern a big difference in salinity levels? Does one seem more compatible with your body? Could you imagine yourself drinking a small cup of the 0.9 percent solution each day? This 0.9 percent saline solution is what doctors have used for years to cleanse wounds and promote healing. Note: The entire class can share the two liters if this experiment is done as a group. Remember, too, that there is much more to seawater than just water and salts. Real thalassotherapy depends upon the teeming richness of living organisms found in every drop.

Seaweed Body Wrap

Seaweed body wraps completely envelop spa clients in a layer of algae in the form of a sea mud, sea clay, reconstituted micronized seaweed, or, very rarely, fresh seaweed (if the spa is located on the coast). A wrap such as this is sometimes referred to as a **cocoon** or a **body masque**, as are many full-body envelopments using other products in addition to seaweed, such as fango mud and desert clay. Seaweed wraps are not considered heat treatments because they do not include the application of heat to the body. However, clients may become quite warm while wrapped up, because their own body heat is being trapped by the surrounding layers of blankets, sheets, or plastic and reflected back to them (Figure 7–4).

Seaweed wraps are often applied in a wet room, and the product is showered off after the wrap, either in a shower stall or on the table using a Vichy shower or a handheld showerhead operated by the therapist. The technique described and illustrated in this section is for use in a dry room, however, because many

cocoon

term used to describe a spa body wrap in which the client is covered first with a spa product such as seaweed or mud and then enveloped within several layers of blankets and sheets

body masque

French spelling of the word "mask;" an application of seaweed or other spa product to the body, usually entailing wrapping of the body as well

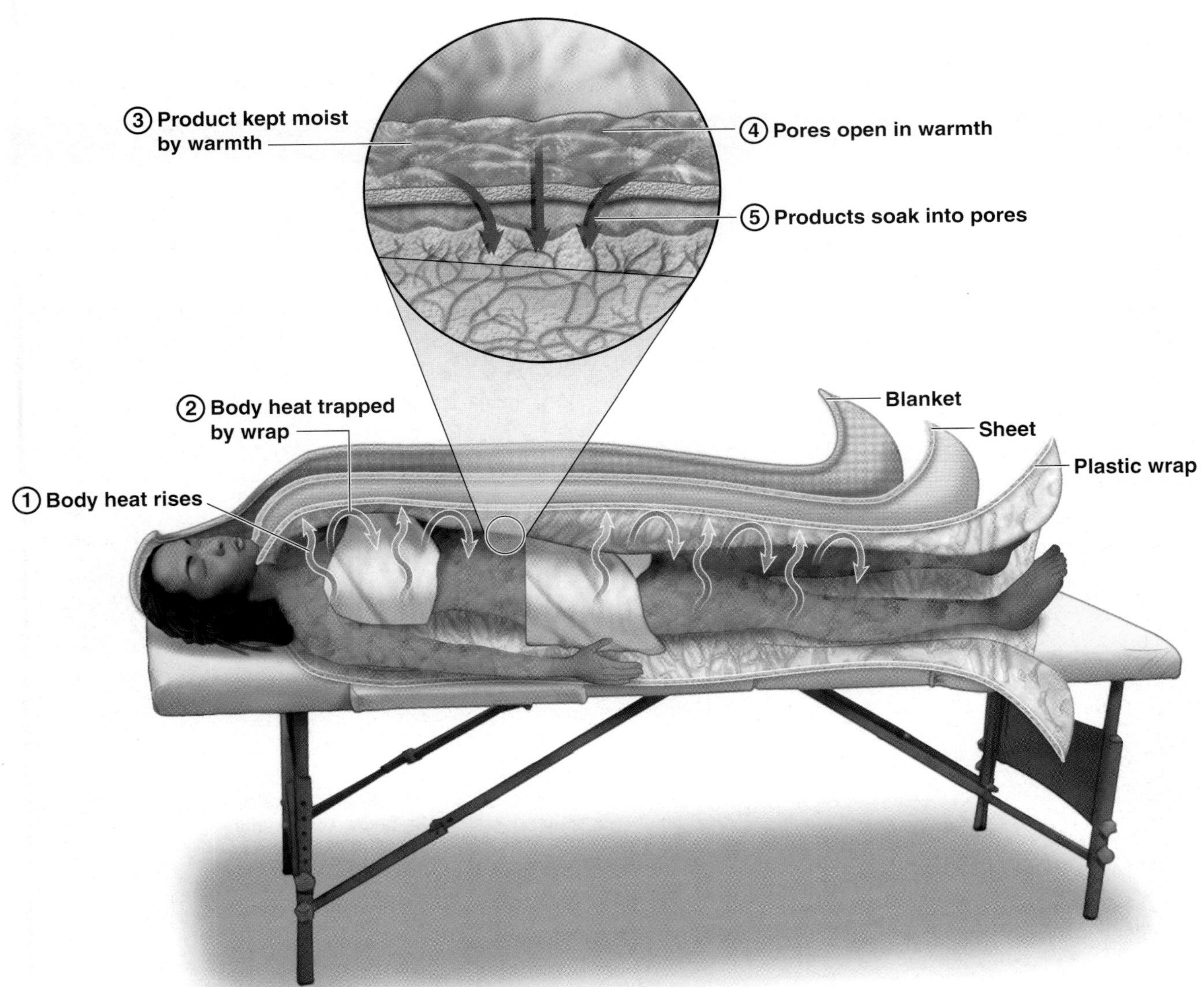
③ Product kept moist by warmth
④ Pores open in warmth
⑤ Products soak into pores
② Body heat trapped by wrap
① Body heat rises
Blanket
Sheet
Plastic wrap

FIGURE 7–4 Even though it is not a heat treatment, clients may become hot in the seaweed wrap.

SPA CAUTION

When using a showerhead or Vichy shower to remove product after a wrap, assure that the water is at the correct temperature range, between 110°F and 120°F, prior to applying the water to the client's skin. Temperatures above that may be uncomfortable or even scald the client.

students do not have access to wet room facilities. When these facilities are available, the procedure is exactly the same, except a shower is used instead of towels to remove product from the body. In a wet room equipped with a wet table and a Vichy shower or handheld shower, the product is washed from the client's skin while she remains on the table. The plastic wrap protects sheets and blankets beneath from getting wet. After the shower, the client either rolls to one side to have the plastic slipped from beneath her body, or steps off the table briefly while the plastic is taken off. In a wet room equipped with a wet table and traditional shower stall, the client is covered with a drape and steps off the table into the shower to wash off the product while the therapist removes the plastic wrap and prepares the table for the lotion application. The client dries off, then returns to the table to complete the treatment. Regardless of whether the wrap is performed in a wet room or a dry room, the same basic six-step procedure is followed:

1. Exfoliate first.
2. Apply product.
3. Wrap.
4. Treat the head or feet while the client is wrapped.
5. Remove product with shower or towels.
6. Apply finishing product.

TREATMENT: SEAWEED BODY WRAP	
Wet Room/Dry Room	dry room
Table Setup	blanket, sheet, plastic wrap, draping
Treatment Duration	60 to 90 minutes
Needed Supplies	exfoliation tool, ¼ cup to ½ cup seaweed or sea mud product, spa bowl, heating unit, a minimum of 4 hot, wet towels, plastic body wrap, optional brush to apply seaweed, optional essential oils to add to reconstituted seaweed, finishing cream or lotion, bolster
Contraindications	claustrophobia, sensitivities to essential oils and additives
Draping	traditional massage draping
Treatment Order	after exfoliation, prior to massage
Safety, Sanitation Issues, & Clean-Up	Seaweed reconstituted in the treatment room can spoil quickly. Dispose of extra product or seal and refrigerate for use within one week. Thoroughly clean product from surfaces to avoid forming mold. Floors can become slippery in wet rooms and shower stalls. Care should be taken when stepping on these surfaces. Rubber mats or non-skid surfaces provide extra safety.
Body Mechanics & Self-Care	same body mechanic considerations as massage therapy
Product Cost	$3 to $5 for seaweed, finishing product, and plastic
Treatment Price	$100 to $150
Physiological Effects	Seaweed soaks into the pores, moistens skin with polysaccharides, and provides minerals and phytoelements which contain antibiotic, bacteria-inhibiting, and anti-viral substances. Although not a heat treatment, the wrap is warming because the client is enveloped in layers.
Pregnancy Issues (information provided by Elaine Stillerman, LMT, author and developer of MotherMassage)	All heat-inducing treatments must be avoided throughout the entire pregnancy. Wait three months postpartum before applying warm or hot body wraps.

Seaweed Body Wrap Preparation

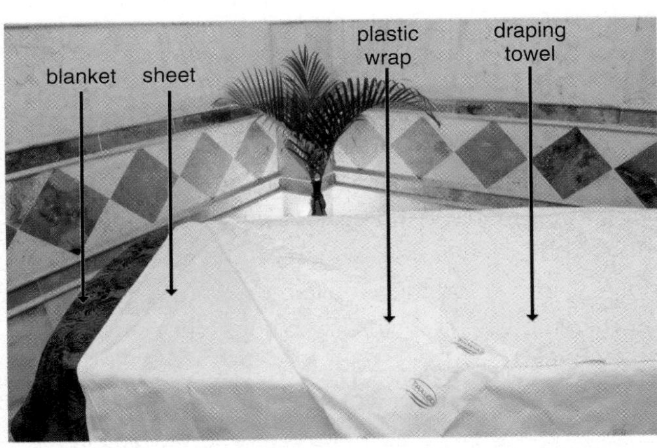

FIGURE 7–5 Table setup for seaweed wrap. Note blanket hangs over head of table, with towel placed over it to match ends.

1. Prepare the table by layering first a blanket, with the top hanging 12 inches over the head of the table, with a bath towel across the top, then a sheet, plastic wrap, and finally draping towels (Figure 7–5).
2. If seaweed is reconstituted for each treatment, mix with adequate water and add 6 to 8 drops of essential oil blend per treatment. Common blends include heating, drainage, detoxifying, and energizing combinations of oils. This improves effectiveness and the aroma of freshly blended seaweed.
3. Place seaweed in a spa bowl and warm in a roaster, hydrocollator, or similar unit.
4. Wring out four hand towels and keep them hot in a roaster or hot towel cabbie. Or, wearing insulated gloves, wring them out in very hot water and place them in an insulated container directly before removing the seaweed from the body.

Seaweed Body Wrap Procedure

1. Start with the client prone and exfoliate, first the back of the left leg, then the right leg and up over the gluteal muscles to the back (Figure 7–6). Then ask the client to roll over, and exfoliate the skin of the front of the legs, abdomen, arms, and shoulders (Figure 7–7). This exfoliation lasts only 5 to 10 minutes and can be accomplished using a dry loofah, exfoliating gloves, or a dry brush. Alternatively, the seaweed wrap can be administered immediately after a full-body exfoliation service as described in Chapter 6, in which case this step is skipped.

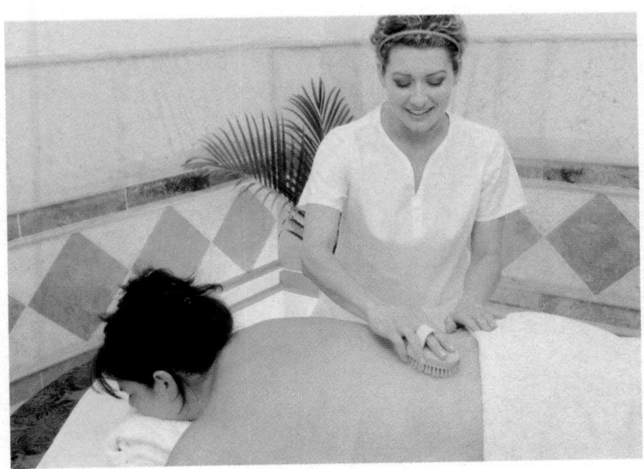

FIGURE 7–6

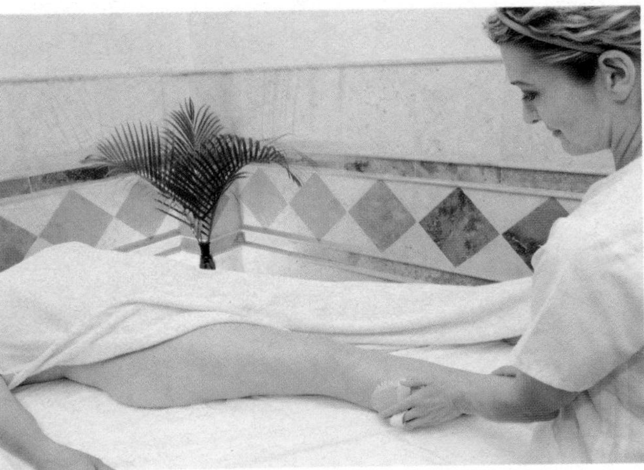

FIGURE 7–7

2. Apply the seaweed, starting on the back. This requires that the client either sit up (Figure 7–8) or roll slightly to one side, then the other (Figure 7–9). Either of these alternatives is preferable to applying seaweed to the entire back and back of legs and having the client turn over, which can be messy and uncomfortable. You can use your hands or a natural-bristle brush to apply the seaweed. Both methods work fine, and it is simply a matter of taste and spa policy as to which method you use. The brush allows a more even and thinner layer of seaweed to be applied, while some therapists prefer the more massage-like feeling of applying product by hand.

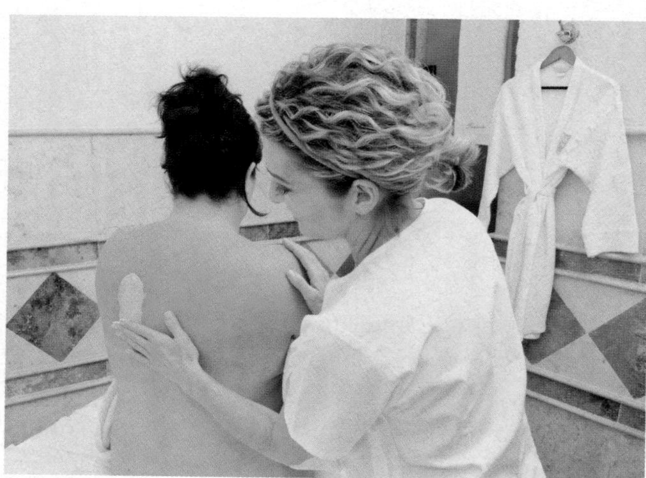

FIGURE 7–8

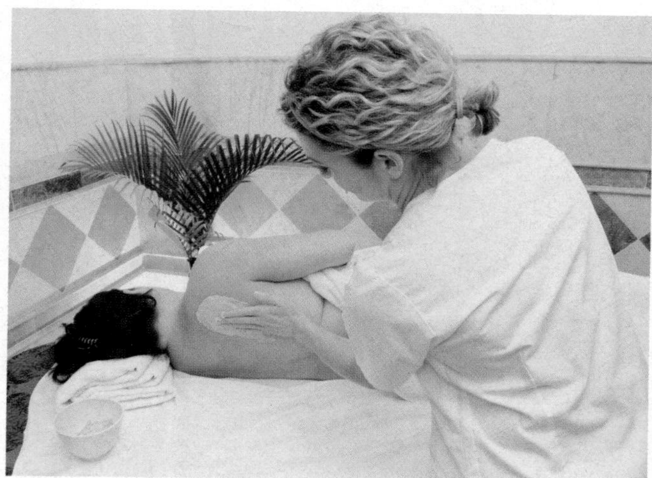

FIGURE 7–9

3. Next, apply seaweed to the left leg. Instruct the client to lift her knee and place her foot flat on the table, rolling slightly to the opposite side. Apply seaweed starting at the ankles; avoid feet if they are going to be treated as part of the service. Move up over the front and back of the leg to the buttock (Figure 7–10). Then have the client lower her leg to the table, and wrap it in plastic.

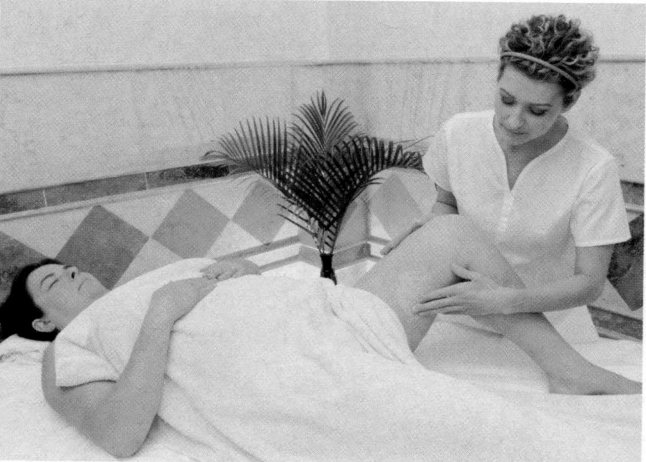

FIGURE 7–10

4. Repeat on the right leg.
5. Apply seaweed to abdomen and décolleté. First, place a breast drape over the chest and slide the main drape out from underneath it down to the hips. Then apply seaweed to the abdomen using clockwise, circular movements (Figure 7–11). Move above the breast drape to apply seaweed to the décolleté area (Figure 7–12).

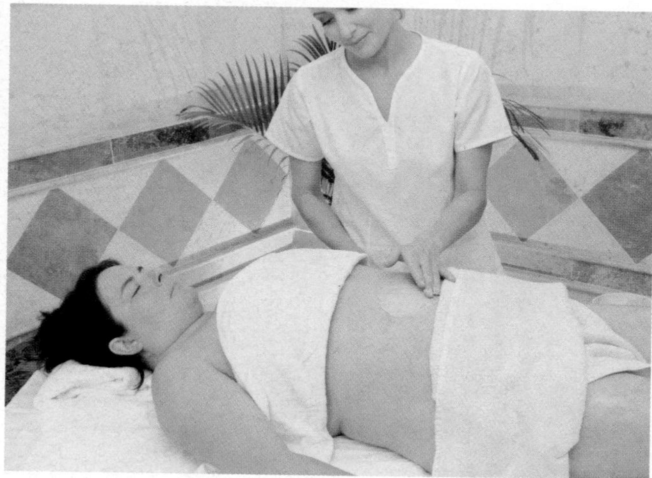

FIGURE 7–11

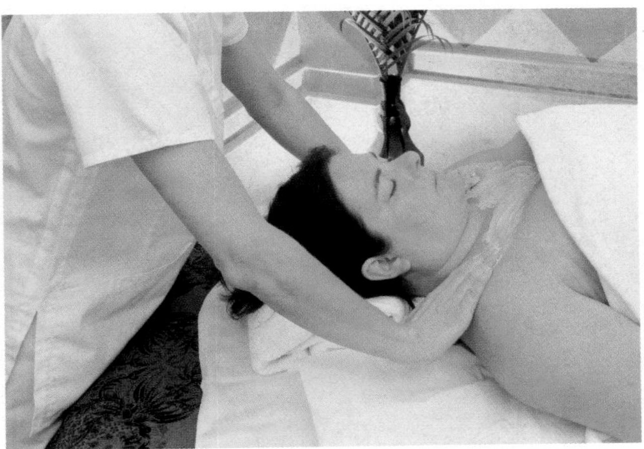

FIGURE 7–12

6. Apply seaweed to the right arm, beginning at the hand and moving up to the shoulder (Figure 7–13). You can instruct the client to lift her arm to apply seaweed to the triceps area if necessary. Cover the arm and the right side of the body in plastic.

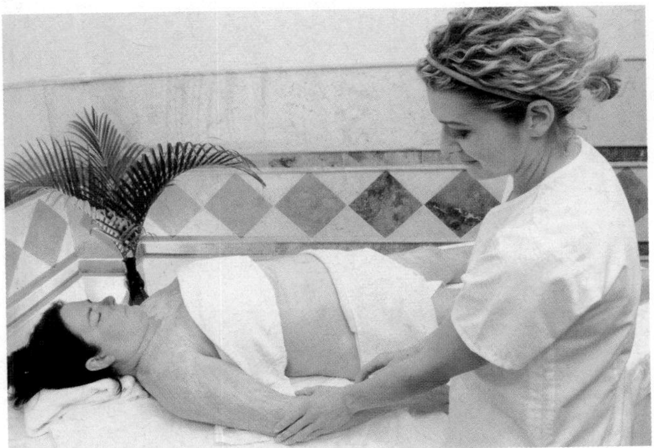

FIGURE 7–13

7. Repeat on the left arm, then cover the arm and the left side of the body in plastic.
8. Standing at the head of the table, grasp the top of the blanket and the lengthwise bath towel in both hands (Figure 7–14). Quickly flip both sides of the blanket up over the client (Figure 7–15). Move down the table and cover the legs and feet. Make sure the blanket is comfortably wrapped around the entire body, then place a bolster beneath the knees. Ask if the client needs anything.

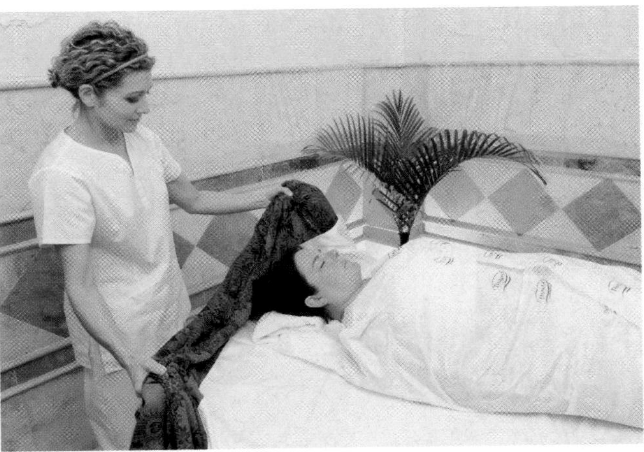

FIGURE 7–14

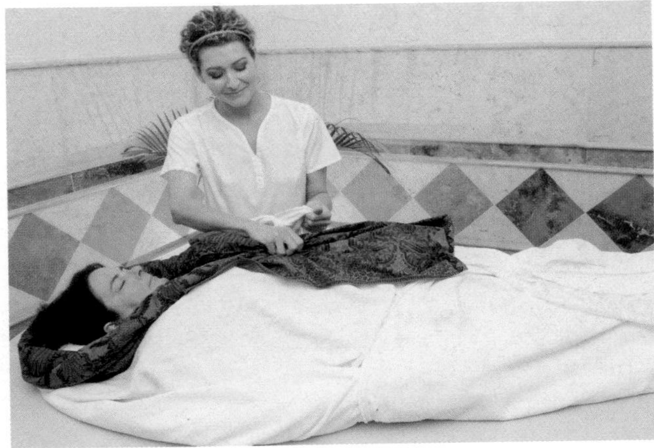

FIGURE 7–15

9. While the client is wrapped for 20 to 25 minutes, apply head, neck, and scalp massage or a mini-face treatment as described in Chapter 13 or a mini-reflexology routine as described in Chapter 9 (Figure 7–16).

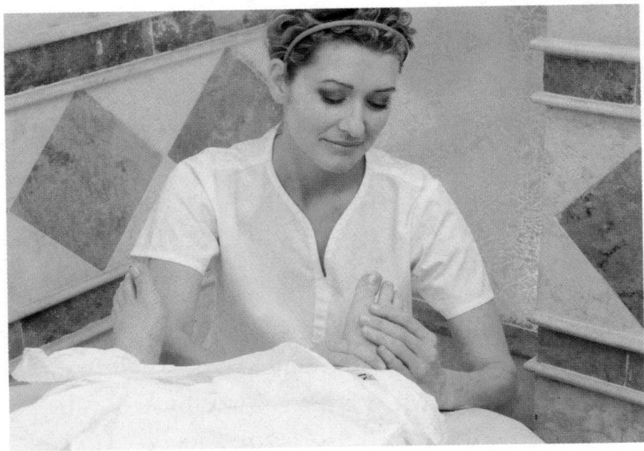

FIGURE 7–16

10. Remove product from the skin. Starting with the left leg, unwrap the blanket and plastic, leaving the rest of the body wrapped to keep the client warm. You can use a rubber spatula to remove excess product from the skin if necessary (Figure 7–17). Then take the first hot towel and wipe the seaweed away from the ankles up to the hips and buttock (Figure 7–18).

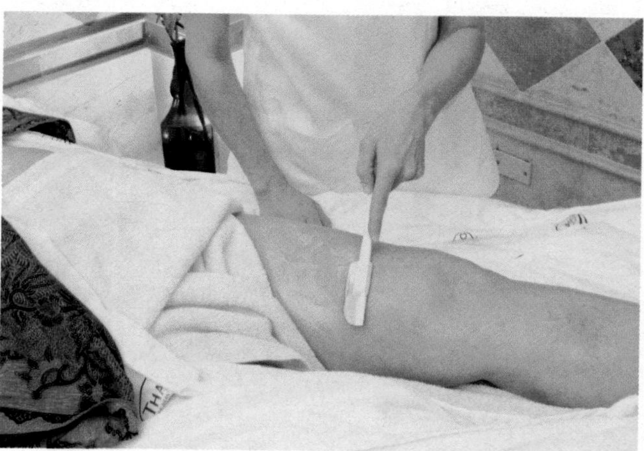

FIGURE 7–17

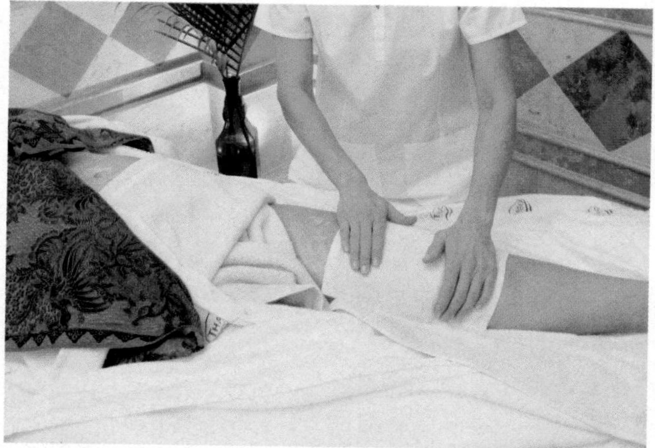

FIGURE 7–18

11. Unwrapping the blanket from the client's left upper body and having her roll slightly to the right, use the second hot towel to remove seaweed from the left arm, shoulder, and left portion of the back (Figure 7–19).

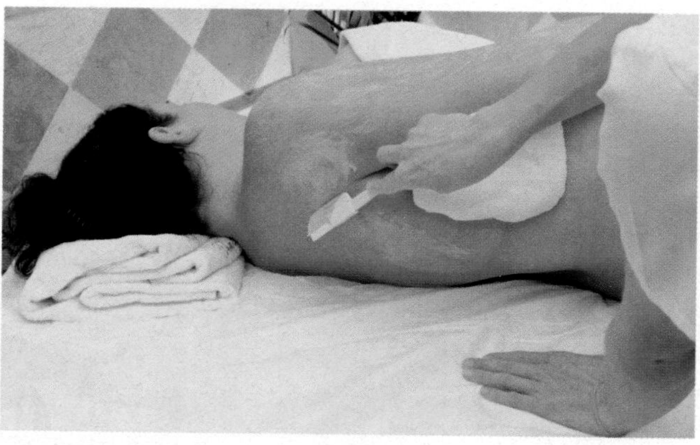

FIGURE 7–19

12. Before the client rolls back down onto her back, tuck the plastic wrap as far underneath the body as it will go so the client lies back down on the clean sheet (Figure 7–20).

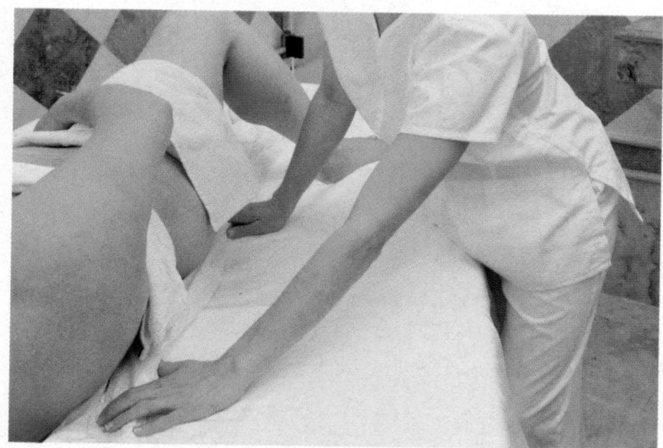

FIGURE 7–20

13. Repeat the previous two steps on the right side of the body, using the third towel, this time completely removing the plastic wrap from beneath the client (Figure 7–21).

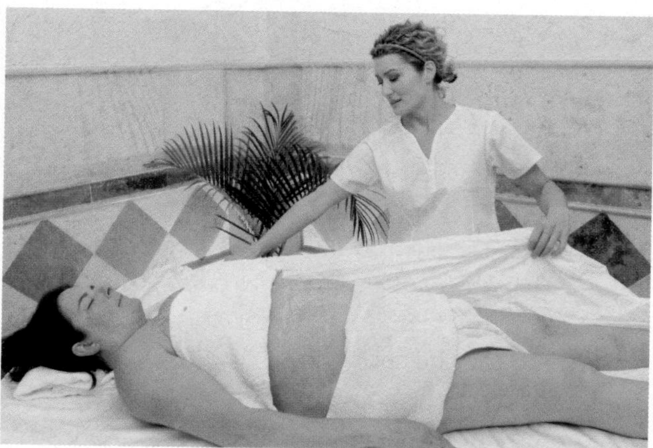

FIGURE 7–21

14. With the last towel, remove the seaweed from the abdomen and décolleté (Figure 7–22).

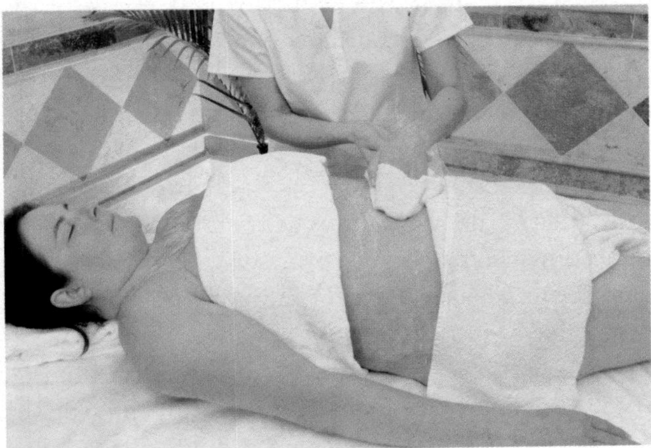

FIGURE 7–22

15. Lastly, apply a finishing product to the skin, a seaweed-infused massage oil, an emollient lotion, a seaweed massage gel, or a spray with seaweed extracts in it. Apply first to the front of the body, retracing steps used to apply the seaweed itself, then have the client roll over and apply to the back of the body. This can be a quick five-minute application or the start of a longer half-hour or full-hour massage.

Seaweed Body Wrap Cleanup

1. Dispose of plastic wrap.
2. Clean the seaweed from the spa bowl and spatula.
3. Launder the towels and sheets.
4. Sanitize the shower stall floors and all surfaces where clients walk barefooted.
5. Properly store and refrigerate any seaweed that has been reconstituted for the treatment.

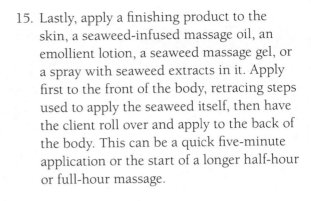

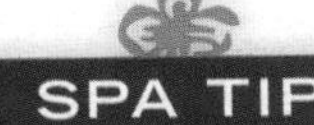

SPA TIP

Do not apply seaweed too thickly in a dry room seaweed wrap treatment, because it will be too messy to remove with towels. A thin layer smoothed onto the skin like paint is enough to allow the seaweed's effects to soak into the client's pores.

Thalassotherapy Bath

Thalassotherapy baths can be administered in a regular bathtub, but their effects are enhanced when done in a jetted tub or, ideally, a hydrotherapy tub with an underwater massage hose. These tubs add mechanical massage effects to the therapeutic effects of the seawater or seaweed product. Traditional thalassotherapy centers offer baths in fresh seawater that has been warmed, but most spas simply add seaweed or seawater extracts to a municipal water source. At these centers, thalassotherapy baths are often given two or three times a week, for a total of 20 or more treatments, often with progressively increasing temperatures. Typical temperatures range from 97°F up to 102°F, with a duration of 10 minutes up to 25 minutes.

SPA ETIQUETTE

Adding Value

Always offer something extra, such as reflexology or a scalp massage, while the client is wrapped in a seaweed wrap. Clients pay well for this service and feel shortchanged if they are left alone for 20 to 25 minutes while the therapist attends to other matters.

SPA TIP

Feeling the Ocean Far from Any Shore

Spa therapists can bring the ocean to their clients, even if those clients are far from the sea, through the application of thalassotherapy treatments. In order to add more of a seashore ambience to these treatments, some spas add special touches such as a wave machine to reproduce the sound of the surf, or a CD with a seashore soundtrack. Some spas dedicate an entire room to these treatments, with murals, ocean-hued paint on the walls, sea shell decorations, and other embellishments that evoke the sea.

A brief exfoliation with a dry bristle brush, loofah pad, or exfoliating gloves is recommended prior to a seaweed bath in order to let the body more readily absorb the ingredients in the seaweed. This can be done by the therapist or the client immediately before entering the bath, or a full exfoliation procedure can be incorporated into the seaweed bath routine. Many spas, however, skip this step. In place of an exfoliation, clients can take a brief shower and rub a soapy wash cloth over the skin.

Seaweed baths sometimes include other components, such as essential oils, which add to the beneficial effects of the seaweed or seawater. They can also increase the pleasure experienced by clients because pure seaweed smells like—well, pure seaweed. Essential oils mask that odor while adding pleasant aromas of their own. In addition, they may have therapeutic benefits. Often, combinations of oils are used to elicit specific effects such as calming, revitalizing, detoxifying, or slimming. These oils can also be included in any finishing lotions or creams applied after the bath. Even if a finishing product is not applied, it is usually recommended that clients do not rinse off, in order to leave active ingredients on the skin and prolong the beneficial osmotic effects of the treatment. The following protocol for a thalassotherapy bath is based on the general outline for therapeutic baths covered in Chapter 4.

TREATMENT: THALASSOTHERAPY BATH	
Wet Room/Dry Room	wet room
Tub Setup	bath tub filled with warm to hot water, therapeutic ingredients already added or nearby, bathmat at entrance, bowl of ice water
Treatment Duration	10 to 25 minutes
Needed Supplies	bath mat, 2 bath towels, hand towel, bowl of ice water, wash cloth, thalassotherapy bath additives
Contraindications	high blood pressure, heart disease, arteriosclerosis, pregnancy, sensitivities to essential oils and additives
Draping	Depending on local laws, clients can be nude in tub when being treated by a therapist of the same sex, or they can wear bathing suits. See Bath Entry Draping Protocol in Chapter 4.
Treatment Order	usually given before massage/body treatments to soften and relax tissues
Safety, Sanitation Issues, & Clean-Up	The tub is sanitized after each use by wiping down entire interior surface with disinfectant. Clients need to be assisted into and out of tub and be warned about feeling weak after treatment. Floors and other surfaces can become slippery.
Body Mechanics & Self-Care	Therapists need to protect lower back while bending over tub and be careful to avoid slipping on wet floors.
Product Cost	generally low, under $3, for seaweed extract or powder to add to bath
Treatment Price	$35 to $75
Physiological Effects	remineralizes body, moisturizes skin, heat in water increases osmotic exchange of nutrients in seaweed while underwater massage hose in hydrotherapy tub relaxes tissues
Pregnancy Issues (information provided by Elaine Stillerman, LMT, author and developer of MotherMassage)	Thalassotherapy is contraindicated during the entire pregnancy. It is safe after three months postpartum.

Thalassotherapy Bath Preparation

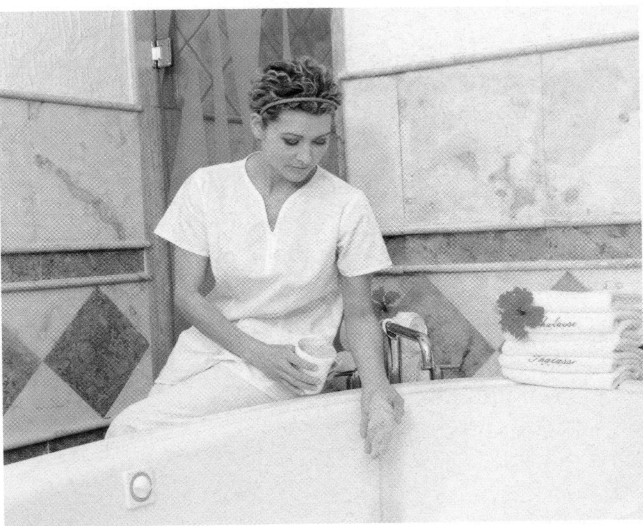

FIGURE 7–23

1. The area is prepared by placing bath mats, non-slip surfaces, towels, ice water, wash cloth and therapeutic ingredients within easy reach.
2. Draw the bath before the client enters the room, setting the temperature to achieve the intended outcome (see Table 4–1), with seaweed bath temperatures averaging 102°F for assimilation and relaxation. Lower temperature and shorter duration can be applied for clients unaccustomed to hydrotherapy treatments.
3. Seawater extract, micronized seaweed powder, or other concentrated sea ingredient is added to the bath while the tub is filling or after the client has entered the room so he can see the products (Figure 7–23). Follow instructions from the manufacturer regarding the amount of product to be added. Some products come in single-use containers.

Thalassotherapy Bath Procedure

1. The procedure, duration, and intended effects are explained to the client prior to entering the tub.
2. The client is assisted into the tub. See the Bath Entry Draping Protocol in Chapter 4.
3. If the bathtub is jetted, the therapist will need to explain to the client how to turn the jets on and off.
4. Have cold compresses available to apply to the client's forehead if needed or desired.
5. The thalassotherapy bath lasts 10 to 25 minutes, depending upon the client's age, health, tolerance for heat, and desired experience. Maximum time for hot baths (100°F or above) is usually 15 minutes, but therapeutic baths cool down over time, as compared to Jacuzzis, hot tubs, hot springs, and whirlpools, which maintain a constant high temperature. Therefore, clients can remain in therapeutic baths longer.
6. Assist the client out of the tub. Offer a bathrobe, slippers, and a glass of water. Help the client into a nearby chair or lounger to relax afterward, or guide him to the next spa treatment.
7. Optionally, a finishing product may be applied to the skin, such as a seaweed-infused massage oil, an emollient lotion, a seaweed massage gel, or a spray with seaweed extracts in it. Apply it first to the front of the body, then have the client roll over and apply it to the back of the body. This can be a quick five-minute application or the start of a longer half-hour or full-hour massage.

ACTIVITY

Thalassotherapy Bath

Experience a thalassotherapy bath for yourself. If your school has a hydrotherapy tub, that is the best place to experience a seaweed-based bath. But if no hydrotherapy tub is available, you can use a regular bathtub at home. Do this: Take two baths, one with micronized seaweed powder or another seaweed extract added to the water, and one with just plain water. What are the differences you note in the way your skin and body feel when the seaweed is added? Are there any powerful effects? Subtle ones? None at all? What senses do you use to tell the difference? Touch? Smell? Sight? In one or more paragraphs, describe the main differences between the two baths.

Thalassotherapy Bath Cleanup

1. The tub must be sanitized after every treatment with a disinfectant spray.
2. Floors must be dried between bath treatments to maintain a safe environment.
3. Towels and wash cloths are laundered, bowls cleaned, products stored, and the room tidied for the next treatment.

CELLULITE

cellulite

dimpled appearance of the skin created by deposits of subcutaneous fat, treated by several spa modalities including targeted massage and hydrotherapy featuring seaweed and essential oils

Cellulite is a normal physiological condition affecting a majority of women who have passed puberty, and yet millions of women treat cellulite more as a pathology than an acceptable fact of life. Many women come to spas seeking treatment for cellulite, and spa therapists need to be knowledgeable and honest about the options available. Cellulite services on spa menus vary in effectiveness, and the surest way for therapists to learn about them is to either experience these treatments for themselves or witness first-hand their effects on clients. Many spa cellulite treatments include some aspect of massage in the form of intense, targeted manipulations to the affected areas, along with lymphatic drainage techniques. Thousands of products and a wide range of specialized equipment has been developed to address cellulite, but one of the most trusted applications remains thalassotherapy in combination with massage and sometimes hydrotherapy.

Cellulite can be defined as a normal condition created by deposits of subcutaneous fat within fibrous connective tissues, especially on the thighs, hips, and buttocks, that give a puckered and dimpled appearance to the skin (Figure 7–24). Cellulite can also affect the upper arms and abdomen in some individuals. There are a number of colorful terms used to describe the condition, including "orange peel skin" and "cottage cheese skin." Some other scientific terms used include *adiposis edematosa*, *dermopanniculosis deformans*, *status protrusus cutis*, and *gynoid lipodystrophy*. Cellulite is not related to cellulitis, which is an infection of the skin and underlying connective tissue that affects both men and women. A number

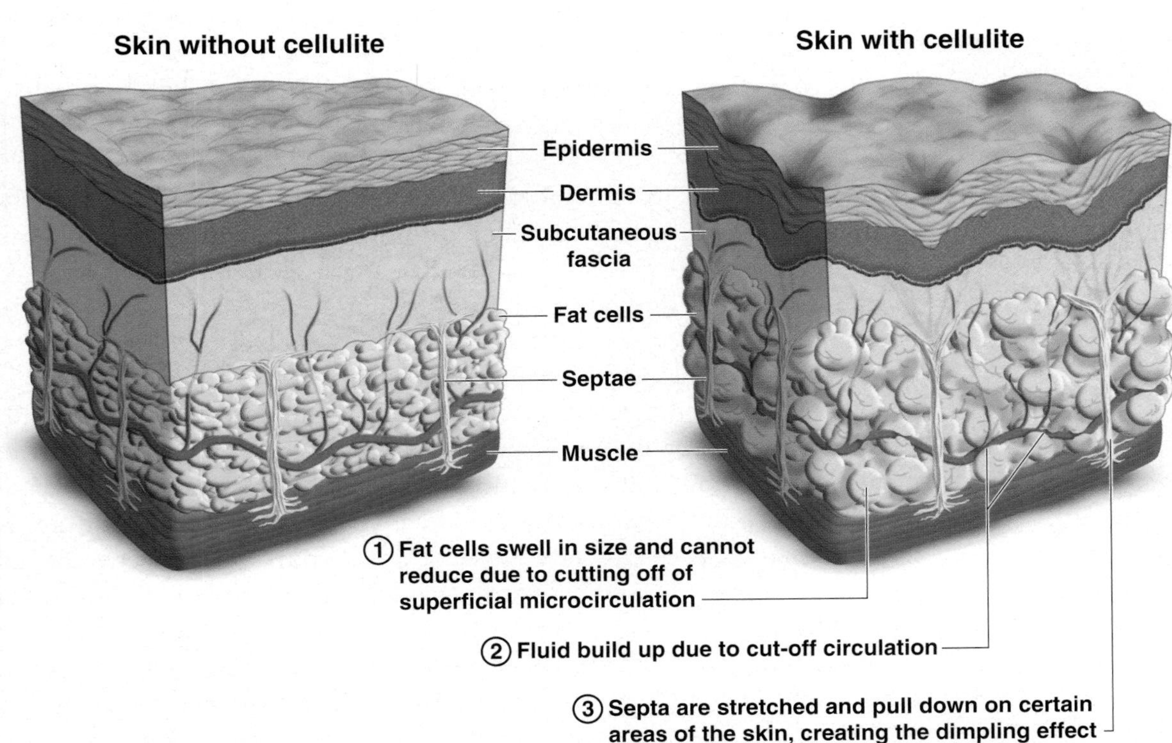
Skin without cellulite
Skin with cellulite
Epidermis
Dermis
Subcutaneous fascia
Fat cells
Septae
Muscle
① Fat cells swell in size and cannot reduce due to cutting off of superficial microcirculation
② Fluid build up due to cut-off circulation
③ Septa are stretched and pull down on certain areas of the skin, creating the dimpling effect

FIGURE 7–24 Cellulite is caused by a number of factors affecting subcutaneous deposits of fat couched within connective tissues. It is formed when connective tissue called *septa* hold down skin that is being pushed up by fat deposits and excess interstitial fluids.

of conditions contribute to the development of cellulite, including the following 10 factors:

1. Growing fat cells found between connective tissues in the subcutaneous layers push up against the skin.
2. At the same time, **septa**, which are the vertical bands of connective tissue connecting the skin to the superficial fascia below in women, begin to harden, holding the skin down in spots while the fat cells push it up.
3. High estrogen levels in the body can stimulate **collagenase** production in **fibroblasts**, which weakens collagen fibers, contributing to cellulite.
4. Fluid imbalances in the body can worsen the appearance of cellulite. Insufficient hydration decreases the body's ability to flush waste from the system, while excess interstitial fluid retention bloats the skin surface.
5. Poor microcirculation and lymphatic elimination create excess pooled fluids and wastes in the superficial tissues.
6. Certain drugs and medications, especially those that affect hormone levels, can have an impact on cellulite.
7. Genetic factors come into play, predisposing some women to retain more superficial fat.
8. Poor diet contributes to the growth of fat cells in the subcutaneous layer.

septa

vertical bands of connective tissue between the skin and the superficial fascia; they can harden and pull down the skin, which is pushed up by fat cells, contributing to the appearance of cellulite

collagenase

enzymes that decompose collagen, which can worsen the appearance of cellulite

fibroblasts

cells that secrete collagen to form the connective tissue matrix of the body

SPA TIP

Men do not exhibit signs of cellulite for two main reasons:

1. Men's connective tissue is not organized into vertical bands as it is by the septa beneath women's skin, so even though their fat cells may grow like women's, they do not push up against the skin in the same uniform way. On top of this, women, in general, have a higher percentage of body fat than men.
2. Men do not have the same levels of estrogen in their bodies. These levels fluctuate in women and may exacerbate the appearance of cellulite. Men who undergo estrogen therapy for prostate cancer sometimes develop cellulite.

9. Inadequate exercise further contributes to the growth of these fat cells.
10. High stress levels can affect hormones and lifestyle habits negatively, leading to more cellulite formation.

It is important to remember that no spa treatment, and no procedure of any kind, actually, will eliminate cellulite. Any technique that promises such should be held suspect. The FDA has never cleared a single product or procedure for the elimination of cellulite, but it has cleared several for this one claim: a temporary reduction in the appearance of cellulite. Notice the two key words in that phrase: temporary and appearance. No procedure, product, or technique in use today will eliminate cellulite, which is, after all, a natural part of the body. When speaking with spa clients about cellulite treatments and programs, always remind them that the results they can expect to achieve are temporary and only affect the appearance of cellulite, not the underlying causes of its existence. This, of course, is perfectly adequate for a large number of women whose goal is, after all, to look better, at least for a while.

It is useless to offer a spa client just one cellulite service. One service will achieve nothing and leave the client feeling that the treatment is ineffective. A series of services over time, usually one or two per week for a total of 10 to 20 treatments, is recommended in order to achieve observable results in the reduction of the appearance of cellulite. At the same time that the spa client is undergoing cellulite treatments, she must agree to follow guidelines regarding nutrition and exercise. Any benefits provided by the treatments will be negated by a sedentary lifestyle and ingestion of fat-laden foods. In addition, clients need to monitor water intake and consume two liters per day in order to help the body flush impurities. And finally, a home-care regimen should be followed, including the self-application of topical products to aid in the ongoing increase of microcirculation and metabolism.

Cellulite treatments are not restricted to overweight spa clients. In fact, underweight and average weight women also get cellulite. Even extremely active triathletes have the condition, and no amount of exercise seems to reduce it. Liposuction, the suctioning of fat deposits from within the body, will not reduce cellulite, because the fat removed is from deeper layers than cellulite, which is found exclusively in superficial subcutaneous areas. The most appropriate candidates for spa cellulite services are women who are willing to lead a healthy lifestyle during the treatment program and who are slightly overweight, with a moderate amount of cellulite. These clients have the best chance at experiencing noticeable results, but these results will be, to reinforce the point, a *temporary* reduction in the *appearance* of cellulite only.

lipolysis

the breakdown of fat stored in fat cells during which free fatty acids are released into the bloodstream; said to occur during spa cellulite treatments

pinch test

self-examination to determine degree of cellulite present in the body

How can a spa seaweed treatment actually affect cellulite? Three main processes are involved. First, specialized massage techniques stretch the septa, which opens the interstitial spaces where fat cells are stored. Then, seaweed promotes local vasodilation, with increased blood and lymph flow. As a result, the increased space and circulation allows the body to re-engage its natural ability to break down fat cells, a process known as **lipolysis**. This "kick-starting"

Did You Know?

The Stages of Cellulite

While 80 to 90 percent of women exhibit some signs of dimpling or orange peel skin, many are confused about the degree or severity of cellulite they have. Some overestimate their amount of cellulite, assuming that the slightest bump signals an all-out infestation. To clarify things, a simple self-exam called the **pinch test** has been devised. To perform this exam, pinch the skin on your outer thigh between your index finger and your thumb. You can also try this on other areas, especially the buttocks and abdomen. Then, once you have the tissues firmly in hand, look for the telltale signs of cellulite—dimpling, bumps, and "cottage cheese." It is best to do this in front of a mirror and with no clothes on (Figure 7–25). A rating called the **Nurnberger–Muller scale** has been devised to classify cellulite, or lack of cellulite, into four stages, beginning with unaffected skin and progressing through to advanced cellulite. The stages are as follows:

- Stage 0 : No dimpling is seen on the skin when you are standing naked in front of the mirror. When the skin is pinched no orange peel effect is seen.
- Stage 1: No dimpling is seen on the skin when you are standing, but when you pinch your skin you have bumps and lumps.
- Stage 2: You can see dimpling or the orange peel effect without pinching the skin when standing naked in front of the mirror, but not when you lie down.
- Stage 3: You can see dimpling both when you are standing and lying down, with no skin pinching necessary.

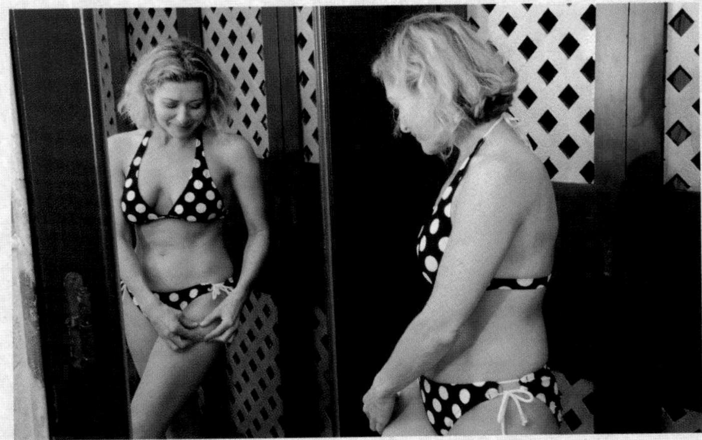

FIGURE 7–25 The "pinch test" is a self-exam for cellulite done before a mirror, normally disrobed.

of lipolysis creates a state in which the body can, for a time, clear some of the fat and excess fluid buildup from superficial areas, improving the appearance of the skin.

Seaweed Cellulite Treatment

Myriad cellulite treatment options have been offered to spa clients, such as laser, ultrasound, **mesotherapy**, **Endermologie®** and others. Anti-cellulite creams, ointments, and elixirs abound, touting their ability to counteract this condition. Among the many natural substances known to affect the rate of lipolysis, improve microcirculation, and facilitate lymphatic drainage are ivy, butcher's broom, ginkgo biloba, arnica, green tea, sweet clover, horse-chestnut, grapes, and evening primrose, among others. Though seaweed is not the only substance said to have a positive impact, it is one of the most respected traditional therapeutic products commonly used in spas today and probably the most widely applied. Another substance many therapists find helpful is paraffin wax, which forms a natural barrier between the skin and the environment, aiding in heat

Nurnberger–Muller scale
breakdown of the visible signs of cellulite into four distinct stages, 0 to 3, ascertainable by self-testing

mesotherapy
injection of fat-dissolving compounds into the skin to treat cellulite and sculpt the body

Endermologie®
mechanical massage using two motorized rollers and suction to mobilize skin and subcutaneous tissues for the treatments of cellulite, scars, burns, and other conditions

lypossage

non-mechanical massage treatment intended to reduce the appearance of cellulite

retention and enhancing the effects of any products applied. More information about paraffin applications can be found in Chapter 13.

The type of massage applied in this treatment is vigorous and intense. It is not meant to be a relaxing experience. A type of cellulite-specific massage used by some therapists is called **lypossage**, which features similarly intense manipulations. When a hydrotherapy tub is available, it can be used to add to the effects of these manipulations by targeting cellulite prone areas with the high-pressure underwater massage hose. An optional step explaining the use of the hydrotherapy tub in cellulite treatments is included in the following procedure.

Some spa therapists have reacted negatively when asked to apply cellulite treatments because they believe them to be superficial and not truly therapeutic. However, when looked at from another perspective, these treatments can be considered among the most life-changing and profound offerings in the spa. Because diet and exercise considerations must be taken into account when undergoing a cellulite treatment program, this creates a perfect opportunity for the therapist to encourage clients to embrace the entire spa philosophy of wellness, fitness, beautification, and self-care. It is a chance for the therapist to act as mentor, motivator, coach, and confidant, helping people make a fundamental change in lifestyle and attitude, which is one of the most satisfying aspects of a spa therapist's job. Also, the therapist can recommend a home-care program for the client, increasing the likelihood that she will benefit in the long term from the lifestyle changes made at the spa. In addition, cellulite services offer plentiful opportunities for the therapist to make retail sales. See Chapter 16 for more information on retail.

TREATMENT: SEAWEED CELLULITE TREATMENT	
Wet Room/Dry Room	wet room or dry room
Table Setup	blanket, sheet, plastic wrap over target area, draping
Treatment Duration	60 to 90 minutes per treatment, 15 to 20 overall program plus home care
Needed Supplies	exfoliation tool, ¼ cup seaweed, spa bowl, small container for massage cream, heating unit, 4 hot wet towels, plastic body wrap, optional brush to apply seaweed, finishing massage cream, essential oils to add to seaweed and cream, bolster
Contraindications	sensitivities to essential oils and additives, easily bruised skin
Draping	traditional massage draping
Treatment Order	stand-alone, usually applied separate from other spa treatments
Safety, Sanitation Issues, & Clean-Up	Seaweed reconstituted in the treatment room can spoil quickly. Dispose of extra product or seal and refrigerate for use within one week. Thoroughly clean product from surfaces to avoid forming mold. Floors can become slippery in wet rooms and shower stalls. Care should be taken when stepping on these surfaces. Rubber mats or non-skid surfaces provide extra safety. If the optional hydrotherapy tub step is used, help clients in and out of the tub, watching for dizziness or weakness. The tub needs to be sanitized afterwards by wiping down interior surface with disinfectant.
Body Mechanics & Self-Care	Intensive skin rolling can be hard on the therapist's hands. Take breaks between applications. Stretch hands afterwards and use strengthening exercises found in Chapter 9.

(Continued)

TREATMENT: SEAWEED CELLULITE TREATMENT	
Product Cost	$3 to $5 for seaweed, finishing product and plastic
Treatment Price	$100 to $150, almost always offered as a package discounted 10% to 20%, minimum 10 treatments, average 15 to 20 treatments; a spa charging $100/treatment could charge $1,200 to $1,350 for a package of 15, for example
Physiological Effects	targeted massage combines with effects of seaweed and essential oils to increase local circulation, mobilize interstitial fluids, flush toxins, and increase lipolytic action; simultaneously remineralizes body and moisturizes skin; inspires overall health and fitness
Pregnancy Issues (information provided by Elaine Stillerman, LMT, author and developer of MotherMassage)	Since lymphatic drainage on the legs is the most appropriate bodywork during pregnancy and for three months postpartum, all treatments that incorporate deep or vigorous strokes on the legs must be avoided. This treatment is contraindicated throughout pregnancy and for the first three months postpartum.

Seaweed Cellulite Treatment Preparation

1. Offer a consultation before the first service in which the spa's cellulite treatment program, including lifestyle modification, is explained and a plan of action is instituted. Assess specific areas to be treated on each client.
2. Optional: If a hydrotherapy tub is available, fill it with 102°F water and add seaweed extract.
3. Cut plastic wrap to fit across table from client's chest down to the knees. Prepare the table by layering first a blanket, with the top hanging 12 inches over the head of the table, with a bath towel across the top, then a sheet, the plastic wrap, and finally draping towels (Figure 7–26).
4. Dip four hand towels in hot water, wring out, and keep hot.
5. Add 6 to 8 drops active, circulation-enhancing essential oil to ¼ cup seaweed in the spa bowl. Single oils or a blend can be used. See Chapter 11 for more information about essential oils. Warm this mixture in a hydrocollator, roaster, or other heating unit.
6. Add 4 to 6 drops of the same essential oil to 1 tablespoon of massage cream in a separate container (Figure 7–27).

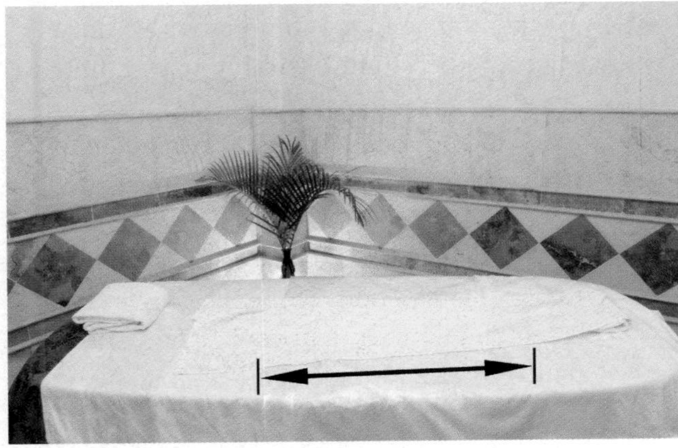

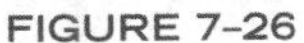

FIGURE 7–26

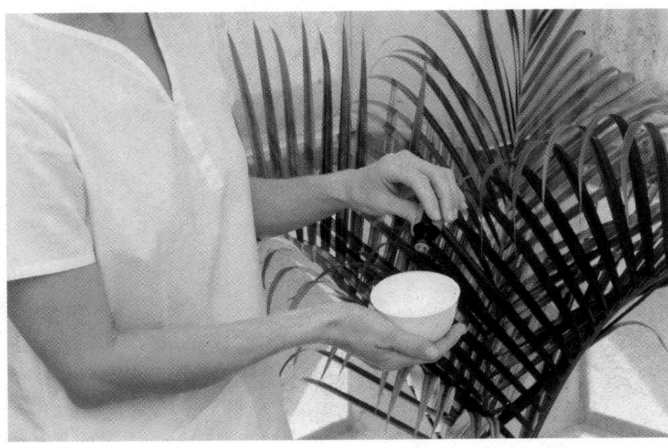

FIGURE 7–27

Seaweed Cellulite Treatment Procedure

1. Start with the client in a prone position and exfoliate the skin in the targeted area with a dry bristle brush or loofah. This should be an invigorating and firm exfoliation meant to strongly stimulate circulation and thoroughly cleanse the skin prior to application of the product (Figure 7–28). Request the client to roll over and repeat the exfoliation to targeted areas on the front of the body (Figure 7–29).

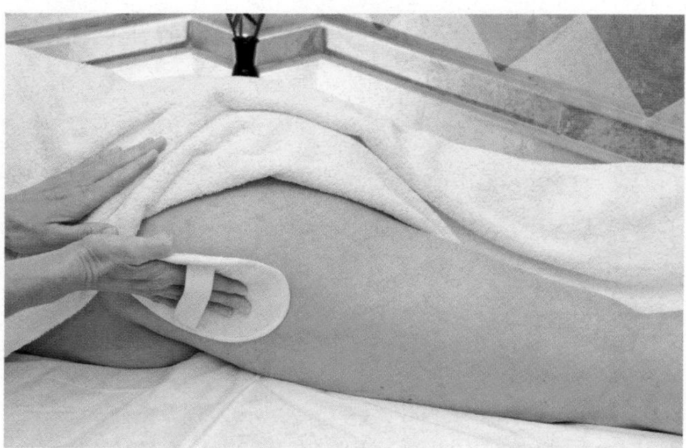

FIGURE 7–28

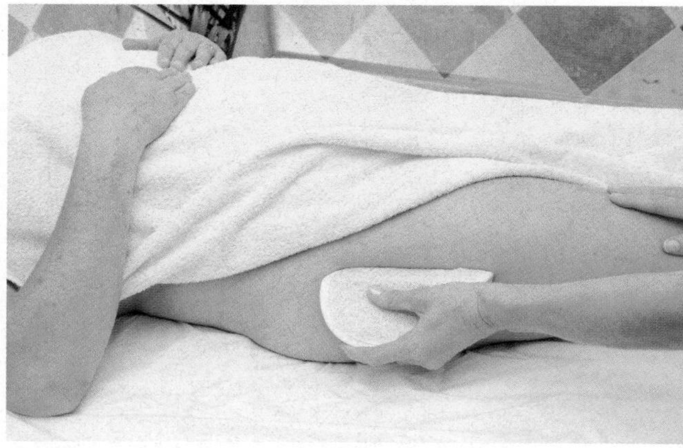

FIGURE 7–29

2. If a hydrotherapy tub is available, use the high-pressure underwater manual massage hose for 10 to 15 minutes, following the procedure in Step 4 of the Hydrotherapy Tub Procedure in Chapter 4. However, concentrate exclusively on targeted areas, including thighs, hips, buttocks, and arms (Figure 7–30). Note: some spas charge 10 percent to 30 percent more for the addition of hydrotherapy.

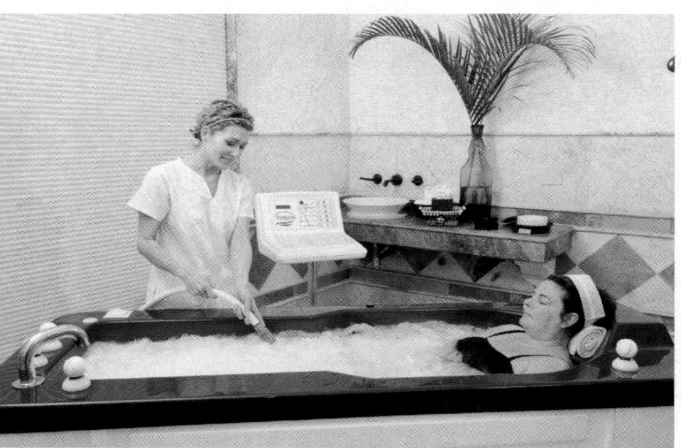

FIGURE 7–30

3. If optional hydrotherapy tub massage is performed, instruct the client to dry her skin and lay supine on the table under drapes afterward.
4. Apply the seaweed/essential oil mix to target areas with your hands or a natural bristle brush, instructing the client to roll to one side, then the other, in order to apply product to the buttocks and back of thighs (Figure 7–31).

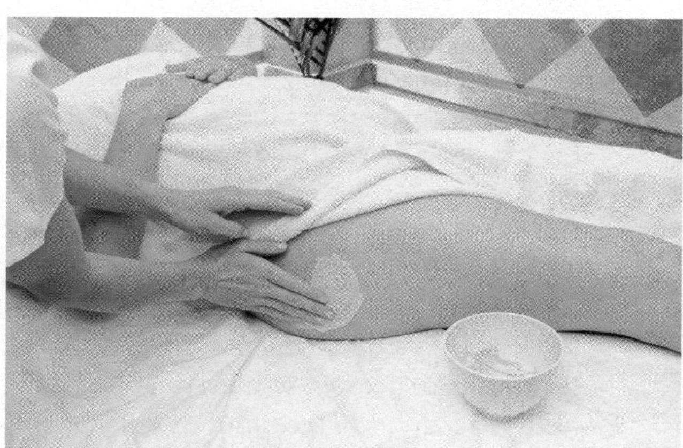

FIGURE 7–31

5. Wrap the client in sheets and blanket and allow her to rest for 20 minutes with a bolster beneath knees. This is a good opportunity to apply a short reflexology routine.
6. Unwrap and remove the seaweed following the same procedure outlined in the Seaweed Body Wrap earlier in this chapter.
7. When the client's skin is free of seaweed, take a small amount of the massage cream/essential oil mixture in your hands, rub your hands together rapidly, and begin a vigorous massage to targeted areas using the following techniques. Apply all five of the techniques in sequence for approximately three minutes

to each area before moving to the next area. Instruct the client to roll into a prone position if necessary. A typical cellulite massage routine will cover eight target areas: fronts of both thighs, medial surface of both thighs, lateral surface of both thighs, and both buttocks. Additionally, the triceps area, abdomen, and waist may be treated if necessary. On the abdomen, use long strokes and skin-rolling only. Avoid knuckle effleurage and percussion. All movements can be applied to the triceps when the client is prone.

a. Apply cream/essential oil mixture with several long effleurage strokes (Figure 7–32).

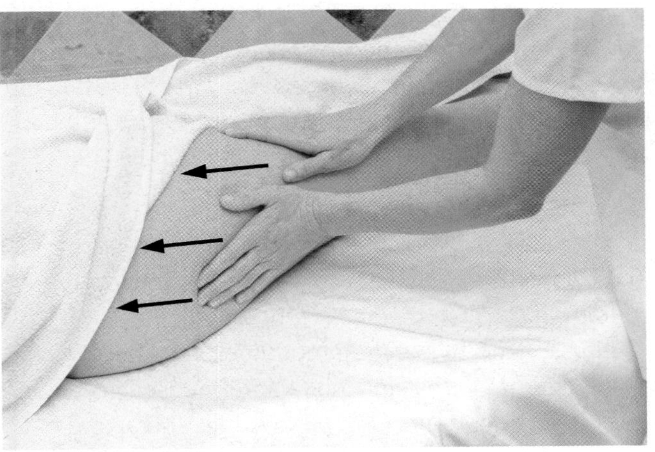

FIGURE 7-32

b. Next, use knuckle effleurage in long strokes until the cream is completely absorbed into the skin (Figure 7–33).

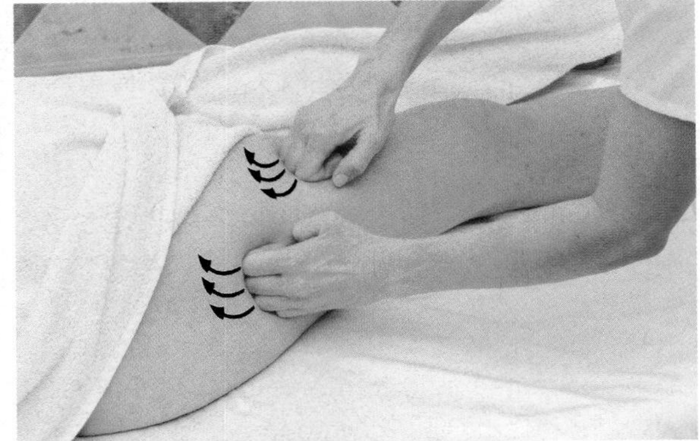

FIGURE 7-33

c. Then apply skin-rolling to stretch the septa and encourage microcirculation and drainage. Push the tissues forward with the thumbs while pulling back with the fingers, moving over the target area (Figure 7–34).

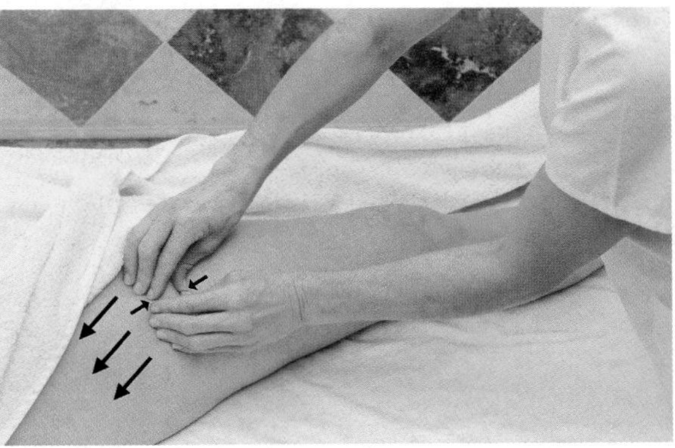

FIGURE 7-34

d. Use finger and hacking tapotement to stimulate circulation (Figure 7–35).

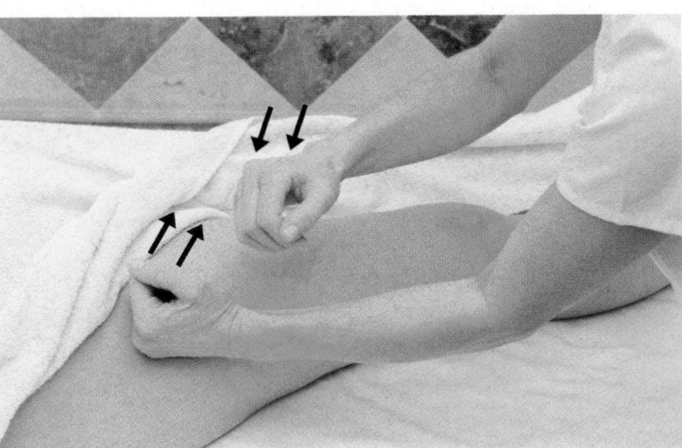

FIGURE 7-35

e. Finish each area with light, lymphatic drainage movements (Figure 7–36).

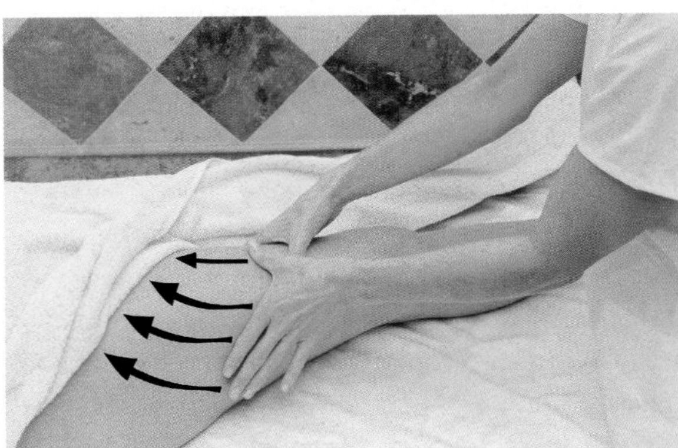

FIGURE 7-36

8. Finish treatment with a full-body application of a seaweed-infused massage oil, a seaweed massage gel, or the massage cream/essential oil mixture. Apply first to the front of the body, then have the client roll over and apply to the back of the body.

Seaweed Cellulite Treatment Cleanup

1. Dispose of plastic wrap.
2. Clean the seaweed from the spa bowl and spatula.
3. Launder the towels and sheets.
4. Sanitize floors and all surfaces where clients walk barefooted.
5. Properly store and refrigerate any seaweed that has been reconstituted for the treatment.
6. Disinfect the hydrotherapy tub if one was used.

parabens

a group of chemicals widely used as preservatives in cosmetics and personal care products, including some spa products; because they are synthetically produced, some spa clients and therapists avoid them

SPA PROFILE *The Ocean Within*

Dan Fryda, President, Spa Technologies

In 1980, Dan Fryda headed to France to study acupuncture. While there, he found himself even more fascinated by the field of thalassotherapy or, as he puts it, "the whole concept of taking the outer ocean and using it to treat the ocean within." He has even written a book about it, called *The Ocean Within*. This ocean within to which he refers is the same seawater-like milieu inside our bodies that French biologist René Quinton studied at the turn of the last century. Fryda knew he wanted to do something that would help popularize this work and give a large number of people the opportunity to experience the therapeutic powers of the sea. So, in the 1980s, he began importing thalassotherapy products from France to the U.S., and in 1992, he opened his own company, Spa Technologies.

"I wanted to import the best European thalassotherapy products, but ones that consumers in the American market would find appealing," he says. "For instance, I knew Americans preferred little or no preservatives or chemical ingredients in their body products, so I chose not to import those with **parabens** to preserve them or fragrances to enhance them, although these additives are popular in Europe. Our raw materials come from France and Iceland, and we have a laboratory here in New York to assemble the finished products. Any spa can incorporate these products on its menu. The seaweed we use is processed in such a way so as to preserve as much of its natural potency as possible. After harvesting, the seaweed is placed in a centrifuge to be sheared of its cellulose walls under cold pressure. The resulting nutrient-dense material is then micronized to a size of 40 microns. It is neither freeze-dried nor treated with chemical solvents. What we end up with is a purée of pure seaweed. This purée contains the elements we find in nature, in the same balance that we find them in our own bodies."

This balance between the body and the sea, the inner ocean and the outer ocean, is a key concept for Fryda. "Every element in seaweed is found within the body in the same proportion," he explains, "and this is the proportion that I believe to be optimal for assimilation and effectiveness. This is an important point for massage therapists to understand when they are applying sea products to their clients in a spa. Seawater, blood plasma and lymph are chemically identical, and the nutrition seaweed delivers is 100 percent compatible with the body, or **biocompatible**, as we say. The effects of seaweed are holistic as compared to reductionist. In **holism**, we use an entire naturally occurring substance to treat the body, and in **reductionism** we extract just one ingredient. For example, a reductionist perspective on pain relief would be to apply salicylic acid, which comes from the willow tree and which constitutes the main ingredient in aspirin. A holistic practitioner, on the other hand, would use a product that contains more components found in the willow so that they can all work together as they do in nature. This is what thalassotherapy offers the practitioner, a way to utilize one of the most holistic of all substances.

(Continued)

not new. For centuries, spas in Europe have promoted the practice of "taking the kür," which involves a series of treatments that use natural ingredients including muds, clays, essential oils, and herbs. (Information on the use of essential oils and the application of aromatherapy treatments is found in Chapter 11). This chapter focuses on the therapeutic benefits of herbs, muds, and clays in spa treatments such as wraps and baths. Because baths have already been discussed in Chapter 4, this chapter starts with an overview of body wraps and then explains specific treatments using muds, clays, and herbs.

BODY WRAPS

Spas offer many types of body wraps for various purposes. Some are for heating the body and detoxification, such as the herbal wrap. Some are meant primarily to relax and improve mood and well-being, such as the aromatherapy wrap. Some are meant to nourish, cleanse, and improve the superficial contours of the skin, such as cellulite wraps. Mud and clay wraps have multiple effects, such as purging and drawing impurities out through the pores, softening the skin, and improving joint elasticity when heated. Seaweed wraps remineralize the skin and entire body as the micronutrients and sea-borne minerals soak in through the pores, as already discussed in Chapter 7. Cold wraps can soothe sunburn pain and improve circulation, especially for sore, tired legs. Less frequently in spas, weight-loss or inch-loss wraps are applied for purely cosmetic purposes, as explained in the sidebar, Slimming Wraps.

Spa body wraps can be categorized into two main types: those that apply heat to the body and those that do not. Heat is a necessary ingredient for some types of purging wraps, such as the herbal wrap. As with all heat treatments, it is important to remember the main contraindications for heated body wraps: high blood pressure, heart disease, and pregnancy. Non-heated wraps include the aromatherapy wrap and many seaweed and mud wraps, which rely upon the body's own heat to keep the client warm during the treatment. See Figures 8–2 and 8–3 for a visual explanation of the effects of body wraps.

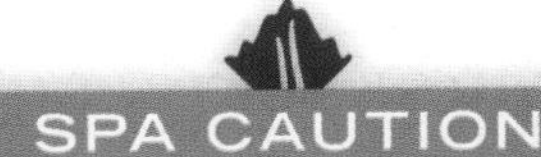

SPA CAUTION

Slimming Wraps

The chances of permanently losing weight in a slimming wrap are slim to none, and most resort and destination spas do not feature slimming wraps on their menus. Some day spas, however, find a demand for these services among their clientele, and they do offer them. Slimming wraps are claimed to aid in weight loss and inch loss. While these results can, in fact, occur as a consequence of these treatments, the effects are temporary and caused primarily by fluid loss. In addition, before-and-after measurements are taken on a multitude of sites on the body and are added together to present a cumulative inch loss that appears greater than it actually is. Clients are wrapped quite tightly, often with elastic bandaging material soaked in minerals that promote fluid loss.

None of the wraps in this chapter or this entire book refer to this type of wrap. While temporary slimming is a welcomed side effect of several therapeutic treatments, such as the herbal wrap, it is not the intended outcome. As a spa therapist, you should caution clients who are expecting weight loss during classical spa treatments. Educate them about the benefits to their well-being and overall health in these treatments, and reinforce the fact that appropriate diet, exercise, and lifestyle are the only methods to achieve true slimming. If appropriate, refer them to other professionals on the spa staff for help with these issues.

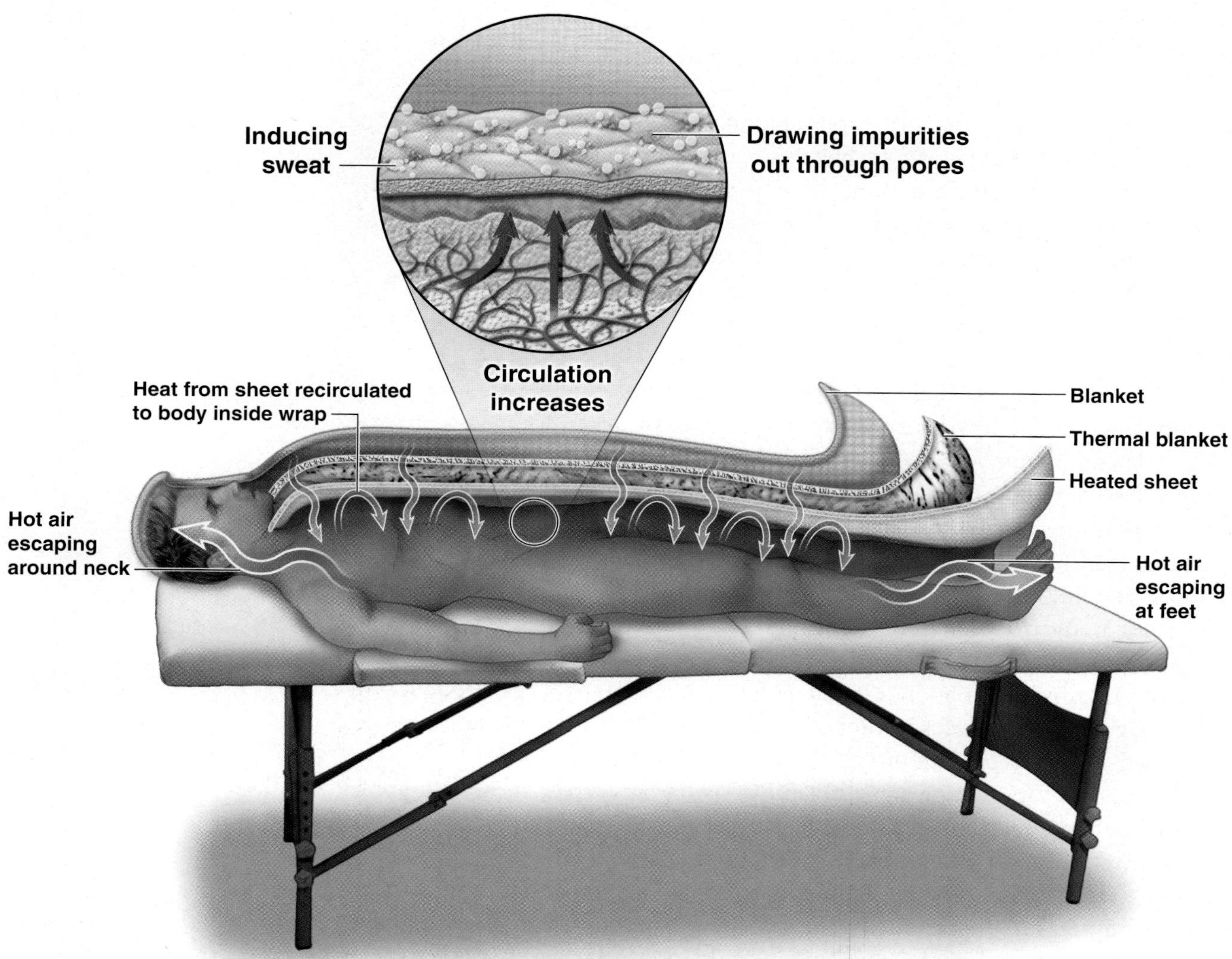

FIGURE 8–2 Heat wraps have a profound effect on the body.

SPA TIP

Adding Value

Offer something extra, such as spa reflexology or a scalp massage, while the client is enveloped in a full-body wrap. Clients pay well for this service and feel shortchanged if they are left alone for 20 to 30 minutes while the therapist attends to other matters. Note, however, that it is not necessary to offer clients this value-added service while in an herbal wrap because the heat normally induces deep relaxation and clients usually prefer to be left alone. Also, it is best if heat does not escape during the herbal wrap, which will happen if you unwrap the head or feet to work on the area. You can offer extra service in other ways, such as getting drinks and cool compresses.

Body wraps can be further differentiated as either *loose* or *tight*, and *partial* or *whole*. Thus, a therapist could perform a loose torso wrap with mud for purification, or a tight full-body wrap with seaweed for remineralization. Partial wraps include leg wraps, foot wraps, hand wraps, and torso wraps. There are also treatments, such as the "back facial," that do not actually wrap around the

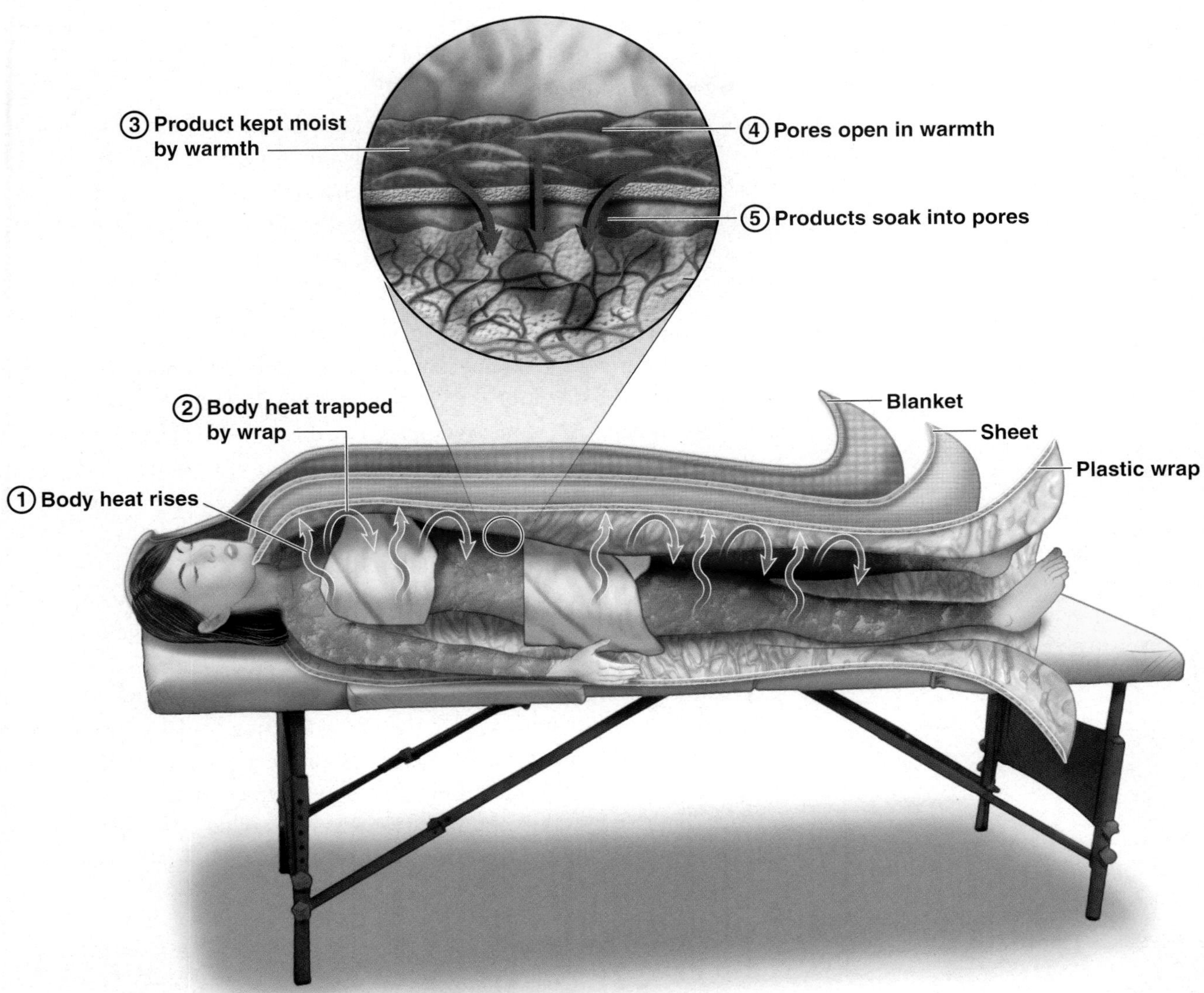
③ Product kept moist by warmth
④ Pores open in warmth
⑤ Products soak into pores
② Body heat trapped by wrap
① Body heat rises
Blanket
Sheet
Plastic wrap

FIGURE 8–3 Non-heated body wraps rely on the client's own body heat to keep product moist and the client warm and comfortable.

entire body or body part but still involve the use of blankets or other coverings to retain heat.

Though the purpose for each type of body wrap varies, they all have certain characteristics in common, those being:

- **Comfort and Security:** People generally experience a sense of safety and of being protected when they are wrapped up. It is a comforting sensation of being "tucked in" that is not generally available to adults except in the spa environment.
- **Warmth:** Whether applied externally or created as a process of body heat, warmth is an integral part of all body wraps, offering a sense of nurturing and engendering deep relaxation.
- **Enclosed Environment:** The enclosed warm environment of body wraps offers ideal conditions for spa products of all types to act upon the body in an effective manner, absorbing through the pores rather than dissipating into the air.

All body wraps are similar in that they envelope the client inside various layers while products are acting upon the skin. Each wrap is unique, however, in the particular manner in which it is applied. Some, for example, call for multiple layers of blankets, sheets, and towels to be wrapped around the client. Others, such as the aromatherapy wrap, may call for only one blanket and one sheet. Still others, such as the drying clay wrap, require only a thin layer of gauze on the skin that is heated by an infrared lamp. As stated earlier, some wraps are tight, while some are applied more loosely. Regardless of the wrap being performed, certain general protocols apply:

- **Communicate:** It is important to communicate verbally with the client about the nature of the wrap. Clients sometimes complain that they are unsure of what to do while the wrap is being performed or while they are lying in the room, alone, wrapped up. Always let the client know that you are available, even while out of the room. Inform the client how long the wrap will last and what he might expect to experience during the wrap. Offer water, a cold compress for heat wraps, and anything else that can make the client more comfortable.
- **Use a Bolster:** Because of the extra weight load on the legs created by most wraps, it is important to always place a bolster under the knees so that the client's lower back does not become hyperextended.
- **Exercise Caution:** All wraps, especially heat wraps, can cause certain clients to feel claustrophobic. See the Did You Know? sidebar regarding how to avoid claustrophobia in wraps for most clients. With heat wraps, it is important not to apply sheets or products that are overly hot in order to avoid burning sensitive skin. The mouth and nose, of course, must remain unwrapped at all times. Always check for allergies or sensitivities to products before applying a wrap.

Fear of Being Wrapped

Did You Know?

Dealing with Claustrophobia during Body Treatments

Many people experience a sense of claustrophobia when they are wrapped up rather snugly in sheets and blankets, especially hot sheets and blankets, as they are in various spa treatments. Some spa therapists suggest that as many as 25 percent of the population feel at least a little claustrophobic under these circumstances. This does not mean, however, that 25 percent of all spa clients need forgo body wrap treatments. Using a simple technique, 99 percent of all those reporting claustrophobia can overcome the sensation.

1. First, before wrapping, you should reassure the client about this issue, letting the client know that she will be able to exit the wrap at any time with no help from anyone else.
2. Then, when you are actually wrapping the client, instruct her to leave her arms unwrapped over her head when the initial layers are being applied (Figure 8–4).
3. Have the client lower her arms onto the wrap that is already around her body (Figure 8–5).
4. Wrap only the topmost blanket over her arms, then allow the client to lift her arms, and see how easy it is to get out of the wrap (Figure 8–6). Place the topmost blanket over the client once again.
5. Reassure the client again that you will monitor her to make sure she is comfortable and to help her should she need anything.

(Continued)

Did You Know?

Fear of Being Wrapped *continued*

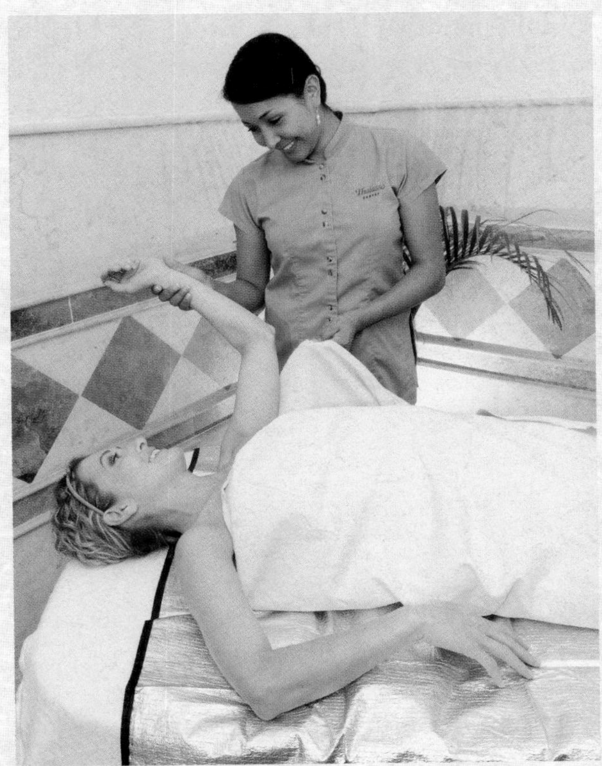

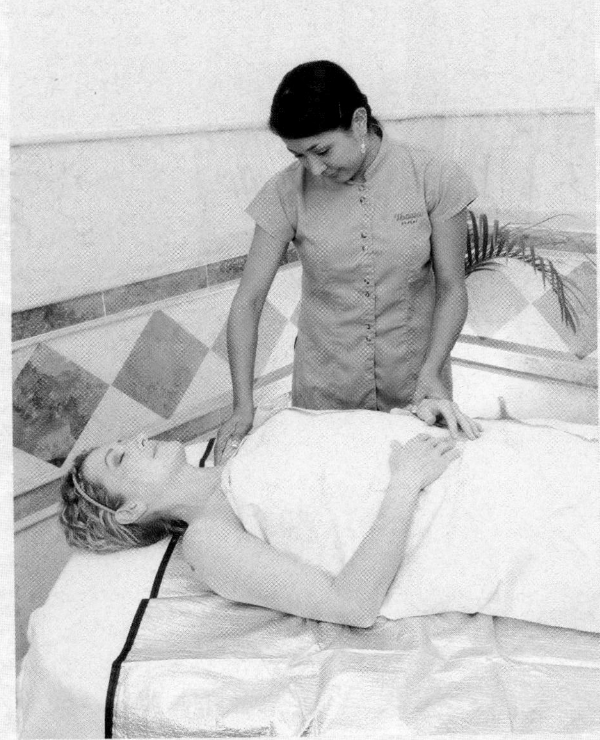

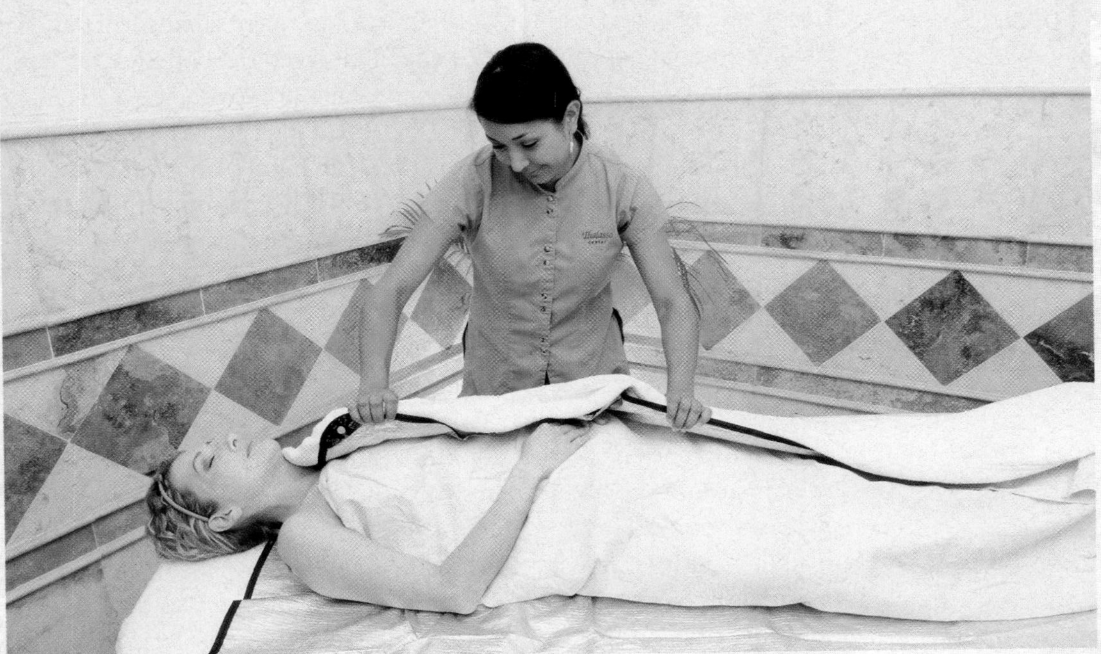

FIGURES 8–4, 8–5, 8–6 Almost all clients can comfortably receive body wraps with no sensation of claustrophobic using this technique.

Body Wrap Protocol

Although spa clients are wrapped up with a wide variety of products applied to their skin, the actual wrapping technique itself remains quite similar from treatment to treatment. While observing the precautions and recommendations already cited in this chapter, you can safely perform many different body wraps using the 10-step protocol explained below. Remember that each spa will have specific guidelines regarding its procedures, and it will be up to you to follow them diligently, but these 10 steps are common to most:

1. Set the table
2. Prepare the product
3. Prepare the skin
4. Apply the product
5. Wrap the client
6. Attend to the client
7. Perform value-added services
8. Unwrap comfortably
9. Remove products
10. Finishing procedure

Set the Table

Each wrap will require several layers of material on the table. The outermost layer of the wrap will be placed on the table first and subsequent layers placed on top of it. Most typically, the outermost layer consists of a blanket. In the past, many spas used wool blankets exclusively for this purpose, but that is becoming less common today. Now, several types of blankets are used, including those made of cotton and other fabrics. This blanket provides the cocoon-like feeling of body wraps and should be comforting in texture, color, and weight. Double- or queen-size blankets work best. Larger blankets can make clients feel suffocated, while smaller ones do not insulate well enough to keep the body warm. This outermost blanket should hang over the head of the table approximately 12 inches so that the blanket can be easily wrapped over the top of the client's head to retain warmth. If the blanket does not fully cover the client, an extra blanket or towel can be placed over the gap between the two ends of the blanket on top of the client.

Often, the next layer is an insulating blanket of some kind, such as the thermal blanket mentioned in Chapter 3. This is wrapped a little more snugly around the client and is meant to retain the client's body heat or the heat produced by an application of hot sheets, as in the herbal wrap. This layer does not have to hang over the top of the table, but rather should leave just enough room for the back of the client's head on the table above it.

Often, a sheet is placed atop the insulating blanket. Its purpose is to provide a clean surface on which to lie when the client emerges from the wrap and the plastic is removed.

The next layer is a sheet of plastic wrap that provides a clean barrier directly on the skin. Formerly, a metallic product called *Mylar* was used for this purpose, but most spas opt for thin, disposable plastic, often of biodegradable quality. This plastic sheet is cut to a five- or six-foot square and draped directly over the top of the insulating blanket. It is disposed of after each treatment, and its cost is factored into the price of the treatment along with any product applied. Occasionally, spas forgo the use of the plastic wrap and wrap a normal sheet against the skin with the product applied. This is a messier option that requires the laundering of heavily soiled sheets, but some people claim the texture of a sheet against the skin is preferable to that of plastic.

Finally, drape sheets or towels are placed atop the various layers so that they are ready to be used when the client arrives. Draping is slightly more challenging for body wraps than it is for massage therapy because of the application of products and the wrapping of layers. See the Did You Know? sidebar for details of a common body wrap draping protocol.

Did You Know?

Body Wrap Draping Protocol

Draping clients during body wraps can be slightly cumbersome because of the product being applied and the non-draping layers of sheets and blankets and plastic that have a tendency to get in the way. However, it is important to keep clients comfortable and adequately draped during these treatments and the protocols suggested here will help you to achieve that. Certain spas may have their own protocols for body wrap draping, in which case you should follow the guidelines of your employer. The general principles outlined here can be applied in most settings.

1. Arrange draping materials atop all wrapping layers prior to the client's arrival. Towels in a diaper-draping configuration are usually the best choice, because sheets cover too much surface area, making product application difficult. For women, a bottom bath towel drape and upper hand towel breast drape are appropriate. Instruct the client to lie down supine and pull the bottom drape up between her legs to cover her torso. For men, you can use a smaller bath towel that does not cover the entire torso.
2. Leave the room while the client disrobes and gets onto the table beneath the drape.
3. Apply product to the back and back of the legs while the client is either sitting up or rolled over slightly to one side while still on her back (Figure 8–7).
4. Apply product to the front of the body (Figure 8–8).
5. When wrapping, leave draping towels in place (Figure 8–9).
6. When unwrapping, three options are available:
    a. Leave the draping towels in place and wipe off product with hot, wet towels (Figure 8–10). Tuck the plastic wrap underneath the body as each area is cleaned.
    b. Leave the draping towels in place and use the handheld shower or Vichy shower to remove product (Figure 8–11). After the entire body is cleaned, remove the plastic wrap by having the client roll from side to side.
    c. Leave the draping towels in place and ask the client to sit up, holding the breast drape in place (for women). Drape another large bath towel over the client's shoulders and assist her to the shower (Figure 8–12). While the client is in the shower, clean the table and prepare it for the final cream or lotion application.
7. If the drape becomes dirtied, place a clean bath towel over the client and have the client lift his or her hips to remove the original drape.
8. Apply finishing product using customary massage draping procedures.

(Continued)

Body Wrap Draping Protocol *continued*

Did You Know?

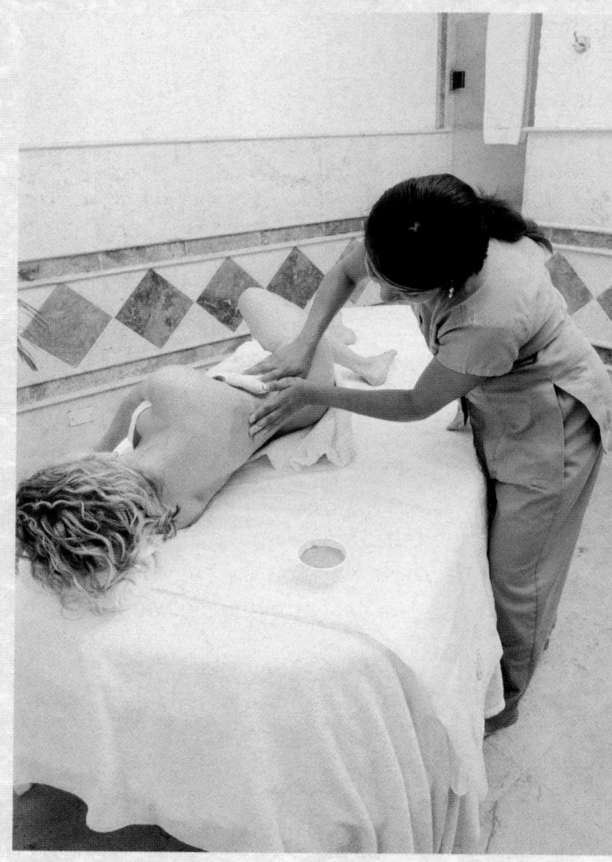
FIGURE 8–7

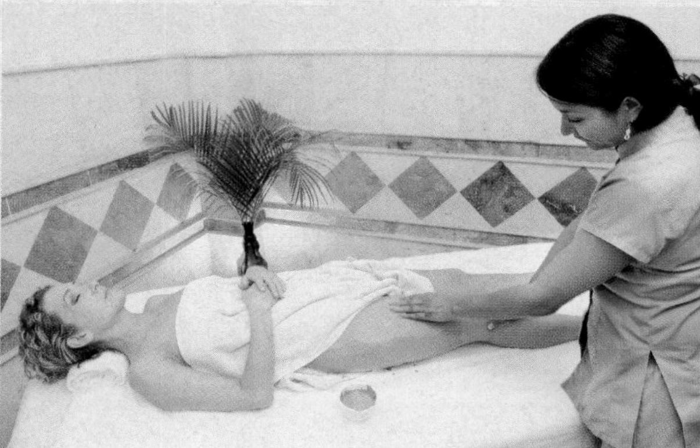
FIGURE 8–8

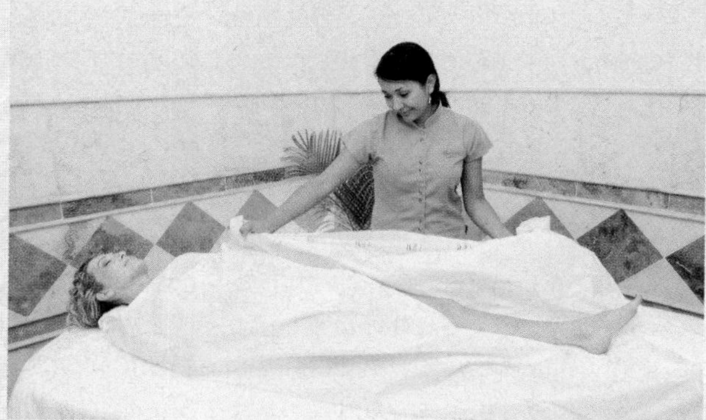
FIGURE 8–9

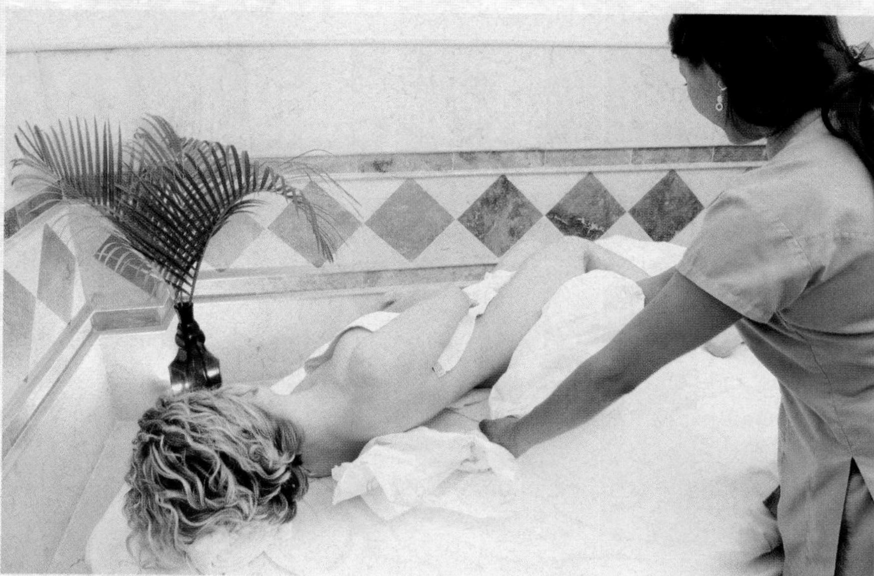
FIGURE 8–10

(Continued)

Body Wrap Draping Protocol *continued*

Did You Know?

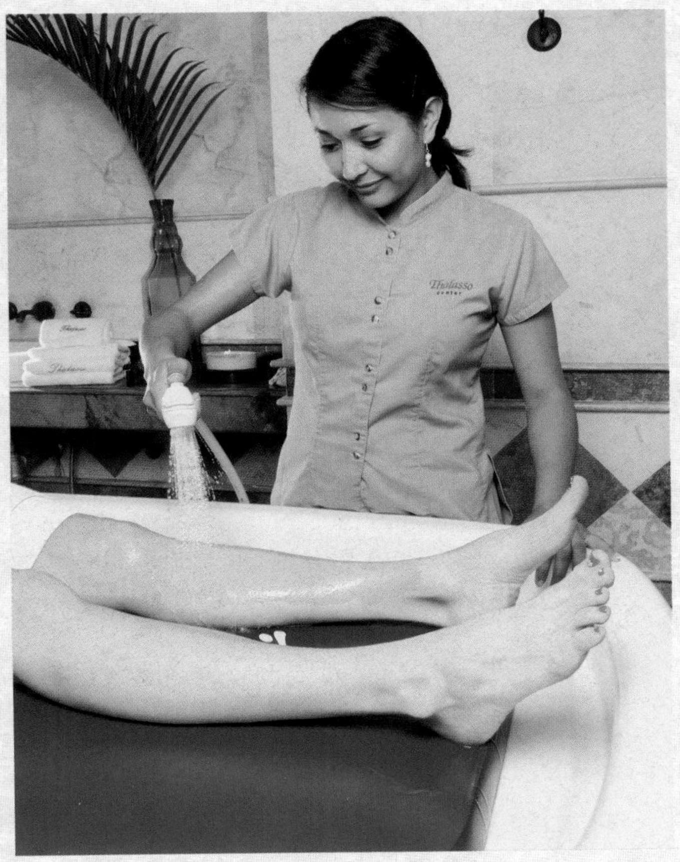

FIGURE 8–11

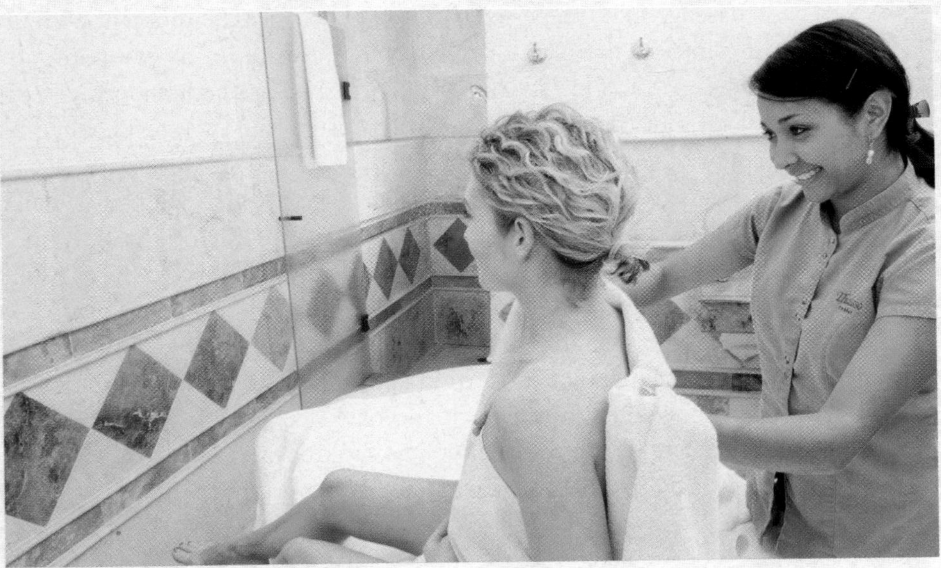

FIGURE 8–12

ACTIVITY

Body Wrap Draping Protocol Practice

Without using any actual products applied to the skin, practice the draping techniques for body wraps in a series of dry runs. Place all wrapping layers on the table as if for an actual wrap, then wrap your partner using proper draping several times in sequence, until you become comfortable with the procedure.

Prepare the Product

Therapists usually prepare body wrap products prior to the arrival of the client in the treatment room, mixing and warming ingredients if necessary. However, some protocols call for the client to give some input regarding which products will be used, as in a customized aromatherapy wrap, for example. In this case, the various ingredients are displayed, ready to be used, near the treatment table or on a tray that is brought to the client prior to the treatment. Various methods are used to keep product warm. Rubber spa bowls are often used for this purpose, with the prepared product being placed in the bowls and floated in warm water or nestled between hot towels. Many spa body wrap products are organic and all-natural. As such, they are prone to oxidization and spoilage. Therapists need to be careful regarding storage and proper handling of these products. Bottles and jars need to be recapped securely and consistently. Certain products need to be refrigerated.

Prepare the Skin

Prior to applying products during a body wrap, most protocols call for an exfoliation of the skin. This can be a cursory two-minute brushing or a full 30-minute exfoliation procedure that precedes the body wrap. Therapists use a dry bristle brush, loofah, scrubbing gloves, body scrub, sea salt, or other exfoliating products or devices. If a product is used, an extra layer must be added to the table, usually a sheet, that catches the excess product and can be removed from beneath the client prior to the actual wrap. Clients can also enter a steam bath or sauna prior to a body wrap in order to open and cleanse the pores. The purpose of these preparations is to allow the skin to more readily absorb the benefits of the products that are applied to the skin.

Apply the Product

There are two main methods to apply spa body wrap products: with the therapist's hands directly and with a brush. Each has its own advantages. Some therapists prefer the feel of using their hands, believing it extends the sensation of massage into the performance of the wrap. The problem with this method is that it requires more product to cover a given area as compared to when a brush is used. With a brush, the product can be applied smoothly, evenly, and in a thin layer, but the hand-feel aspect is lost. Some therapists, when using their hands, wear disposable gloves for sanitary purposes.

As each part of the body is covered with product, it is usually a good idea to protect the area with plastic wrap, draping it atop the skin lightly to avoid chilling, because clients quickly become cold when they have product applied, even if the product is initially warm.

Some spas have a distinctive protocol that they favor regarding this application. For instance, at certain spas, clients will begin facedown and the product will be applied to the back and backs of the legs first. Other spas have the client lay faceup for the entire application process. Some spas start at the feet and move upwards. Other spas start at the neck and move down.

Wrap the Client

Clients are usually wrapped layer by layer for the sake of creating a uniform, snug fit of the various layers over the body. First, the plastic wrap is placed around the body, then the extra sheet and the thermal blanket, then the outer blanket. A bolster is placed beneath the client's knees for comfort and to help support the extra weight placed on the lower back by the wrapping materials. The areas around the head and the feet can be tucked closed with bath towels. When reflexology is going to be applied during the wrap, the feet can be loosely covered.

Attend to the Client

Just because a client is fully wrapped on the table does not mean the therapist is no longer performing a treatment. It is important to let clients know that you will be there for them, attending to their needs and comforts. Some clients report feeling anxious or vulnerable when wrapped, and it is up to you to calm their fears. Before the treatment begins, reassure them that you will be monitoring their comfort throughout the treatment. Then, once they are wrapped, once again tell them that you are there for their comfort. Offer to assist them with a sip of cool water through a straw. Apply a cold compress to the forehead or neck during heat wraps. You may even need to scratch an itch on the face that the client cannot reach while wrapped. Some clients prefer to be left alone to relax or meditate while wrapped. In this case, ask their permission before leaving and reassure them that you will check back periodically.

Perform Value-Added Services

Spa clients pay high prices for body wraps, and yet some spas offer no additional modalities while the client is wrapped, leaving them alone while the therapist steps out to take a break. It is greatly preferable to perform an appropriate allied modality while the client is in the wrap. The most popular choice for this purpose is spa reflexology, which is explained in Chapter 9. Face, head, and neck massage and mini-facial treatments are also good choices to offer guests while they are wrapped. Some spas choose to charge extra for these **value-added services**, while others include them in the price of the treatment.

value-added services

a treatment, usually of short duration, that is offered in addition to the main spa modality being performed, in order to increase its value

Unwrap Comfortably

Getting unwrapped can be an uncomfortable experience for clients because they tend to cool off quickly after being cocooned in the warmth of the wrap. It is important, then, to keep the body covered as much as possible during the unwrapping procedure and to expose only one area at a time to the cooler air of the treatment room. Also, be sure to preserve clients' modesty with proper draping while removing the wrapping layers.

SPA TIP

Spa wrap rooms, like exfoliation rooms, should ideally be kept a few degrees warmer than massage rooms, because clients' skin is periodically exposed to the air with product applied, which makes them feel chilled. Some spas install infrared lights in body wrap rooms to counteract this chilling effect.

Remove Products

In a wet room, clients either enter the shower to remove products from their skin or, less commonly, the therapist will use a Vichy shower or a handheld shower to wash away products while the client is still on the table. The unwrapping protocol in a dry room calls for the use of hot towels. Occasionally, a spatula or other device is used to wipe away excess product before the hot towels are applied. Clients then either dry themselves after a shower or the therapist can pat the skin dry with a fresh towel.

SPA TIP

Muds and clays have had a long history of use in soothing minor insect bites. Have a store of powdered therapeutic clay at hand, and the next time a bee or other pests have stung you or one of your clients, quickly mix up a paste and apply a small amount directly over the sting as people have been doing in various cultures for centuries. Let it dry in place for half an hour and then gently wash away.

peloids

mud prepared and used for therapeutic purposes

peat

partially carbonized vegetable matter saturated with water

moor

nutrient-rich black silts formed by the decomposition of excess plant life in eutrophic lakes, used in spas for its purifying and chelating properties

specific heat

the heat required to raise the temperature of one gram of a substance one degree centigrade

thermal indifference

the temperature of the body (93°F to 95°F) at which there is no change in the production or giving off of heat and little or no effect on the heart or circulation, used to describe various substances applied to the body in spa treatments such as water and peloids, which have different temperatures of thermal indifference

Finishing Procedure

Most body wrap procedures call for the application of a finishing lotion, cream, gel, or specialty product to the skin after removal of the wrap. If they have taken a shower, clients get back on the table at this point. If they have had their skin cleansed by the therapist while still on the table, clients lay upon a fresh sheet at this point, which was layered for this purpose beneath the plastic wrap in the table setup, as you will recall. All plastic and other traces of the wrap are removed by this time, and the therapist applies the product to the skin. This is not a massage, just an application, usually lasting five minutes or less. If the client has booked a massage after the wrap or as part of a package of services, the therapist can begin the massage at this time, using the finishing product as a lubricant, if appropriate. Otherwise, a massage lotion or cream can be used.

MUD USE IN SPAS

It is perhaps counterintuitive to think that applying something as "dirty" as mud to one's skin will beautify and improve it, but this is indeed the case. In addition, the application of mud to parts of the body or the entire skin surface has been proven to have beneficial effects for people suffering from rheumatic conditions, muscle aches, and other complaints. Since pre-history, people have applied various types of muds to wounds, insect bites, and minor trauma. Modern spas take the application of mud to new levels of sophistication with specially designed warmers, blankets, immersions, and packs. The muds used are sourced from specific locations that have been proven to contain high concentrations of beneficial compounds. Mud dug up in your backyard, in other words, would not produce the same effects. Some spas have been built on the site of natural mud baths such as Calistoga in the U.S. and Terme de Saturnia in Europe. When used properly, muds can easily be prepared and applied in the spa setting with minimal mess.

All the different types of muds used in spas are classified under the heading of **peloids**, which also include clay, **peat**, **moor**, and even coastal slime. See Table 8–1 for a list of peloids commonly used in spas. Peloids do not create the same aggressive heating sensation that water does because their **specific heat** is lower, which means they do not conduct heat as well as water does. The point of **thermal indifference**, at which the body feels neither heat nor cold when subjected to an application, is 93°F for water but 100°F for peloids. The layer of mud closest to the client in a mud bath creates a barrier through which further heat must be transmitted. Higher temperatures can therefore be used, and yet the mud will not feel too hot to the client. High temperatures used for mud applications are approximately 110°F to 120°F. The most important therapeutic property that peloids offer spa clients is their ability to transmit heat.

The heat from the mud penetrates into the tissues, stimulates blood circulation, relaxes muscles, slackens connective tissues, and eases minor pains. When applied over the entire body, a heated mud pack or mud immersion increases body temperature, causes profuse perspiration, and increases heart rate. Blood pressure falls. Peripheral vessels dilate, creating hyperemia and increasing local metabolism, which speeds the activity of chronic inflammatory processes and aids healing. The heat also creates a reflex reaction in certain inner organs (see Chapter 5, Reflex Effects of Heat).

PELOID	DESCRIPTION	USES	POPULARITY
Clay	*Clay* is a general term used for many substances in the spa, including fango and sea-based products. See Table 8–2 for descriptions of some clays.	Primarily used for drawing impurities from the skin. Certain types are also moisturizing.	medium
Fango	Fango is a specific type of clay created from volcanic ash, high in mineral content, especially found in Battaglia, Italy.	Used in a pure reconstituted form or mixed with paraffin to create Parafango, this clay offers deeply penetrating heat in spot applications or full-body wraps.	medium
Moor	Moors are formed in eutrophic lakes and other shallow bodies of water. The excess plant life formed dies off, creating nutrient-rich silts of a deep black hue used in spas.	Many brands of moor mud are used in spas for face, body, hand, foot, and other specific applications.	high
Mud	*Mud* is a general term for products that range widely from "sea muds" to moor mud to clays.	Most spa menus feature some sort of body mud pack, wrap, or spot application.	high
Peat Bog	Peats are mostly plant life, from the *Sphagnetalia* family, such as sphagnum or bog moss. Peat bog absorbs excess dead skin cells and provides heat.	Sometimes used in wraps in Europe. The sulfur, iodine, ferrum, and humic acids in the peat provide anti-inflammatory effects to help ease arthritis pain.	rare

TABLE 8–1 Types of Peloids Used in Spas.

One of the main active substances in mud is humic acid, which is known to aid in the purification of the body through the process of **chelation**. It is believed that the chelating humic acid, which is especially prevalent in moor muds, can help draw impurities through the skin. Moor mud comes from **eutrophic** lakes and other shallow bodies of water and is primarily composed of the silts built up over time as vegetable matter dies off, decays, and sinks. Moor is rich in nutrients and has a deep black color (Figure 8–13). The moor mud from each separate lake has distinct properties, and some providers claim that the **silts** from certain lakes have a higher concentration of beneficial humic acid compounds.

chelation

the process of removing a heavy metal from the bloodstream by means of a substance such as those found in certain spa muds that bond to the metals and draw them

eutrophic

of a lake or other body of water rich in nutrients which cause a dense growth of plant life, the decomposition of which depletes the supply of oxygen in the water, leading to the death of animal life and the creation of sediment known as *moor mud*, which is used in spa therapy

silts

sedimentary mud deposited by a river or lake; moor mud used in spa treatments is an example

Clays

Clays are a special type of peloid and are particularly absorbing. They come from many different sources around the world, in a wide variety of forms, colors, textures, and properties. See Table 8–2 for a list of several popular clays used in

SPA TIP

More Squares and Rectangles

Mud therapy offers yet another squares and rectangles analogy for the spa. Mud typically refers to the entire general category of earth-based products applied to the skin in spa therapies. Clay, peat, moor, sea mud, sea clay, fango, and all other such products are types of muds. Therefore, in the same way that all squares are rectangles but not all rectangles are squares, it is true that all clays are muds but not all muds are clays. Going further into this analogy, you will discover that fango is a certain sort of clay from volcanic sources in Italy. As such, all fangos are clay but not all clays are fango (Figure 8–13).

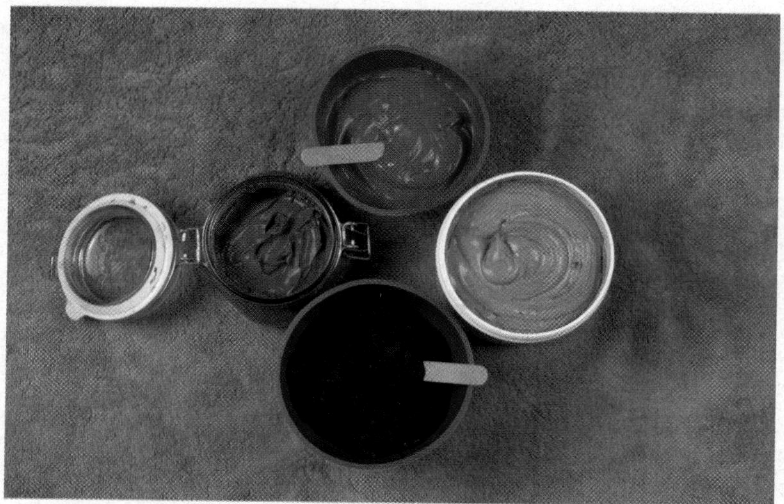

FIGURE 8–13 Moor mud (bottom), Sedona clay (top), rose clay (right), fango (left).

spas. Spa clays include Sedona clay, which is a rich, dark, reddish-brown clay from the desert that is used to draw impurities from the skin (Figure 8–13). In contrast, a rose clay compound from France has been formulated with massage oils for use by therapists and is actually moisturizing (Figure 8–13). All clays, of course, contain the natural minerals and other elements found in the earth where they are mined.

Spa clay applications range from the somewhat rustic, such as Glen Ivy, where clients literally wallow in a large outdoor clay pit and then let the clay bake into their skin in the sun, to the highly stylized, such as the exotic Rasul chambers found at high-end resorts. In the Rasul, clients enter a steam-filled chamber and apply various-colored muds to their own bodies or their partner's body during the treatment. Steam gradually fills the chamber, creating an exfoliation effect as the clients rub the moistened mud into their skin. After the steam, showers built into the ceiling are turned on to wash the mud away. Rasul chambers are elaborate affairs, festooned with decorative tiles and twinkling lights that represent the starts in an Arabian sky. The experience can be quite relaxing but also fun if clients enjoy the treatment with friends.

CLAY	DESCRIPTION	USES
Bentonite Clay	From volcanic ash, this clay is highly drawing and detoxifying.	used for its drawing properties in body mask recipes
Green Sea Clay	Green clay is extracted from dried sea beds, often in the Mediterranean. It contains algae, phytoplankton, and nutrients.	Green clay has been widely used for centuries in Europe and Asia for masks and scrubs. Draws impurities from the skin when applied topically or from the intestines when taken internally.
Kaolin	a light, fluffy clay used mostly for its absorptive qualities	Used as a binder for scrub grains in exfoliants and for body masks, kaolin is suitable for dry, aged skin. It draws impurities from the skin when applied topically or from the intestines when taken internally.
Rhassoul Clay	Used for over 1,400 years as a soap, shampoo, and skin treatment in Morocco, this clay has the ability to absorb oil and impurities from both the skin and hair, reducing dryness and improving skin texture.	Rhassoul can be used as a soap, skin conditioner, shampoo, and face and body mask.
Rose Clay	an attractively colored, medium-weight clay	Used as a coloring for soaps and spa products, it is sometimes blended with oils to provide moisture to the skin in wraps.
Sedona Clay	a dark-brown clay, usually in powdered form, then mixed with water for use in spas; highly drying and drawing	Used in back facials and in full-body applications where plentiful shower facilities are available because it hardens on the skin.

TABLE 8–2 Some Clays Used in Spas.

One of the most popular forms of clay used in the spa setting is known as **fango**. *Fango* is the Italian word for mud. In particular, the fango used in spas is a grayish clay created from the volcanic rock known as **phonolite**. This was once molten lava, which hardened in the Miocene Epoch, from 13 million to 25 million years ago. Today, it exists as solid rock beneath a layer of fine-grained clay, which is known as **loess**. This rock is mined, processed at high temperature, and ground into a fine powder called *volcanic fango*, the main mineral component of which is **zeolite**. Volcanic clay has been used therapeutically for centuries, and Plinius (23–79 AD) mentioned the use of the fango mud from the thermal ponds of Battaglia, near Padua in North Italy. Battaglia sits on the shore of a volcanic lake, where extensive Roman bathing facilities stood at one time. The occasional use of this thermal mud from Battaglia can be dated back hundreds of years, but it has been used on a larger scale only in modern times.

Parafango is a combination of fango and paraffin wax. This product was developed by a professor in Hamburg, Germany, and introduced as a spa treatment in the 1950s. It has since become quite popular, especially in Europe. Sometimes referred to as "Parafango Battaglia" after the famous source in Battaglia, Italy, this substance contains dried fango, paraffin wax, and small amounts of talcum and magnesium oxide to improve workability and consistency. The combined product usually comes in bars that are melted at 140°F into a paste that is poured onto a plastic sheet and applied to the body in a 1-inch-thick layer. Clients are then wrapped with a thermal blanket and an outer blanket as in a regular mud wrap application. The most important therapeutic benefit of an application of hot Parafango is thermal, not chemical, since most of the compounds in the substance cannot penetrate the pores.

fango

mud, especially a clay mud from hot springs at Battaglia, Italy, that is warmed and used in therapeutic spa applications

phonolite

compact igneous rock of volcanic origin; a primary source of fango for spa treatments

loess

a fine-grained unstratified accumulation of clay and silt deposited by the wind

zeolite

a family of glassy minerals analogous to feldspar containing hydrated aluminum silicates of calcium or sodium or potassium; formed in cavities in lava flows and used as the basis of volcanic fango powder for spa treatments

parafango

a combination of fango and paraffin wax developed in Germany and used therapeutically in spa treatments, creating powerful thermal effects; sometimes referred to as "Parafango Battaglia" after its source in Italy

Peloid Treatments—Mud Wrap

Peloids are used for a wide range of spa services, as demonstrated in Table 8–3. Certain spas specialize in these treatments and have gained fame primarily due to their muds or clays, while other spas simply include mud or clay services on their menus among many other options. Treatment types are normally broken down into services that cover different areas of the body, including face, foot, hand, back, and whole body. A mud bath protocol can be found in Chapter 4, and back facial, foot, and hand treatment protocols in Chapter 13. In this chapter, we look at the full-body mud wrap.

The chemical constituents of mud do not pose any major contraindications. When the peloids are heated for application, however, certain precautions are advised. Also, it must be remembered that certain clays and muds are extremely drawing and drying. Therefore, care should be taken when working with clients who have overly sensitive, delicate, or dry skin. All muds must be from a pure source and uncontaminated. Hot peloids applied directly to the skin carry the following contraindications:

- acute inflammation
- local eczema—specific areas need to be avoided
- bleeding or open wounds
- heart disease
- severe hypertension

SPA MUD AND CLAY TREATMENTS			
TREATMENT	**DESCRIPTION**	**BENEFITS**	**CONTRAINDICATIONS**
Back Facial	mud application exclusively to the back after cleansing and exfoliation, with additional cleansing and moisturizing techniques	meant to draw impurities from the skin of the back and is especially beneficial for people suffering from acne on the back and shoulders	open sores, cuts, abrasions, severe acne, skin conditions on the back
Bath	mud, usually powdered, is added to hot water to make a solution in which the client immerses the body	therapeutic for stiff joints and arthritis, relaxing, and purifying through the effects of humic acid	high blood pressure, heart disease, arteriosclerosis, open sores or cuts, pregnancy, sensitivities to certain muds
Body Wrap	clients' skin is exfoliated first, and then a layer of warmed mud is applied to the entire body before being wrapped, usually in plastic sheeting and blankets	depending on type of mud used, can be nourishing, remineralizing, purifying, moisturizing, or cleansing; induces relaxation	acute inflammation, eczema, bleeding, open wounds, heart disease, severe hypertension, overly sensitive skin, diabetic peripheral neuropathy, sensitivities to certain muds
Face Mask	mud is applied to the face after cleansing; emollient lotion or cream is used after the mud is removed	helps draw impurities from the skin, can be drying or exfoliating depending on type of mud	open sores, cuts, abrasions, severe acne, skin conditions on the face, sensitivities to certain muds
Foot Soak	mud, usually powdered, is added to hot water to make a solution in which the client immerses the feet	soothing, relaxing, purifies and cleanses the skin of the feet	open sores, cuts, abrasions, skin conditions on the feet, sensitivities to certain muds
Hand Pack	mud is warmed and applied to the hands, which are then wrapped in plastic; after unwrapping, emollient lotion is massaged into the area	soothes minor aches and pains caused by overwork or inflammation; as a side benefit, mud hand packs are excellent for sore, tired therapists' hands	open sores, cuts, abrasions, skin conditions on the hands, sensitivities to certain muds
Immersion	clients immerse in 100% strength mud or peat contained in tubs at elevated temperatures, often at or near the source	benefits of systemic heat application plus humic acid's chelating properties and nutrients/minerals inherent to specific muds used in immersion	acute inflammation, eczema, bleeding, open wounds, heart disease, severe hypertension, overly sensitive skin, pregnancy, diabetic peripheral neuropathy, sensitivities to certain muds
Parafango Pack	a true heat treatment involving the application of volcanic fango blended with paraffin wax and heated to melting point	benefits of systemic heat application, tones circulatory system	acute inflammation, eczema, bleeding, open wounds, heart disease, severe hypertension, overly sensitive skin, diabetic peripheral neuropathy, sensitivities to certain muds
Rasul Chamber	chamber inlaid with mosaic tiles in which clients self-apply muds that are later steamed and washed off	creates an exotic environment to apply the benefits of therapeutic muds and steam	high blood pressure, heart disease, open wounds, arteriosclerosis, pregnancy, sensitivities to certain muds

TABLE 8–3 Mud and Clay Spa Treatments.

- overly sensitive skin
- diabetic peripheral neuropathy
- pregnancy

Even though the mud in a full-body wrap is applied warm, the body does not undergo a systemic reaction to the application because the mud is not hot enough. The only true heat treatments involving mud are baths, Parafango packs, and full immersions. For the treatment described in this chapter, any type of mud may be applied, depending on the results desired. The protocols remain the same. It is important to note that certain muds are more difficult to remove without a shower, such as Sedona clay and moor. The treatment outlined here is performed in a dry room. If a wet room is available, it is of course simpler to use a shower stall, handheld shower, or Vichy shower to remove the mud, as demonstrated in the Body Wrap Draping Protocol earlier in this chapter. Many spas opt to add a single-note essential oil or blend to the mud prior to application to improve the aroma and add to effectiveness.

TREATMENT: MUD WRAP	
Wet Room/Dry Room	dry room
Table Setup	blanket, sheet, plastic wrap, insulating blanket, large bath towel or another sheet, draping
Treatment Duration	50 minutes
Needed Supplies	choice of body mud, clay or fango, spa bowl, heater, spatula, plastic body wrap, bolster, minimum 4 heated moist hand towels, optional essential oils to add to mud, finishing lotion
Contraindications	acute inflammation, eczema, bleeding, open wounds, heart disease, severe hypertension, overly sensitive skin, diabetic peripheral neuropathy
Draping	diaper draping with breast covering for women; see Draping sidebar in this chapter
Treatment Order	after exfoliation, prior to massage
Safety, Sanitation Issues, & Clean-Up	Be careful not to overheat the mud as it could burn the skin if it is too hot. Darker muds such as moor can discolor certain light-colored fabrics over time; dark sheets and draping should be used for services using these products. Peloids can drain into most sewage and septic systems with no problem.
Body Mechanics & Self-Care	same body mechanic considerations as massage therapy
Product Cost	Depending on the quality of the product applied, muds can range from one dollar to several dollars per treatment, plus the cost of plastic wrap.
Treatment Price	$80 to $120 for wrap alone, more if exfoliation and/or massage is included
Physiological Effects	Different muds have varying effects. The main properties of clay are drawing and purifying, while the main properties of moor mud are chelating through the effects of humic acid. Fango offers minerals and heat. Some popular muds such as rose clay are nourishing and moisturizing.
Pregnancy Issues (information provided by Elaine Stillerman, LMT, author and developer of MotherMassage)	Contraindicated during pregnancy and for three months postpartum.

Mud Wrap Preparation

1. Place approximately ½ cup of mud in a spa bowl. Add 6 to 8 drops of essential oil to mud per treatment if desired. See Chapter 11 for information on effects of specific essential oils. Warm the mixture by floating in hot water or placing in a roaster or double boiler.

2. Prepare the table by layering first a blanket, with the top hanging 12 inches over the head of the table, with a bath towel across the top, then a sheet, plastic wrap, and finally draping towels.
3. Wring out four hand towels and keep them hot in a roaster or hot towel cabbie. Or, wearing insulated gloves, wring them out in very hot water and place them in an insulated container directly before removing the mud from the body.

Mud Wrap Procedure

1. Start with the client prone, and exfoliate, first the back of the left leg, then the right leg, and up over the gluteal muscles to the back. Then ask the client to roll over, and exfoliate the skin of the fronts of the legs, abdomen, arms, and shoulders (Figure 8–14). This exfoliation lasts only 5 to 10 minutes and can be accomplished using a dry loofah, exfoliating gloves, or a dry brush. Alternatively, the mud wrap can be administered immediately after a full-body exfoliation service as described in Chapter 6, in which case this step is skipped. Note that no finishing lotion is applied after exfoliation if it directly precedes a wrap.

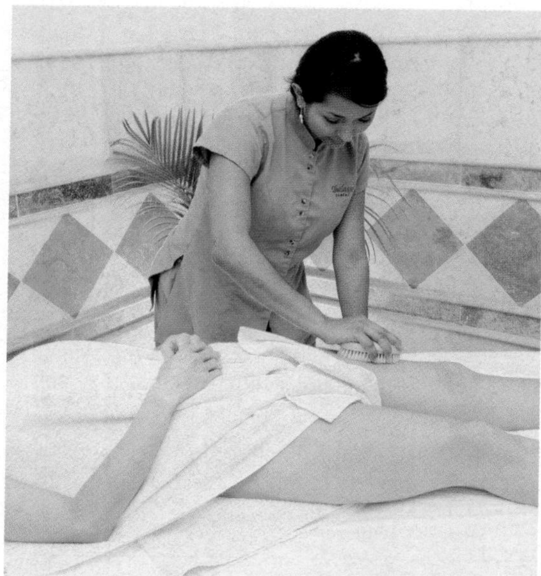

FIGURE 8–14

2. Using your hands or a natural-bristle brush, apply the mud starting on the back. This requires that the client either sit up or roll slightly to one side, then the other (Figure 8–15).

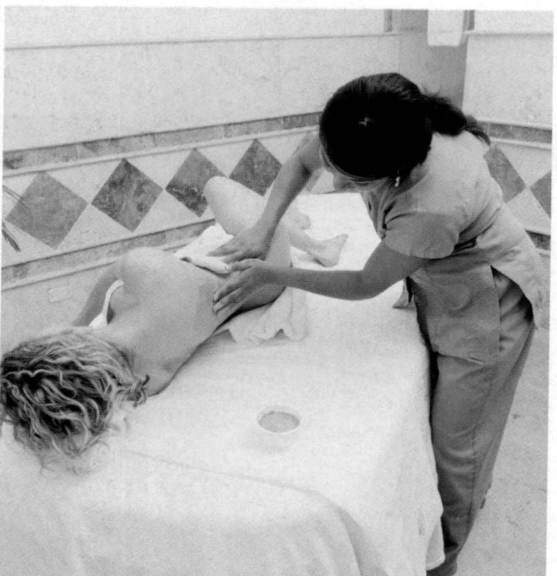

FIGURE 8–15

3. Apply mud to the left leg. Instruct the client to lift her knee and place her foot flat on the table, rolling slightly to the opposite side. Apply mud starting to the ankles; avoid feet if they are going to be treated as part of the service. Move up over the front and back of legs to the buttock (Figure 8–16). Then have the client lower her leg to the table and wrap it in plastic. Repeat on the right leg.

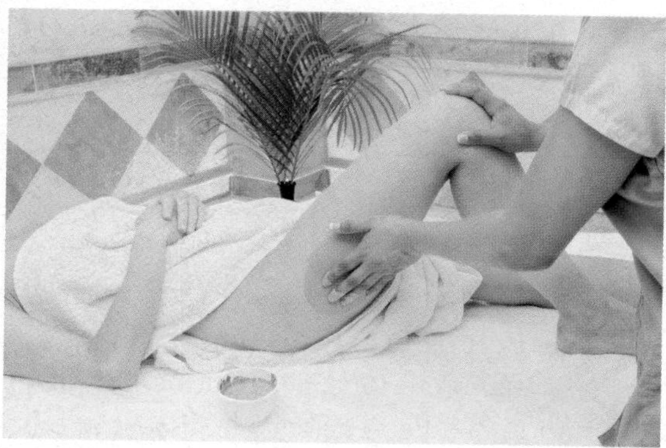

FIGURE 8–16

4. If the mud is particularly drying, like Sedona clay, add water to the application with a spray bottle as you proceed.
5. Apply mud to the abdomen and décolleté. First, place a breast drape over the chest (for women) and slide the main drape out from underneath it down to the hips. Then, apply mud to the abdomen using clockwise, circular movements. Move above the breast drape to apply mud to the décolleté area (Figure 8–17).

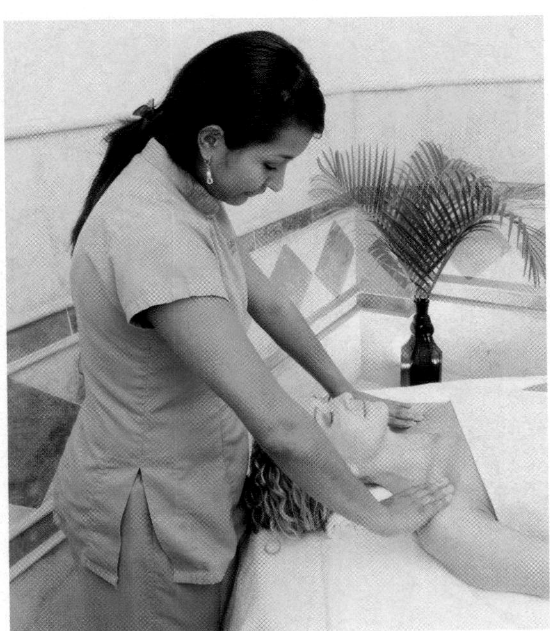

FIGURE 8–17

6. Apply mud to the right arm, beginning at the hand and moving up to the shoulder. You can instruct the client to lift her arm to apply mud to the triceps area if necessary. Cover the arm and the right side of the body in plastic, then repeat on the left side.
7. Wrap the client layer by layer, first plastic, then extra sheet and thermal blanket, then outer blanket, leaving an opening for the feet. Place bolster under the knees. Ask if the client needs anything.
8. While the client is wrapped for 20 to 25 minutes, apply head, neck, and scalp massage or a mini-reflexology routine as described in Chapter 9 (Figure 8–18).

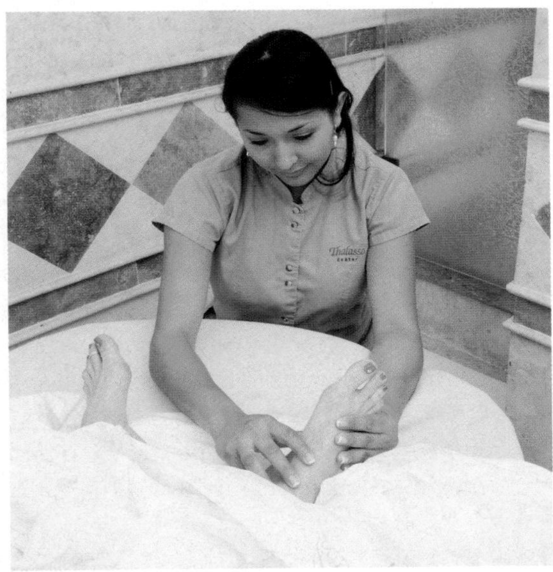

FIGURE 8–18

9. Remove mud from the skin. Starting with the left leg, unwrap the blanket and plastic, leaving the rest of the body wrapped to keep the client warm. You can use a rubber spatula to remove excess product from the skin if necessary (Figure 8–19). Then, take the first hot towel and wipe the mud away from the ankles up to the hips and buttock (Figure 8–20).

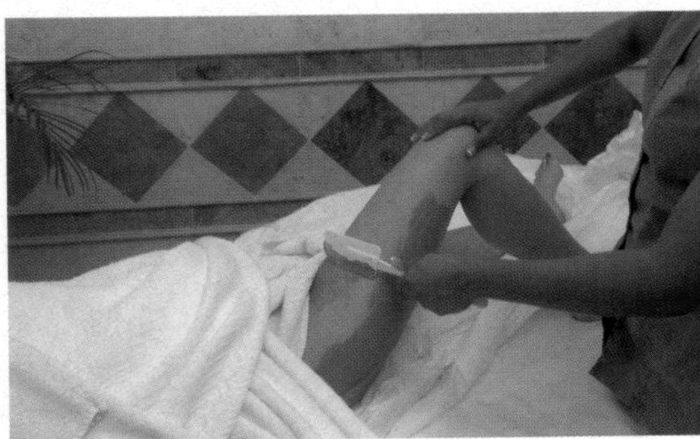

FIGURE 8–19

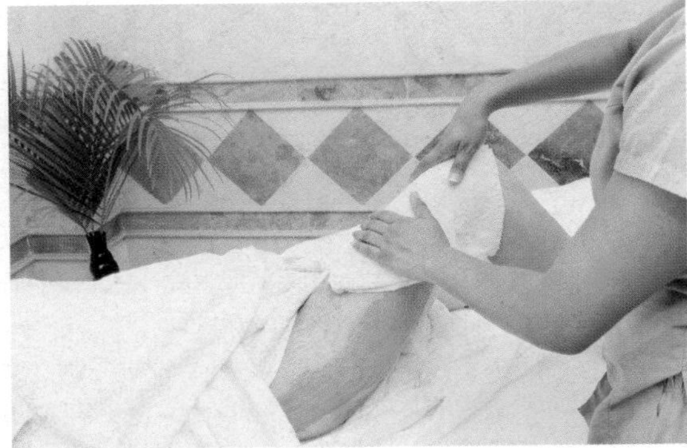

FIGURE 8–20

10. Unwrapping the blanket from the client's right upper body and having the client roll slightly to the left, use the second hot towel to remove mud from the right arm, shoulder, and right portion of the back.
11. Before the client rolls back down onto his back, tuck the plastic wrap as far underneath the body as it will go so the client lies back down on the clean sheet.
12. Repeat the previous two steps on the left side of the body, using the third towel, this time completely removing the plastic wrap from beneath the client (Figure 8–21).
13. With the last towel, remove the mud from the abdomen and décolleté.
14. Lastly, apply a finishing product such as a cream or an emollient lotion to the skin. Apply first to the front of the body, then have the client roll over and apply to the back of the body (Figure 8–22). This can be a quick five-minute application or the start of a longer half-hour or full-hour massage.

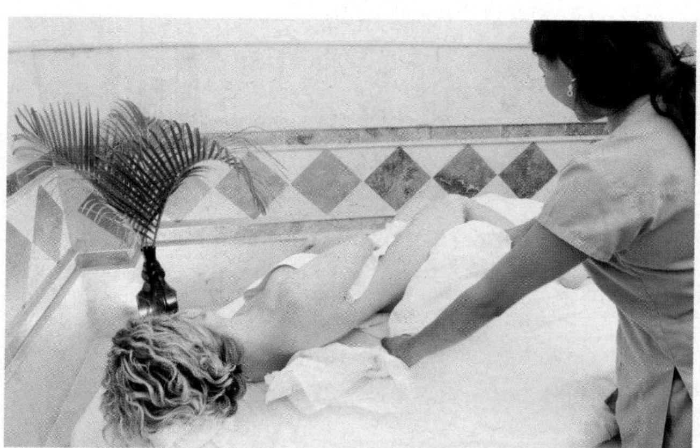

FIGURE 8–21

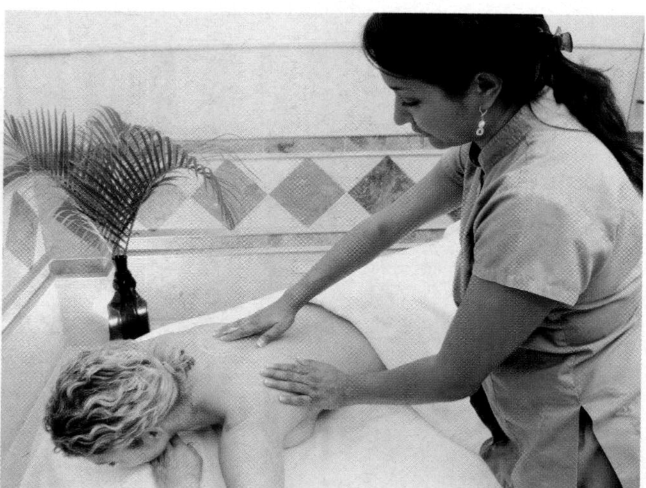

FIGURE 8–22

Mud Wrap Cleanup

1. Dispose of plastic wrap.
2. Clean mud from the spa bowl, brush, and spatula.
3. Launder the towels and sheets.
4. Sanitize and dry all surfaces where clients walk barefoot.

SPA TIP

Different Mud Strokes

Though messy by nature, mud can be applied in a relatively neat manner if the following tips are taken into consideration.

1. First, try using just one hand for the application; keep the other hand free and clean.
2. Keep a moist towel nearby to wipe up excess mud.
3. Apply only a thin layer of mud to the skin, just enough to obscure your view of the skin through the layer.
4. Moisten mud during application, especially if it is a particularly drying type such as Sedona clay.
5. Use a paint brush for application if you wish and the spa allows it, but be sure to choose a natural bristle brush to avoid irritating the skin.

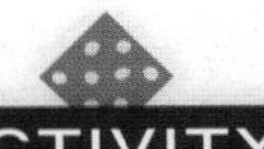

ACTIVITY

Experiencing Body Wrap Products

Investigate the body wrap products available at retail stores and spas in your area, including muds, clays, and fango. Choose one that you find most appealing and use it for body wrap practice with one or more partners from your class. If the product is expensive, you can share the cost with your partners. Perform some research regarding the active ingredients in the product. After your research and test wraps, write a one-page report about your experience with this product and its potential benefits for spa clients.

HERBAL THERAPIES

Herbs have been used by humans for thousands of years to treat disease and improve health. Many modern medicines are derived originally from compounds found in plants, such as aspirin, for example, which is sourced from salicylic acid found in the willow. In spas, the most common forms of herbal application include full-body herbal wraps and herbal compress therapy. Some spas also offer herbal baths, for which the therapeutic bath protocol in Chapter 4 can be used. A somewhat less common spa treatment is the herb-based exfoliation as is sometimes used in Ayurvedic protocols. Many spas also offer their guests the benefits of herbs through the ingestion of herbal teas. The herbs used in spas are either cultivated for human use or **wildcrafted**, and most spas buy the herbs they use. However, some spas, such as the Golden Door, actually grow the herbs on-site, which, they believe, add to the potency of the treatments they provide. See Table 8–4 for a list of popular herbs used in spas. The herbs are most often used in their dry, bulk form (Figure 8–23), with which spa therapists make an **infusion** for use in treatments. One important active ingredient in herbs that makes them useful in spa services is the class known as **phenols,** which serve as the plants' defense against

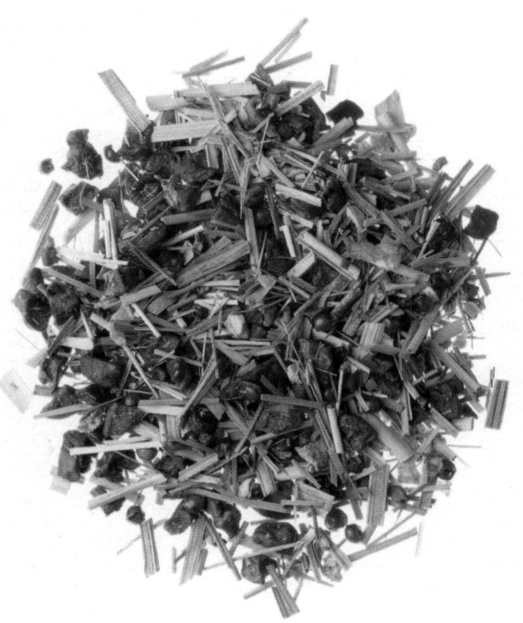

FIGURE 8–23 Dried herbs are the most popular form used in spa treatments.

SPA TIP

Although most muds wash out easily and can be rinsed down any drain, you may want to avoid using white linens as they can become discolored over time, especially if exposed to darker muds such as moor. Many spas opt for earth-toned, green, or brown towels and sheets for use during mud treatments.

wildcrafted

plants that are harvested from their natural or "wild" habitat for food, medicinal, or other purposes; often used regarding herbs gathered for spa treatment applications

infusion

a solution obtained by steeping or soaking a substance, usually in water

phenols

any of a class of weakly acidic organic compounds; many phenols occur in the herbs used in spa treatments and are a contributor to their effectiveness

HERB	BOTANICAL NAME	BENEFITS	CONTRAINDICATIONS	TREATMENTS
Arnica Flowers	*Arnica montana*	sports injuries, bruises, strains, sprains, anti-inflammatory	sensitive or broken skin	Use arnica-infused oil as a massage oil, adding 60 drops to 8 oz warm water; soak a cloth in it and apply to the affected area. Cover with a dry cloth and leave 20 to 60 minutes.
Calendula Flowers	*Calendula officinalis*	skin soothing, anti-inflammatory, helps with slow-healing and difficult wounds, surgical incisions and burns	none	Make a tea infusion for compressing. Use as an addition to herbal body wrap formulas. Apply salves made with infused calendula oil.
Chamomile Flowers	*Matricaria recutita*	soothing to skin irritations and ulcerations, itching, and inflammations; calming and relaxing to the emotions.	possible reactions if allergic to plants of the daisy family such as ragweed and asters	Create compresses with cloths soaked in tea. Use in herbal body wrap formulas. Apply gauze pads soaked in tea to the eye area during a massage or body treatment.
Eucalyptus Leaves	*Eucalyptus globulus*	for bronchial congestion, coughs, infections, muscle aches, and pains	caution for gall bladder and liver conditions	Place herbal tea infusion in compresses for sore muscles. Add to detoxifying body wrap formulas.
Ginger Root	*Zingiber officinale*	stimulates circulation and perspiration, warming herb for indigestion, relieves cramps, comforting during colds and flu	caution for gall bladder conditions	Apply compresses with the hot tea across the abdomen for cramps, or on sore muscles. Add to herbal body wrap formulas for detoxification and to help raise body temperature.
Lavender	*Lavandula officinalis*	relaxing and calming for the nervous system, healing for many skin conditions, excellent for muscle spasms and cramps	none	Use the infusion in baths, facial steams, herbal body wraps, foot baths, and compresses. Apply gauze pads soaked in tea to the eye area during a massage or body treatment. Wash wounds with the tea infusion.
Lemongrass	*Cymbopogan flexuosus*	invigorating, strengthening, and cleansing, appetite stimulant	possible skin irritation	Often used in Thai-themed treatments with ginger, sandalwood, vetiver, patchouli, and ylang ylang. Use an infusion in baths, or the powdered herb in body scrubs.
Peppermint	*Mentha piperita*	refreshing and stimulating, used for headaches, congestion, and muscle pain	none	Use an infusion in hand and foot baths. Add a very small amount to herbal body wrap formulas for stimulation. Compress sore muscles or bruised areas with a tea infusion-soaked cloth. Serve the tea for headache, nausea, and after body wrap treatments.

TABLE 8–4 Popular Herbs Used in Spa Treatments (courtesy Rae Dunphy Aromatics). *(Continued)*

HERB	BOTANICAL NAME	BENEFITS	CONTRAINDICATIONS	TREATMENTS
Rose	*Rosa damascena* or *centifolia*	soothing and uplifting	none	Add rosebuds to foot soaks. Make a face or body mist with the tea infusion for a luxurious finishing treatment.
Rosemary	*Rosmarinus officinalis*	for bronchial conditions, muscle aches and pains, bruises; diaphoretic and stimulating	pregnancy	Add to herbal body wrap formulas for stimulation and detoxification. Make a very strong tea for a foot bath during colds and flus.
St. John's Wort	*Hypericum perforatum*	anti-inflammatory for nerve injuries, muscular bruising, varicose veins, and burns	possible photosensitivity if applied externally	Used in massage or skin treatment preparations as an infused oil, especially for burns.

TABLE 8–4 Popular Herbs Used in Spa Treatments (courtesy Rae Dunphy Aromatics).

microorganisms, insects, and herbivores. Phenols and other constituents of herbs create myriad effects, and several of these effects are highly sought after for use in spa treatments, as listed below:

antipyretic: Herbs that help lower fever. Also known as *febrifuge* herbs, they help reduce production of heat in the body. Examples include black pepper and sandalwood. These are especially good in baths when clients are overheated or have been overexposed to the elements.

antispasmodic: Herbs that help reduce muscle tightness. Calendula and willow are examples of the type of herb that help soft tissues release and relax. Effectively used in compresses and baths.

demulcent: Herbs that have a softening or soothing effect. Aloe is one example of these herbs, which can be combined with others to create a secondary soothing effect to the skin during cleansing and purifying treatments such as the herbal wrap.

diaphoretic: Herbs that increase perspiration. Ginger and peppermint are two examples, often used in the herbal wrap to promote detoxification.

diuretic: Herbs that induce loss of fluid through the urinary system, helping to cleanse the vascular system, kidneys, and liver. Examples are green tea and dandelion.

nervine: Herbs that soothe the nervous system. Examples include chamomile and valerian. Often used in teas or capsules for ingestion, or as part of body wrap blends to calm clients during intense treatments.

stimulating: Herbs that uplift and energize. Some examples are lemongrass, ginger, and peppermint, which most often affect the respiratory, digestive, and circulatory systems.

antipyretic
preventing or alleviating fever

demulcent
having a softening or soothing effect, especially to the skin

diaphoretic
used to induce perspiration

diuretic
a substance that tends to increase the flow of urine

nervine
having the quality of acting upon or affecting the nerves; quieting nervous excitement, as do several herbs and oils used in spa treatments

SPA TIP

Creating Herbal Body Mists

You can create an herbal infusion by soaking teabags or bulk herbs in hot water. Try chamomile for a relaxing mist, lavender for a healing mist, and peppermint for a refreshing mist. Remove the teabag or strain out the herbs, cool the water overnight in the refrigerator, and place in a spray bottle. Use the cool mist on clients' skin after a hot herbal bath or massage during the summertime.

Herbal Wrap

The herbal wrap is one of the most effective treatments in the spa therapist's arsenal. When used properly, it can have a real impact on clients' well-being. A true heat treatment, the herbal wrap uses special sheets soaked in a near-boiling herbal infusion to induce intense sweating. The effectiveness of this wrap is attained by inducing a false fever in the body, which triggers a release of impurities through the pores, just as when you are experiencing a real fever due to an infection and the body is trying to rid itself of the invading organism. This heightened body temperature is known as *hyperthermia*, as noted in Chapter 5. In order to achieve this state, the treatment protocol must be followed precisely, and several key instructions must be kept in mind.

1. The client must be warmed prior to being wrapped. This warming can only be achieved through immersion in a heating environment, including steam, sauna, or hot bath. Hot showers are not true immersions and do not warm the body sufficiently.
2. The client should be warmed internally as well as externally prior to the wrap through the ingestion of some herbal tea.
3. The wrap should be snug and not offer avenues for cool air to penetrate and lower the effectiveness.
4. The sheets need to be well-soaked in the hot herbal solution, ideally at 165°F to 195°F.
5. The sheets must be wrung out extremely well so that no excess moisture remains. Sheets with excess moisture can potentially harm clients. Also, water cools down more swiftly than the sheet itself. Therefore, an overly wet sheet can scald someone and then become a cold, ineffective wrap—not a good combination.

Herbal wraps are normally administered every other day during an extended spa stay, for a total of three times per week. Clients wishing to go on a cleansing program while at the spa will find that the herbal wrap is a powerful tool to aid them. For instance, if a client comes to the spa trying to lose weight, he can increase his exercise load, follow the spa's recommended diet program, and receive a series of herbal wraps along with other services such as massage. Or, if a client is trying to kick the nicotine habit, he can stop smoking while receiving a series of herbal wrap treatments. The wraps, properly performed, will help leach the tissues of compounds built up in the body through smoking. The "false fever" stimulates the body to release nicotine and other substances from the body in the same way that a real fever helps purge a virus attacking the body.

In addition to detoxification, herbal wraps also help soothe sore, aching muscles and relax muscular tension that may be causing pain. Due to the nature of being wrapped and lying quietly during the treatment, a state of deep relaxation will be reached by most individuals. Although the heat and the snug fit of the herbal wrap cause approximately 20 percent of clients to experience a sense of claustrophobia, this sensation can be avoided and the wrap performed successfully on almost all clients if the protocols for dealing with claustrophobia found earlier in this chapter are followed.

muslin

a type of finely woven cotton fabric, used in spa treatments and specifically in the herbal wrap

The sheets used for herbal wraps are special. It is best to use unbleached, organic, canvas-grade **muslin** sheets. Muslin is a type of cotton fabric that was

Herbal Sheet Folding Technique

Did You Know?

Fold the sheets in the following way (Figure 8–24):

Step 1: Fold both edges into the center, lengthwise.
Step 2: Fold both edges into the center again.
Step 3: Fold this in half to create a strip.
Step 4: Fold the strip in thirds.
Step 5: Fold it in half.

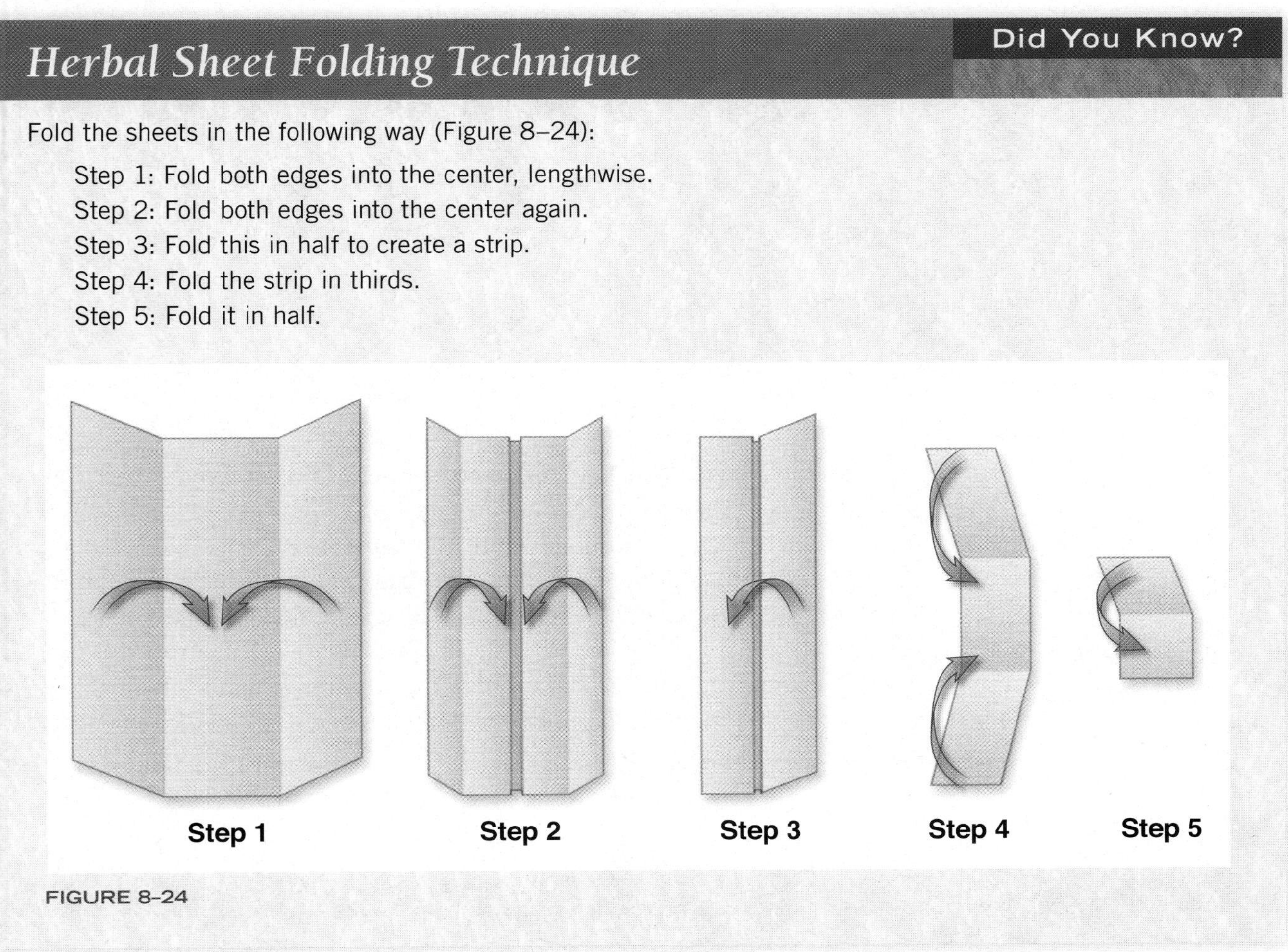

FIGURE 8–24

introduced to the West in the seventeenth century. It was named for the city where Europeans first encountered it, Mosul, in present-day Iraq, but the fabric originally came from Dhaka in what is now Bangladesh. Regular bed sheets just do not compare to this material and are not effective because they do not absorb enough herbal solution and cool too quickly. Make sure to launder new sheets prior to first use, as they will not absorb herbs as well until washed once. Wash in hot water with a small amount of mild detergent. These sheets must be folded in the proper manner for three important reasons:

1. When all sheets are folded alike, they also unfold in the same manner, making it simple for all therapists on a spa staff to quickly and economically maneuver the sheets onto the table and around the client when they are hot and speed is of the essence.
2. Properly folded sheets fit well inside heating units such as hydrocollators.
3. Sheets folded in this manner stay hot longer because they can be kept compact while being unfolded.

It is best to use natural, organic herbs for your solution if possible. A large number of herbs and herb combinations are appropriate for an herbal wrap, and spas customize their blends according to season and client needs. In general, the herbs in combination should stimulate circulation and produce diaphoretic

HERB	BENEFITS IN HERBAL WRAP
allspice	analgesic, for bronchial conditions, joint pain
calendula	skin soothing, anti-inflammatory
Clove	antiseptic, antispasmodic
eucalyptus	for bronchial congestion, coughs, muscle aches, and pains
Ginger	stimulates circulation and perspiration, relieves cramps
oatmeal	skin protection, **antipruritic,** moisturizing, anti-inflammatory, skin cleanser
rosemary	diaphoretic and stimulating; for bronchial conditions, muscle aches and pains, bruises

TABLE 8–5 Detox Blend Herbs.

and diuretic effects. This is to augment the main purpose of the herbal wrap: detoxification. However, the wrap can serve other purposes as well, and some spas offer relaxing, soothing, or uplifting versions of the herbal wrap as well as the traditional detoxifying. One combination of herbs used in hundreds of spas is called the *detox blend*, consisting of allspice, calendula, clove, eucalyptus, ginger, oatmeal, and rosemary, the effects of which are highlighted in Table 8–5. A small muslin bag with a half-cup of herbs is sufficient for a full day of herbal wrap services. The bag is left in the heating unit and the water is replenished as needed throughout the day.

antipruritic

a substance that relieves or prevents itching

SPA CAUTION

It is best to wear two pairs of rubber gloves while wringing out herbal sheets in order to keep your hands from getting burned. The inner pair are shorter and fit snugly, while the outer pair are large and long, reaching half way up the forearm (Figure 8–25).

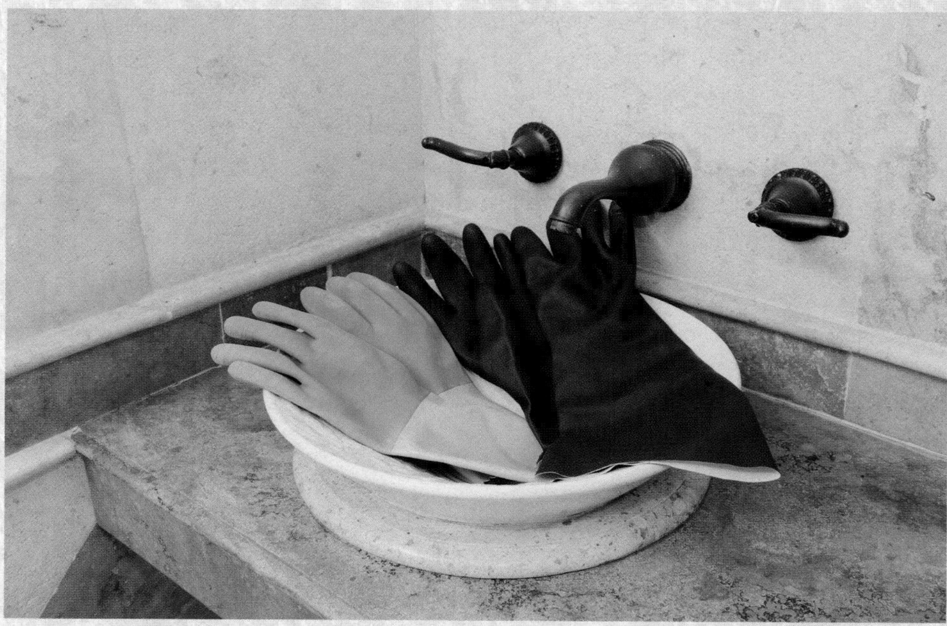

FIGURE 8–25

THAI HERB	BOTANICAL NAME	PART OF PLANT USED	EFFECTS
Lemongrass	*Cymbopogon citratus*	stem	anti-inflammatory for sprains, bruises, and sore muscles
Plai	*Zingiber cassumunar*	rhizome	helps bronchial; anti-inflammatory for contusions, sprains, or joint inflammation; antiseptic, soothes, and heals the skin
Turmeric	*Curcuma longa*	rhizome and leaf	cleansing, antiseptic, soothing, anti-inflammatory for bruises, joint pain, sprains, or muscle pain
Kaffir Lime	*Citrus hystix*	leaves	treatment of colds, congestion, astringent
Camphor	*Cinnamonum camphora*	crystals derived from the gum of the tree bark	stimulating and dilating effects on respiratory system, calms anxiety, anti-inflammatory and analgesic for muscle stiffness, sprains, strains, bruises, or swelling.
Tamarind	*Tamaridus indica*	leaves	astringent values draw out the oils and toxins to cleanse and purify the skin, while the antiseptic properties soothe and heal the skin

TABLE 8–6 Herbs Used in Thai Compresses.

Herbal compress therapy creates four distinct benefits for clients based on the effects of aromatherapy, herbal therapy, heat therapy, and massage therapy. The compresses can be custom blended to treat specific complaints, but the blend of herbs used in most Thai compresses is based on a recipe from the Wat Po temple in Bangkok, where a massage clinic and school are located. This blend is said to have an invigorating effect, while also soothing sore and over-worked muscles. The major herbs used in the traditional recipe are those listed in Table 8–6. Other herbs also used include mango ginger and *Curcuma comosa* from the turmeric family, sweet sage, orange skin, patchouli, and the shikakai shrub, the bark of which contains high levels of **saponin**.

Herbal compresses are soaked and then steamed for 10 to 15 minutes prior to use before being applied directly to the skin. Larger compresses are used for the body and smaller ones for the face. Two compresses are used for each treatment so that one is always kept hot in the heating unit, which can be a steamer or roaster, the same as that used for heating spa stones. Contraindications for the treatment include fever, heart disease, hypertension, diabetic peripheral neuropathy, pregnancy, open cuts, wounds, sores, and abrasions.

saponin

an agent, found in several herbs used in spa treatments, that forms soapy lather when mixed with water

SPA CAUTION

The following safety precautions must be taken while performing herbal compress treatments.

- Take special care when lifting the lid off the steamer, as hot water may drip onto your skin. Lift the lid away from the face and body.
- Handle the herbal ball with a towel or piece of cloth when removing from the steamer and during the first few minutes of application.
- Always test the temperature of the herbal ball on your own inner forearm when it comes out of the steamer and before applying it to the client's skin.
- When first making contact, stamp the herbal ball on the client's skin with light rapid motions until it begins to cool down after 30 to 60 seconds.

A complete herbal compress service includes stimulation of many points along the energy pathways according to Thai tradition, plus some Thai massage stretches. A complete signature service as performed in spas is quite involved, yet the basic maneuvers used with the herbal balls are simple. They are:

Stamping:	the first maneuver used when the herbal ball is hottest, it consists of light, rapid touching of ball on the skin while moving it constantly over the body, usually along a sen sib pathway (Figure 8–35)
Rocking:	a steady rocking of the ball back and forth on one spot and then lifting it up and moving it to the next spot to repeat (Figure 8–36)
Rolling:	pivoting the ball in a circular motion on one spot (Figure 8–37)
Stationary:	steady downward pressure of the ball on just one point (Figure 8–38)
Dragging:	steady pressure into the body while dragging the ball over the skin (Figure 8–39)

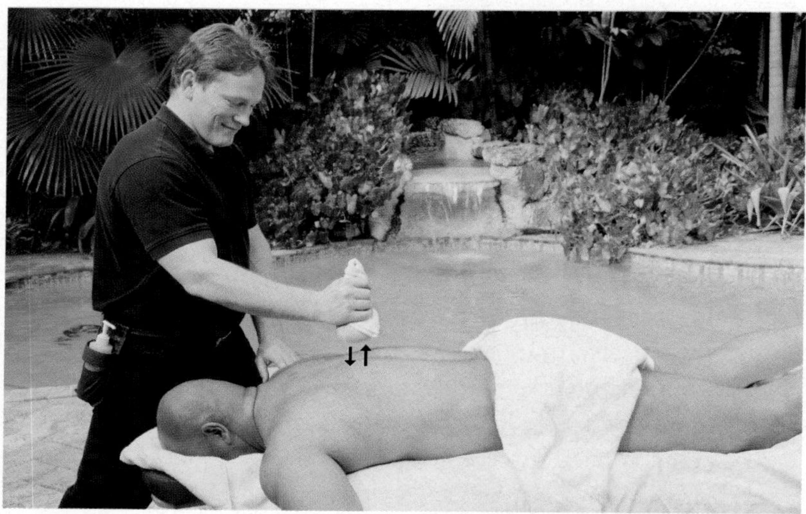

FIGURE 8–35 Light, rapid touching of ball on the skin while moving it constantly over the body, usually along a sen sib pathway.

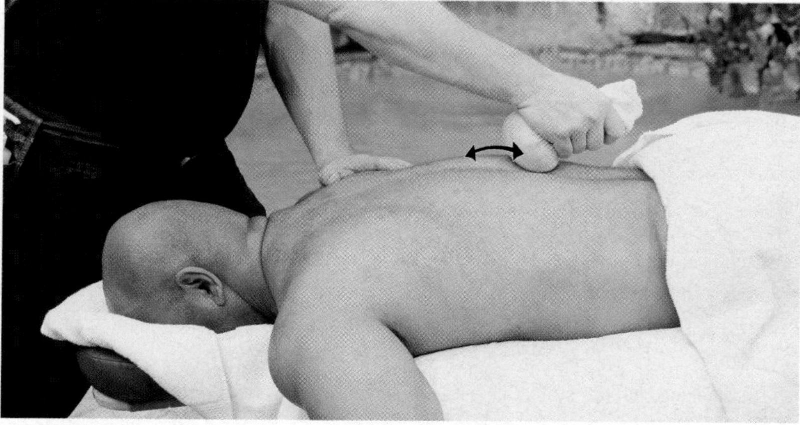

FIGURE 8–36 Steady rocking of the ball back and forth on one spot and then lifting it up and moving it to the next.

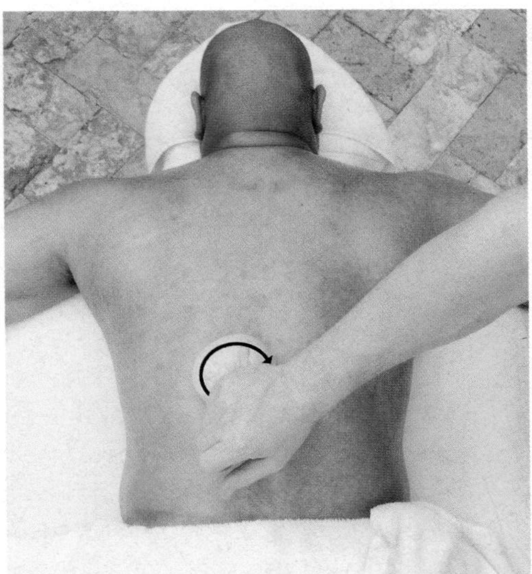

FIGURE 8–37 Pivoting the ball in a circular motion on one spot.

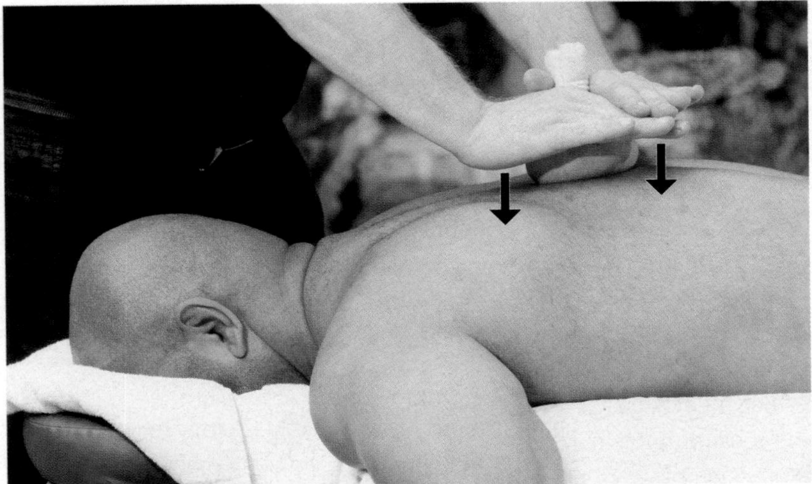

FIGURE 8–38 Steady downward pressure of the ball on just one point.

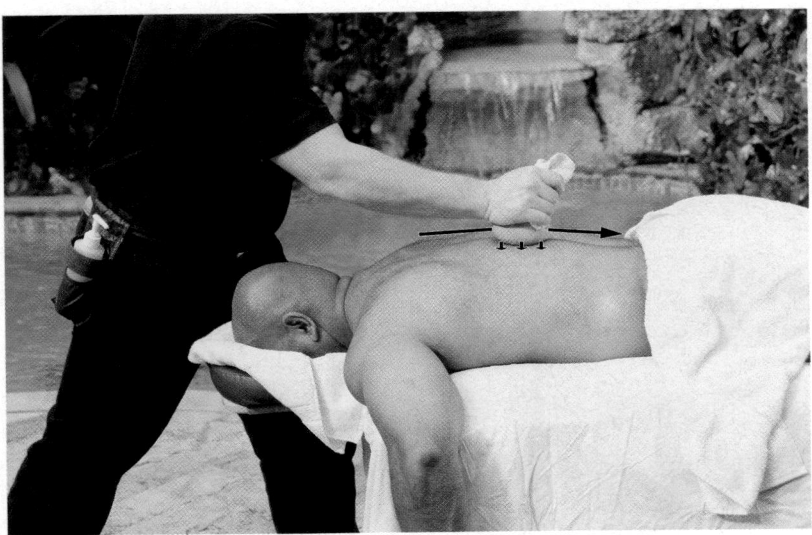

FIGURE 8–39 Steady pressure into the body while dragging the ball over the skin.

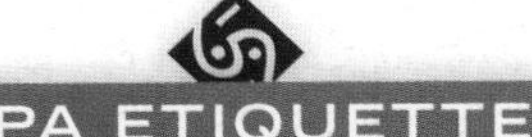

SPA ETIQUETTE

After use, seal herbal compasses in a plastic bag or container and offer to the client for home use. This proves that the compresses are used only once and allows the client to continue to experience the benefits of the herbs at home, where they can be used in a bath.

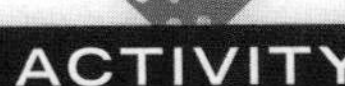

ACTIVITY

Basic Herbal Compress Maneuvers

Observing all safety precautions and contraindications, practice the five basic maneuvers using Thai herbal compresses. Use dry herbal compresses that have not been steamed yet to practice the maneuvers first before trying them with heated compresses.

RESEARCH

Choose one herb that is used in spa therapy and write a one-page report about it, including its origins, history of use, benefits and applications in the spa setting.

SPA PROFILE

Rae Dunphy, Owner, Rae Dunphy Aromatics

In 1971, Rae Dunphy enrolled in an herbology course taught by a Latvian woman whose mission was to bring Old World herbal knowledge to the new world. The training lasted for four years, with plenty of self-directed study and an intensive residential component each summer. The experience changed her life.

"I finished my course in 1974," recalls Dunphy, an energetic mother of four girls with a passion for her work. "Soon after, I opened a bulk herb shop in Calgary, Alberta, the first of its kind in that area, modeling it after a traditional apothecary shop."

After 12 years, Dunphy turned the store over to other people to run. "I was reading about aromatherapy at the time," she says, "and as I dove further into the subject, I became more and more single-minded about the application of essential oils. Some of my herbal roots got shelved as I went more deeply into aromatherapy, but over the years I've come to realize that the two go hand in hand. Much of aromatherapy is about reminding people that what is in the little bottle is the ethereal aspect of the plant. In a sense, aromatherapy is liquefied herbology. People usually don't make that mental jump from the plant to the oil for some reason, but to me, it's like essential oils are an expression of the plant's hopes and dreams, distilled from their essence. Women have intuitively known this for millennia, and that's why they have been burned at the stake—it was the women who carried that knowledge of natural self-care from plants and were sometimes labeled as witches. They passed the knowledge down from generation to generation, though much of it has been lost, which is a shame. Women used to have distilling rooms or 'Still Rooms' in their homes, and they would harvest the wonderful herbs from the garden and put up essentials for the winter."

One of Dunphy's missions is to support massage practitioners in the success of their businesses. "I think that there's a tendency for massage practitioners to come out of their massage training with a single-minded point of view," she says. "They focus on the muscles, on physical tension, spasms, adhesions and so on, which is fine, but what I've tried to do through my products, workshops, and writings is to show ways that they can incorporate new ideas into their practices. One critical area therapists need to focus on, for example, is retailing of related products. They miss such an opportunity to increase their sales without expending hands-on energy, and provide healthy products that will extend the benefits of the treatment. I try to show them that a massage practice is an all-encompassing business and that they need to think of creating an experience for customers the moment they come in the door. Some therapists are uncomfortable with that. They prefer to stick with a plain white clinical setting and offer massage only. But after spending a little time with me, they begin to see the beauty of creating a space filled with the rich, healing aromas of herbs. The retail success these therapists encounter is really just a side benefit to their love of the herbs and the great properties they offer."

Dunphy's enthusiasm for herbology extends to the spa industry, and she sees many possibilities there for spas to expand the efficacy of their herbal programs. Unfortunately, she sees most spas as being somewhat deficient when it comes to the full and proper use of herbs. "It's not to say a lot of spas aren't already implementing herb-based treatments," she says. "They are. Ayurvedic spas focus on herbal treatments, for example. At the Hills Health Ranch Spa in British Columbia, all the treatments are built around pressed rosehip seed oil. And many other spas use herbal-inspired products. But the concept of creating their own customized herb-based treatments is still in its infancy."

As far as the herb-based treatments that are being most successfully used by massage therapists in

(Continued)

massage, sports massage, deep tissue massage, couples massage, four-handed massage, topical heating and cooling massage, and chair massage.

MASSAGE PRACTICE IN THE SPA SETTING

First and foremost in the spa come your duties as a massage therapist. Massage is what you have trained for and what you have been hired to do. Statistically speaking, you as a spa therapist will be spending the majority of your time performing massage, which is the most popular modality when compared to all other spa treatments, as demonstrated in Table 2–5 in Chapter 2. Therefore, it is natural for a newly hired therapist to feel that all she need do to successfully fulfill her duties is to get behind that closed door as quickly as possible and begin the massage. When you practice massage therapy in a spa, however, you will need to remain aware that you are operating within a larger structure that encompasses and helps to define what it is you are doing in the treatment room.

By definition, a massage given at any particular spa facility must stay within certain boundaries involving time limit, style, pre- and post-massage protocol, etiquette, and other criteria. Some spas, though not many, even insist that therapists follow a set massage routine in order to create a uniform experience for their clients. It is important to follow spa guidelines, of course, but to be an excellent massage, your treatment must somehow transcend these boundaries and limitations. Normally, when performing massage, you have four components of the experience to concentrate on: yourself, your client, your technique, and your schedule. In a spa, you will have five components: yourself, your client, your technique, your schedule, and the spa's particular way of doing things. This is important. Each spa has developed its own protocols and standards when it comes to implementing massage on its premises, and it will be up to you as an employee to master these protocols and adhere to them while on the job.

Taking into account the wide variety of bodywork administered in spas, it is difficult to arrive at one simple definition for "spa massage." However, when people use this term, they most often mean a spa's basic massage offering, which is commonly Swedish massage. For many therapists working in spas, it is challenging to give high-quality spa massage sessions consistently. This is true for several obvious reasons, including fatigue, boredom, and injury. Three other main reasons that many therapists overlook are:

- *Low Expectations*: Many spa clients arrive with no particular complaints or pains, and they do not expect the massage therapy session to help them very much beyond simple relaxation.
- *Time Constraints*: It is difficult for therapists to retain enthusiasm and high energy levels when doing many massages each day, all within the same time guidelines.
- *Inexperienced Clients*: Many spa clients are first-time massage recipients or casual recipients who have not formed an appreciation for bodywork and need to be educated about its effects and benefits.

With these constraints in mind, it is still possible for spa therapists to make their massage sessions fresh and effective, giving each client a customized

The Real Meaning of "Relaxation Massage"

Did You Know?

The literature at many spas refers to something known as a "relaxation massage," which sounds relatively benign, if not bland, but what exactly is it? The standard response to this question is that a relaxation massage is a Swedish massage, not one of the advanced modalities, but as you have no doubt learned in school, a Swedish massage can also be invigorating, stimulating, therapeutic, and downright intense. Is "relaxation" simply a code word for "fluffy spa-type massage with no therapeutic value"? Are spas doomed forever to suffer from this stigma as places where relaxation equals substandard?

Seen from another angle, all massages should be a relaxation massage, shouldn't it? Even deep structural integration, which may be intense in the moment, leads eventually to a relaxation of tissues and holding patterns in the body.

The problem here is that we are looking at the terminology from a massage therapist's point of view. The real meaning of the term "relaxation" as it is used in terms of spa massage is correctly understood when seen from the client's point of view, as it probably has more to do with easing clients' fear than anything else. It is a way to let spa clients know that they are not going to be mauled by a rough Russian or Turkish character like those depicted in old movies. Over the years, the term has ended up being applied to any massage that is gentle and non-threatening. This may be unfair, however, because Swedish massage can actually be much more than simply "relaxing."

If the spa where you work uses the term "relaxation massage" in their literature to signify basic Swedish massage, you may have to help educate clients about what this means and about the many other ways in which Swedish massage can benefit them beyond mere relaxation.

experience in spite of the fact that many of the massage moves and timing may be the same from massage to massage. This requires discipline and enhanced skill on the part of the spa therapist. Far from being easier to perform than massage administered in other venues, spa massage can be, in a certain fashion, more challenging, and therapists who master it can rightfully feel proud. In order to achieve this, therapists working in spas profit by paying particularly close attention to the following points: scope of practice, intake procedures, optimal number of massages per day, timing of services, preparation, and cleanup.

Scope of Practice

The massage therapist in a spa setting is of course subject to all of the same limitations to scope of practice as are massage therapists in any professional setting. Additional points to consider in a spa are these:

- Many spa clients are receiving massage for the very first time, and it is important to be sensitive to this. Often, it is appropriate to use light pressure over the entire body at first, until a level of comfort and rapport can be established. Even if you specialize in deep bodywork and are willing to share it with spa clients, they are often unprepared for it and may react adversely. With first-time recipients, keep the pressure light and limit massage strokes to basic Swedish maneuvers unless the client has requested otherwise after clear communication on the subject. You must also stay aware of the spa's restrictions on this subject and refrain from offering any modalities or manipulations that are not allowed.

- Because people are often on a quest for better health while visiting a spa, they are especially open to suggestions about diet, fitness, nutrition, and lifestyle. It must be remembered that these are not your areas of expertise. It is allowable to offer general positive encouragement for spa clients, inspiring them to take part in the spa's full list of healthy activities and practices, but it is not your place to suggest specific advice in these areas unless you have been trained and credentialed in them.
- Some people visit spas in order to address long-term physical conditions ranging from addictions to obesity to heart disease and many others. It is tempting to want to help people with these conditions, showing them how the combination of massage, detoxification, and improved diet and lifestyle offered at the spa will help heal many ills. However, it is important not to promise any benefits that cannot be substantiated or that are not sanctioned by the spa. In general, the benefits you can rightfully claim for the spa services that you personally offer include those created by heat, special products such as herbs, clays, and seaweeds, and massage therapy.
- Because so many spa treatments involve the use of hot water, you must be thoroughly conversant with all contraindications for the use of heat.

Spa Massage Intake Procedures

Each spa has its own unique intake procedures. Some employ an extensive screening process that may even involve a doctor's visit, stress test, and thorough physical examination. Some have well-trained **intake specialists** who spend a half-hour or longer molding the client's experience, recommending treatments, and gleaning much important information that therapists can use in their sessions. These facilities usually fall into the destination spa, medical spa, or mineral spa categories. Some resort and club spas have extensive intake procedures as well. Other spas, however, have a bare-bones intake form that perhaps asks for emergency contact information and the client's reason for requesting massage. Many day spas require little screening for a massage session, and some require none at all.

intake specialists

also referred to as *hospitality specialists* in some spas; see Chapter 15; these employees are responsible for helping clients decide which programs and treatments to experience while at the spa

As you study **S.O.A.P. notes** and charting during your massage education, you will no doubt see the value in these procedures, and the lack of such documentation in many spas may come as an unwelcome surprise. It is important, then, to use your own discretion when working with a client for the first time. Whenever an intake form of any kind is available, use it to full advantage, and if the spa does not use one, it is permissible to ask the client verbally about medical conditions and possible contraindications.

S.O.A.P. notes

(acronym for subjective, objective, assessment, and plan) method of documentation employed by massage therapists to write out notes in a client's chart

Some spas, especially hair- and esthetics-based day spas, focus their intake procedures on the skin rather than overall health, because their main business consists of cosmetic procedures and the sale of cosmetic products. This paradigm works well for many spas. Some therapists, new to the industry, perceive the type of intake procedures at these spas as an insult to their therapeutic integrity, and this can lead to tension between management and massage staff. If this is the case, it is permissible for the therapist to suggest to spa management that they institute a massage-specific intake procedure, but if one is not implemented, it is best for the therapist to either accept this or seek employment elsewhere rather than create ill will among the staff and clients. The section entitled "Liability and Risk Management for the Spa Therapist" in Chapter 3 discusses this topic further and offers an example of an intake form to which therapists can refer when treating spa massage clients.

Greetings

Prior to a spa massage, you will have only a few minutes to put the client at ease after the initial greeting and before the treatment actually begins. This short time span is crucial for setting the tone of the treatment. It is important to do all you can during this brief period in order to make the client comfortable and to usher him into the therapeutic environment. In addition to filling out or reexamining an intake form, some therapists practice some of the following simple techniques to make this greeting phase effective.

- Shaking hands firmly and making eye contact when first meeting will put the client at ease.
- Most spas encourage therapists to address each client by name as Mr., Mrs., Ms., or Dr. ________________. It is permissible to ask the client for his name if you do not have the name already.
- Some therapists touch the client gently on the shoulder while directing him down the hallway toward the treatment room, thus initiating a sense of reassuring contact.
- Many clients appreciate a thorough explanation of the draping procedure used at the spa, along with some words about the process of getting undressed and how the therapist will leave the room, allowing them plenty of time and privacy.
- A minute or two spent in dialogue after the client is on the table and before the massage actually begins helps to initiate first-time clients into the massage experience. More experienced clients may prefer to begin the session immediately.

For more information about these and other appropriate behaviors when interacting with spa clients, see the section entitled "The Seven Main Customer Service Skills for a Spa Therapist" in Chapter 15.

Number of Massages

Because massage therapy is the most popular service in spas, it is often necessary for therapists to perform several sessions back-to-back. What this means differs from spa to spa, however. Many spas maintain a strict break of at least 15 minutes between treatments, with some going as high as 30 minutes. Other spas offer very little break at all, as little as 5 minutes, but these are increasingly rare because spa owners are seeing the benefit of keeping their employees healthy. It is not good for business to have therapists out of work and receiving workers' compensation due to carpal tunnel syndrome and other injuries.

For the same reason, it is customary for spas to limit their therapists' total number of massage treatments each day. The number varies, but the norm is five massages per day. Many factors contribute to altering this number in particular spas. For example, some spas have therapists perform only two or three massages in a row, with less taxing spa treatments interspersed throughout the day. Thus, a therapist can perform eight total treatments, but three of them might be body scrubs, wraps, or specialty services.

On-call therapists not employed full-time by the spa are often called upon to perform more back-to-back services. When client demand is at its peak, these therapists can sometimes perform eight massages or more. Attempting heroics by performing this number of full-hour sessions day after day is a sure way to cause injury. Though the lure of immediate income is strong, it is best to take a long-term point of view and pace oneself. Many therapists have enthusiastically entered the spa industry, only to leave disillusioned a few short years later due to disability.

Spas that force therapists to perform too many massages, with no regard for their welfare, usually experience high therapist turnover and lowered client satisfaction. These spas are the least enjoyable to work for. While there are no laws limiting the number of massages a spa can ask employees to perform, those spas that overwork their therapists soon build a poor reputation in the industry.

Over an extended period of employment at a spa, therapists find a rhythm that both satisfies client demand and preserves their health. This rhythm is different for each therapist, with some choosing to perform only three or four services of any kind on a given day or 20 in a given week. Others can perform several more as long as the massage services are interspersed with other spa treatments. And there are a few—usually young—therapists capable of performing many massages a day for weeks on end.

For more information on staying healthy while working as a spa therapist, refer to the "Self-Care for the Spa Therapist" section in Chapter 3.

Timing of Spa Massage

Massage therapists sometimes find the strict time limitations imposed in the spa setting onerous. Constantly watching the clock, they feel, drains value from the massage, and the same massage given over and over again within a certain number of minutes becomes stale and rote. Therapists who work in spas need to overcome this challenge and find ways to make their work fresh within the confines of the spa's necessary structure. Meeting this challenge is the essence of giving a good spa massage.

Some therapists, wanting to give each client the best service possible, habitually overrun the allotted time for each treatment, running in a perpetual state of slight delay. This can undermine the smooth running of the entire spa, from reservations to the front desk to the locker room. And, of course, it is not fair to the next client who has arrived on time for her appointment. It is necessary to end the massage several minutes before the next treatment is scheduled to begin. Certain services such as body wraps and scrubs require more time to prepare than massage, and this needs to be taken into consideration.

If a client arrives late to an appointment, it is the therapist's responsibility to inform him that the treatment needs to end on time and will necessarily be curtailed. However, if the spa allows it and no appointment is scheduled afterward, the therapist may perform the full service. Even if both therapist and client have free time directly after the scheduled service, it is usually not a good idea to run over or intentionally give a longer treatment because clients given an extra-long massage or spa service may tell other clients and create jealousy.

Spas usually prescribe the length of each massage and spa service on the menu, and clients expect that this time will not include preparation and cleanup. Thus, an 80-minute massage is scheduled on the books in a 90-minute block, allowing for time before and after the actual hands-on treatment. The typical time frame for a full-body massage is 50 minutes at most spas, with an 80-minute extended option. It is rare for a spa to offer a 20- or 25-minute massage, unless it is localized and confined to one area, such as the neck and shoulders, or the feet.

Most spas have a cancellation policy in effect and will charge clients fully or partially for skipped services. In this case, the therapist may or may not be compensated, depending upon the compensation structure and internal policies of the spa. If the therapist is paid, it is his responsibility to find some productive work in the spa to fill the hour, such as stocking and tidying the treatment room, working on client notes, or cleaning.

Creating Timelessness

One of the biggest challenges when giving a spa massage is to create a sense of timelessness within the very strict time structure imposed in the spa setting. The three main ways to do this are to slow down, internalize your timing, and focus on the moment.

Slow Down: Paradoxically, when you slow down your movements during a massage and perform fewer maneuvers with greater concentration and focus, from the client's point of view, the massage actually seems longer and more luxurious. Rushing to get in all of the massage moves you know you are capable of actually makes the massage seem shorter. Choose three or four key techniques on each area, then focus on them in a slow, methodical manner and see what kind of results you achieve.

Internalize Your Timing: A spa massage should be a well-paced session that is soothing and relaxing but at the same time has specific therapeutic goals. To achieve this, spa therapists need to develop a heightened awareness of their own, as well as their clients', internal sense of rhythm. Instead of watching the clock constantly, feeling the deadline of the 50- or 80-minute time frame looming ever closer, it is possible to end the massage right on time yet rarely—if ever—glance at the clock. After performing hundreds of massages within the spa's tight time frame, your mind will become accustomed to the time needed for each area, and you will know spontaneously when to move on. Learn to trust this inner clock.

Focus on the Moment: Think about what you are doing, not what you are going to be doing next. Once your spa massage routine becomes second nature, it is easy to think in terms of the next step, instead of the step you are presently performing. Several times throughout the massage, remind yourself to focus on the tissues beneath your fingers, and let that guide you to a new next step, which may surprise you. When you surprise yourself, you are in tune with the client, and he will experience a longer-lasting, more thorough massage.

Transitions during Spa Massage

In the same way in which the moments of silence between musical notes help define the music, the movements between massage strokes, between segments, and between treatments are as important as the massage itself, especially when working within the limited parameters of a spa massage.

Between Strokes: Pay particular attention to and spend more time on maintaining physical contact with the client and developing a creative sequence during a spa massage. Focus on those movements that connect the separate strokes during a massage, making them flow and become part of a graceful whole rather than disjointed, which is especially important in the time-pressed environment of a spa (Figure 9–1).

Between Segments: By focusing on graceful transitions from one part of the body to the next, the therapist can avoid creating a hurried sensation

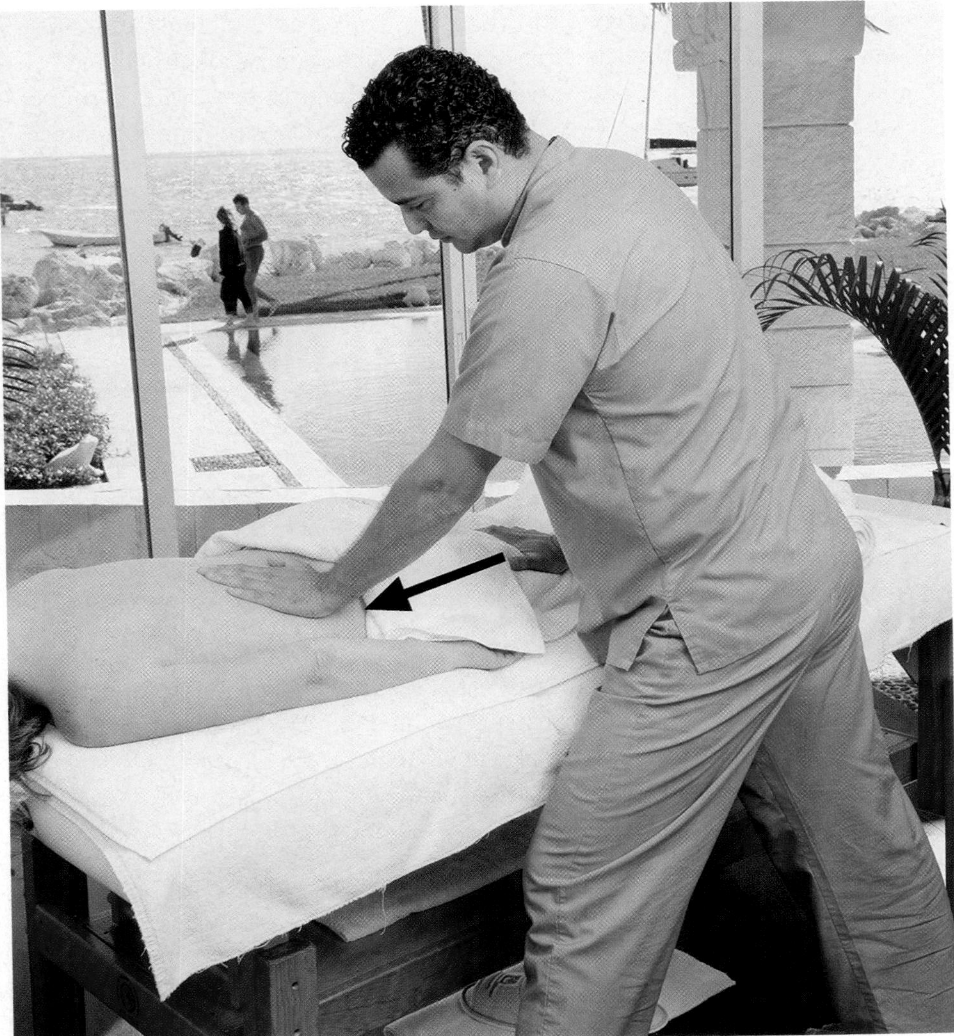

FIGURE 9–1 Slow, gradual transition strokes make spa massages flow more smoothly.

while covering the entire body in a shorter time. Make the first stroke and the last on each area especially relaxing. Even while adjusting the drapes, use slow, deliberate movements to augment the client's sense of ease and timelessness.

Between Treatments: Between treatments is the one time when it is better to speed up. Refresh yourself. Get the blood flowing. Move around. Rapidly clean the treatment room and set up for the next client so that you will not be rushing once it is time to start again.

Making a Spa Massage Unique

In the spa setting, it is important to remember that each client is unique, even though she may have the same expectations as many other clients and even though the setting, protocols, and routine are the same for each. All of your clients on a given day may be receiving the "same" massage, yet each treatment should be slightly different and geared to that client's needs. In order to achieve this, it is helpful to (1) target problem areas, (2) use the breath as a tool, and (3) use techniques to avoid burnout.

Target Problem Areas: A relaxing spa massage is made even better when the therapist applies targeted work to those areas holding tension. Using trigger point and other therapies, problem areas can be identified and techniques applied to relieve tension and holding patterns. These will be different for each client. After leaving the spa massage routine temporarily and focusing on such areas, move on seamlessly to the next step of the routine.

SPA ETIQUETTE

The Therapeutic Sound of Silence

To speak or not to speak during a massage? The answer to this question is often provided in spa rules and regulations. Some spas even go so far as to insist on complete silence during treatments. Some therapists believe this to be the best practice as well, and they routinely ask clients to remain silent during treatments. Regardless of what spa management insists or what other therapists do, you will have to make this decision for yourself when you are alone in the treatment room with a client.

The golden rule of silence for spa therapists is: Do not speak unless it is necessary. During a massage, only speak about the treatment itself, to give instructions, or to ask questions. If the client speaks to you first, it is appropriate to respond, but do not continue the conversation. It is also appropriate, if the client talks to the point of distraction, to suggest silence or steer the conversation in a therapeutic direction.

Insisting on complete silence can be as distracting as constant chatter. Make it a practice to guide clients back toward stillness without forcing the issue, and you will contribute to the wellness, stress-relief, and rejuvenation that they have come for in the first place. With no chatter in the treatment room, clients can then focus on soothing music or therapeutic sounds such as waterfalls, white noise, and wind chimes.

Use the Breath as a Tool: You can use the breath as a guide to tune into each client's unique tension-release patterns. Do not make your own breath too conspicuous, but rather just focus on the client's breath. Observe. Make subtle adjustments when you notice a change in rhythm or depth.

Use Techniques to Avoid Burnout: Make sure to take care of yourself physically and mentally so that you are fresh enough to offer each client a unique experience. This means receiving periodic bodywork, getting adequate rest, and limiting yourself to giving the number of treatments you can safely perform for your own particular age, body type, and situation. See the "Self-Care for the Spa Therapist" section in Chapter 3 for more information on this topic.

Preparation and Cleanup

The time periods immediately before and after a massage hold particular significance in the spa environment. Viewed from the perspectives of the client and the spa owners, a massage is actually more than just a massage. It is a coordinated experience meant to evoke certain sensations and results. In order to achieve this, spa therapists must be willing to work diligently at both preparing the treatment room for the massage and cleaning up afterward in anticipation of the next treatment. Experienced spa therapists engage in the following practices prior to and after massages in order to create the best overall experience: folding, tidying, stocking, mood setting, and centering.

Folding: A never-ending flow of towels and sheets streams into the massage room, and in order to preserve best appearances, these need to be folded correctly and kept in the proper area. Some spas determine exactly where these linens will be kept, while others leave it up to the therapists. In either case, a neat, organized appearance is important.

Tidying: Because the massage rooms in a spa are often communal property, used by more than one therapist, it is important to keep the rooms clean for fellow employees as well as clients. Make it a habit to perpetually be tidying, straightening, shining, wiping, aligning, and uncluttering all surfaces in the massage room.

Stocking: In addition to linens, all of the products used in the massage room need to be kept at optimal levels. Therapists need to use the time before their shift and between massages to make sure all products are available in the treatment room at all times. In addition, some spas have therapists check inventory in a central dispensary as part of their duties.

Mood Setting: Lighting, music, ambient sound, candles, water fountains, and other details that add to the massage experience can be modified by therapists during the shift. Maintaining the exact same environment for all clients is not always advisable, as weather, time of day, day of the week, and other factors come into play. Unless the spa has rules governing the preferred ambience in the room, it is advantageous for therapists to experiment, as long as they stay within the spa's guidelines.

Centering: Before shifts and during the day, it is helpful to refocus your intentions and center yourself in preparation for each new client. Because spa therapists see so many clients in a row, taking just a few moments for this centering can make a big difference in the quality of the massage and the client's overall experience.

Practicing Elements of Spa Massage

You have already learned massage in school, or you are in the process of doing so now. The purpose of this chapter is not to reeducate you in massage technique, but rather to augment your training with some skills that are specific to massage in the spa environment. You can determine which pieces of information are valuable to you and incorporate those into your own massage routine to make it particularly suitable for spa work. Typically, the 50-minute massage routine is the shortest time frame offered in spas, and therefore it is recommended that you incorporate the following suggestions into a 50-minute practice session. Focus on creating a sense of flow, even though you know you are on the clock. Try to avoid cookie-cutter performances while making this spa-styled massage both deeply therapeutic and relaxing. As an aide, Table 9–1 condenses key points about spa massage and lays out the details so you can keep them in mind while performing the treatments.

Product Use Problems

Did You Know?

As a therapist, you will soon become familiar with the costs of massage oils, lotions, pain relieving gels, and other products used on clients' skin. Although these products are not cheap, they are considered part of doing business, and most therapists do not mind paying premium prices for premium products, rather than buying bulk vegetable oil at the local food warehouse. However, in larger spas, where many therapists are giving multiple treatments every day, the cost of these products adds up very quickly. Spa managers have found that some therapists have the tendency to overuse these products, especially when they do not have to pay for them out of their own pockets. In order to counteract this overuse, spas have implemented a number of conservation measures, with the two main ones being rationing and self-supply.

Spas that ration product give their therapists only enough to complete each treatment, or one shift's worth of treatments. The product is portioned out in containers for this purpose. Some therapists react negatively to this restriction, but it has proven effective in controlling costs, especially in larger spas.

One way in which smaller spas choose to contain product cost is to require therapists to purchase their own product for use on clients. Thus, if therapists choose to use more than the recommended amount of product, it is at their own expense. The potential disadvantage of this practice is that therapists, when given the choice, prefer to use their own favorite products. If the spa forces them to purchase a certain product they do not like, at their own expense, it may create ill will.

The lesson here is simply to be extra-aware when working in a spa that the amount of product used is a real issue. Spa managers and owners are not trying to make therapists' lives harder. They are trying to maintain thriving businesses and thus continue to provide jobs for the therapists themselves.

TIMING	SPA MASSAGE ELEMENT	POINTS TO REMEMBER
Pre- and Post-Massage	Preparation and Cleanup	1. Folding 2. Tidying 3. Stocking 4. Mood setting 5. Centering
Intake and Greetings	Scope of Practice	1. Be sensitive to first-time massage recipients. 2. Do not offer guidance outside professional expertise. 3. Claim only direct benefits of massage.
	Greetings	1. Shake hands firmly. 2. Address clients by name. 3. Make contact. 4. Explain draping. 5. Dialogue about treatment.
	Intake Procedures	1. Follow spa guidelines while assuring client safety. 2. Chart and document treatments when appropriate. 3. Ask questions when no intake form is available.
During Massage	Creating Timelessness	1. Slow down. 2. Internalize timing. 3. Focus on the moment.
	Transitions	1. Between strokes 2. Between segments 3. Between massages
	Uniqueness	1. Target problem areas. 2. Use breath as a tool. 3. Use techniques to avoid burnout.

TABLE 9–1 Elements of a High Quality Spa Massage.

Massage Preparation

1. Neatly fold sheets, towels, and any other linens for storage in the treatment space.
2. Tidy the area in general, arranging all equipment neatly.
3. Assure that all necessary supplies and products are fully stocked.
4. Set appropriate mood with music levels, lighting, ambient noise, etc.
5. Center yourself and prepare to greet the client.

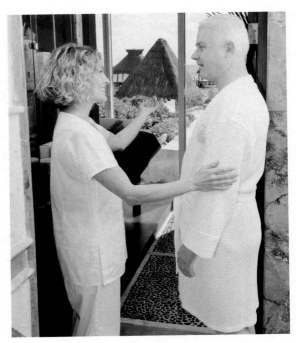

FIGURE 9–2 A therapist's touch can be reassuring even before the massage begins.

Intake and Greetings

1. Shake hands firmly, address the client by name, and lead her to the treatment room, making contact with a light touch on the shoulder or elbow (Figure 9–2).
2. Review intake form and dialogue about the treatment.
3. In the treatment room, explain draping procedures and protocol for undressing.
4. Leave room while the client undresses and lies on the table supine.

Massage Procedure

1. Wash and dry your hands.
2. Begin the massage. Follow the routine you have learned in massage school.
3. During each part of the massage, engage in the following techniques:
   a. Slow down.
   b. Do not look at the clock. Try to internalize the timing of the massage. Your ability to do this will improve with practice.
   c. Focus on what you are doing in the moment, rather than the next step called for in the massage routine.
   d. When moving from one massage stroke to the next and one body part to the next, create a bridge by slowing down and connecting the two areas, touching both at the same time for a moment if possible, and taking your time adjusting the draping.
   e. Stop routine maneuvers and target any tight muscles found for a full minute.
   f. Tune into the client's breath for subtle clues about how the massage is affecting her.
   g. During the massage, constantly remind yourself about proper body mechanics to avoid burnout; between massages, you can stretch, move, and rest.
   h. Especially take your time and slow down at the end of the massage, potentially spending a full minute in a gentle cradling position or light touch to finish.
4. Wash and dry your hands at the end of the massage.

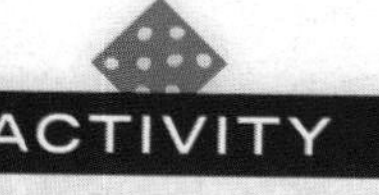

ACTIVITY

Practicing Elements of Spa Massage

Give and receive three massages in a row that are each precisely 50 minutes long, with no more than 10 minutes before each massage for preparation, cleaning, intake procedures, and greetings. Using techniques outlined above, strive to make the experience feel as leisurely and timeless as possible for the recipients. Also, when possible, recreate conditions found in a real spa: Walk clients from the greeting area to a separate treatment room, use intake forms, and set up the treatment room as it would be in a spa.

Massage Cleanup

1. After saying farewells to the client, speed up your movements as you get ready for the next client.
2. Practice your self-care techniques.
3. Then, coming full circle,
   a. Neatly fold sheets, towels, and any other linens for storage in the treatment space.
   b. Tidy the area in general, arranging all equipment neatly.
   c. Assure that all necessary supplies and products are fully stocked.
   d. Set appropriate mood with music levels, lighting, ambient noise, etc.
   e. Center yourself and prepare to greet the next client.

BASIC MASSAGE MODALITIES IN THE SPA SETTING

Although the majority of requests for massage therapy services in spas are for Swedish massage, many other types of massage are playing an increasingly important role on spa menus. Popular basic modalities include chair massage, couples massage, deep tissue massage, four-handed massage, pregnancy massage, reflexology, sports massage, and topical heating or cooling massage. Details about each can be found in Table 9–2 and in the following sections. Sometimes,

MASSAGE NAME	DESCRIPTION	HOW USED IN SPAS	BENEFITS FOR SPA CLIENTS	PROBLEMS WITH DELIVERY
Chair Massage	Massage administered while client is seated in a specially constructed supportive chair.	Chairs placed in public areas to attract clients in for full-body massage. Some spas, especially in busy areas such as airports, offer chair massage as a main service.	No need to get undressed. Quick turnaround time. No lubricant used in treatment.	At some spas, chair massage is not considered high-end enough, and is therefore not used.
Couples Massage	Massage given to two people, often husband and wife, simultaneously in the same room by two therapists.	Often promoted in spas billed as romantic that cater to honeymooners and other couples. Sometimes used by friends, mother/daughter, etc.	Offers clients a rare chance to experience and enjoy spa massage together.	Extra care with draping and modesty must be applied.
Deep Tissue Massage	Massage ranging from slightly firmer than Swedish all the way to deep structural integration.	Many spas list deep tissue as an alternative to Swedish, for those clients who like firmer pressure. Other spas, however, use the term in its more traditional therapeutic meaning, which is something more akin to Rolfing.	Deeply therapeutic. Addresses serious somatic issues. Can be rehabilitative, especially for long-term spa clients during a stay of 2 weeks or more.	Often just deep Swedish and not understood by clients. Spa clients are sometimes not ready for true deep tissue. Requires a specially qualified therapist. One session is not fully effective.
Four-Handed Massage	Two therapists work on one client at the same time, usually using Swedish techniques.	Offered as a premium service or in conjunction with an advanced modality or treatment package.	Extremely luxurious sensory experience. If the therapists are highly skilled, four-handed massage can be deeply therapeutic as well.	Needs to be well-choreographed to be good. Prohibitively expensive for many clients. Takes a high number of therapist-hours.

TABLE 9–2 Spa Massage Menu Descriptions. *(Continued)*

MASSAGE NAME	DESCRIPTION	HOW USED IN SPAS	BENEFITS FOR SPA CLIENTS	PROBLEMS WITH DELIVERY
Pregnancy Massage	Massage for pregnant women.	Sometimes part of a nurturing wellness program for mothers-to-be.	Soothes pregnant clients' tired legs and sore lower back muscles. Nurturing. Can complement overall wellness program for women at a time when they need to remain most healthy.	Bolstering can be an issue if the spa is not properly prepared. Some spas are reluctant to assume any responsibility and refuse to offer pregnancy massage. Therapists need to be highly trained.
Reflexology	Massage of the feet to stimulate reflexes that correspond to all areas of the body.	Offered as an *à la carte* service or in conjunction with many spa services, such as when a client is wrapped in a body wrap or is receiving a scalp treatment.	No need to undress. Can affect entire body. Can be administered in public areas such as waiting rooms.	Therapists sometimes use reflexology as a diagnostic tool, which is outside their scope of practice.
Sports Massage	Massage meant to aid in performance and recovery from sports-related discomfort or minor injury.	Offered as an advanced modality, often targeted toward men, sometimes in conjunction with particular sports popular at the spa such as golf or tennis.	Clients at destination spas and resort spas quite often engage in more exercise than they are used to, and sports massage helps them stay flexible, lessening soreness and muscle fatigue.	Techniques used in spas are sometimes not true sports massage but rather deep Swedish.
Topical Heating/ Cooling Massage	Application of topical cooling agents, such as those containing menthol and camphor.	Added at the end of massage sessions for additional pain relief or cooling. Often incorporated into other services such as sports massage and foot treatments. Sometimes used as stand-alone pain relief treatment for targeted areas.	To soothe local area and relieve minor pains.	Some clients may be overly sensitive to the products used and feel chilled or a burning sensation.

TABLE 9–2 Spa Massage Menu Descriptions.

clients do not actually know what kind of massage they want or need, and this is when something more than just fancy menu descriptions are called for. It is important for key members of the spa staff, including front desk personnel, receptionists, managers, fitness trainers, and nutritionists, to be familiar with these massage treatments in order to speak knowledgeably about them. It will be up to the spa staff to educate clients in as concise a way as possible. Note that only basic massage modalities are listed here. Many other specialized spa services, such as Ayurvedic treatments, for example, include massage as well. These and other bodywork styles found in spas, like craniosacral and shiatsu, are explained in Chapter 12, "Advanced Modalities."

Pregnancy Massage in the Spa

Whether to offer massage to pregnant clients has been a contentious issue in spas for many years. Spa owners and directors do not want to be liable in the event a pregnant client experiences problems or complications while at the spa or after visiting. This is unfortunate, because pregnant women can benefit greatly from massage throughout their entire pregnancies. The discomfort and pain they experience, especially in the neck, lower back, legs, and feet, can be greatly alleviated by skilled massage specifically targeted to these areas. In addition, mothers-to-be benefit from the nurturing touch offered by a therapist who has been trained in pregnancy massage techniques. Several teachers offer advanced courses and workshops in these techniques, notably Elaine Stillerman, creator of the MotherMassage system of massage.

In order for spas to safely offer massage to their pregnant clients, it is imperative that every therapist who works on these clients be trained and certified in pregnancy massage techniques. This can be accomplished at the spa itself with in-house training, or individually by therapists who seek training outside the spa. This training focuses on safety above all else. In particular, trained therapists learn how to properly bolster and support pregnant clients to avoid putting undue stress on muscles, joints, and blood vessels (Figures 9–3 and 9–4). They also learn about

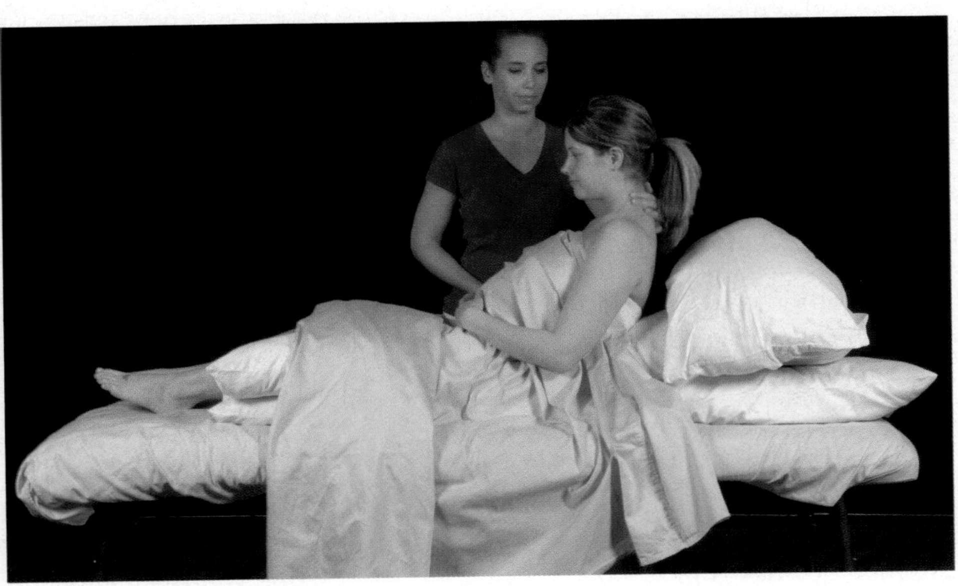

FIGURE 9–3 It is important to provide plenty of support and comfort for pregnant clients with bolsters, pillows and blankets.

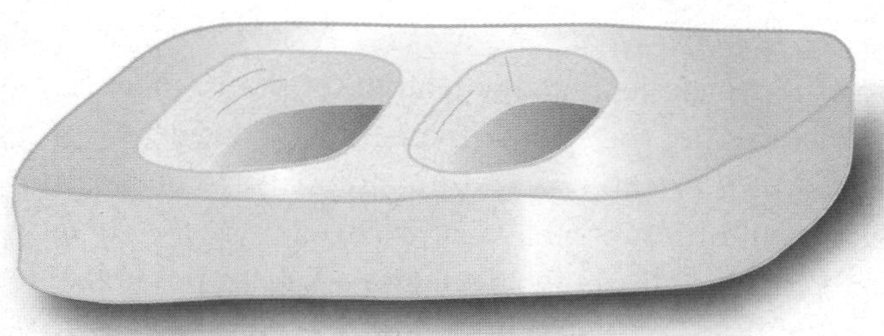

FIGURE 9–4 Specially constructed pillows can help support pregnant clients.

common contraindications for pregnancy, which areas and conditions to avoid altogether, and which areas and conditions warrant a lighter touch.

Some spas avoid massage for pregnant clients because of a prevailing myth that massage is contraindicated for all women in the first trimester. This is absolutely not the case. Massage is safe and supportive, as long as all proper precautions are observed, and all appropriately trained therapists are familiar with these precautions. In the later stages of pregnancy, it is recommended that women do not lie completely supine because this may put excess weight from the fetus onto the aorta and inferior vena cava, thus cutting off some circulation to the placenta. These clients need to be propped up at a 45- to 70-degree angle using pillows or assume a side-lying position to receive massage.

edema

swelling caused by excessive accumulation of fluid in tissue

pitting edema

edema in which pitting results in a depression in the edematous tissue that disappears only slowly

preeclampsia

a serious condition developing in late pregnancy that is characterized by a sudden rise in blood pressure, excessive weight gain, generalized edema, severe headache, and visual disturbances; may result in convulsions and possibly coma if untreated

zone therapy

a theory hypothesizing that the entire body can be divided into different zones and that stimulation to one part of a zone affects other parts of the zone as well; a key component in *reflexology*

Edema is a common problem during pregnancy, and **pitting edema** is a contraindication which should be referred to a physician. Normal swelling, though, especially in the lower limbs, reacts favorably to lymphatic drainage massage, a technique that is highly recommended throughout pregnancy and for several weeks postpartum. The pressure should be 10 to 30 grams, affecting the lymph vessels of the skin. Of course, it is important not to apply direct pressure in the abdominal area itself, but light effleurage and light petrissage here are soothing and beneficial. One contraindication that does warrant concern during pregnancy is **preeclampsia**. Though rare, this condition can lead to serious consequences and should be referred to a physician immediately.

Always remember to keep pregnant clients' comfort foremost in mind. Be ready to help clients onto and off the table, providing a stepping stool if necessary. Make sure that the client avoids "jack-knifing" off the table, and rather turns to her side and pushes herself up using her arms and abdominal muscles. Proper draping and a respect for modesty must be maintained, even though it may be challenging for the therapist. Some spas have treatment rooms that are some distance from the nearest restroom, and the extra pressure exerted against the bladder by the developing fetus can create a need for more frequent urination. Be sure to suggest a visit to the bathroom before beginning a massage, and keep robes and skid-proof slippers or socks handy for those mid-treatment bathroom visits. During the massage, ask often about comfort, temperature, and pressure. Some pregnant women find it uncomfortable to remain lying down for more than 45 minutes. A change of position may be enough to remedy the situation.

Spa Reflexology

Reflexology is a type of massage that typically concentrates on the feet. It is meant to stimulate reflexes that correspond to all areas of the body. The application of reflexology is based on a theory, called **zone therapy**, and a full

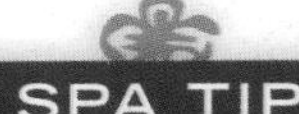

SPA TIP

Foot Massage for Pregnant Spa Clients

Many spas are enlightened enough to offer much-needed massage for mothers-to-be, but they still do not allow therapists to touch the feet of pregnant clients at all. This stems from the belief that stimulating certain reflexology and acupuncture points on the feet, specifically those points on the ankles corresponding to the uterus and ovaries, might precipitate a premature delivery or some other complication. While scientific data on the likelihood of this actually occurring is unavailable, it is still wise to avoid deep, protracted pressure on these areas. It is a shame and completely unnecessary to avoid massage to the feet entirely, however, because this is a part of the body that most definitely needs massage. The bottom line: Foot massage for pregnant spa clients is safe and greatly appreciated, as long as appropriate care is taken to avoid pressure on the specific areas illustrated in Figure 9–5 and the massage encourages lymphatic drainage with light pressure.

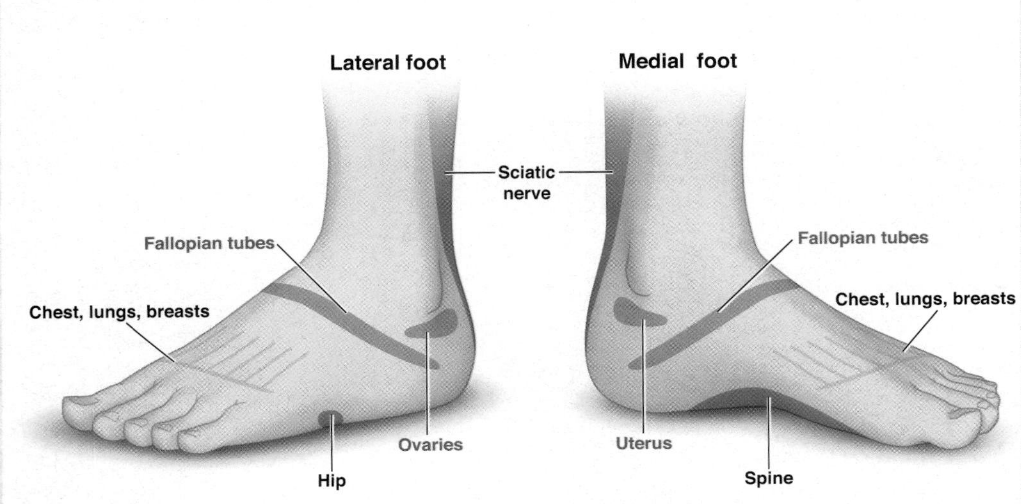

FIGURE 9–5 Avoid the uterus, ovary and fallopian tube reflex points on pregnant clients.

scientific explanation of the mechanisms behind its effectiveness has never been offered. However, it has been proven effective time and time again in treating a wide range of conditions. Ancient Egyptians used some form of reflexology, as can be seen in their artwork. Modern applications of the technique are based on the work of Dr. William H. Fitzgerald, who first introduced the concept of zone therapy to the American medical profession in the early 1900s. According to the theory outlined in zone therapy, the entire body can be divided into various zones. Anything that affects the body in one area also affects other parts of the body within the same zone. By applying pressure to an area in a distant part of a zone, such as the feet, relief can be brought to a distant part of the body that lies within the same zone.

Reflexology is sometimes administered in spas as a stand-alone therapy, in 30- or 45-minute sessions. Often, though, this modality is incorporated into other spa services as a value-added benefit, at times for an additional fee and at times incorporated into the price of the service. Most spa goers are familiar with reflexology and feel comfortable requesting it. However, some clients have come to regard the technique primarily as a diagnostic tool, which can be dangerous. For instance, a client who experiences soreness in a particular area on the foot

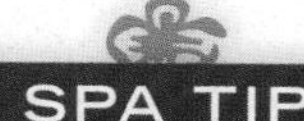

SPA TIP

When applying spa reflexology, keep the following points in mind:

- Use either a steady "walking" movement or a smooth gliding movement of the thumbs over the area indicated. The classic reflexology movement, thumb walking, uses forward motion and downward pressure into the foot as the knuckle is bent and straightened continuously in an "inchworm" movement (Figure 9–6).
- Do not press hard enough to cause any pain, but do press hard enough so that the client experiences the pressure. Reflexology is not a light, feathery maneuver.
- Keep hands relatively oil-free in order to provide the friction needed in reflexology. One or two drops of essential oil can work, while some therapists avoid lubricants altogether and instead use a teaspoon of cornstarch as a medium.
- Do not use massage tools, pencil erasers, or other objects to stimulate the reflexology points, as they may cause damage.
- Unlike a full reflexology routine, which treats one foot first and then the next, both feet are treated simultaneously in spa reflexology. Alternate between feet, or work on both feet simultaneously, then continue onto the next step.

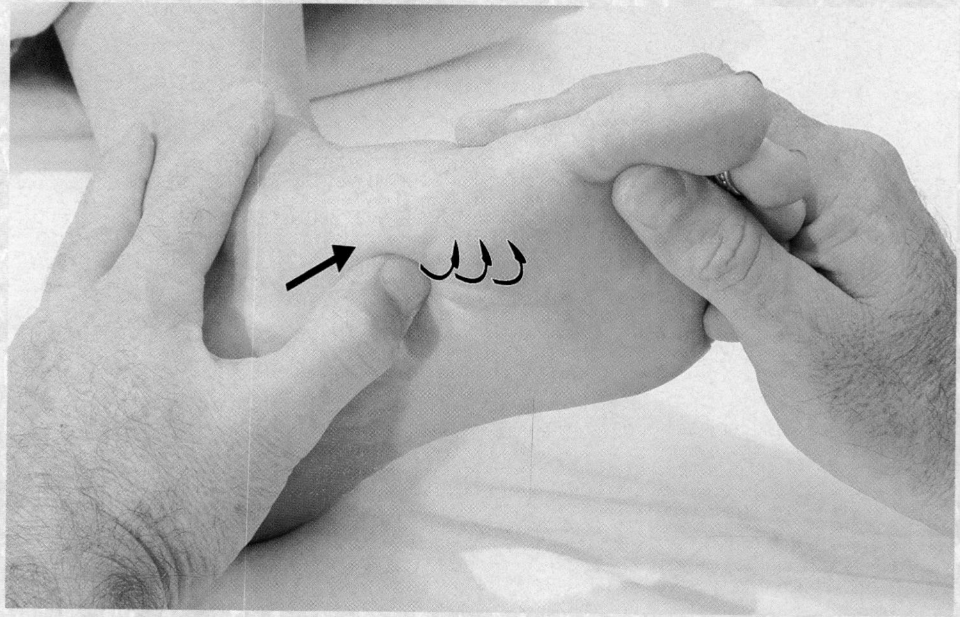

FIGURE 9–6 Thumb walking is a classic reflexology movement.

may be told that she must have a problem with a corresponding area on her body according to the zone map of the feet. You as a spa therapist need to be aware of this. It is not within your scope of practice to diagnose conditions or prescribe medical treatment.

The main benefits of reflexology as it is applied in the spa setting include:

- Clients can receive the treatment while still dressed, in a waiting room or other public area, thus freeing up valuable treatment room space.
- The technique is targeted to just one easily accessible area, but addresses the entire body.
- Reflexology can be performed while the client is wrapped during spa services.

Some spas feature a few highly trained, certified practitioners who perform reflexology treatments exclusively. However, with the growing popularity of this modality, an increasing number of spas have developed a pool of therapists trained in basic spa reflexology, which is a simplified, shortened version of the full technique. While a full reflexology session lasts on average 45 minutes, spa reflexology can be completed in 10 minutes. In spa reflexology, maneuvers meant to affect reflex points on the feet are condensed so that several points are stimulated at once. Also, both feet are treated at the same time, rather than consecutively. The following is a simple spa reflexology routine that can be performed by any licensed massage therapist, as long as no diagnostic claims are made for the technique. It can be learned in minutes. A significantly higher amount of training is required to become a professional reflexologist.

TREATMENT: SPA REFLEXOLOGY	
Wet Room/Dry Room	dry room
Table Setup	flat or tilted table with raised head or chair with foot support
Treatment Duration	10 minutes
Needed Supplies	hot towel or sanitary wipe to clean feet, cornstarch
Contraindications	broken skin, infected sores, lesions, pregnancy
Draping	Clients can remain clothed. No need for draping. Often, they are wrapped in spa products and blankets during spa reflexology.
Treatment Order	usually given during another spa service
Safety, Sanitation Issues, & Clean-Up	Make sure feet are clean prior to reflexology. Make sure feet are dry after service to avoid slips and falls.
Body Mechanics & Self-Care	Therapist is often seated or kneeling for this service. Take care to avoid stooping over while working on feet. Adjust seat to proper height.
Product Cost	none
Treatment Price	usually free, added into the price of spa service
Physiological Effects	According to the theory of zone therapy, points stimulated on the foot will have therapeutic effects on other areas of the body in corresponding zones.

Spa Reflexology Preparation

1. If the client has not come from the shower, cleanse the client's feet with hot towels or sanitary wipes.
2. Optionally, have cornstarch or foot powder available for use on feet. This is not necessary, and most therapists apply reflexology with clean, dry hands or small amounts of residual products from the spa treatment they are performing at the moment, such as essential oil.
3. Have the client recline on a chair or massage table. They can be dressed or draped for warmth if necessary. Often, clients will be wrapped as part of a spa treatment during the reflexology application.

Spa Reflexology Procedure

1. Start by applying light pressure over both feet and squeeze gently to familiarize the client with your touch.
2. Slide your thumb and index finger up from the base of each toe to the tip, holding the tip in traction for a moment before moving to the next (Figure 9–7). Corresponds to: sinus and head reflexes.

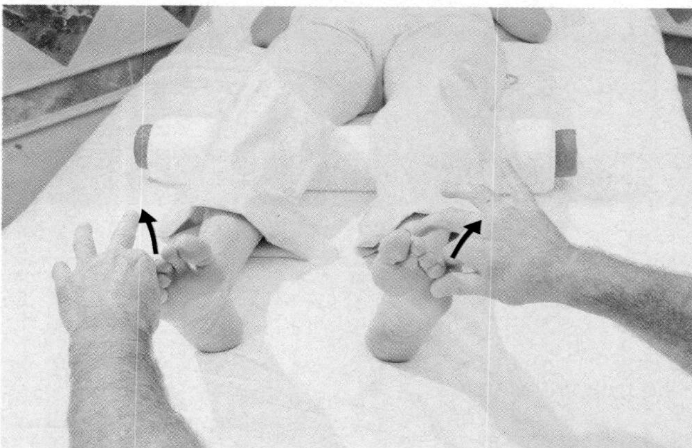

FIGURE 9–7

3. With the fingers of one hand grasping the toes, use the knuckles of the other hand to stroke briskly back and forth across the tops of the toes (Figure 9–8). Corresponds to: sinus and head reflexes.

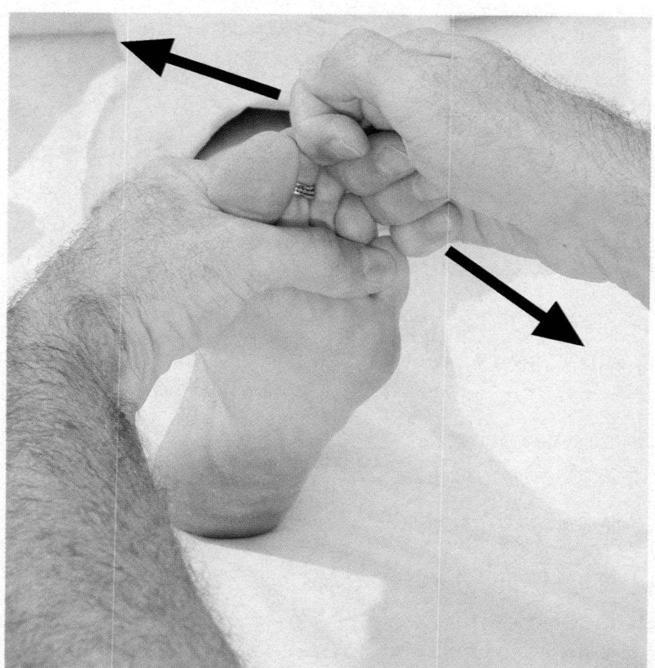

FIGURE 9–8

4. Stretching the toes back toward client's head, place your knuckles in between the toes at the base and rock your hand from side to side (Figure 9–9). Corresponds to: eye and ear reflexes.

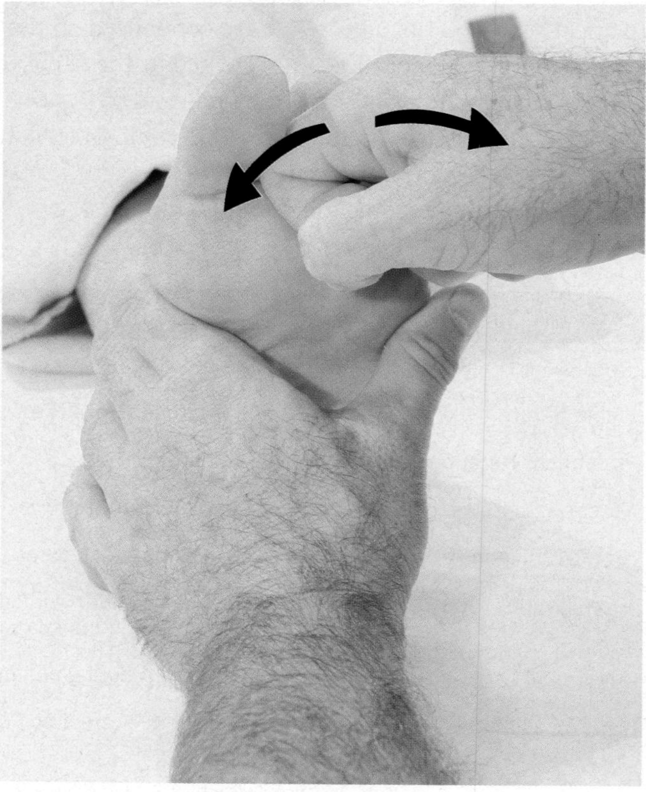

FIGURE 9–9

5. With your index finger on top of the foot and thumb beneath, push between the metatarsal bones and hold the pressure while twisting the foot medially and laterally (Figure 9–10). Corresponds to: lung and chest reflexes.

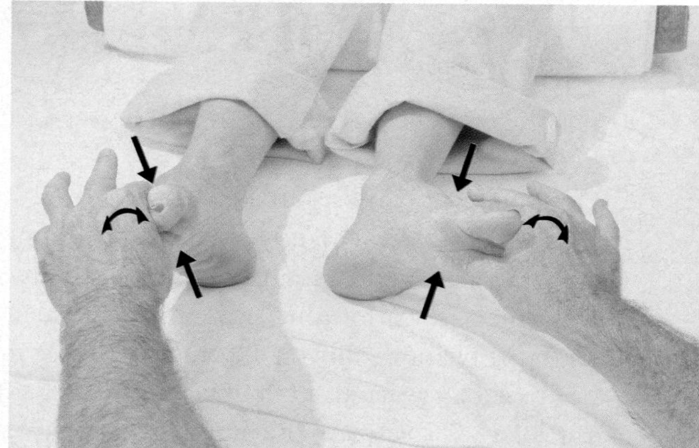

FIGURE 9–10

6. With both thumbs in the center of the foot, spread them out toward the borders of the foot, making a windshield wiper movement (Figure 9–11). Corresponds to: internal organ reflexes.

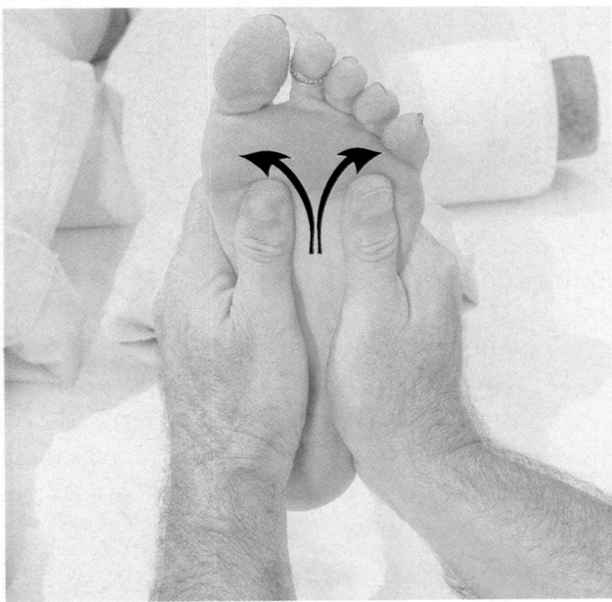

FIGURE 9–11

7. Starting at the lateral border of the right heel, make thumb-walking motions up the outside of the heel and across the foot at the lateral protrusion of the cuboid bone. Continue across the same line onto the left foot and go down the lateral border of the heel, finishing off toward the center of the foot (Figure 9–12). Corresponds to: large intestine reflex.

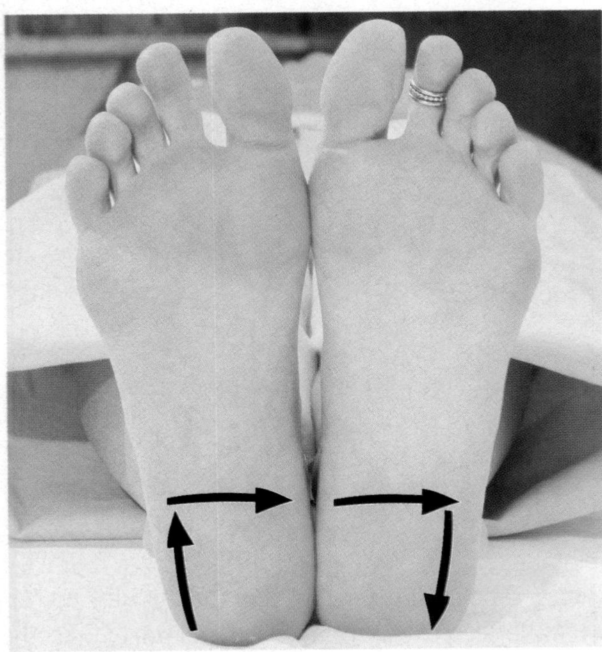

FIGURE 9–12

8. Use the knuckles of your index and middle fingers to squeeze the bottoms of the heels and twist in both directions (Figure 9–13). Corresponds to: small intestine reflex.

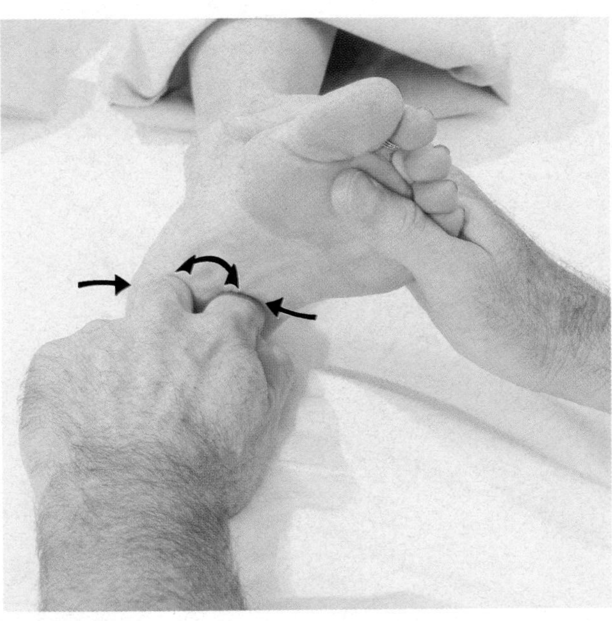

FIGURE 9–13

9. Make a sawing motion with the edge of both hands back and forth over the arch of the foot (Figure 9–14). Corresponds to: spine reflex.

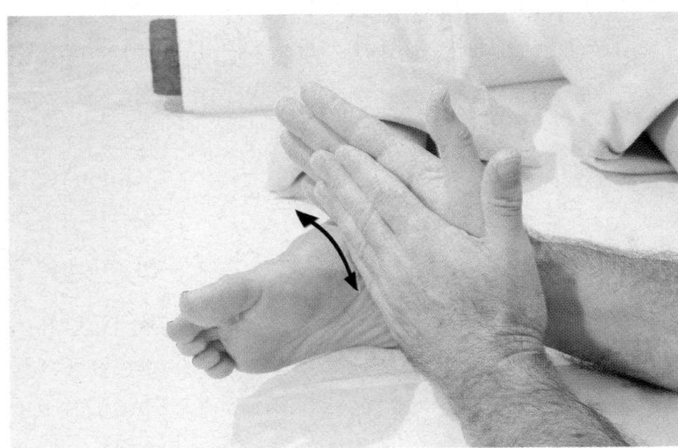

FIGURE 9–14

10. Cupping the medial and lateral malleolus bones in each palm, jiggle both borders of the foot at the upper ridge of the heel, releasing

lower back and hip areas (Figure 9–15). Corresponds to: hip and lower back reflexes.

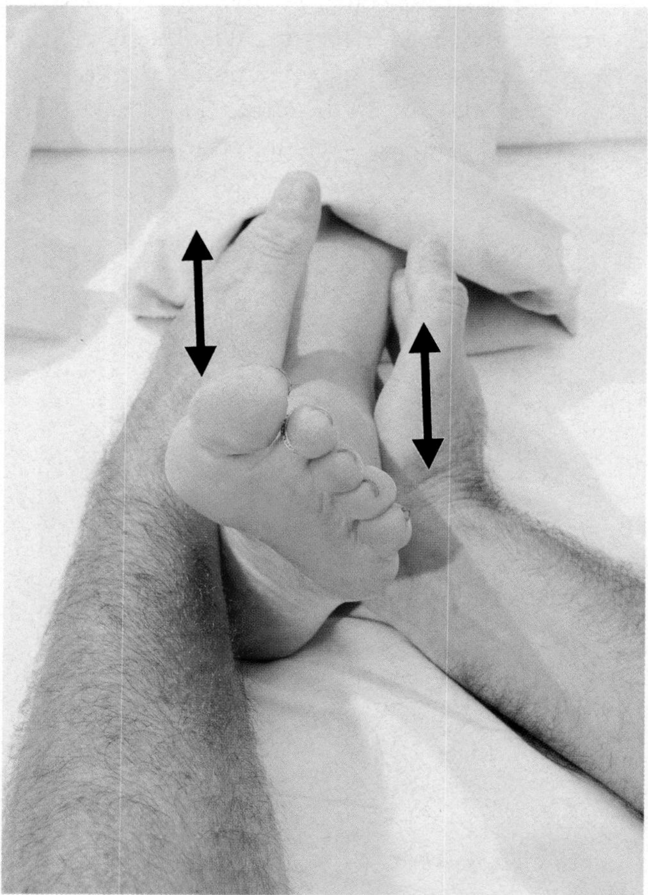

FIGURE 9–15

11. Stroke up the front of the foot and up the back of the ankle, moving toward the heart, then rotate and stretch the ankle, helping to circulate lymph fluid through the leg (Figure 9–16). Corresponds to: lymph reflexes.

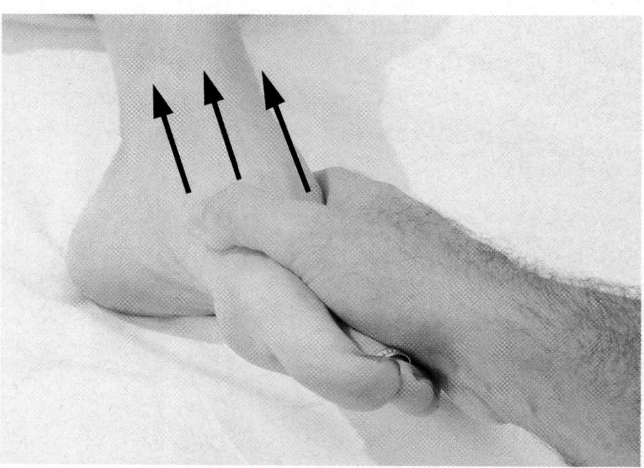

FIGURE 9–16

12. Slide your thumbs down the arch of the foot from the kidney point to the bladder point near the heel (Figure 9–17). Corresponds to: kidney and bladder reflexes. Encourage the client to drink plenty of water after treatment.

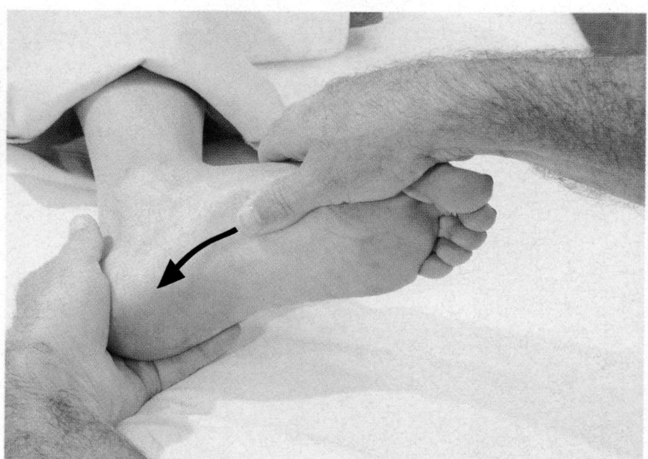

FIGURE 9–17

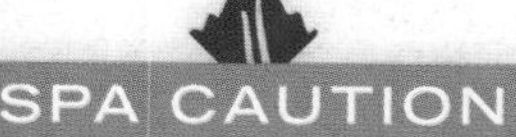

SPA CAUTION

Never use reflexology to attempt to diagnose a disease or a problem. If an area of the foot is particularly sore, it is appropriate to tell the client which part of the body this area corresponds to. Do not, however, suggest that soreness in the area means a medical condition is necessarily present.

Spa Reflexology Cleanup

1. Pat the client's feet dry with a hand towel to make sure they are dry before she stands up.
2. Launder the towels and any draping, if used.

Deep Tissue Massage

Deep tissue is an item often listed on spa massage menus, but there is little consensus among spa patrons as to what they can expect from such a treatment once they sign up for it. Therefore, it is important to educate clients about this modality. The true definition of deep tissue massage refers to techniques that affect the deeper tissue structures of the muscles and especially the fascia. In a deep tissue treatment, the fascia connecting muscles and organs is affected, sometimes resulting in a rearrangement of fascial layers and holding patterns in these tissues. The techniques can be so deep that they foster psychological as well as physiological releases in clients. One popular example of a deep tissue massage technique is Rolfing.

Obviously, most clients do not visit a spa in order to receive Rolfing sessions. Even though deep tissue massage is listed on the menu, some spa clients who sign up for it may not be fully aware of what the term implies and are actually looking for a slightly less superficial Swedish massage. Perhaps they have received an extremely light Swedish massage at another spa and are just seeking a level of pressure that you, as an experienced recipient of massage, would consider quite moderate. You will be able to tell by clients' body language in the first few seconds if they are actually prepared to receive a true deep tissue treatment. Any flinching, tightening or withdrawing is a sign to lessen pressure, even if the client claims the pressure is okay. In general, it is a good idea not to press too deeply into the soft tissues when first beginning a spa massage, even if the client has requested a deep tissue massage.

When you work at a spa, you will need to know the precise definition that the spa attaches to the term "deep tissue" and the policies guiding you during its application. If you one day run your own spa, you will be responsible for defining what "deep tissue" means for your therapists and clients. Does the term refer to a deep Swedish massage, a vigorous sports-style massage, or true deep tissue bodywork that affects the fascia on profound levels? All of these alternatives are represented on the menus of reputable spas, which adds to clients' confusion. It is up to each individual spa to clarify this issue for its therapists and clients.

Sports Massage

Sports massage can be defined as the application of massage techniques, hydrotherapy, range of motion evaluation, flexibility protocols, and strength training principles on people engaged in sports and physical activities in order to achieve a specific therapeutic goal. It is uncommon for spas to offer a full sports massage program that includes all of these elements over a period of time. More typically, spas include a single sports massage item on the menu that incorporates massage, stretching, and perhaps strengthening principles designed to benefit clients engaging in an increased level of physical activity. Sports massage is most often found at resort and destination spas where a heightened level of physical activity is common. Some spas offer massage targeted toward those conditions and muscle groups affected by specific activities engaged in at the resort. For instance, sports massage for golfers and sports massage for tennis players are two common modalities on the menus at spas that offer clients the use of golf and tennis facilities. In addition, spas offer sports massage to support the fitness programs of clients who begin or augment weightlifting or cardiovascular exercise programs.

Confusion is caused at times when spas make no clear distinction between sports massage and deep tissue massage. Sports massage includes vigorous movements such as compression, direct pressure, and cross-fiber friction, but these techniques are not specifically intended to affect the fascia, as in deep tissue massage. Sports massage mainly treats the muscles involved with specific physical activities. Further, sports massage is categorized by intent and timing, and is broken down into several subtypes, including:

- *Pre-Event*: at an event site just before competing
  - assists warm-up
  - increases circulation
  - maintains flexibility
  - enhances athletic performance
- *Intra-Competition*: at an event site between competing
  - assists warm-up
  - increases circulation
  - maintains flexibility
  - enhances athletic performance
- *Post-Event*:at an event site after competing
  - relieves cramping
  - reduces soreness
  - enhances venous return
  - promotes lymphatic drainage
- *Recovery*: post-competition/not at event site (up to three days later)
  - reduces soreness
  - enhances venous return
  - promotes lymphatic drainage
  - reestablishes balance
- *Maintenance*: during light training or in off season
  - addresses chronic injuries
  - relieves stress patterns
  - increases flexibility
  - increases strength
- *Injury Maintenance*: any time after an injury has occurred
  - eliminates spasm
  - promotes proper scar formation
  - restores flexibility
  - rebuilds strength

The outcome-specific sports massage administered in all of these circumstances can vary widely regarding pressure, tempo, and maneuvers. It is difficult to recreate the full palette of sports massage possibilities in one hour of treatment in a spa. However, spa therapists who have been trained in sports massage techniques can work individually with each spa client to provide the most appropriate type of therapy for the circumstances.

Couples Massage

Many higher end spas reserve one or more rooms for couples massage, which entails placing two massage tables near each other and performing massage simultaneously on two people (Figure 9–18). The two clients do not necessarily

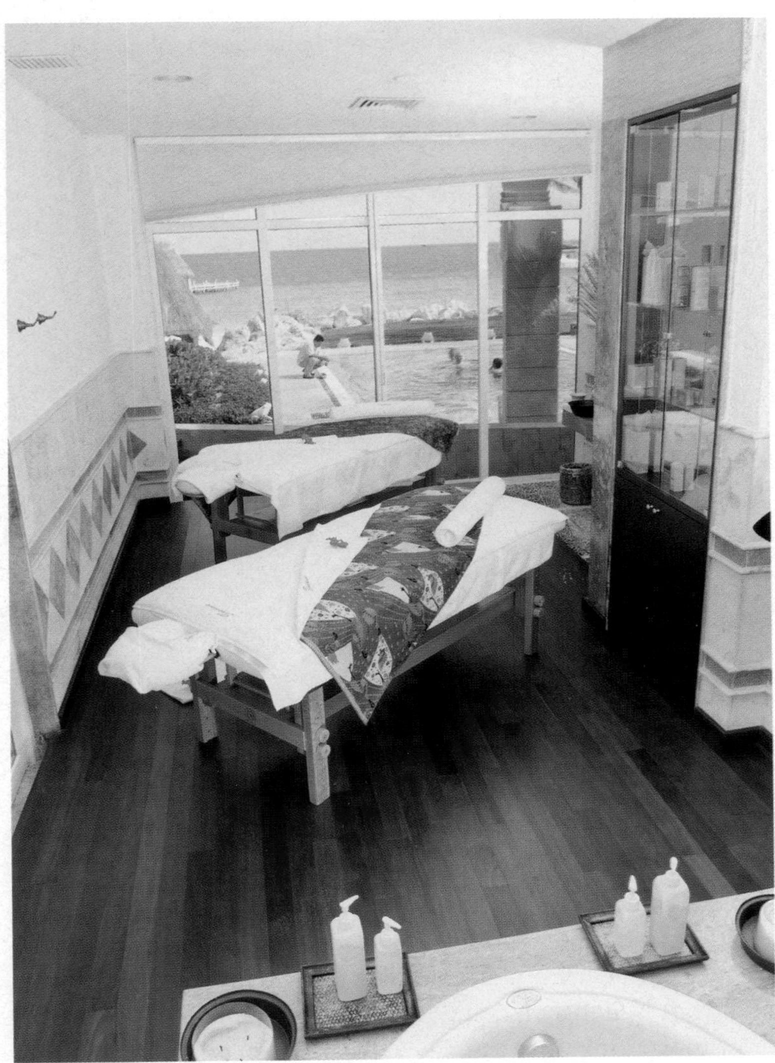

FIGURE 9–18 Couple's massage is a big part of many high end spas.

have to be a couple, but that is usually how this higher-end, expensive service is marketed. Other combinations of potential clients include mother–daughter and girlfriend–girlfriend for bridal parties and similar events.

Spas in popular destinations for couples such as Napa Valley and the Caribbean are most likely to install a couples massage room. Other spas, in less romantic locales, follow suit hoping to attract this niche clientele. According to industry experts, though, these rooms are only used 7 percent of the time on average. The other 93 percent of the time, they represent a wasted investment. Wise spa owners and developers have begun creating multipurpose couples' rooms with a moveable wall or partition that can divide the room into two separate single massage areas.

Some spa therapists work on couples in a choreographed manner, with the massage moves devised in advance. Others work independently from each other but usually try to at least start and finish the session at the same time. Spas that offer this service will often feature it in their brochures and on their Web sites because it is appealing and is one of the more expensive items on the menu. Therapists are paid their normal rate and sometimes more for performing this service.

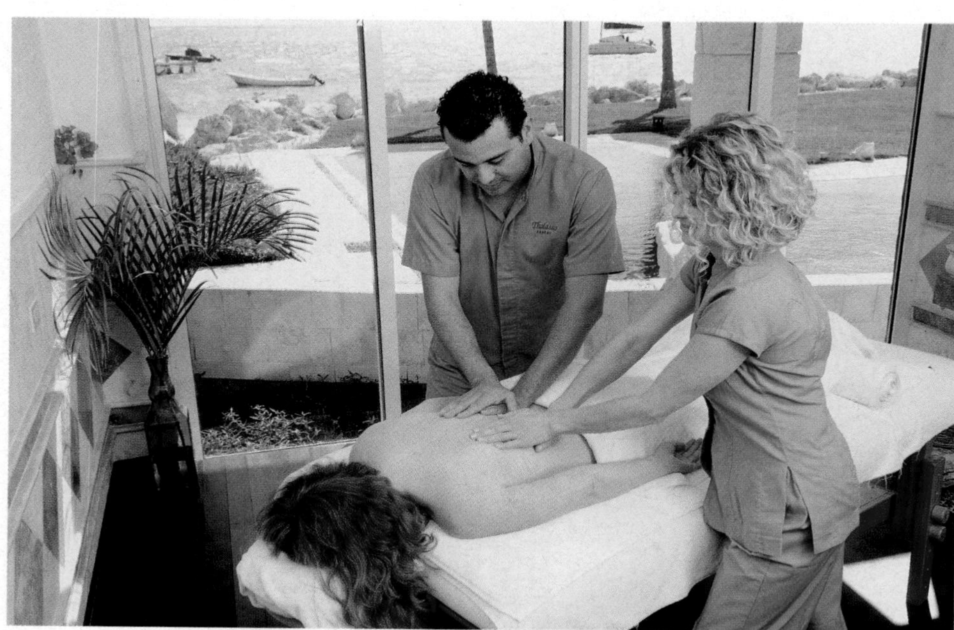

FIGURE 9–19 Four-handed massage is a luxury at high-end spas.

SPA ETIQUETTE

Draping can be more of an issue when there are two therapists' eyes watching from different angles in the room. At the very least, getting on the table, draping, and turning clients over must be planned and choreographed in advance on the part of both therapists in order to avoid any embarrassment.

Four-Handed Massage

Some spas offer a four-handed massage, which involves two therapists working on one client for the entire session (Figure 9–19). This is often billed as the ultimate luxury, and it can indeed feel indulgent to have two therapists working over you at the same time. On the other hand, if it is not performed skillfully, the experience can be uncomfortable. The two therapists have to have a good rapport and work well together, and they need to map out the main steps of the session prior to working on a paying client, including draping, moving the client, changing positions themselves, applying lubricant, and adjusting tempo and pressure. Some spas make this treatment even more luxurious with the addition of a four-handed exfoliation service prior to the massage. Specialized therapies such as Ayurveda and Balinese massage feature four-handed treatments as part of their tradition. See Chapter 12 for more details.

ACTIVITY

Choreograph a Four-Handed Massage

Choreograph your own four-handed massage routine with a classmate. Starting from the basic concepts you have learned in this section, design a complete 50-minute four-handed massage that you would be proud to offer in a luxurious spa. Each stroke does not need to be thought out beforehand, but the massage should be broken down into steps that can be followed by another pair of therapists. Write a one-page instruction sheet outlining these steps, along with special products or supplies needed, such as oils or exfoliating tools. Remember to include a description of how draping will be handled during the massage.

Chair Massage

Chair massage is an important adjunct modality in many spas, primarily for its marketing value. It can be used to promote massage in other parts of the spa outside traditional treatment areas, such as the exercise facilities, reception area, or hair salon. When clients see massage being given in these areas, it reminds them to sign up for treatments. It can also be effectively used outside the spa to promote the business at events for the general public such as health fairs, farmer's markets, supermarkets, community events, and other occasions. While all spas can benefit from the promotional aspects of chair massage, certain spas specialize in the modality and feature it as one of their main services. Most typically, smaller day spas and salon spas will offer the service for clients who do not wish to undress or only have a short period of time available to receive a service. Some spas offer manicures to clients seated in massage chairs, incorporating massage into the service. Some spas located in airports and other highly travelled locations feature chair massage for its ease of application.

The areas most often treated in chair massage include the head, neck, shoulders, and, of course, the back. These are the sites most often complained about by spa clients, and in this sense, chair massage can target the majority of specific complaints quite effectively. Even at times when people are wearing heavier clothing, therapists can use massage tools such as the Magic Massager™ massage cloth to rub over clothes and create a sensation of working directly on the skin with a lubricant (Figure 9–20).

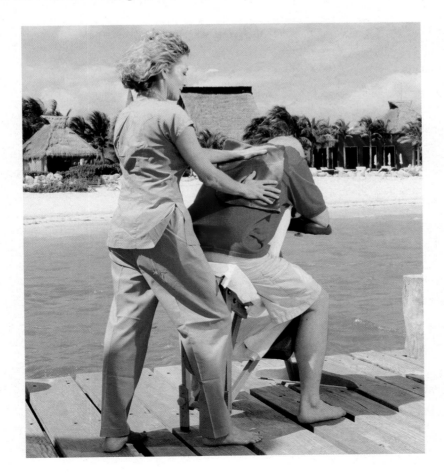

FIGURE 9–20 The Magic Massager™ makes chair massage easier to apply.

analgesic
a substance that relieves pain

compression
a rhythmic straight-in-and-out pumping movement on muscle, intended to spread muscle fiber

paraspinal
adjacent to the spinal column

effleurage
the application of gliding strokes that follow the contour of the body

Topical Cooling/Warming Massage Treatments

Many spas have begun offering topical cooling and heating treatments on their menus. The treatments include the application of a gel, oil, or cream that contains ingredients such as menthol, camphor, and ilex, among others. Certain essential oils such as peppermint can have profound effects also and should be used with caution. You will learn more about essential oils in Chapter 11. The primary purpose of these treatments is **analgesic** as they offer pain relief to clients.

The Back Refresher treatment described here is designed to relieve tension, stress, and discomfort in the muscles of the back. It is on the treatment menu at several top spas and uses two popular therapeutic products. Prossage™ Heat is an area-specific warming ointment that enhances the blood flow and oxygenation in tight and stressed soft tissue. Biofreeze® is a pain-relieving gel that is applied to localized areas of tenderness and pain at the end of this treatment to leave the back refreshed with a cooling effect that also helps reduce pain and inflammation. This treatment is designed for individuals who request a deeper massage to the back muscles and is recommended for those who suffer from chronic pain.

TREATMENT: PROSSAGE™ HEAT/BIOFREEZE® BACK REFRESHER	
Wet Room/Dry Room	dry room
Table Setup	Drape two sheets, one on top of the other, folding top sheet partway down with a diagonal fold.
Treatment Duration	30 minutes
Needed Supplies	massage table, bolster, massage oil, Biofreeze, Prossage Heat, 2 hand towels
Contraindications	sunburn, skin rashes or conditions, open sores, fractures to the spine, fever or infections, pregnancy
Draping	Client is draped with top sheet. Have several hand towels available if needed for additional draping.
Treatment Order	This treatment is scheduled after other treatments and can even be added onto the end of a full-body massage.
Safety, Sanitation Issues, & Clean-Up	Therapists must take care when handling the heating and cooling products so as not to get them in clients' eyes or their own. Also avoid mucous tissues, nasal passages, etc., as the products may be irritating. Thoroughly wash hands afterward.
Body Mechanics & Self-Care	The same body mechanics apply as for massage therapy.
Product Cost	less than $1
Treatment Price	Normal markup is a 10 to 20% premium over a regular massage service of the same duration. Some spas include the cost of the product in the treatment price and give the client a container to take home with them.
Physiological Effects	stress relief, reduction of muscle spasms, reduction of discomfort and pain, increased circulation, improved range of motion, overall invigoration
Pregnancy Issues (information provided by Elaine Stillerman, LMT, author and developer of MotherMassage)	Prossage Heat and Biofreeze Back Refresher are contraindicated during pregnancy. This treatment can be modified during postpartum recovery: avoid entirely while client's bleeding continues; once the discharge stops, avoid use on the legs for the first three months after childbirth.

Prossage™ Heat/Biofreeze® Back Refresher Preparation

1. Prepare the massage table. If the room is cool, a table warmer is helpful because clients can become chilled when cooling products are applied.
2. Moisten and heat two hand towels. Keep them warm in an insulated container.
3. Have all products near the massage table on an easily accessible surface.
4. After greeting the client, ask about sensitivities to analgesic products and explain the sequence of the treatment and benefits to be derived.

spinous process

bony protuberance directed backward and downward from the junction of the laminae, where muscles and ligaments attach

Prossage™ Heat/Biofreeze® Back Refresher Procedure

1. Position the client prone on the massage table using a face cradle, and place bolsters for comfort.
2. Apply a warm towel to the back and use **compression** on top of it to cover the entire back. Remove the towel.
3. Place 6 to 8 drops of Prossage Heat in the palm of your hand. Rub palms together briskly to activate ingredients.
4. Apply effleurage strokes to warm the tissue of the back.
5. Standing at the head of the table, apply hands to upper traps of both shoulders, anchoring the tissue with pressure, and glide hands down the **paraspinal** muscles to the sacrum (Figure 9–21). Repeat three times.
6. Use the knuckles and backs of the fingers in deep gliding movements down the paraspinal muscles from the upper traps to the sacrum (Figure 9–22). Repeat three times.

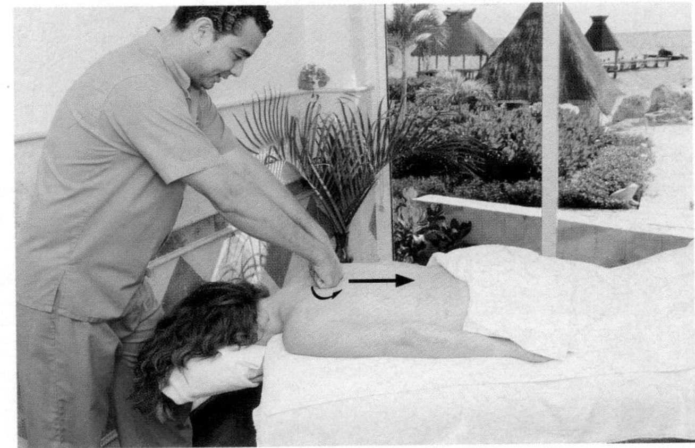

FIGURE 9–22

7. Apply **effleurage** down the paraspinal muscles and out the iliac crest and repeat three times.
8. Using the fleshy part of your elbows with the forearm positioned vertically, start by pressuring the traps in on top of the shoulders (Figure 9–23). Then, lifting the traps and pushing them down over the back, turn your forearm horizontal after passing the scapula and continue down the back to the iliac crest (Figure 9–24). Repeat three times. Use caution and stay off the **spinous process** while using your elbow.

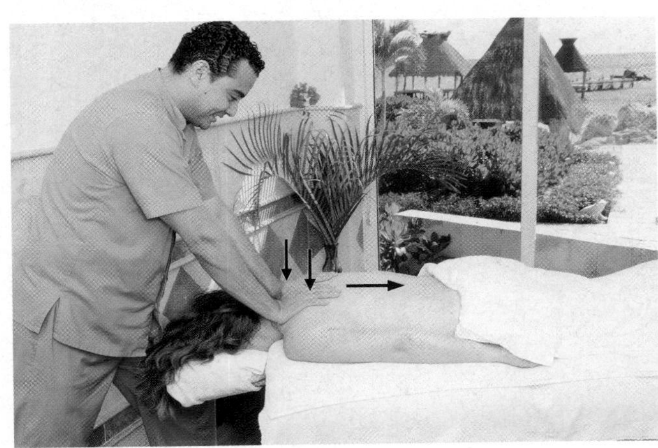

FIGURE 9–21

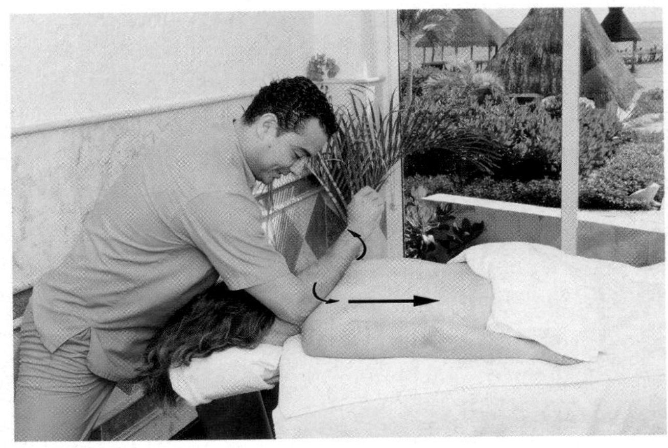

FIGURE 9–23

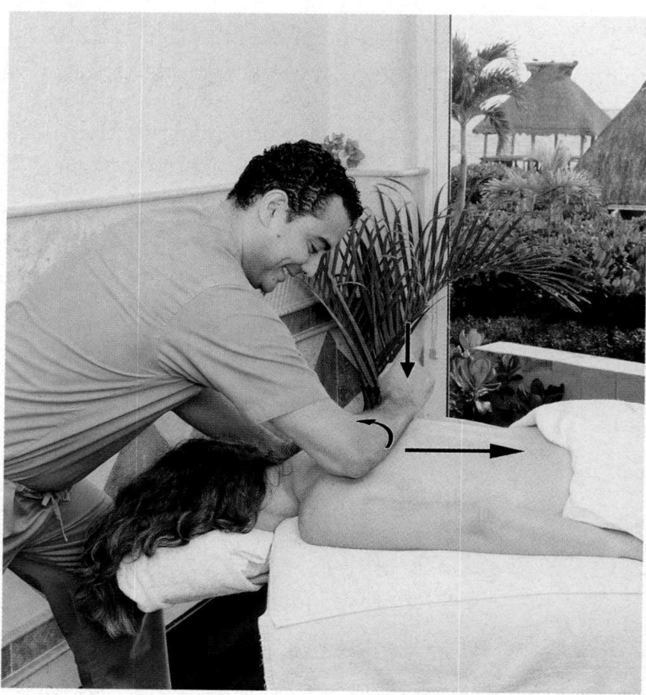

FIGURE 9–24

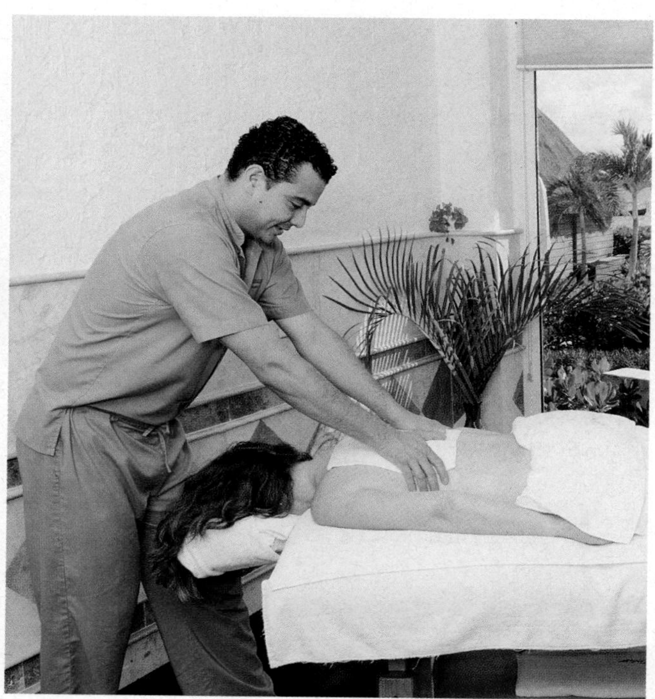

FIGURE 9–25

9. Starting at the shoulders, perform skin rolling on both sides of the spine to sacrum. Then skin roll down one side of the spine at a time to the sacrum.
10. Apply **direct pressure** for 8 to 12 seconds with the thumbs on either side of the spine, starting at the sacrum and moving up a few inches at a time to the shoulders. Repeat three times.
11. With both hands, apply **petrissage** to neck and shoulders.
12. Apply circular **friction** with both thumbs, starting at the **mastoid process** and working toward the midline of the head. Repeat three times.
13. Apply direct pressure for 8 to 12 seconds along the paraspinal muscles of the neck.
14. Apply effleurage strokes from the neck to the sacrum and back up, ending at the shoulders.
15. Apply another hot, moist towel to warm the muscles and remove the oil (Figure 9–25).
16. Apply Biofreeze gel to any localized areas of tenderness, but not to the entire back, as this may be too chilling. Use information you gain when you **palpate** the client's soft tissues to determine where tender areas are. Also ask for the client's feedback.
17. Apply a cross-body stretch, holding at the hip and opposite shoulder for 8 to 12 seconds (Figure 9–26). Repeat on the opposite side.

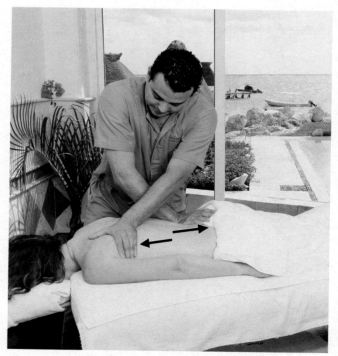

FIGURE 9–26

18. End with several light effleurage strokes up and down the back.

Prossage™ Heat/Biofreeze® Back Refresher Cleanup

1. Be especially careful about washing your hands because they have products on them that can irritate the eyes and other sensitive tissues.
2. Securely cap products and wipe down bottles with a wet towel after use.
3. Launder the sheets and towels.

direct pressure

the application of compression of tissue with static pressure

petrissage

the application of lifting, squeezing, and kneading strokes to tissues of the body

friction

the application of compression to tissues while adding movement

mastoid process

prominence of the temporal bone behind the ear at the base of the skull

palpate

examine by feeling an area to determine the state of the tissues there

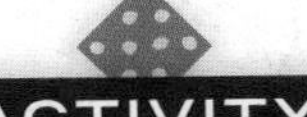

ACTIVITY

Biofreeze Hand & Foot Treatments for Therapists

Use Prossage Heat and Biofreeze to perform a hand or a foot version of the back treatment explained in this chapter. Follow each step, but apply them to hands, wrists, and forearms or feet, ankles, and calves, respectively, modifying the movements when necessary to conform to the area being worked on. These procedures are especially beneficial for working therapists who spend many hours on their feet, working with their hands.

RESEARCH

Head to your massage school's supply store or look in a distributor's catalogue to find topical heating or cooling products. Choose two products and use them on a partner while trading a targeted massage such as the one described above. What is the difference in the sensations created? Is one product more analgesic than another? Which do you find most effective? Note how your perception of a given product affects the experience of your client.

SPA PROFILE: Spa Massage in the Medical Setting

Brent Bauer, M.D., Director of Mayo Clinic's Complementary and Integrative Medicine Program

Dr. Brent Bauer has been intrigued by the spa industry for a long time. After his residency and a year-long fellowship, he officially joined the staff of Mayo Clinic at their Arizona facility in 1992, where he immediately noticed that a large percentage of the patients coming through the door were self-treating with many of the alternative therapies offered at spas such as yoga, herbs, massage, meditation, and nutritional advice. Patients brought him literature about these therapies, and one even sent him to a Jin Shin Jyutsu class. "This set my inquisitive nature into high gear," he remembers. "I learned a lot from my patients in Arizona. When I returned to the Mayo facility in Rochester, Minnesota, in 1996, I felt I knew a good deal about the topic, which led me to propose that the clinic institute a complementary and integrative medicine program."

It was not until 2001, after building his case gradually over time, that he was able to convince enough people that the time was right. During that period, the National Institutes of Health (NIH) put some serious money into researching the realm of complementary therapies, which helped his cause.

"At the same time," he recalls, "I got to know Ruth Stricker, founder of the Marsh Spa, which is also in Minnesota. She was the one who got me involved

(Continued)

SPA PROFILE Spa Massage in the Medical Setting *continued*

with the International Spa Association. Over the past 10 years, I've watched what she's been doing at the Marsh, and I've seen how it helps people. Most patients are not going to go to Mayo Clinic or to their doctor's office five times a week for exercise, Pilates, yoga, massage or acupuncture, but they will go to a spa for these purposes. I realized that it's crucial for our patients to know about and take advantage of the spa resources available. What's important now is that those patients need to hear a uniform voice on this topic, from the medical world and the spa world. They need to know it's okay to use meds when needed, but it's equally important to go to the spa for cooking classes, massages, and so on. The connection between spa and conventional medicine is still relatively unexplored even today, but Ruth saw that connection 20 years ago. Conventional medicine is only now beginning to catch up."

Dr. Bauer is a board member of the ISPA Foundation, and he believes that part of his mission is to create a bridge between the two communities of spa and medicine. To do this, he must provide his fellow physicians good, evidence-based information about the effectiveness of what goes on in spas. "Most physicians in leadership roles today trained long enough ago that the whole field of alternative therapies was not part of their vernacular," he says. "They are not so much resistant to it as they are curious about its effectiveness. Their attitude is 'we need to learn more,' and that's why my staff and I have focused so much on research. Once we show excellent results, it is no longer a question about *if* we will incorporate complementary and integrative modalities into our medical model, but *how* we can do it. We now realize that patients are not trying to supplant conventional medicine with alternatives but rather just take better care of themselves. Physicians have come around. It is no longer a good-versus-bad scenario, but rather the question now is—how do we work together?"

Dr. Bauer's research studies at Mayo Clinic have primarily focused on the effectiveness of massage. "Our cardio surgeons and nurses held meetings to discuss what we could do to help patients through the experience of cardiovascular surgery," he says, "and the one aspect of the program that has received the widest acceptance is massage.

"We have an excellent occupational therapist in the area who owns a massage school, and she runs our massage program. She took a look at the entire process of cardiovascular surgery and implemented protocols tailored to patients' needs. We offer treatments on days 2 and 4 post-surgery, and what we found is that, on day 3 patients ask, 'Where's my massage today?' Some of them even prolong their stay just to make sure they receive their second massage. If patients want to stay in the hospital longer just to get a massage, it tells you how valued that is for them. In a way, it's ironic; we give them this therapy so they feel better and can go home earlier, and it looks like it's working, but then the patients want to stay longer to get their massage!

"We conducted one 60-patient study and found that the group receiving massage had a statistically verifiable reduction in anxiety and pain. And we know that if you reduce pain and stress while in the hospital, wounds heal better, which is important because if you're in pain you take narcotics, you don't move, you can't eat, and you can't get out of the hospital. A vicious circle forms around the pain. So when a non-toxic therapy like massage can achieve such good results, it's really helpful.

"Our colorectal surgical group undertook a similar program that ended up being so successful that patients started coming all the way from California because they heard massage would be included in their healing process. Other medical centers call wanting to know how to implement their own programs, which is great. We want to be as transparent as possible, and we're always happy to share. We're looking at how we might credential providers so other people do not have to start from scratch with programs like this, to create a model that can be broadly available.

(Continued)

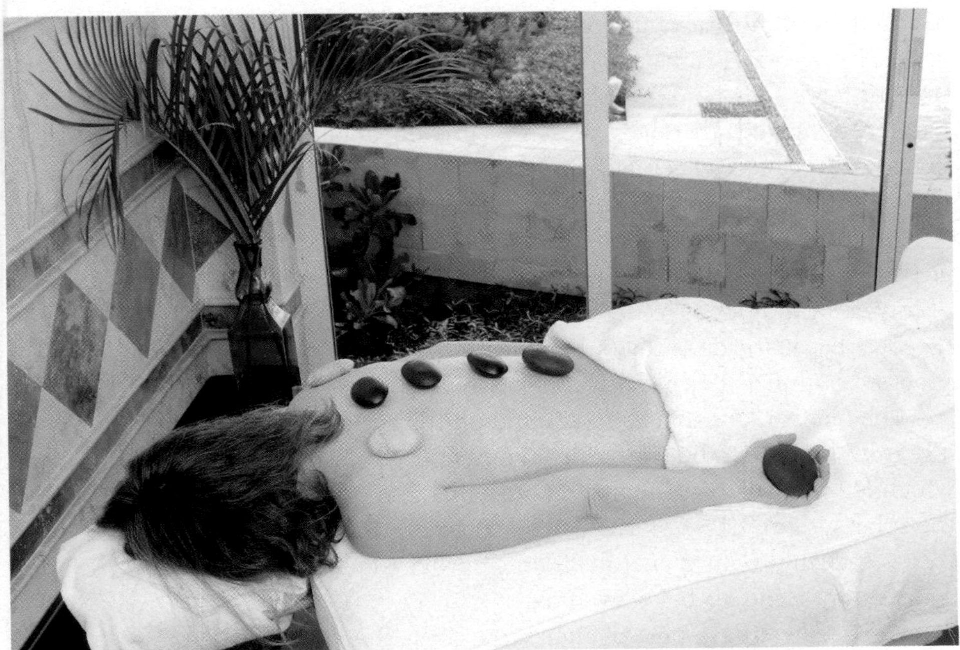

FIGURE 10–1 Stone massage is deeply relaxing and a popular treatment on many spa menus.

formed, seemingly custom-made for its use in stone massage. The rocks have been tumbled by rushing rivers and pounding surf into rounded, smooth, dense objects that fit snugly in a therapist's hands and against a client's body.

The study of these massage stones forms a part of the discipline of **petrology**, the study of rocks. Basalt is the most plentiful type of **igneous** rock, meaning it erupts from the Earth's crust in the form of molten lava. Because this mineral-rich lava cools very quickly on the planet's surface or in the ocean, it forms crystals that are especially small, which makes it particularly smooth and appropriate for massage. Rocks that form this way, as lava that has cooled outside the crust, are known as **extrusive**. In comparison, **intrusive** igneous rocks are formed from magma that cools quite slowly, over a period of many years, while still trapped under the earth's surface. This rock is exposed only much later, and it is much coarser. Granite is a form of intrusive stone. The entire Sierra Nevada mountain range in California is an example of intrusive igneous rock that has been forced to the surface. Basalt is the most common form of igneous rock. In fact, it covers the entire ocean floor, which comprises over two-thirds of the Earth's surface.

The other two primary forms of rock on the planet, in addition to igneous, are **sedimentary** and **metamorphic**. Sedimentary rock is formed by the compacting, cementing, and hardening of existing rocks, shells, bones, and bits of organic matter. This compacting process is called **lithification**. Metamorphic rock is created from other forms of rock when it subjected to intense pressure and heat. Each type of rock always transforms into the same type of metamorphic rock. Marble, for example, which is

intrusive

igneous rock that has crystallized from molten magma while still below the surface of the Earth, solidifying underground before reaching the surface

sedimentary

one of the three main forms of rock, along with igneous and metamorphic; forms over time in a layering and cementing process called *lithification*

metamorphic

rocks that have been formed under great pressure and heat

lithification

the process through which sediments compact under pressure, lose fluids, and gradually turn into stone; the final stage in the process of petrification and creation of sedimentary rocks

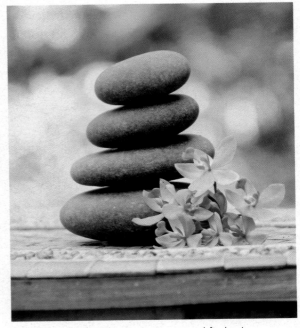

FIGURE 10–2 Black basalt stones used for heat application.

chondrites

stony meteorites formed by the accretion of dust and small grains present in the early solar system

paleomagnetism

science that studies the intensity and direction of residual magnetization in ancient rocks

mafic

of, relating to, or being a group of usually dark-colored minerals rich in magnesium and iron, as are basalt stones used in stone massage

magnetite

a black isometric mineral that is an oxide of iron and an important iron ore

piezoelectricity

electricity produced by mechanical pressure on certain crystals, notably quartz, or a change in the linear dimensions of the crystal caused by electrostatic stimulation

used for the cold stones in many stone massage treatments, is a metamorphic rock, always being transformed through natural forces from limestone into its present form. The cold marble stones are chalky white, compared to the dark basalt, giving an esthetically pleasing yin-yang appearance to the overall treatment (Figure 10–3). The marble stones are cooled in a refrigerator, ice water, or freezer, and applied to the skin to complement the effects of the heat.

All three kinds of rock—igneous, sedimentary, and metamorphic—are created from the same basic building blocks, which are minerals. It is the process of formation that determines the resulting type of stone. All rocks start out as igneous, because that is the only process that creates completely new rock. This process continues today, as is visible in locations like the Hawaiian Islands.

The oldest rocks that can be found on the surface of the Earth are not actually from the Earth, but rather from outer space. These are called **chondrites**, which fell to Earth as meteors and are some of the oldest objects to be found in the solar system, having formed approximately 4.5 billion years ago. The oldest rocks to form on our planet itself are approximately 3.8 billion years old, with some extant minerals being even older.

One interesting aspect of ancient basalt is the fact that the rapidly cooling lava records the Earth's magnetic field as it was at the time of formation. This means that a massage stone that is one billion years old contains the imprint of a different energy field than the one present on the planet today. Scientists theorize that the orientation of the magnetic poles has actually switched many times through the ages. The North Pole used to be the South Pole, and vice versa, over and over again. Thus, according to the precepts of **paleomagnetism**, this means that the massage stone you hold in your hand and apply to your client's skin may contain energy patterns quite different than those we experience today, and can therefore have a powerful energetic effect on the body. Basalt is a **mafic** rock, meaning it is comparatively rich in iron and magnesium. It also contains the mineral **magnetite**, which is so strongly magnetic that it can locally distort compass readings. This is the reason basalt imprints the earth's magnetic field so well.

In addition to the main basalt and marble, other specialized materials are sometimes applied to the body or held near it for therapeutic purposes during stone massage, including quartz crystals and semi-precious stones such as amethyst, sodalite, lapis lazuli, turquoise, rose quartz, tiger's eye, jasper, bloodstone, and others (Figure 10–4). These stones are not applied for their thermal effects and are therefore not heated or cooled. Rather, they are meant to have a subtler influence and are used to align clients' energies. Quartz crystals, in particular, emit a form of energy called **piezoelectricity** which can affect the body when the crystals are struck while in contact with the skin. Often, these stones are placed on clients' **chakras** (Figure 10–5). Regular basalt stones can also be struck in this manner because of their crystalline content.

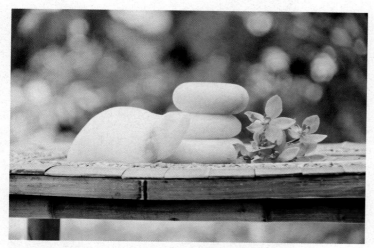

FIGURE 10–3 White marble stones used for cold application.

SPA TIP

Some therapists claim that the effectiveness of stone therapy derives from the energy or "personality" of the stones themselves. Because the stones were formed millions of years ago and are a fundamental part of the Earth, they are believed to emanate vibrations that connect the recipients of stone massage directly to the "soul" of the planet. Therapists should exercise discretion when speaking in these terms with clients, as some spa goers prefer a more straightforward explanation of the benefits of the therapies they receive. Whether the esoteric benefits of stone massage really exist is a matter of debate, but the therapeutic benefits of massage plus temperature therapy are undeniable. The stones, as noted in this chapter, seem to offer paleomagnetic benefits as well. At the very least, it can be accepted that modern stone massage offers spas a simple way to add an exotic form of heat and cold therapy to the menu and put clients back in touch with a piece of the natural world.

chakras

literally translated as "wheel" in Sanskrit, any of several (usually seven) points of physical or spiritual energy in the human body as described in yogic philosophy, sometimes referred to as vortexes, where semi-precious stones are placed during some stone massage treatments

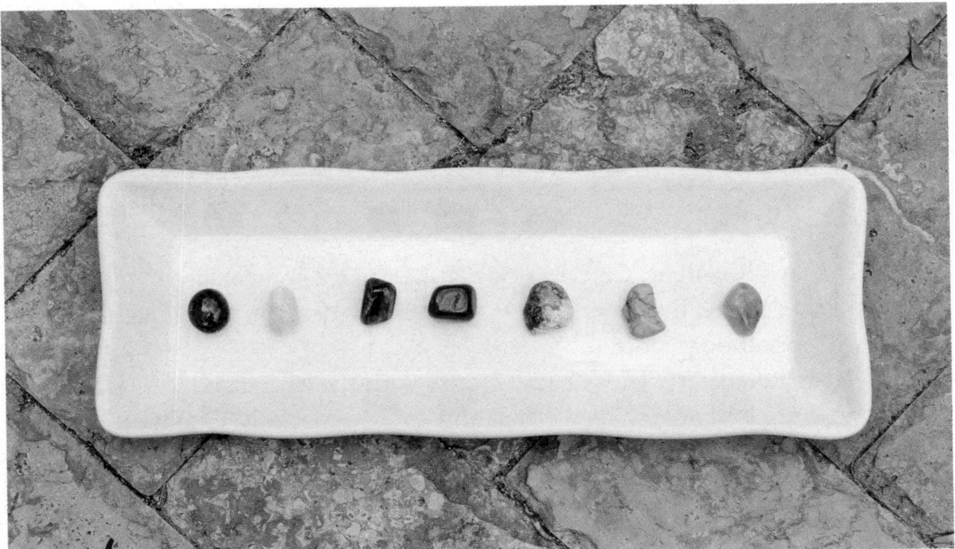

FIGURE 10–4 Semi-precious stones used for stone massage.

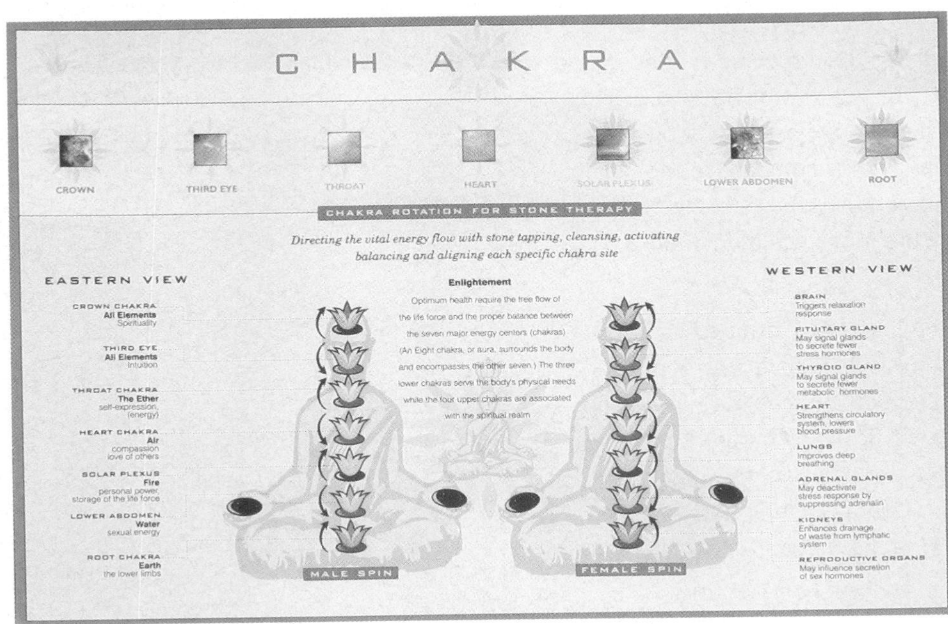

FIGURE 10–5 The chakras treated in some forms of stone massage.

Harvesting Stones

Typically, massage therapists purchase stones from a supplier or use the stones provided by the spa where they are employed. The suppliers obtain the stones from three main sources: quarries, river beds, and rocky coastlines. Some practitioners are able to choose the stones themselves, if they have access to an appropriate source. Therapists sometimes refer to the gathering of stones for massage as "harvesting," which they perform with appropriate respect for the environment and the energies of Mother Earth. Unlike basalt stones, which come ready-made from the Earth, marble has to be mined and then carved and polished. Thus, it is not possible for therapists to harvest marble in nature.

Four main determining factors are considered when choosing stones for use in massage:

1. **Magnetic Energy:** The initial imprint of magnetic energy formed at the time that basalt was extruded from underground determines much of the invisible energetic component of the treatment. Some therapists claim to be able to sense this energy, which they say is more pronounced in certain stones, making them more valuable as therapeutic tools.
2. **Mineral Content:** Certain stones have higher percentages of quartz or other specific minerals such as olivine, magnesium, iron, magnetite, pyroxene, and labradorite.
3. **Heat Retention:** Those basalt stones with the highest concentration of iron are best able to retain heat and so are especially sought-after for stone massage.

Mohs scale

a scale of relative hardness devised by Friedrich Mohs in 1812, used as an aid to identify minerals

The Mohs Scale

Did You Know?

Some rocks are harder than others, and the rocks used for stone massage are chosen partly for their specific hardness, which is measured on something called the **Mohs scale**. This scale of mineral hardness was devised by Friedrich Mohs in 1812, and classifies all minerals as they compare to the classic list of ten that Mohs devised. Table 10–1 shows some typical minerals and where they fall on the Mohs scale, including basalt at a very hard 8.

To determine the hardness of a mineral, it is rubbed against a known mineral. The harder mineral will leave a scratch on the softer one. If both scratch each other, they have the same hardness. Certain everyday objects fit neatly on the Mohs scale and can be used to test minerals. A fingernail, for instance, is 2½. A penny is just under 3. A knife blade is 5½. Glass is 5½. A steel file is 6½. Diamond is the hardest and will scratch every other substance.

HARDNESS	MATERIALS
1	talc, graphite
2	gypsum, rock salt
3	chalk, marble
4	dolomite
5	apatite
6	feldspar
7	quartz
8	basalt
9	ruby, sapphire
10	diamond

TABLE 10–1 Hardness of Minerals Measured on the Mohs Scale.

4. **Smoothness and Shape**: The stones can be used on every flat surface and curve of the body and thus need to be chosen for their ability to fit the body as well as the therapist's hands. Also, the smoothness of the stones is important for client comfort and pleasure.

After the stones are gathered, they are cleaned and grouped into sets for use in massage. Some suppliers polish the stones, though others claim that this makes them slippery and harder to use.

Shapes and Sizes of the Stones Used

The size and shape of the stones chosen during each part of the treatment depend on the area of the body the therapist wishes to access, the size of the client, the size of the therapist's hands, and also on the modality being practiced, whether it be deep tissue, Swedish, aromatherapy, lymphatic drainage, or others. The main sizes and shapes of the stones, along with uses and the number of each found in a typical set, are illustrated in Figure 10-6 and explained in Table 10-2.

Therapists must become adept at using the right stone at the right time on the appropriate area of the body. This particular skill can only be developed with practice, but it quickly becomes second nature once the therapist has become accustomed to handling the heated stones. Each set of stones used in a spa contains enough of each size and shape for at least one complete treatment, and a wide variety of sets are available for different uses. Some therapists, for example, use the stones primarily for placement on the body, not for use as massage tools, and the number and type of stones in their sets will reflect that. Other sets have been created specifically for therapists who focus on deep tissue stone work. Still others are for use during manicures, pedicures, or facials.

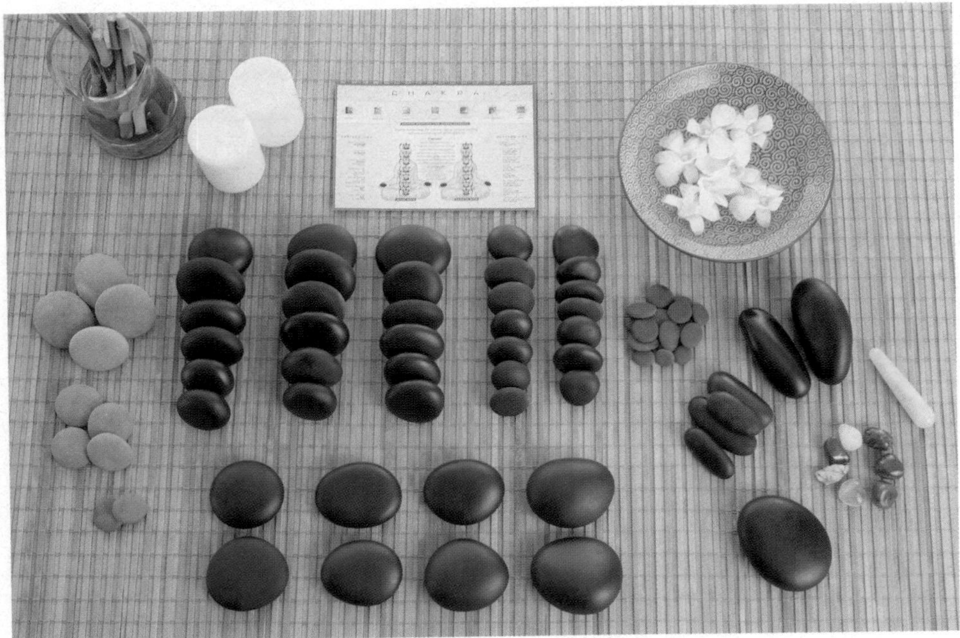

FIGURE 10-6 Massages stones have a variety of purposes. Courtesy of TH Stone.

TYPE OF STONE	# IN SET	SHAPE	USAGE
Extra-Large	1	oval, flattish, heavy, the largest stone in the set	These stones are typically used on the abdomen or solar plexus while the client is supine and the sacrum when the client is prone.
Large	8	rounded, fills up therapist's hand	These stones are used for massaging larger muscle groups such as the quadriceps, hamstrings, gluteals, and pectorals.
Medium	8	rounded	These stones are used on smaller muscle groups such as the hands, arms, and lower legs.
Small	8	rounded	These smaller stones are used to massage delicate or bony areas such as the forehead, neck, and face.
Spinal	8	round but flatter than the other body stones	These stones are placed beneath the erector spinae when the client is lying supine, or on top of the erector muscles when the client is prone.
Neck	1	large, oblong, thick	This stone is used as a pillow of sorts under the occipital area when the client is supine.
Trigger Point	4	oblong, slightly sharper ends and edges	These stones can be used as massage tools on meridians, trigger points, and adhesions.
Contour	2	oblong, medium-sized	These stones are placed on the soles or in the palms for a sense of comfort and to relieve minor aches in those areas.
Toe	8	extremely small, flat	These stones are placed between the toes and removed once they cool down.
COLD STONES			
Small	2	small, oval, and flattish	These stones are used on the face and more delicate areas to soothe and cool. Two especially small stones are often reserved for use on the eyelids, usually atop a protective cloth.
Large	2	same size as small basalt stones but usually flatter	These stones are used for trigger points, to cool down overheated areas and create contrast therapy effects.
CRYSTALS AND SEMI-PRECIOUS STONES			
Crystal Wand	1	approximately six inches long, oblong	This, often quartz, crystal stone is not heated but rather used to align and balance clients' subtle energies. Sometimes called an attunement wand.
Chakra Stones	7	small irregular nuggets	Semi-precious, unheated stones that are placed on clients' chakras to affect subtle energies.

TABLE 10–2 Types of Stones Used for Massage.

Effects of Stone Massage

For spa clients, the effects of stone massage are immediate and often quite powerful. The result of the combined effects is luxurious and somehow liberating. As the mind and body are brought back gradually into a state of reconnection with the Earth, many recipients describe experiencing a release of preoccupations and tensions. The end result is one of grounding and deep relaxation. The physiological effects that combine to create such profound reactions to stone massage fall into three main categories: thermal, energetic, and mechanical.

Hot stones create all the effects and benefits of local heat application, while cold stones offer clients the benefits of local cold application. And, when used in conjunction for contrast therapy, hot and cold stones create a stimulating effect on the circulation, which pumps more blood to the tissues being treated. See the section on Effects of Hot and Cold Contrast Therapy in Chapter 5 for more information on this pumping effect of contrast therapy.

The **specific gravity** of basalt is approximately 3, making it one of the heaviest types of common stone on the planet. The thermal effects of stone massage are transmitted so effectively to the client's body precisely because the stones have such a heavy mineral content, especially iron, as already mentioned. The iron absorbs and retains heat particularly well.

The human body has a bioelectric field that is influenced by that of the stones. Some therapists claim that this influence extends to clients' chi or prana, which runs in energy pathways, or meridians, throughout the body. And when therapists place semi-precious stones on chakras or wave a crystal **attunement wand** in a spiral pattern over a client's body, their aim is to affect this energetic system as well. Therapists' claims for these energetic effects are often difficult to prove empirically; however, it is known that crystals conduct energy and basalt stones carry magnetic fields, and that therefore the human body must be affected in some way by coming into contact with them. The single most important factor determining the quality of a stone massage treatment, or any massage, is the focused intention of the therapist. Therefore, if placing semi-precious stones on chakras and invoking the healing powers of quartz crystals while spiraling them over a client's body focuses a therapist's intentions, then it is, in a sense, working. In addition, there can be no doubt that a very real biomagnetic effect is created by the stones' mineral composition.

The mechanical effects of stone massage are produced by the pressure of the stones and the therapist's hands on the client's body, which influences circulation of both lymph and blood, relaxes tight muscles, and can soothe minor aches and pains. The type of massage most often incorporated into a stone treatment is Swedish, though the stones can actually be thought of as an add-on to all massage modalities. For instance, some spas incorporate the use of aromatherapy with the stones, some specialize in treating the face with small stones, some spas use the stones primarily as instruments in deep tissue massage, and others offer reflexology with stones. Stones add to massage, enhancing each modality, rather than replacing it.

Although it may consist of energy work, heat, and esoteric techniques, stone massage is, in the end, massage. The official definition of massage in most state and local laws includes the use of heat, cold, and therapeutic instruments in the treatment of soft tissues. Stones, in this sense, can simply be construed as therapeutic instruments. They are tools.

ACTIVITY

Handling & Placing Stones

Under the close supervision of your instructor, practice handling each different-sized stone and placing them on your partner's body while they are not heated. Note where each stone fits most easily and how the various sizes and shapes affect different areas with their weight, pressure, and edge shape.

specific gravity

the ratio of the density of a given substance to the density of water, when both are at the same temperature; also sometimes referred to as *specific density*

attunement wand

an oblong piece of crystal, often of quartz or rose quartz, used unheated in stone massage to align and balance client's subtle energies

HISTORY OF THERAPEUTIC STONE USE

Stones have been so central to human civilization that they have been used as markers to differentiate between different ages of history. Thus, the Old Stone Age, or Paleolithic, is followed by the Middle Stone Age, or Mesolithic, and finally the New Stone Age, or Neolithic. The Greek root "lithos" means stone.

The Kahuna Stones

Did You Know?

Right in the midst of the tourist destination of Waikiki Beach in Hawaii, four giant basalt boulders, weighing several tons apiece, sit on a lava rock platform behind a protective fence. Although they are seen every day by many thousands of people, most passersby probably do not realize that native Hawaiians have regarded these stones as sacred for generations. They are called the Kahuna Stones (see Figure 10–7), or sometimes the Wizard Stones or Healing Stones, and a legend shrouds their origins in mystery. According to local lore, four great healers arrived in Hawaii hundreds of years ago and performed healings for the local people. Afterwards, they transferred their healing energies into the stones. Today, the stones serve as symbols of Hawaii's spiritual healing tradition and have become well-known and respected by therapists, students, and healers from many lands.

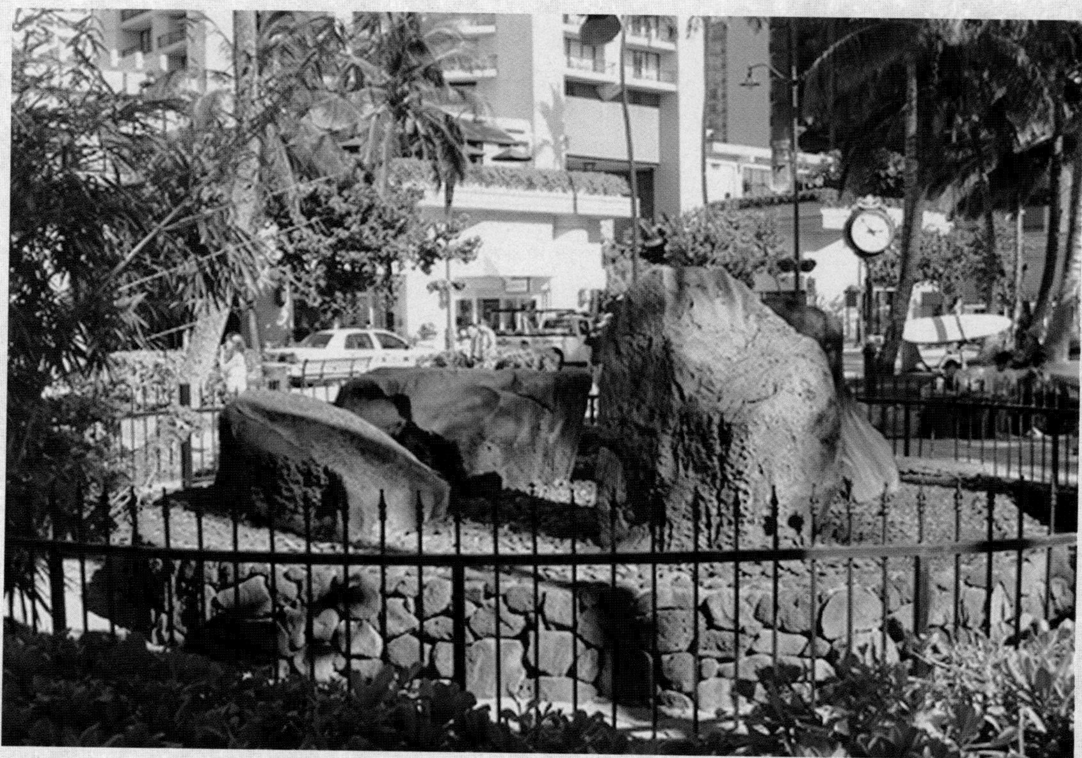

FIGURE 10–7 Hawaii's Kahuna stones.

Stones have been worshipped, prayed to, idolized, and cast into important mythical roles in human spirituality for eons. Entire religions have literally revolved around them. In Islam, the Black Stone, or *al-Hajar-ul-Aswad*, is a small black rock embedded into one wall of the Kaaba, which millions of Muslim pilgrims circumambulate every year, touching or kissing the holy stone as they pass.

sarsen

a type of dense, hard sandstone; the prehistoric builders of Stonehenge used the substance to erect their monument

The **sarsen** megaliths of Stonehenge, erected over 4,000 years ago, were transported more than 40 kilometers from where they were mined to form an ancient ceremonial circle. The stones at this site and others in Great Britain were purported to have healing properties, which led some people to venerate them so fanatically that the church felt it necessary to intercede, issuing many proclamations forbidding stone worship. People, however, persisted in seeing stones

A Stone Massage by Any Other Name . . .

Did You Know?

Although the majority of spas list it as simple Stone Massage or Hot Stone Massage on their menus, this unique treatment is perfectly suited for innovation and creativity when it comes to customizing the client's experience. In some cases, that creativity spills over into the naming of the treatment itself. For example, take a look at the names of the following 10 stone massage offerings on the menus of some innovative spas. Perhaps you will consider a one-of-a-kind name yourself if you ever have the opportunity to coin a new name for your own version of stone massage.

1. Canyon Stone Massage
2. Stone House Stone Massage
3. Native Stone Massage
4. Indo-Asian Hot Stone Massage
5. Bones of the Earth Hot Stone Massage
6. Lomi-LaStone Connection
7. Signature Sage Stone Massage
8. Sacred Hot Stone
9. Sun Baked Stone Massage
10. Warm River Stone Massage

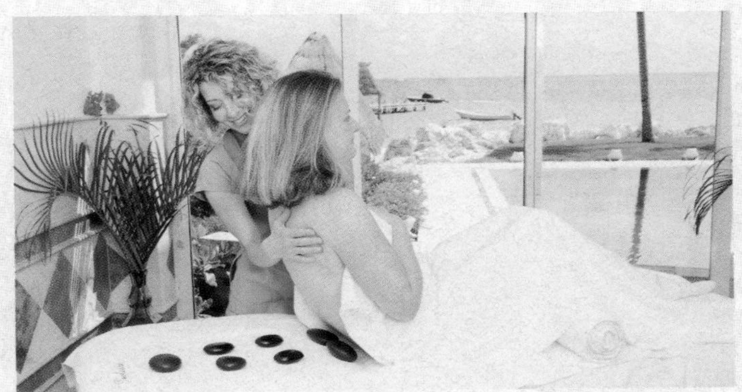

as having healing properties. Another site in southwest England, called the Mên-an-Tol, or Crick Stone, features three standing stones, the middle one having a large hole in it through which countless babies over a span of many centuries have been passed back and forth nine times, naked, in hopes that the stone would cure them of rickets.

Most of the 887 strange and evocative towering moai of Easter Island were carved from compressed volcanic ash, but 13 of them were made from basalt, the same material used for massage stones, and it is these few examples that offer the most intact representation of what the figures originally looked like. The basalt resists weather damage well, and for this reason 6 of the 13 statues removed from the island for display worldwide are basalt. The early inhabitants of Easter Island created the moai to represent deceased ancestors, or perhaps powerful tribal chiefs who were idolized and worshipped.

In China, during the Neolithic age, people used stones for healing purposes, as proven by the unearthing of stones that had been refined into fine needles, ancient precursors to modern acupuncture needles. These were called **bian stones**. It was not until centuries later that metal needles replaced the stones.

bian stones

stones refined into fine needles and used as instruments of healing in ancient China

For centuries, Native Americans have used stones to create heat for their sweat lodge ceremonies, and other people have used stones to aid healing and to heat special chambers such as the Finnish sauna. See Chapter 5 for more information about saunas. The temperatures at which stones are used for these purposes, however, are much too high for direct application to the body. Although many cultures report using warmed stones to heat bedding, provide general warmth, or even soothe pain, the systematic use of the rocks through direct application as part of hands-on therapy appears to be a relatively new innovation.

Though many different forms and philosophies of stone massage are in use in spas today, special mention must be given to a modern pioneer in the technique, Mary Nelson of Tucson, Arizona. In 1993 she developed a unique systemized method of applying hot and cold stones as part of a massage, claiming Native American healers and spirit guides as her inspiration. She called her technique **LaStone Therapy**. This particular form of stone massage is still offered in many spas, but there have been several other variations promulgated by a wide variety of therapists, trainers, and vendors since that time. Nelson and her team conduct workshops to train other massage therapists in the LaStone technique, with its strong and steady focus on respect for the stones, the application of energy work, and a unique blending of Native American points of view into each treatment.

LaStone Therapy

original form of stone-based treatment developed by Arizona massage therapist Mary Nelson in 1993, including energy work, deep tissue stone work, sage smudge stick purification, and the application of hot and cold stones

SAFETY AND SANITATION FOR STONE MASSAGE APPLICATIONS

A stone massage program is easy to set up, requiring only a heating unit, an optional refrigerator or freezer, and the stones themselves. However, caution must be exercised when practicing stone massage. The application of hard hot objects to the skin and tissues below is inherently hazardous. It follows that students must be trained adequately and undergo sufficient practice before using stones on clients. When applying stone massage, the following four safety considerations must be kept in mind.

1. **Water Temperature:** Water in the heating container must be kept at the correct temperature, which is between 110°F and 140°F. Temperatures below 110°F do not generate sufficient warmth for therapeutic application, and temperatures above 140°F make it difficult to handle the stones. Stones heated beyond this temperature may also cause discomfort for the client or even damage tissue if applied directly to the skin. The use of a thermometer to monitor water temperature in the stone warmer is highly recommended. The warmer may be placed on high to heat the stones quickly at first, but then it must be brought down to the appropriate operating temperature for use.
2. **Client Protection:** Stones may be placed directly on the skin, but the therapist must exercise caution when doing so. Often, it is preferable to place sheets, pillowcases, or towels between the stones and the skin in order to protect the client from possible harm or discomfort. The thickness of these protective layers may be adjusted or they may be removed altogether during the course of the treatment as the temperature of the stones cools.
3. **Cleaning Stones and Implements:** Proper sanitation is crucial in order to assure a safe experience for the client. The stones should be cleansed with fresh water and antibacterial soap after each use and rinsed before being placed back in the heating unit. If the stones are sticky from oil, they can be cleansed with alcohol. The water in the heating unit should be changed daily. A sterilizing solution can be added to the heating

unit each day to assure a sanitary treatment. At the end of each work day, the unit should be turned off and the stones removed and placed in hot water with antibacterial soap or a small amount of sea salt. Then each stone should be washed, rinsed, and placed on a towel to dry. The heating bin should be emptied, sprayed with alcohol, and dried. The stones are replaced in the bin, which is left dry until the next work day when it is filled and heated once again.

4. **Depth of Pressure with Stones:** When using stones as tools during massage, some therapists tend to apply excessive pressure as they strive for therapeutic effects. It must be remembered that stones penetrate the tissues much more forcefully than therapists' fingers or thumbs. Extreme caution must be exercised in order not to cause damage.

Contraindications

Stone massage presents several contraindications, including the most obvious one for heat. It is important to keep in mind, however, that stone massage does not create systemic effects in reaction to the heat application, but rather only local effects. Even though a large area of the skin surface, such as the back, may experience a notable temperature increase, the core temperature of the body will not rise in reaction to a local external application. Therefore, clients with high blood pressure, for example, will not be likely to experience the same adverse reactions to stone application as they will for a full-body heat immersion such as the herbal wrap or heated hydrotherapy bath. The heat of the stones can still cause harm, though, and it is crucial for therapists to maintain continuous open communication with the client during a stone massage application regarding comfort and temperature.

SPA TIP

Reenergizing Massage Stones

Some therapists believe that the massage stones become depleted energetically as they are used during treatments and should be reenergized through the use of various techniques. While this belief may be a subjective perception and perhaps will never be proven scientifically, it helps many therapists pay more attention to the care and sanitation of the stones and gives them an increased respect for the effects the stones can have upon clients.

The techniques suggested to reenergize the stones include:

- Placing the stones directly on the Earth. This is believed to realign the stones with the electromagnetic currents of the planet from which they came.
- Bathing the stones in moonlight.
- Bathing the stones in sunlight.
- Washing the stones in seawater.
- Arranging the stones into a medicine wheel or spiral, or other mandala-like patterns.
- Placing stones in a bowl containing organic raw brown rice to absorb negative energies.
- Holding the stones over sage smoke.

In general, the primary contraindications for stone massage are:

- any condition where general massage is contraindicated
- surgery in which nerves have been cut, causing loss of feeling
- nerve damage or neuropathy—avoid specific areas
- use of prescription medications that are adversely affected by heat applications
- infectious skin disease, rashes, lesions, or any skin conditions aggravated by heat

Several conditions warrant the use of caution and should receive a doctor's consent prior to the application of stone massage. These include:

- pregnancy (except by practitioners certified in pregnancy massage; never in the first trimester)
- heart disease and clients prone to blood clots
- high blood pressure
- circulatory problems
- diabetic peripheral neuropathy (decreased skin sensitivity to temperature)
- extreme obesity which puts a strain on the heart
- metal implants (stones may heat implants and cause discomfort)
- cancer
- immediately after chemotherapy or radiation
- Parkinson's disease

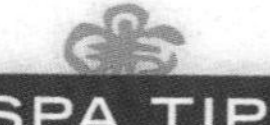

SPA TIP

As your training in stone massage becomes more advanced and you acquire more experience, some of the listed contraindications may no longer be applicable to your work. When you increase your clinical knowledge, you will be able to adapt the treatment for clients with a variety of conditions by lowering temperatures, modifying application techniques, and changing areas covered. As a beginner at stone massage, however, it is important to closely observe all contraindications.

Finally, some conditions are not outright contraindicated for stone massage and do not require a doctor's consent, but they should be approached with caution. These include:

- varicose veins—avoid hot stones directly to the area, but cold stones in moderation with light pressure are permissible
- older thin skin—use light pressure and lower heat
- open wounds, bruises, tumors, hernias, recent fractures—avoid the areas
- acute inflammation—cold stone therapy can be used in these areas

Benefits of Stone Massage

The therapeutic application of stones offers myriad benefits (Figure 10–8). The heat provided by the stones stimulates circulation and helps muscles relax even more quickly than in a traditional massage. This allows therapists to apply deeper pressure more quickly, if desired. Also, the stones offer the benefits of a reflex reaction to the heat and cold being applied to the surface, thus affecting interior organs. Cold stones ease inflammation and offer pain relief. More details about specific benefits of hot and cold stone application are listed below.

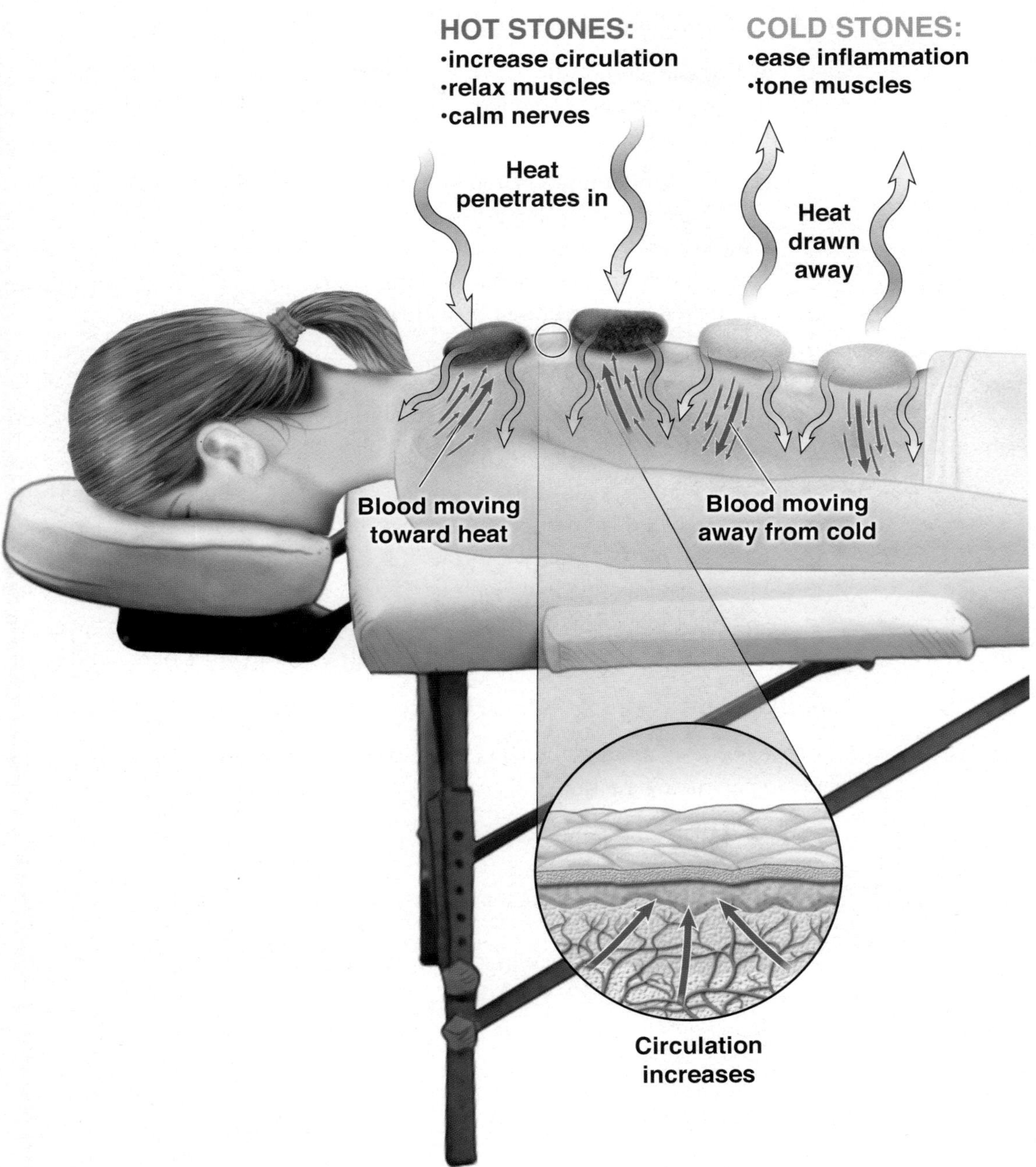

FIGURE 10–8 The application of stones offers many benefits.

Benefits of Hot Stone Therapy

The major benefits derived from the application of hot stones include:

- relaxes muscles and softens connective tissues
- relieves minor aches and pains
- soothes the nervous system
- reduces overall stress
- increases lymph and blood circulation
- can help ease tension headaches
- can help ease menstrual pain

Benefits of Cold Stone Therapy

Some practitioners and trainers claim that stone massage can be fully therapeutic only if cold stones are included. The specific benefits offered by cold stone application are:

- decreases inflammation and swelling
- can help ease sinus congestion
- stimulates the nervous system
- can help ease pain caused by strains, contusions, and soft tissue injuries
- can help ease pain caused by arthritis

Benefits of Alternating Hot and Cold Stone Therapy

When hot and cold stones are used in combination, some of the effects of contrast therapy can be induced, including the following:

- send blood to areas of poor circulation
- remove blood from hyperemic areas
- increase microcirculation by creating a "blood pump"—see Chapter 5, Effects of Hot and Cold Contrast Therapy
- stimulate reflex effects in organs beneath the surface area being treated—see Chapter 5 for more information on the reflex effects of hot and cold

Conditions Benefited by Stone Therapy

All of the above-mentioned benefits make stone massage particularly helpful for clients experiencing a number of common conditions, including:

- muscular aches and pains
- arthritis
- fibromyalgia (with a doctor's consent)
- stress and anxiety
- circulatory problems (with a doctor's consent)
- insomnia
- depression

TECHNIQUES

The techniques used for stone massage applications can be broken down into two broad categories: placing the stones on the body and holding the stones while applying massage maneuvers. Skilled therapists can seamlessly weave these two uses of the stones together to create a treatment that flows smoothly from start to finish. Ideally, the stones will become an extension of the therapist's hands, adding heat and texture to the massage.

SPA TIP

Make sure the stones and your hands are dry before touching the client's skin. Any excess hot water that comes into contact with the client may cause discomfort or pain.

Placing Stones

1. Stones should be placed on the client's body on an exhalation so that the heat and weight of the stone can be more easily accepted (Figure 10–9). This is true for stones placed on the torso or limbs but not necessarily on the head or feet.

2. Stones should be lifted away from the torso and limbs on an inhalation so that it feels as though the body is helping to push the stones up and away (Figure 10–10).

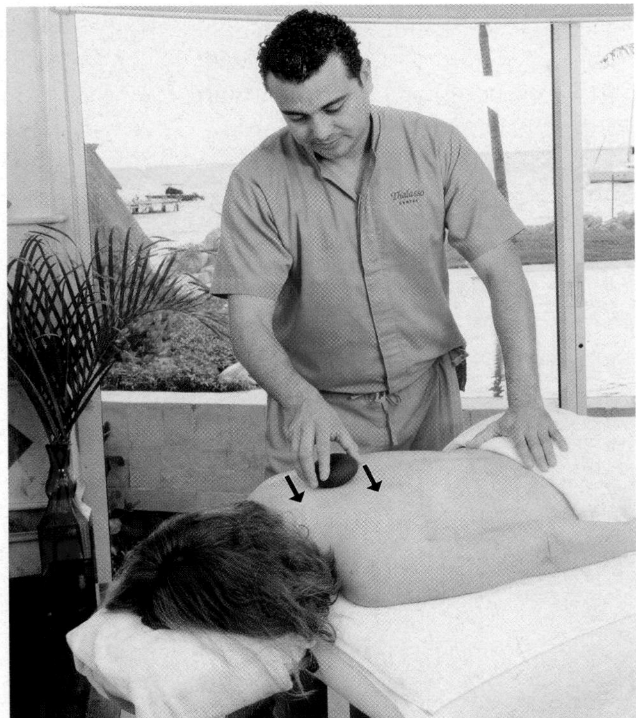

FIGURE 10–9

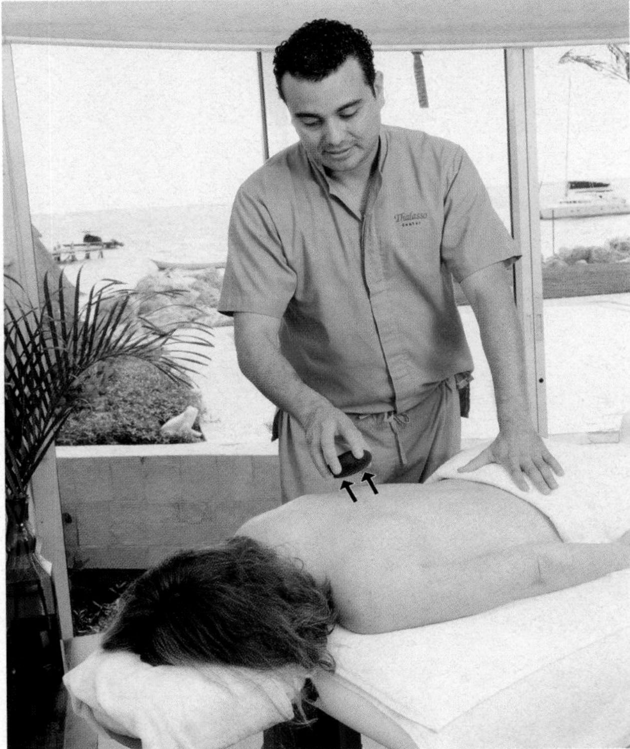

FIGURE 10–10

3. Stones can be tucked beneath the client's body in strategic locations such as gluteals, occipital ridge, shoulder, and thigh (Figure 10–11).
4. Stones can be laid down beneath the client, under a towel, in two rows along the area where the erector spinae will rest, from sacrum to cervical vertebrae. Then, the client is instructed to roll back onto the stones (Figure 10–12). The number of stones depends on the size of the client and the arch of the spine. Experiment until you become proficient in choosing and placing layout stones.

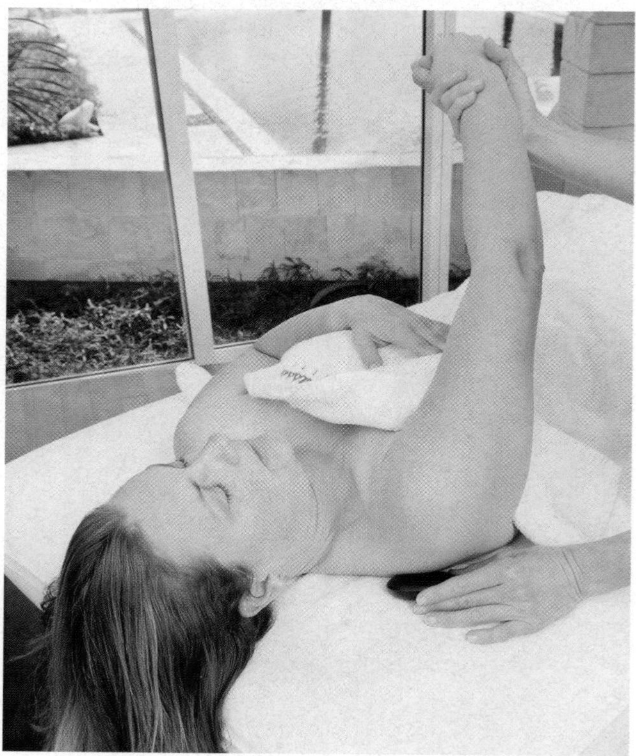

FIGURE 10–11

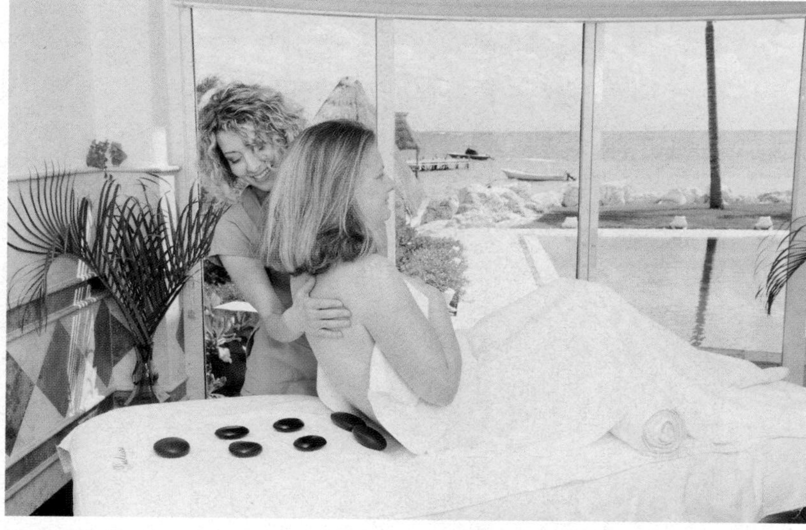

FIGURE 10–12

5. Stones can be placed on energy vortexes, or chakras, atop the body (Figure 10–13).
6. Contour stones can be placed in the client's hand or on the sole of the foot (Figure 10–14).
7. Larger stones can be placed atop the belly, beneath the belly, or on the sacrum (Figure 10–15).

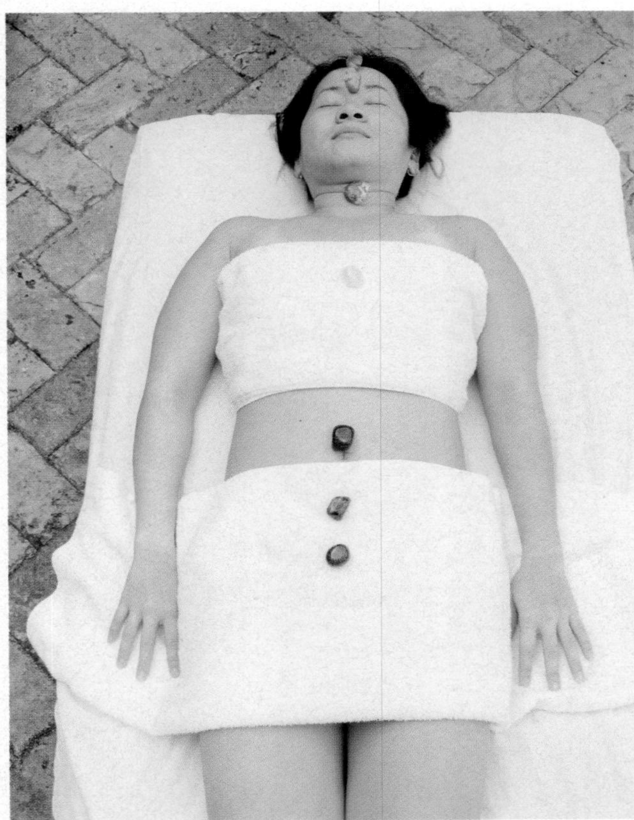

FIGURE 10–13

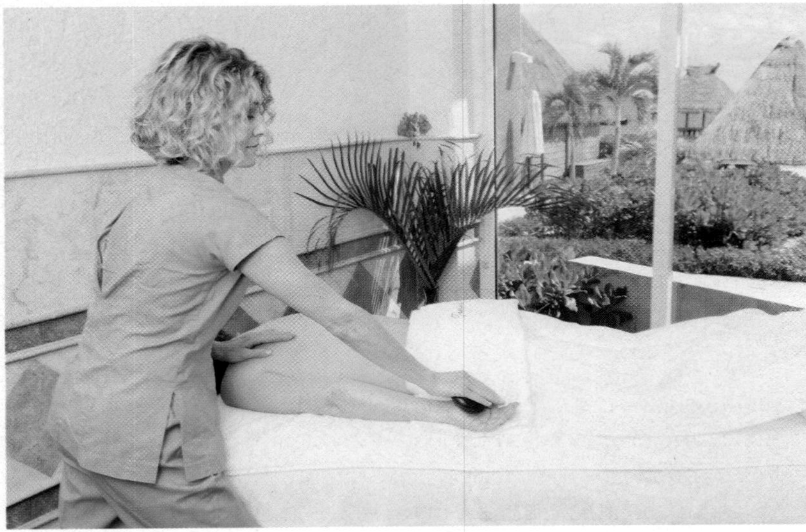

FIGURE 10–14

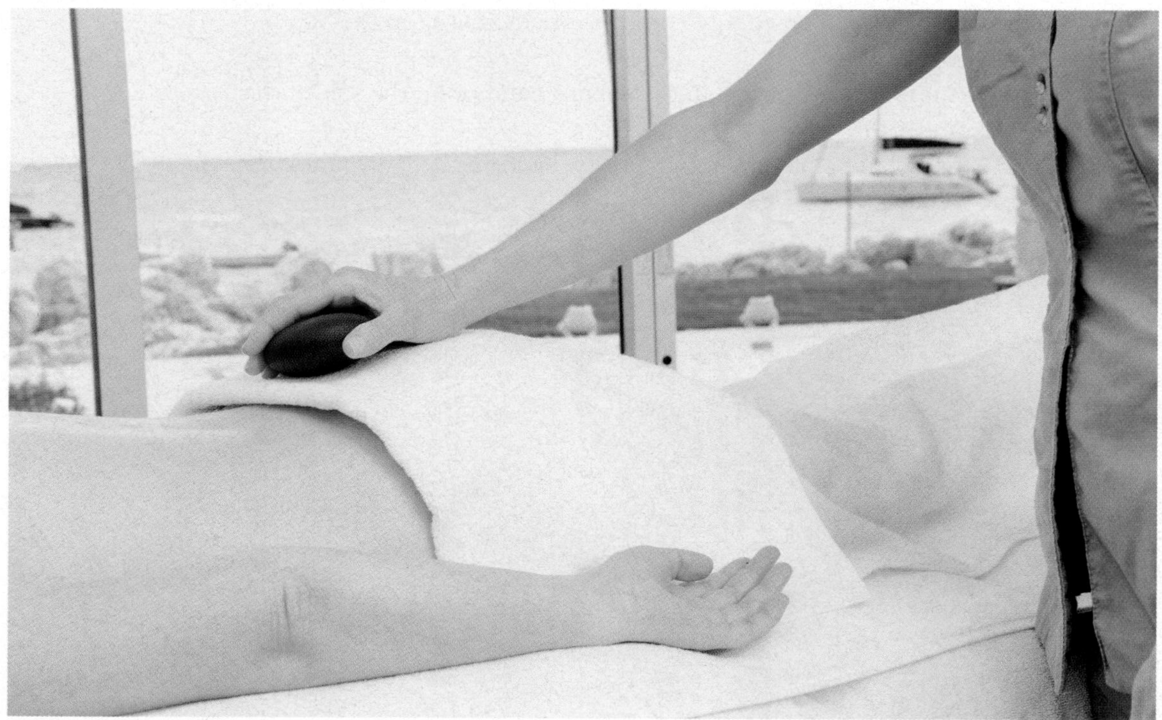

FIGURE 10–15

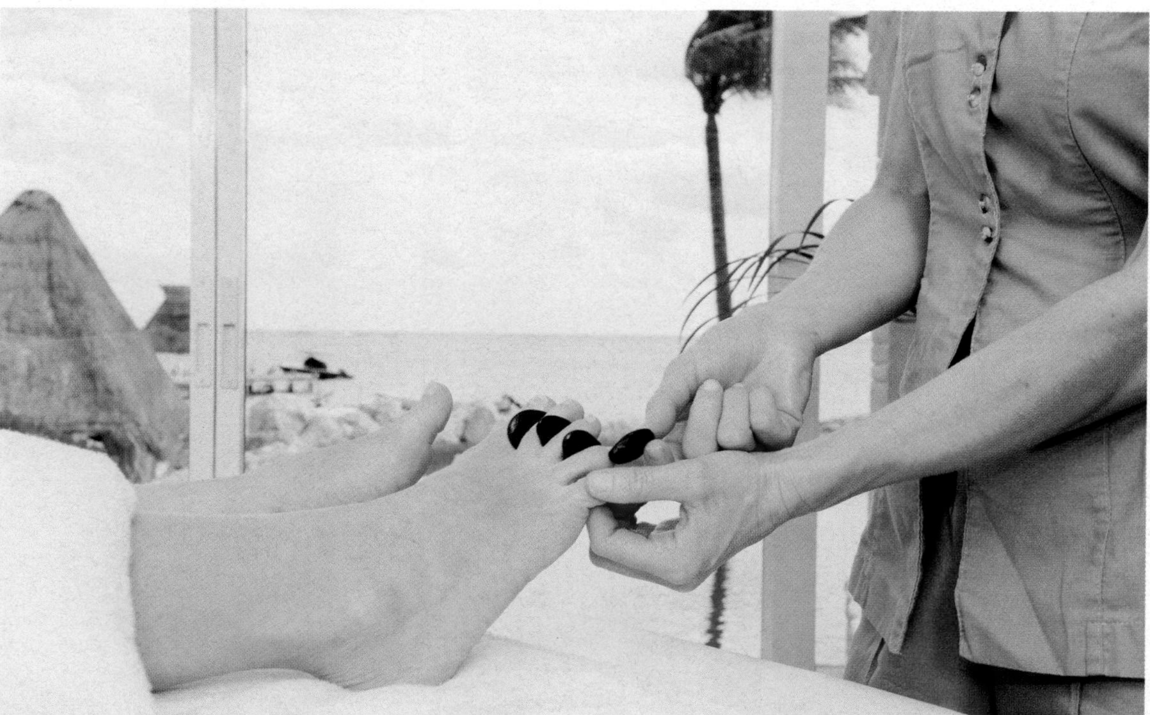

FIGURE 10–16

8. Small flat stones can be placed between the toes (Figure 10–16).
9. Stones already placed on the body can be tapped with another stone to create the effects of piezoelectricity (Figure 10–17).
10. As stones cool, the therapist may remove them or replace them with warmer stones (Figure 10–18).

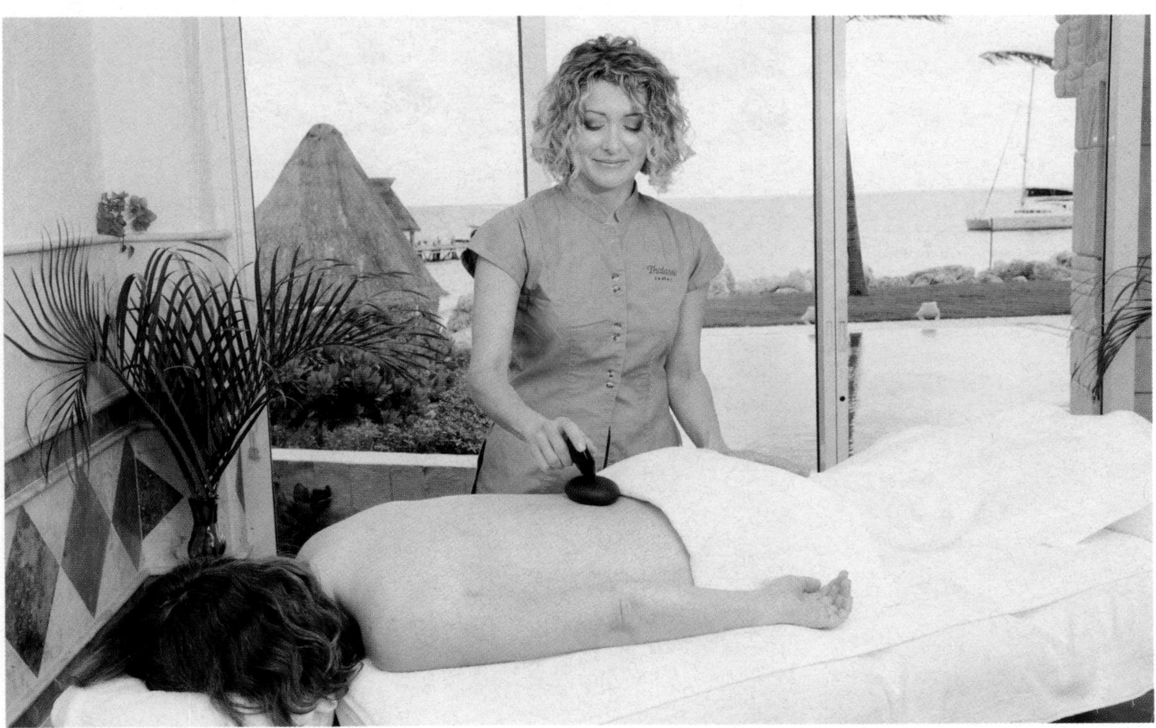

FIGURE 10–17

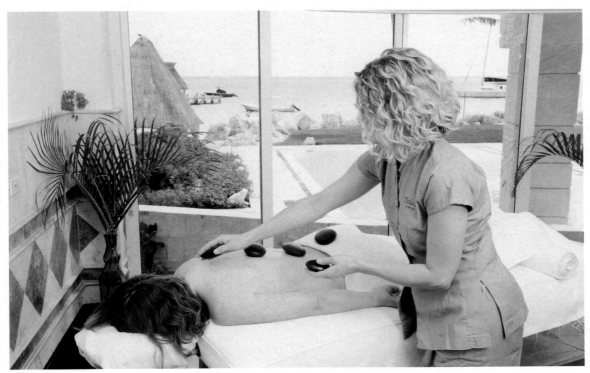

FIGURE 10–18

Massaging with the Stones

1. Initial Contact: Introduce stones to the body gradually by first touching the back of your hand to the client's skin before bringing the stone into full contact (Figure 10–19).

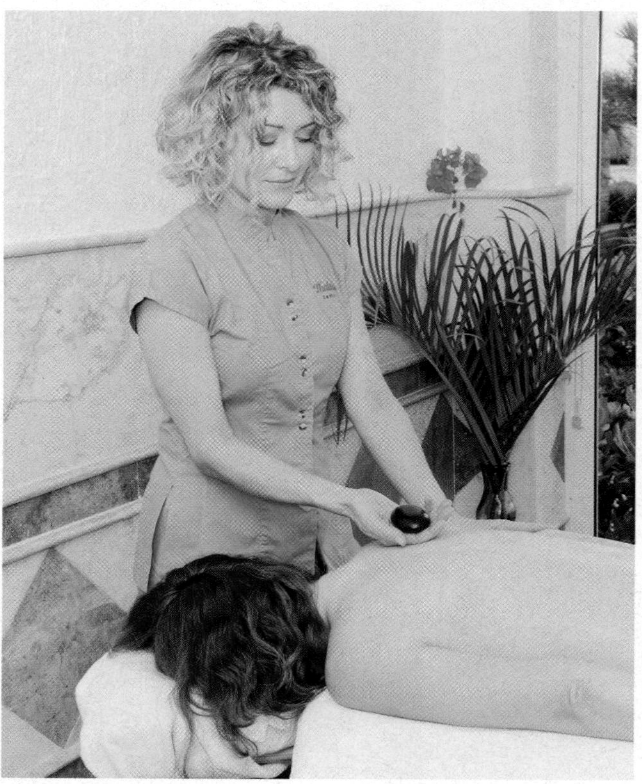

FIGURE 10–19

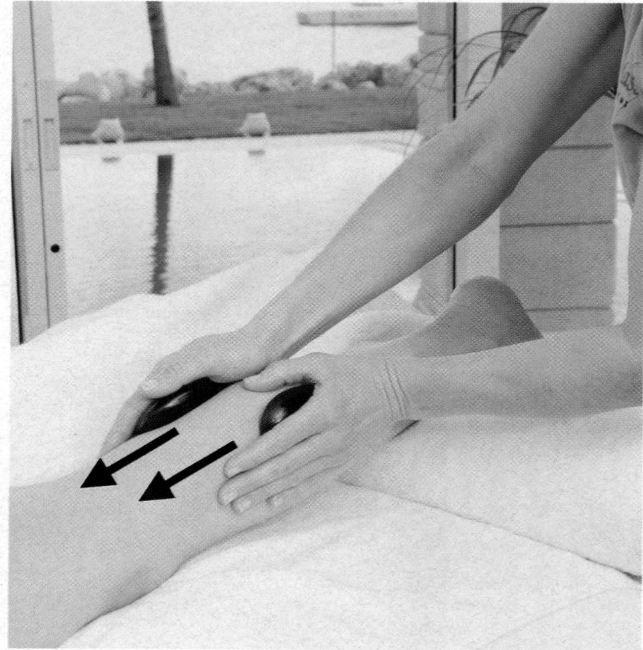

FIGURE 10–20

2. Gliding: Use one or two stones to glide over the skin in a movement similar to effleurage (Figure 10–20).
3. Deep Tissue: Use one or two stones to glide along the skin, pressing in deeper in areas of tension. The stones can also be turned on their edges for this maneuver (Figure 10–21).

4. Kneading: Holding small stones in the palm, it is possible to perform a petrissage-type maneuver against the skin, but it is difficult to keep a grip on the stones at the same time (Figure 10–22).
5. Friction: The stones can be rubbed against muscle fibers to create a cross-fiber friction effect (Figure 10–23).

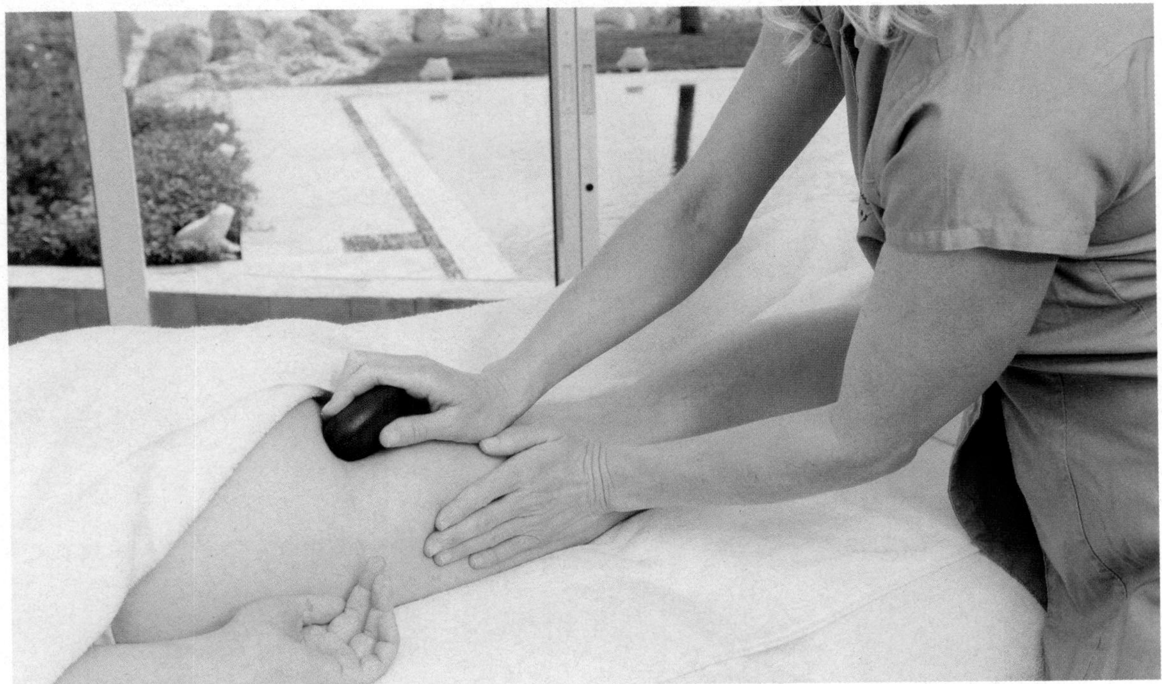

FIGURE 10–21

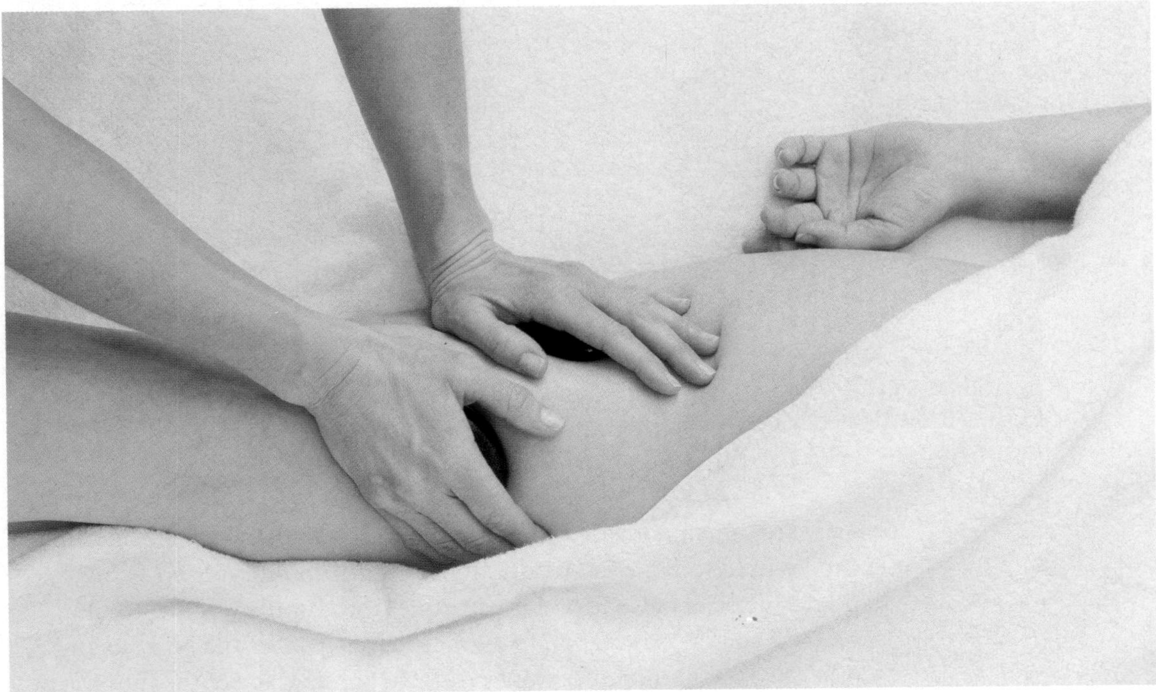

FIGURE 10–22

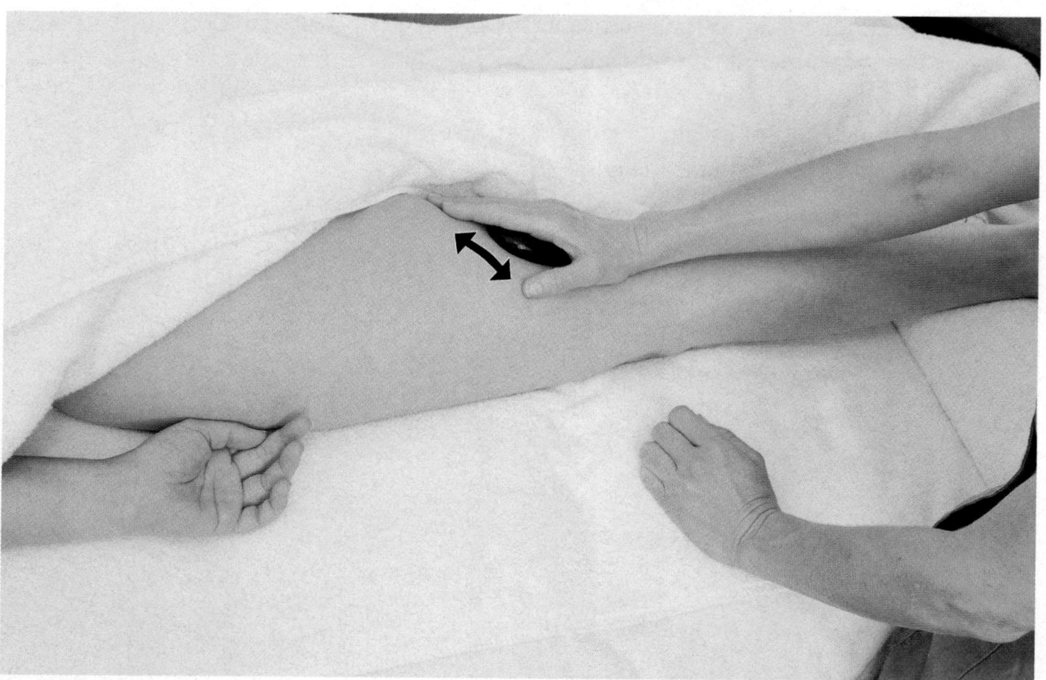

FIGURE 10–23

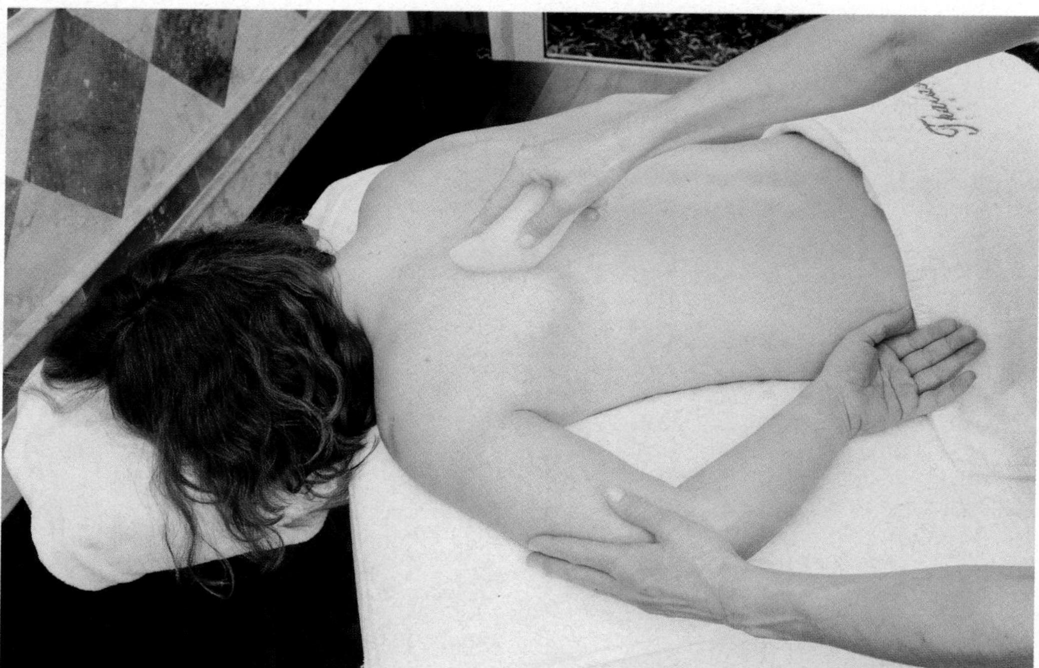

FIGURE 10–24

6. Trigger Points: Elongated rocks with more protuberant edges and tips can be used to hone in on adhesions, trigger points, and pressure points. They are also ideal for use under the scapula (Figure 10–24).
7. Transferring Stones: When moving from one part of the body to another or transitioning from one stroke to another, make the movement of the stones over the body graceful and flowing.

8. Face Massage: Use extra small stones to work on the face, applying gliding, gentle kneading, and light pressure to the temples and jaw muscles.
9. Exchanging Stones: As the stones cool during massage, trade them for heated ones from the warmer.
10. Cold Stones: Chilled stones can be used for any of the massage moves noted above, using the same techniques but moving more slowly. They can also be left in one position to cool the tissues after hot stone massage to the area.

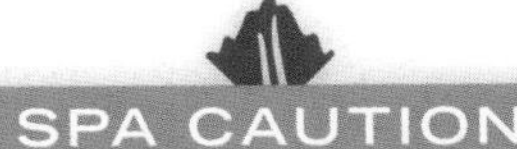

SPA CAUTION

Avoid placing stones on bony prominences such as spinous processes, medial epicondyles, malleoli, and other spots where very little tissue covers the bones. These areas heat more rapidly than others. In addition, applying pressure with stones on them could cause bruising. Always ask the client if the stone temperature is comfortable, especially the first time a stone is applied to an area. During the treatment, adjust temperature if needed by cooling stones down or inserting more layers of cloth between the skin and the stones.

Correct Body Mechanics for Stone Massage Application

When working with stones, it is especially important to use correct body mechanics in order to eliminate unnecessary wear on your hands, wrists, and entire body, thus keeping you healthy and prolonging your career. Whenever possible, it is best to allow the weight, shape, smoothness, and heat of the stones to do the work rather than overwork your own body. In general, all the same concerns facing therapists while performing a Swedish massage are present during a stone massage session as well. Therapists need to keep their knees bent while performing massage with the stones and avoid excessive bending at the waist to save their backs from undue strain. It is also important to employ two specific maneuvers, pinning and flipping, that are specific to stone massage.

Pinning Stones

As stone therapy instructor Bruce Baltz notes, it is important to "pin the stone to the body," which means that the palm of the therapist should close over the stone and hold it to the client's body, as shown in Figure 10–25. In contrast,

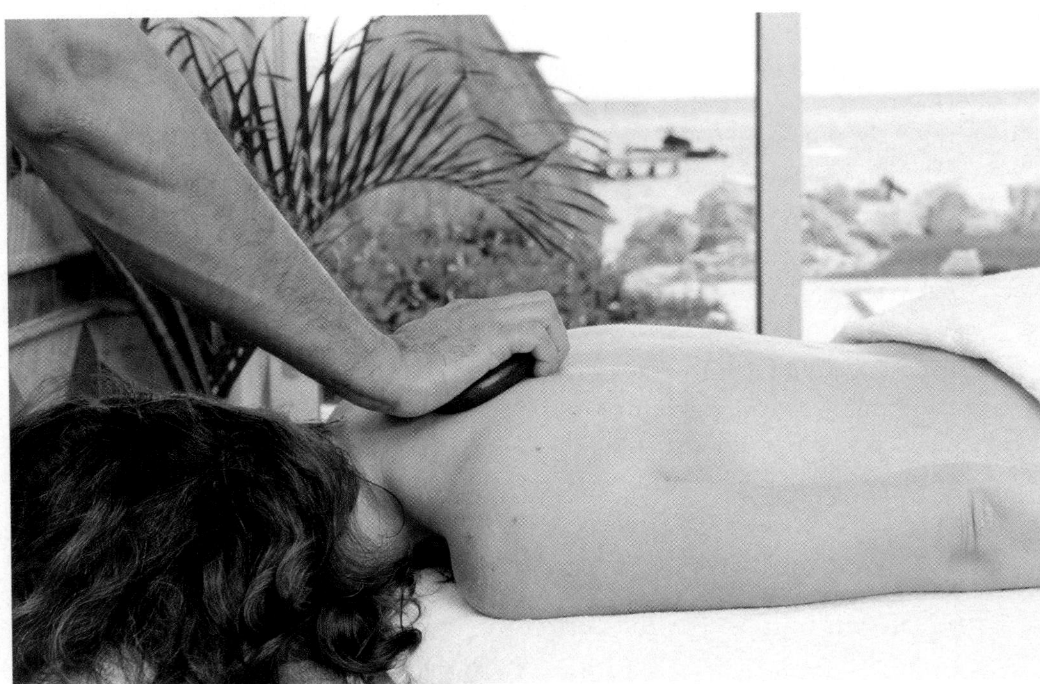

FIGURE 10–25 Correct: pinning the stone to the body.

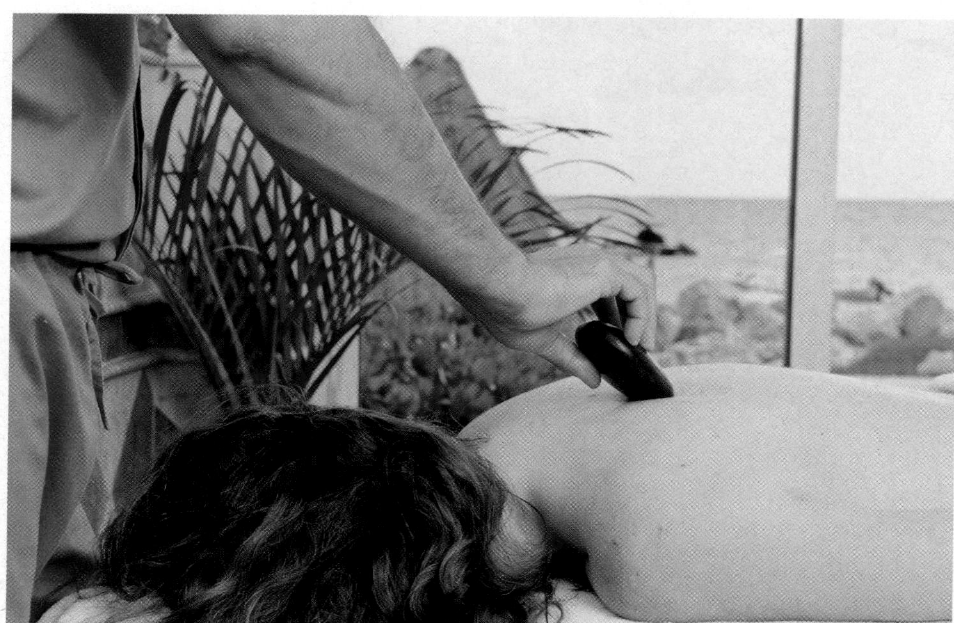

FIGURE 10–26 Incorrect: Grasping the stone with fingers puts strain on therapists' hands.

SPA TIP

To ensure that temperatures are not too high, hold stones in your own hands and touch them against the skin of your inner forearm before placing them on your client's body. When you feel the temperature is comfortable, apply the stone and remember to ask for feedback. Even though the temperature may be good for you, the client may find it too hot. Each client has his own comfort range.

grasping the stone with fingers, as shown in Figure 10–26, puts extra stress on the hands and joints, potentially causing injury over time.

Flipping Stones

Frequently flipping the stones, especially when they are first removed from the water and are at their hottest, saves therapists' hands and provides the optimum temperature level to clients. This technique should be practiced extensively until it becomes second nature. Stones are flipped by quickly turning them over at the end of a massage stroke when they are lifted momentarily from the body (Figure 10–27). This lowers the stone's temperature because it passes through the air and immediately starts to cool through convection. At the same time, this maneuver places the warmer side of the stone toward the client.

Stone Massage Treatment

A complete stone massage treatment can take many different forms and is infinitely adaptable to the style and intention of the therapist applying it. In addition, spas can customize the service by adding modalities and changing auxiliary ingredients such as the oils used. Though the stone treatments at spas vary in many respects, they also have elements in common, of course, all of which are featured in the generic stone massage treatment outlined in this section. Once you have mastered the basics offered here, you can expand your skills through further learning in workshops or at the spas where you work, which will train you in the customized version of stone massage they offer their clients.

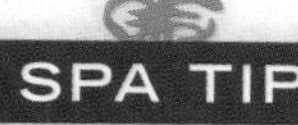

SPA TIP

A great deal of stress will be put on your wrist if it stays in a hyper-extended position while holding a stone during the treatment, so be careful to vary the angle of your wrist as often as possible.

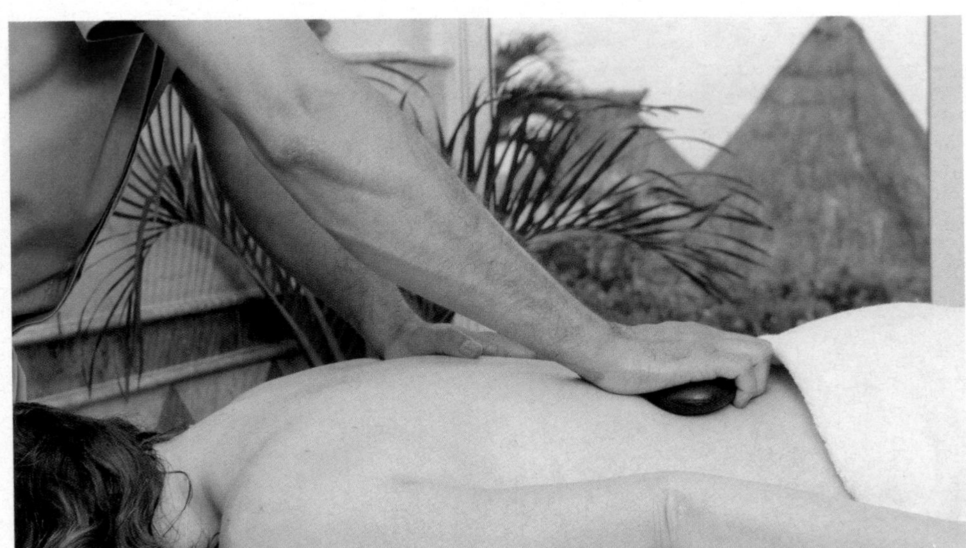

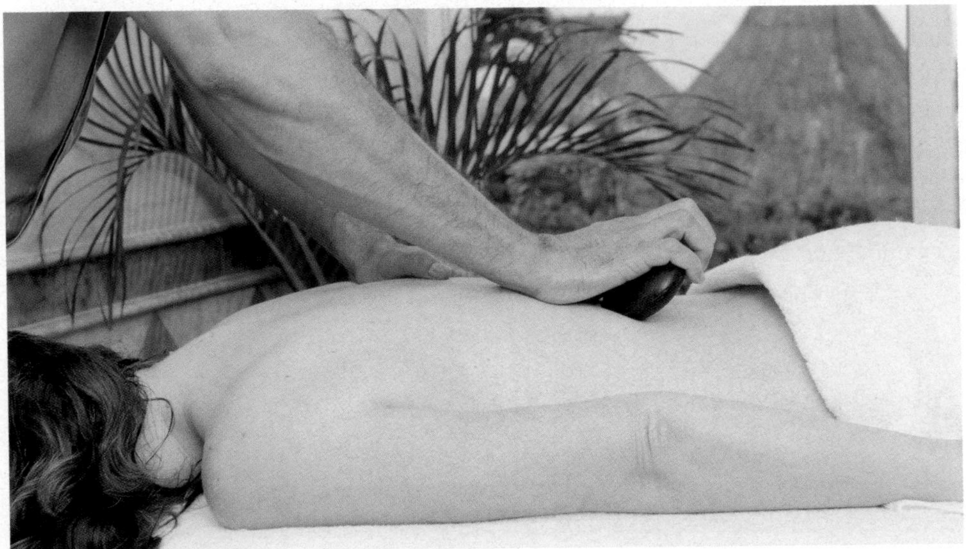

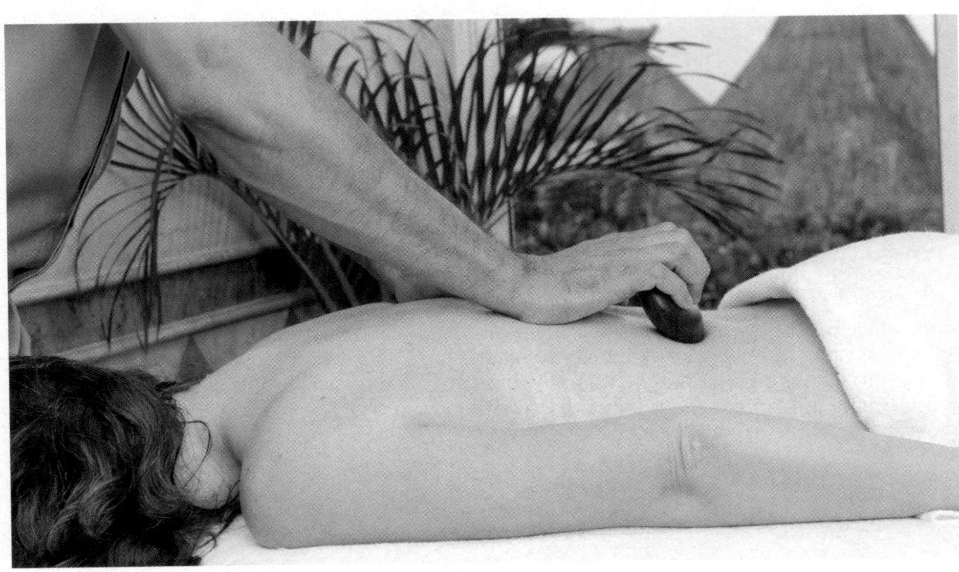

FIGURE 10–27 A–C Flipping stones at the end of massage strokes helps cool therapists' hands.

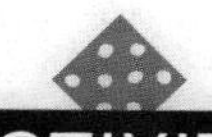

ACTIVITY

Practicing Safety Techniques, Body Mechanics, and Basic Maneuvers

Before attempting a full stone massage routine, spend time practicing the basic stone placement and massage techniques at a leisurely pace under your instructor's close supervision, keeping safety foremost in your mind as you become familiar with the stones.

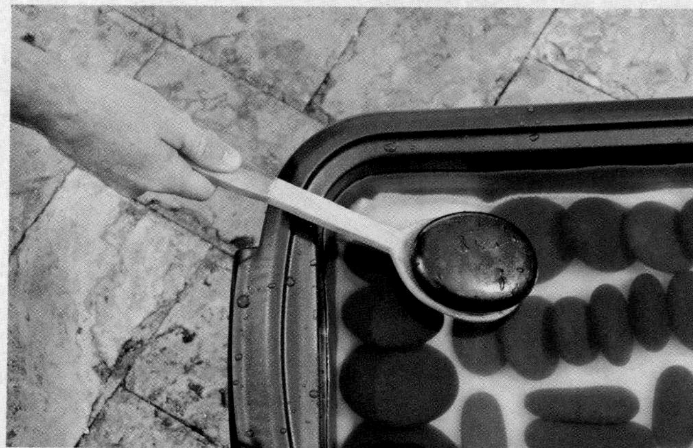

FIGURE 10–28

- Warm a set of stones to the low end of the usage range, approximately 110°F to 120°F, using a thermometer to check the temperature.
- Practice removing stones with a spoon, mesh net, or rubber gloves and laying them on a towel to dry (Figure 10–28). Note how long the stones need to be out of the water until they can be comfortably kept in contact with the skin of your own inner forearm.
- Practice the stone placement and stone massage maneuvers described above one at a time on different areas of the body until you become comfortable performing them.
- Practice locating chakras and placing gem stones.
- Receive the same maneuvers from your partner so you will know what the stones feel like.
- At the end, cleanse and sanitize the stones, along with the equipment you have used.

TREATMENT: STONE MASSAGE	
Wet Room/Dry Room	dry room
Table Setup	sheet to cover table, towels for draping
Treatment Duration	60 to 90 minutes
Needed Supplies	stone heating unit, approximately 40 basalt stones in a variety of shapes and sizes, optional 7 chakra stones and 1 crystal wand, bolster, sheet, draping sheet, or towel, 3 hand towels, massage oil
Contraindications	any condition where general massage is contraindicated, surgery in which nerves have been cut causing loss of feeling, nerve damage, or neuropathy (avoid specific areas), use of prescription medications that are adversely affected by heat applications, infectious skin disease, rashes, lesions, or any skin conditions aggravated by heat; caution for: pregnancy except by practitioners certified in pregnancy massage and never in the first trimester, heart disease, susceptibility to blood clots, high blood pressure, circulatory problems, diabetic peripheral neuropathy, extreme obesity, which puts a strain on the heart, metal implants, cancer, immediately after chemotherapy or radiation, Parkinson's disease
Draping	regular massage draping, with extra-thick draping over certain areas where larger hot stones are left in place

(Continued)

TREATMENT: STONE MASSAGE	
Treatment Order	Stone massage is performed after exfoliation and body wraps. Exception: Done without oil, hot stones can be applied prior to body wraps to open pores, then cold stones applied after wrap to pull excess heat out of body and close pores. Finish with lotion or cream application.
Safety, Sanitation Issues, & Clean-Up	Clean stones with fresh water and antibacterial soap, and rinse. Wipe excess oil off with alcohol. At the end of each day, empty heating bin, remove and clean all stones, spray bin with alcohol and dry, and replace stones in bin. Before next treatments begin, refill, add sterilizing solution, and heat. Exercise caution with hot stones; always use thermometer and ask for client feedback. Be careful with water spills on floor.
Body Mechanics & Self-Care	All body mechanics rules for massage therapy apply, plus the following: vary wrist angles, flip stones to save hands from heat, and pin stones to body to relieve pressure on fingers.
Product Cost	only the cost of oil, cleansers, and electricity to heat stone sets, which cost $100 to $300 with warmers
Treatment Price	ranges from $70 to $190, typically $125
Physiological Effects	thermal effects of heat and cold, energetic effects of electromagnetic fields and piezoelectricity, and mechanical effects of massage and pressure
Pregnancy Issues (information provided by Elaine Stillerman, LMT, author and developer of MotherMassage)	Avoid during the first trimester and use only on the back during the second and third trimesters. This requires use of pillows and cushions to permit safe and comfortable prone positioning. Legs, hip, and pelvic regions should also be avoided. Stones should never be left on the client, but used for stroking purposes. Monitor the temperature of the hot stones; some pregnant clients may prefer cold stones.

Stone Massage Preparation

1. Place sanitized stones in a stone warmer, then cover with water and heat to 110°F to 140°F. Use a thermometer to determine water temperature. The type and number of stones are listed in Table 10–2.
2. Place cold stones in freezer or ice water.
3. Prepare massage table with sheet and towels for draping.
4. Arrange warmer, chilled stones, and massage oil near table for ease of use during treatment. Place a hand towel near the warmer for drying stones as they are taken out.

Do not use a microwave to heat the stones because basalt has traces of iron and magnetite in it, and this may affect the operation of microwaves and could potentially be dangerous.

TYPE OF STONE	# IN SET	SHAPE	USAGE
Extra-Large	1	oval, flattish, heavy, the largest stone in the set	These stones are typically used on the abdomen or solar plexus while the client is supine and the sacrum when the client is prone.
Large	8	rounded, fills up therapistís hand	These stones are used for massaging larger muscles groups such as the quadriceps, hamstrings, gluteals, and pectorals.
Medium	8	rounded	These stones are used on smaller muscle groups such as the hands, arms, and lower legs.
Small	8	rounded	These smaller stones are used to massage delicate or bony areas such as the forehead, neck, and face.

TABLE 10–2 Types of Stones Used for Massage. *(Continued)*

TYPE OF STONE	# IN SET	SHAPE	USAGE
Spinal	8	round but flatter than the other body stones	These stones are placed beneath the erector spinae when the client is lying supine, or on top of the erector muscles when the client is prone.
Neck	1	large, oblong, thick	This stone is used as a pillow of sorts under the occipital area when the client is supine.
Trigger Point	4	oblong, slightly sharper ends and edges	These stones can be used as massage tools on meridians, trigger points, and adhesions.
Contour	2	oblong, medium-sized	These stones are placed on the soles or in the palms for a sense of comfort and to relieve minor aches in those areas.
Toe	8	extremely small, flat	These stones are placed between the toes and removed once they cool down.
COLD STONES			
Small	2	small, oval and flattish	These stones are used on the face and more delicate areas to soothe and cool. Two especially small stones are often reserved for use on the eyelids, usually atop a protective cloth.
Large	2	same size as small basalt stones but usually flatter	These stones are used for trigger points, to cool down overheated areas and create contrast therapy effects.
CRYSTALS AND SEMI-PRECIOUS STONES			
Crystal Wand	1	approximately six inches long, oblong	This, often quartz, crystal stone is not heated but rather used to align and balance clientsí subtle energies. Sometimes called an attunement wand.
Chakra Stones	7	small irregular nuggets	Semi-precious, unheated stones which are placed on clientsí chakras to affect subtle energies.

TABLE 10–2 Types of Stones Used for Massage.

Stone Massage Procedure

1. As the client enters, instruct her to lie beneath the top drape in a supine position, then leave the room as she prepares herself.
2. Upon reentering, set a therapeutic intention for yourself and your client, and begin the treatment by removing and drying the stones to be used for the spinal layout from the warmer.
3. Have your client hold the drape against her chest while sitting up. Arrange stones in a pattern on the table where the erector spinae muscles rest, from the sacrum up to C7, cover stones with a hand towel, and have your client lie back on the stones (Figure 10–29). Avoid placing stones directly beneath the client's spine.

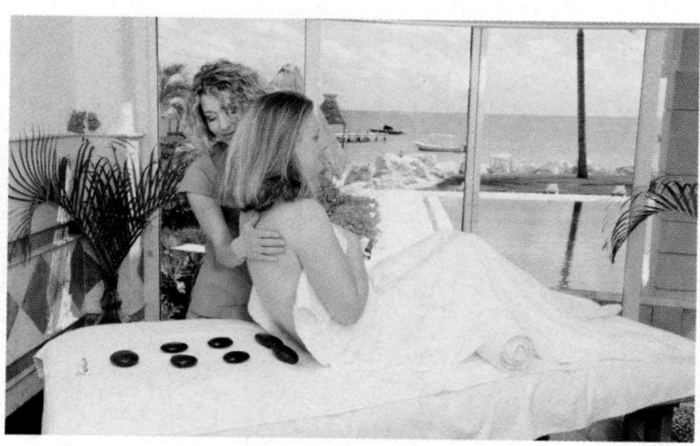

FIGURE 10–29

4. Place a rounded neck stone beneath the client's occipital ridge.
5. Place five large stones atop the chakra areas, over the blanket, including lower belly, belly, solar plexus, heart, and upper chest/throat. Remember to apply each stone while the client exhales. Bring stones into contact with your client's skin slowly and gradually. Communicate extensively with your partner regarding stone temperature and comfort.
6. Place the extra-small flat stones between the toes (Figure 10–30).

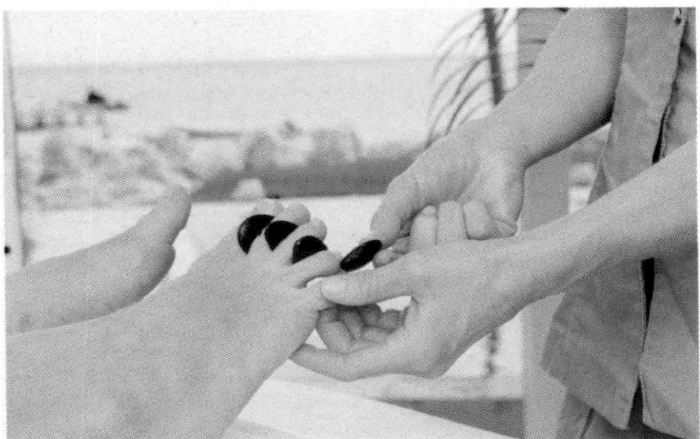

FIGURE 10–30

7. Apply massage oil to the left hand, arm, and shoulder with effleurage strokes, then use two medium-sized stones to apply massage to the area (Figure 10–31). Gliding, deep tissue, friction, and trigger point maneuvers can be applied with the stones to specific areas as you see fit.

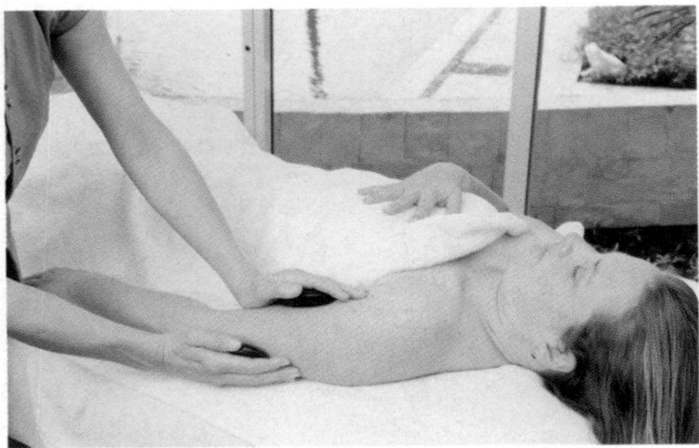

FIGURE 10–31

8. Tuck a medium stone beneath the left shoulder (Figure 10–32).

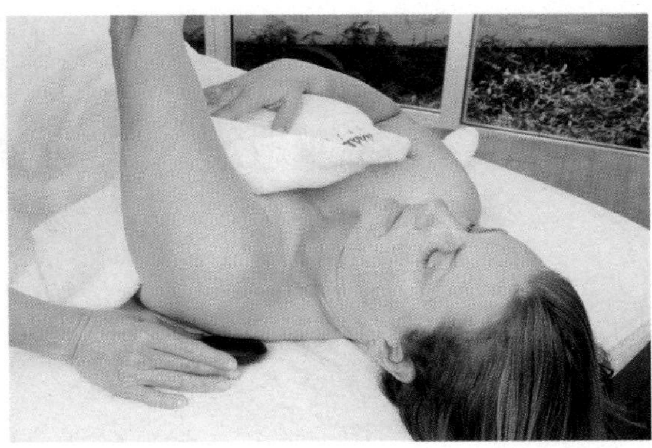

FIGURE 10–32

9. Repeat massage on the right hand and arm, and tuck a medium stone beneath the right shoulder.
10. Sit at the head of the table. Removing the neck stone, apply a small amount of oil to the neck and face with effleurage movements, then use two small hot stones to work the areas (Figure 10–33). Circular pressure over the temples and jaw muscles is especially effective. Stones can also be used over hair to treat the scalp. You may replace the neck stone afterwards if the client feels comfortable with it placed beneath the occipital area.

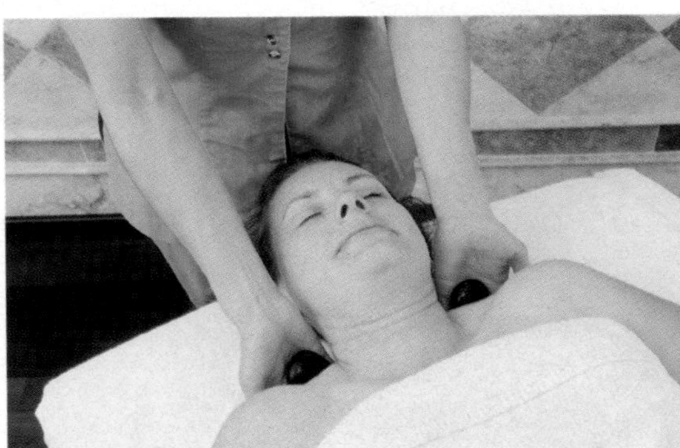

FIGURE 10–33

11. Use two small cold stones to apply effleurage over the face (Figure 10–34). Two extra-small cold stones may also be placed over the eyes, atop small protective cloth coverings.

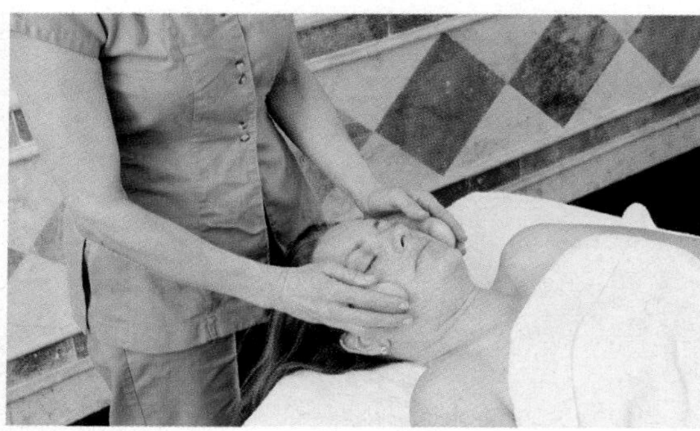

FIGURE 10–34

12. Remove stones tucked beneath the shoulders and stones between the toes.
13. Apply massage oil with effleurage strokes to the left leg.
14. Use two medium or large stones, depending on the size of the client, to massage the left foot and leg. Gliding, deep tissue, friction, and trigger point maneuvers can be applied with the stones to specific areas as you see fit (Figure 10–35).

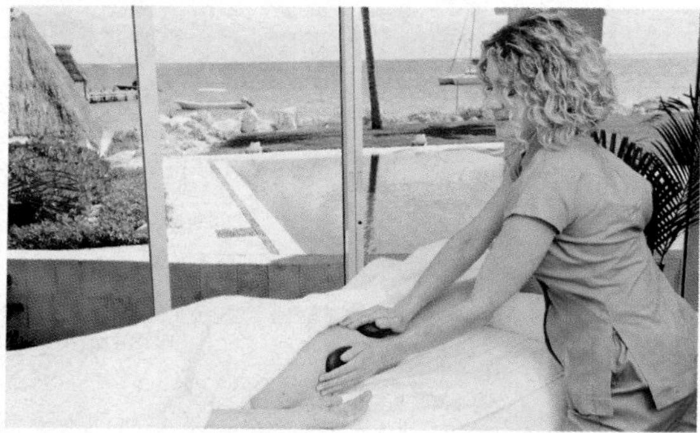

FIGURE 10–35

15. Tuck a medium stone beneath the left gluteal muscles (Figure 10–36).

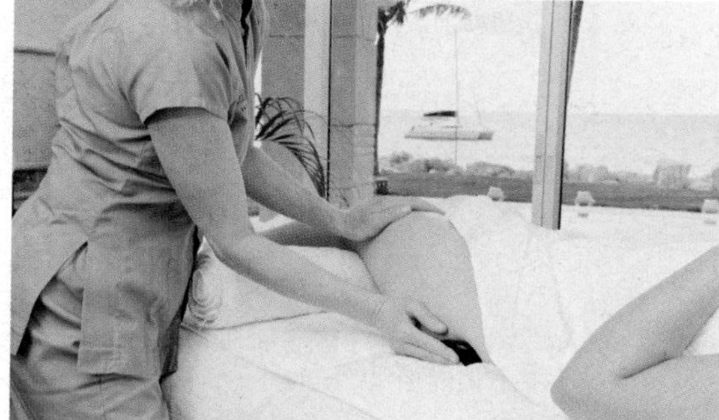

FIGURE 10–36

16. Repeat massage on the right foot and leg, and tuck a medium stone beneath the right gluteal muscles.
17. Click a medium stone against each of the stones placed on the chakra sites to stimulate the effects of piezoelectricity. Remove each chakra stone after clicking it.
18. Remove the stones tucked beneath the gluteal muscles. If small stones were placed on the eyes, remove them now. Then, ask the client to sit up, holding draping in place, while you remove spinal layout stones. Ask the client to turn over, holding the draping sheet over her body as she turns over.
19. Place an extra-large warm stone on the sacrum, atop a hand towel (Figure 10–37).

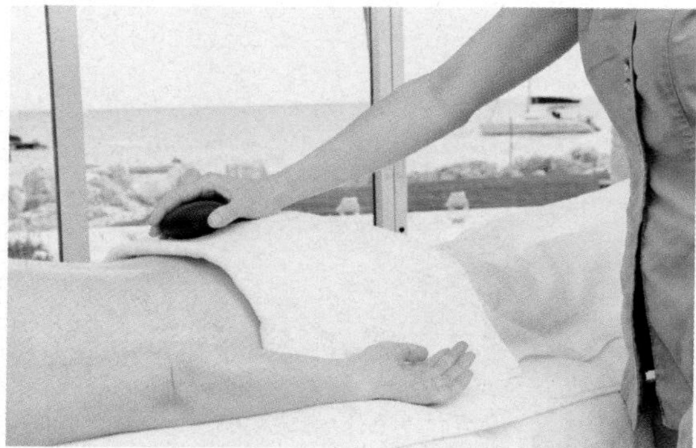

FIGURE 10–37

20. Apply massage oil with effleurage strokes to the back.
21. Run a large stone or contour stone over the back and down the client's left arm, leaving it in her palm as you continue other maneuvers (Figure 10–38). Repeat for the right arm.

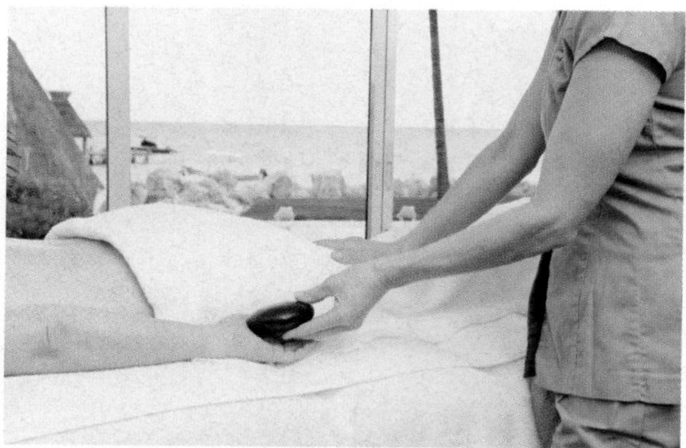

FIGURE 10–38

22. Tuck two medium-sized stones, one beneath each shoulder, beneath the anterior portion of the deltoid muscles.

23. Use two large stones to massage the back, using gliding, deep tissue, friction, and trigger point maneuvers as you see fit (Figure 10–39). Exchange the stones for warmer ones if needed.

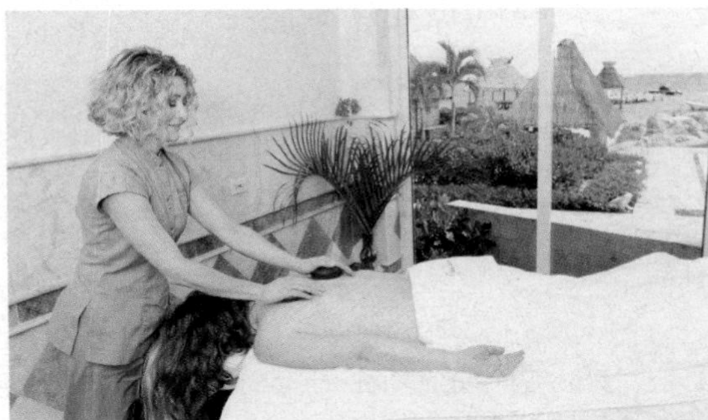

FIGURE 10–39

24. Apply massage oil to the left leg with effleurage strokes.
25. Use two medium or large stones, depending on the size of the client, to massage the left leg (Figure 10–40).

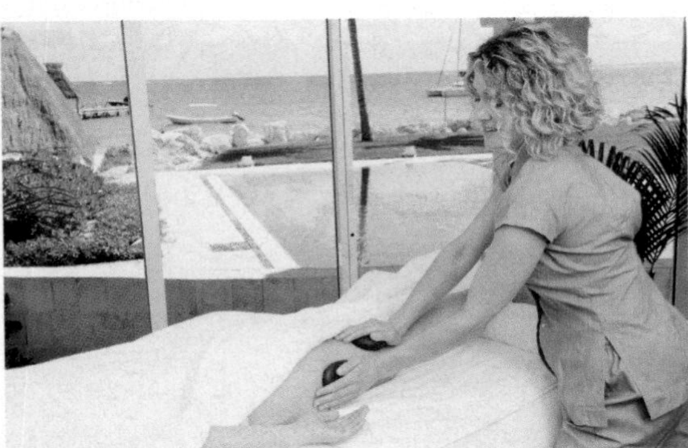

FIGURE 10–40

26. Repeat massage procedure to the right leg.
27. Remove stones from atop the sacrum, from the palms, and from beneath deltoid muscles.
28. Run two large cold stones in effleurage movements over the left leg, up the left side of the back, down the right side of the back, then down the right leg (Figure 10–41).

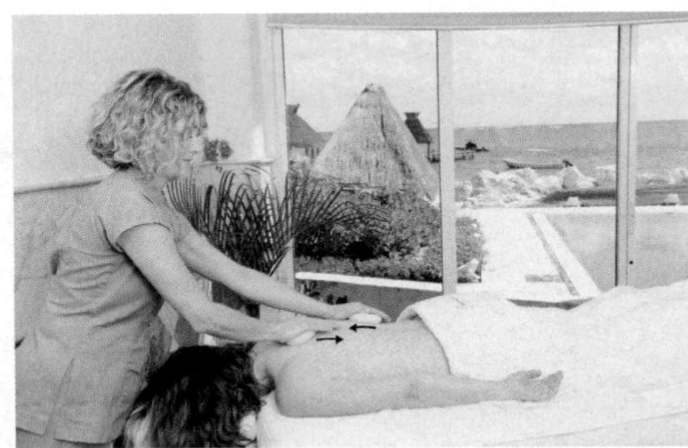

FIGURE 10–41

29. Hold the two cold stones on the soles of the feet for a few seconds, then gently pull them away.
30. Finish with light effleurage up over the backs of the legs and the back to finish with a light touch with a warm stone on the crown point atop the head (Figure 10–42).

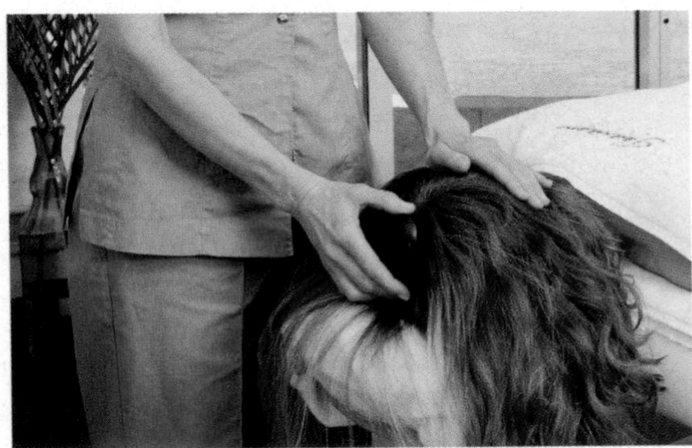

FIGURE 10–42

Stone Massage Cleanup

1. Sanitize stones and replace them in heating unit.
2. Change all table cover and draping linens.
3. Change the water and sanitize the warmer at the end of each day.

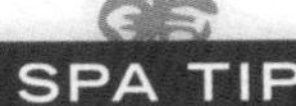

SPA TIP

You can create an interesting sensation for your clients by holding one hot stone stationary against the body while maneuvering a second stone in your other hand using a variety of massage techniques. After a minute, switch the stationary and moving hands. For a more intense contrast of sensations, use one hot stone and one cold.

SPA TIP

Use oil for stone massage, because lotions and creams form a viscous layer on the stones, cooling them more rapidly and making them more difficult to maneuver and clean. A basic carrier oil with chosen essentials added is a good choice.

SPA PROFILE

Bruce Baltz, founder of SpiriPhysical: Deep Tissue Healing, The Art of Stone Massage

Bruce Baltz, LMT, runs his own stone massage training company called SpiriPhysical in Miami, Florida. He teaches workshops across the nation, offers trainings for spa staffs, speaks at conventions, produces educational DVDs, sells stone-related products, and has developed a skin-care line with stone-based ingredients. In 1997, he took his first workshop with the founder of LaStone Therapy, Mary Nelson, in New York City, and he immediately became fascinated. "From the first day of that class, I asked Mary if I could write her deep tissue program," he remembers, "but it was premature at that point. I decided to work with the stones for a while, and about a year later she asked me to write the program. It was called Deep Tissue Healing at that time, which was a three-day class that included muscle testing and clinical application of the stones. "

Baltz worked with LaStone Therapy for about four years, developing their deep tissue program, which was the first specialty class that LaStone Therapy took on. He started SpiriPhysical in 2003 based on the knowledge he had gained from Mary Nelson and techniques he had developed himself. In addition, he forged a friendship with Manny Two Feathers, a man of Native American heritage whom Baltz describes as a spiritual stone healer. "Native American people work with what the Earth provides them," explains Baltz. "They use stones, among many other natural objects, in their healing practices. Manny taught me about the natural world and healing, and along the way he became a very good friend and mentor. He taught me about working with intention. And he understood the healing properties of stones and how to work with them."

Baltz pauses as he remembers his friend, who has passed away now. "Manny came to his understanding through his own spiritual connection to the world. That understanding prompted him to write books such as *Stone People's Medicine and My Road to the Sundance*. He would do stone readings for people, who were amazed at his ability to determine the nature of their problems. In spite of that, he never thought of himself as a clairvoyant, but rather as an interpreter. He called himself a 'stone interpreter,' and he read stones like some people read tarot cards. He had a set of stones with different figures on them—Kokopelli, man in maze, wolf, bear, and other animals—which he used in his interpretations.

"What Manny's work showed me is that the stones have an energy that can help people heal, and when therapists approach the work with the intention of honoring that energy, it takes their egos out of the way. Therapists' healing intentions should also inform their choice of the stones they are going to work with. I encourage people to seek out their own stones and see if they work for them. In general, we do know that the family of basalt stones hold heat better, and marble stones hold cold better, but apart from that, people should use their intuition when finding stones to work with."

As an instructor who shows therapists how to apply heated stones directly to the body, Baltz naturally emphasizes caution. "One of the major safety issues is working with proper equipment, making sure that your heating element is a stone heater and not a kitchen appliance. Most stone heaters have heavier wiring and grounded plugs. In case of any

(Continued)

SPA PROFILE

Bruce Baltz, founder of SpiriPhysical: Deep Tissue Healing, The Art of Stone Massage *continued*

potential lawsuits, insurance companies will not look favorably upon a heating unit that says turkey or ham on it. The average temperature in the stone heater should be kept near 120°F. At that level, most bacteria will not be able to survive. But with temperatures that high, you must be aware of how to apply stones safely to somebody's body so you do not burn them or hurt yourself. The heat must be introduced gradually so the body can get adjusted to the change.

"As my teaching evolved, I realized I needed to put much more emphasis on body mechanics," says Baltz. "This realization was born out of survival because I was hurting my own hands and wrists, but I wanted to keep working with the stones. So, I focused on three simple principles. First, it is important to vary the wrist angle as often as possible and work with both hands equally. Second, you need to be aware of where you are at all times while performing stone massage so you can change things about your body mechanics that are not optimal. And finally, I emphasize taking the shape of the stone with your entire hand and pinning it to the body, rather than holding onto it with your fingers."

Baltz teaches therapists and spa owners alike that stone massage is more than just another modality. "It's an extension of every spa modality that already exists," he says. "Aromatherapy, shiatsu, deep tissue, Swedish—all of them. Stones can be used within any treatment, as a minor adjunct or a major part. And spas can charge 15 to 20 percent more when stones are incorporated into treatments, increasing profitability. Also, they can potentially boost income by adding retail sales with products such as the SpiriPhysical skin care line that has granulated basalt and gem stone extract in it.

"In the end," says Baltz, "using the stones is all about healing. And we know the body heals through change. It doesn't heal through the norm. Change and recover, change and recover; that's how we feel better. That's all we're doing in any modality. Stones are the perfect medium to introduce that change through temperature, pressure and time."

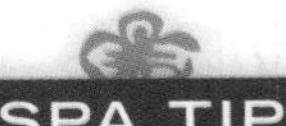

SPA TIP

Regarding the pressure and pace used during stone massage, expert Bruce Baltz says that in most situations, when using heated stones, firm pressure and faster movement of the stone will allow the client to accept greater temperature contrast. Half of the formula is true with the use of cool stones. The pressure will be firm but the pace will be much slower.

RESEARCH

Receive a stone massage at a local spa. Afterwards, write a one-page report about your experience. Include the following information:

1. *Did the spa have you fill out an intake form? What items relevant to heat and cold application were on it?*
2. *Did the therapist explain the treatment to you beforehand?*
3. *Were you comfortable with the treatment throughout, including draping, temperature, pressure, and massage techniques?*
4. *What aspect of the treatment did you like the best?*
5. *Were there any aspects of the treatment that you would change?*
6. *What was your overall impression of stone massage in general and your experience at this spa in particular?*

SPA TIP

When working with stones we have to take into consideration the client's preconceived conditioning to acceptance of temperature. With cold, they often have a preconceived notion of not liking it—it's a mental block. We have to then gradually introduce it through proper education and explain why we use cold. Psychologically, it may be a better idea to have the client see stones being removed from cold water, rather than a freezer, when first receiving a stone massage. Or, you can even remove the stones from the freezer early, before the client arrives, and have them sitting on a towel, so they are not too cold, until the client becomes accustomed to the temperatures used.

— Bruce Baltz

CONCLUSION

Stone massage is a popular part of the experience at many spas and has become an unofficial symbol of the entire spa industry. The image of stones aligned along a spine is shorthand for relaxation, wellness, tranquility, and reconnection to nature. The development of elaborate stone massage rituals that are featured on spa menus has led the public, and even some therapists, to conclude that the stones are a type of modality in and of themselves. What they really are, though, are tools. In the same way that a hydrotherapy tub or a loofah scrub pad are tools, not modalities, stones too are instruments in the spa therapist's arsenal. Used to deliver powerful **thermotherapy**, they are not only esthetically pleasing and exotic, but also deeply therapeutic. Spa therapists who hope to be well-rounded and effective need to be aware of these potent tools and skilled in their use.

thermotherapy

the use of heat to treat pain or improve wellness by applying heating pads, hot compresses, hot-water bottles, hot stones, etc. to promote circulation and relax muscles

REVIEW QUESTIONS

1. What are the three primary forms of rock, and from which are massage stones sourced?
2. What is the main factor that determines any particular basalt stone's heat-retaining capacity?
3. How would a therapist create "blood pumping" action through stone massage?
4. Which massage modality is most frequently used with stones?
5. What is the general temperature range for the use of hot stones? Why?
6. Why do therapists need to monitor the pressure they exert on clients more closely during stone massage than during Swedish massage?
7. Are varicose veins a contraindication for stone massage?
8. What are the two broad categories into which stone massage techniques can be broken down?
9. Describe a good way to keep from shocking clients when a hot stone or cold first comes into contact with the skin.
10. What does it mean to "flip" and "pin" massage stones? Why are these techniques used?

CHAPTER

11

Aromatherapy

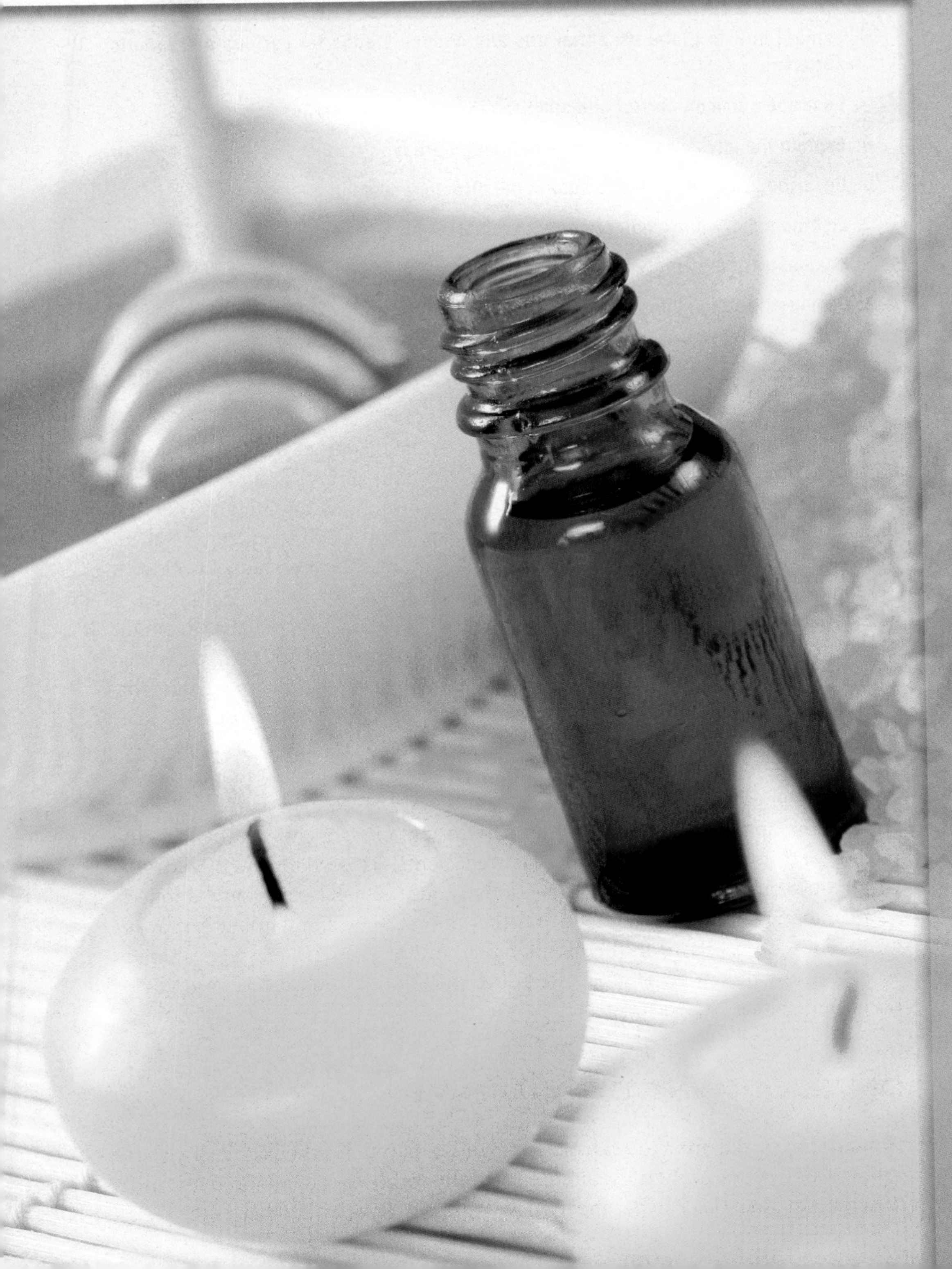

LEARNING OBJECTIVES

1. **Define aromatherapy and explain how it is used in spas.**
2. **Describe the historical development of aromatherapy.**
3. **List key figures in the development of aromatherapy and their contributions.**
4. **Explain what essential oils are and describe the various methods to produce them.**
5. **List popular essential oils used in spas, describing their properties and uses.**
6. **Explain how to blend essential oils and choose blends for various therapeutic purposes.**
7. **Describe common carrier oils and their therapeutic properties.**
8. **Explain the physiological effects of aromatherapy.**
9. **Describe how essential oils impact the olfactory system.**
10. **List the major contraindications for aromatherapy treatments.**
11. **Demonstrate the ability to perform aromatherapy massage.**
12. **Demonstrate the ability to perform aromatherapy baths, exfoliations, and wraps.**

INTRODUCTION

Aromatherapy can be defined as the use of essential oils processed from flowers, peels of fruits, leaves, grasses, needles, stems, wood, and roots through topical application, inhalation, and, rarely, ingestion to affect mood and improve health, beauty, and well-being. Essential oils add sensory depth and therapeutic value to many spa treatments. Some spas offer extensive aromatherapy treatment options on their menus, while others list just a basic aromatherapy massage, but it is rare for a spa to offer no aromatherapy treatments at all. At the very least, in small spas, aromatherapy candles or **diffusers** are used to impart some of the benefits of aromatherapy to guests even if no aromatherapy treatments are offered. From the moment a client walks in the door of a spa, the powerful effects of aromatherapy begin their work on the olfactory organs. See the "Spa Aromas for the Massage Room" section in Chapter 17 for more information about general ambient aromas in spas and their effects on clients.

diffusers

any device or technique that disperses the fragrance of essential oils into an area, either through heating, ventilation, nebulization (also called atomization), dilution in water, or other methods

Spa therapists need to understand why certain oils are chosen, their major effects, and how they work in specific treatments. This chapter will address these topics and give detailed instructions about the most commonly applied aromatherapy-based spa treatments. Further information about aromatherapy is available in books listed in the bibliography. In order to call oneself a trained aromatherapy practitioner, further training and study is required after graduation from massage school.

DEVELOPMENT OF AROMATHERAPY

Humans have used aromatic substances found in nature for thousands of years. People watched as animals gravitated naturally to beneficial compounds, and then followed their lead, experimenting with grasses, flowers, and plants through trial and error to find the ones that could soothe and heal, and to avoid those that could harm or even kill. Ancient Chinese, Persian, and Indian people made extensive use of aromatic plants, and the ancient Egyptians incorporated certain plant extracts, particularly cedar, into their embalming fluids to mummify the dead. The Egyptians, both men and women, also used oils as perfumes.

Several key figures throughout history are credited with advancing the study and use of essential oils. Dioscorides, a first-century Greek physician, pharmacologist, and botanist, was famed for writing his five-volume work, *De Materia Medica*, which described the medicinal uses of approximately 500 plants. His work remained the most authoritative book on herbs for many centuries. Avicenna, a Persian physician, scholar, and philosopher of the eleventh century, invented an advanced distillation method, incorporating a coiled pipe instead of a straight one, which allowed steam to cool down with increased efficiency. The medieval physician and alchemist Paracelsus focused on using plants as medicine and is said to have coined the term "essence" to describe the vital elements in nature. He was also among the first to assert that illness was the result of the body being attacked by outside agents rather than an internal imbalance of humors.

In modern times, the aromatherapy landscape was dominated by René-Maurice Gattefossé, a French chemist who worked in the early twentieth century. He originally focused on the aromatic value of essential oils in perfumery, but then switched his interest to their healing properties when he suffered an accident in his laboratory. After severely burning his hand, he immersed it in a vat of lavender oil and discovered that it healed much more quickly, and with less pain and scarring, than it normally would have. This led him to coin the term "aromatherapy" in a 1928 article, using the word to differentiate between the purely aromatic uses of oils and the curative uses that he experienced firsthand. His 1937 book *Aromathérapie: Les Huiles Essentielles Hormones Végétales* was eventually translated into English as *Gattefossé's Aromatherapy*, and it is still available today. From this time forward, the practice of aromatherapy has included an emphasis on the treatment of both emotional and physical conditions with essential oils.

Another seminal figure in modern aromatherapy was the Frenchman Jean Valnet, who became well-known after using essential oils to treat injured soldiers during World War II. He also wrote a book entitled *The Practice of Aromatherapy*.

Austrian biochemist Madame Marguerite Maury refined the use of aromatherapy through the twentieth century, prescribing essential oils as remedies for her patients. She was the first to recommend using essential oils in massage, as she recognized early on that the oils can be absorbed through the skin and travel through the body to affect distant organs and other tissues. Her book, *The Secret of Life and Youth*, greatly popularized aromatherapy.

In 1977, Englishman Robert B. Tisserand wrote the first aromatherapy book in the English language, entitled *The Art of Aromatherapy*. His work became widely known and eventually introduced thousands of people, including many massage therapists, to the practice and enjoyment of aromatherapy.

The way in which aromatherapy developed in modern times has led to a divide among practitioners. This divide is sometimes referred to as the French versus the British model of aromatherapy. Gattefossé is considered the father of the French model, which is more medically oriented and includes intensive use of full-strength oils, both externally and internally. Jean Valnet's use of essential oils in medical settings is another example of the French model of aromatherapy.

Many Definitions

Did You Know?

Aromatherapy is a word that can have a variety of slightly different definitions, depending upon whom you ask. Here, in the words of some authorities in the field, are a variety of explanations:

> "Aromatherapy is a caring, hands-on therapy which seeks to induce relaxation, to increase energy, to reduce the effects of stress and to restore lost balance to mind, body and soul."
>
> —Robert Tisserand

> "Aromatherapy is . . . the skilled and controlled use of essential oils for physical and emotional health and well being."
>
> —Valerie Cooksley

> "Aromatherapy can be defined as the controlled use of essential oils to maintain and promote physical, psychological, and spiritual wellbeing."
>
> —Gabriel Mojay

> "Aromatherapy is essentially an interaction between the therapist, client and essential oils, working together to bring forth the healing energy which will help the client regain their sense of well being and vitality."
>
> —Jade Shutes

Many physicians in Europe still use aromatherapy in this fashion today. The British model, on the other hand, is more spa-like. It is based on the work of Marguerite Maury and focuses on the use of diluted oils in full-body massage applications and other therapies. The type of aromatherapy practiced in North American spas is based mainly on the British model.

ESSENTIAL OILS

Essential oils are the heart of aromatherapy. They are exotic, expensive when compared with other oils, and, of course, aromatic. Therapists are naturally attracted to these powerful substances packaged so delightfully in tiny little bottles, and they enjoy sharing them with spa clients during treatments. It is important, then, for therapists to understand where these oils come from and how they are processed into the products used in spas around the world.

The word "essential" itself, as it relates to oils, does not mean "important" or "sorely needed," but rather comes from the root "essence" and means something more akin to "inner quality." Use of the term "oil" can be somewhat confusing, because most of these essences are very light and volatile, more like alcohols than oils.

wildcrafting

process of locating, identifying, and harvesting botanicals in their natural environment, with no planting or cultivation involved; said of plants found in nature and used as the basis of certain aromatherapy oils

Essential oils are sourced in two primary ways, either through cultivation (Figure 11–1) or through **wildcrafting**. The cultivation of plants such as lavender for the production of essential oils and floral waters has become big business practiced in many countries around the world. The international center for such cultivation can be found in and around the town of Grasse, in southeastern

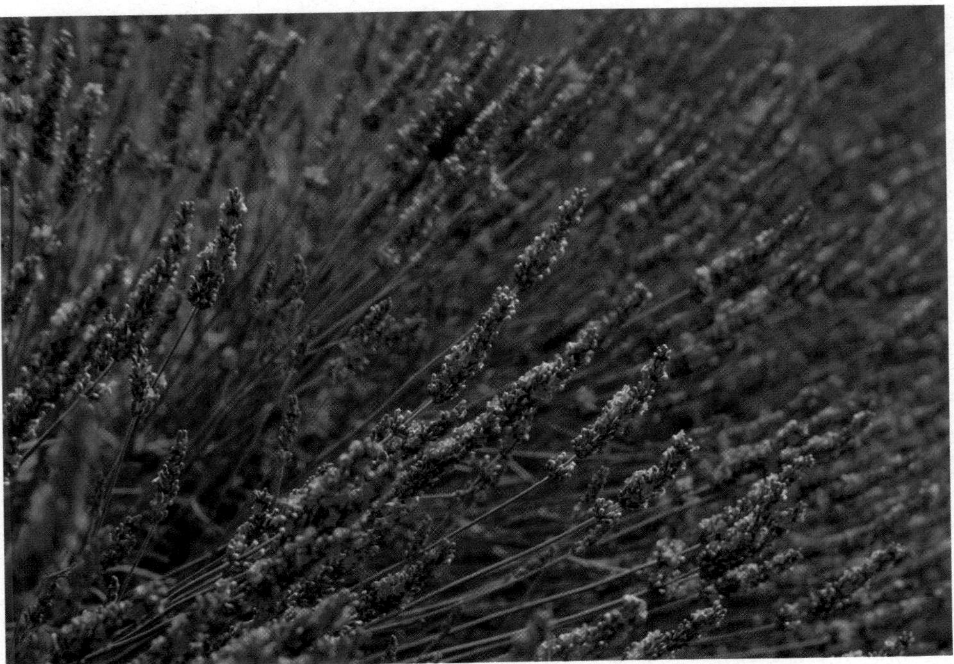

FIGURE 11–1 Lavender fields under cultivation for the production of essential oils.

France, which is known as the perfume capital of the world. The area produces 27 tons of jasmine annually and over two-thirds of all the natural aromas in France. This industry grosses Grasse businesses nearly a billion dollars a year.

Once the plant material has been harvested, it must be processed in order to produce essential oils. The three main processing techniques used to create essential oils are distillation, extraction, and cold pressing. Essential oils are derived from many different parts of plants, and a distinct processing method is appropriate for each part. See Table 11–1 for a list of where each oil comes from and popular processing methods used to produce the oils used in spas today.

All essential oil extraction methods have their advantages and disadvantages, and all can produce oils of good quality, as long as the original plant material is sourced appropriately and extracted skillfully. Some manufacturers cut corners, however, and produce lower-grade oils through dilution or poor plant quality. The only way to tell absolutely if an aromatherapy oil is pure or not is through a range of analytical tests, including **thin-layer chromatography** (TLC), **infrared analysis** (IR) and **gas chromatography/mass spectrometer** tests.

thin-layer chromatography

technique used to separate mixtures and identify compounds present in a given substance, including essential oils

infrared analysis

a spectrometric technique for analyzing the chemistry of materials, including essential oils, by measuring specific wavelengths of light energy

gas chromatography/ mass spectrometer

a method that identifies different substances, including essential oils, by analyzing its molecules

Steam Distillation

Of the several distinct methods of distillation employed to extract essential oils, steam distillation is the most popular. In this technique, heat produces steam that passes over the plant material, causing globules of oil in the plant to burst and the oil to evaporate, lifting volatile chemicals and aromatic compounds away into a condenser which chills the steam, forming a liquid combination of water and oils. The watery part of this combination is known as a **hydrosol**, and what's left floating on top of the water is the essential oil, which is then separated.

hydrosol

water infused with aromatic compounds that condenses after distillation of plant materials; essential oils float atop this water and are removed; also called floral water or herbal water

PART OF PLANT USED	ESSENTIAL OIL	POPULAR PROCESSING METHODS
Berries	allspice, juniper	carbon dioxide extraction steam distillation
Seeds	anise, celery, cumin, nutmeg oil	carbon dioxide extraction steam distillation
Bark	cassia, sassafras	solvent extraction
Wood	camphor, cedar, rosewood, sandalwood, agarwood	water distillation hydrodiffusion
Rhizome	ginger	carbon dioxide extraction
Leaves	basil, bay leaf, sage, eucalyptus, lemongrass, melaleuca, patchouli, peppermint, pine, rosemary, spearmint, tea tree, thyme, wintergreen	water and steam distillation
Resin	frankincense, myrrh	solvent extraction steam distillation
Flowers	chamomile, clary sage, clove, geranium, hyssop, jasmine, lavender, marjoram, orange, rose, ylang-ylang	steam distillation solvent extraction
Peel	bergamot, grapefruit, orange, tangerine	cold pressing
Root	valerian	steam distillation hydrodiffusion

TABLE 11–1 Parts of Plants Used for Various Essential Oils.

still

specialized piece of equipment, consisting of a vessel into which plant materials and heat are added and a device that is used for cooling the resulting steam, used in distilling essential oils

floral water

see "hydrosol"

herbal water

see "hydrosol"

nebulizer

a dispenser that turns liquids, such as essential oils, into a fine mist

hydrodistillation

method used to produce essential oils in which plant material is soaked in water and the mixture is heated to produce steam

In traditional steam distillation, an outside source of steam is piped into the distillation unit, or **still** (Figure 11–2), sometimes at high pressure. The steam passes through the plant material and into the condenser. Many practitioners with a purist bent believe that steam distillation is the best and only form of extraction that should be used. It is important to monitor the entire process carefully so the heat involved does not damage delicate plant materials.

After distillation, the hydrosol is not discarded. It contains the plant's water-soluble aroma and other essences. Sometimes also called a **floral water** or **herbal water**, this substance is used as a cooling spray or cleansing wash that contains some of the same beneficial properties as the essential oil. Some practitioners prefer to use the hydrosol rather than the essential oil because it is a milder version of the oil itself. Hydrosols can be used at 100 percent strength directly on the body and in **nebulizers** to create an aromatherapy-infused atmosphere for a spa. Some of the most popular hydrosols are lavender, rose, jasmine, orange, and other citruses. Hydrosols are chemically distinct from simple solutions in which essentials oils are diluted in water.

Water Distillation

In this method, plant matter is fully submerged in water and the resulting mixture is boiled, producing steam which contains aromatic compounds. This is the oldest method of distillation and is still used in areas with less advanced technologies available. This technique, also called **hydrodistillation**, is particularly appropriate for spices, wood, roots, nuts, and other tough materials.

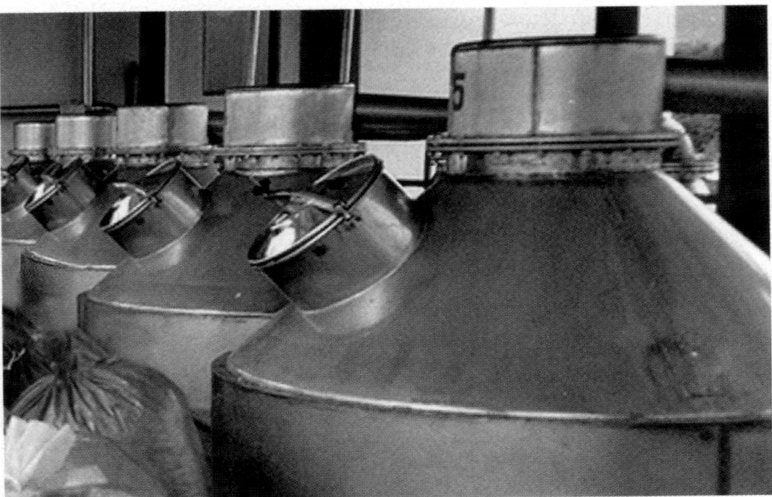

FIGURE 11–2 Steam distilling of essential oils.

Water and Steam Distillation

In this method, water is boiled beneath plant matter, which is suspended above it. Steam passes through the plant matter, releasing the aromatic compounds. The steam condenses and is collected and then separated into its hydrosol and essential oil components. This is a cruder method than pure steam distillation, in which the steam is introduced into a separate chamber containing the plant material. It can be compared to a kitchen steamer basket filled with herbs placed over a pot of boiling water.

maceration

softening by soaking or steeping a substance in a medium such as water or oil; used for making herbal-infused massage oils

extract

a solution obtained by steeping or soaking a substance in water or another medium such as oil

Maceration

Maceration is a technique that creates a type of infused oil, as compared to an essential oil. In the technique, plant material is soaked in a medium, often oil, heated, and then strained. The resulting liquid is a type of **extract** that contains some of the plant's aromatic compounds but in a different strength and consistency from essential oils produced in other manners. The resulting oil can be strained and used at full strength as a massage oil.

absolute

a highly concentrated aromatic extract derived from plant material which has undergone at least two extraction processes by chemical solvent and is free from waxes and other by-products; similar to a regular essential oil but more highly concentrated

Solvent Extraction

Using chemical solvents to extract essences from plant material yields a product similar to essential oils but more highly concentrated. A concentrated oil created in this manner is called an **absolute**. To create an absolute, the plant material is subjected to at least two extraction processes. First, the material is placed on a perforated tray and washed with a solvent, often hexane, which dissolves the aromatic compounds plus pigments and non-aromatic waxes. The solvent is then filtered out, and the remaining waxy substance, which contains the aromatic compounds, is called a **concrete**. The concrete is then further processed by warming it and stirring in a second solvent, usually ethanol,

concrete

waxy aromatic substance created through solvent extraction of plant materials, which can be further processed to form an absolute which absorbs the aromatic compounds in the wax. Finally, this alcohol solution must be frozen, then cold-filtered to precipitate out any remaining wax. After the concrete has been processed in this manner to create an absolute, another usable product is left behind called **floral wax**, which has a light scent and can be used in making candles, creams, and lotions in place of beeswax. The solvent extraction method is often used for delicate petals and blossoms that could be damaged through traditional steam distillation, such as jasmine, rose, lavender, and lotus. Absolutes are more concentrated and richly fragrant substances than essential oils and as such are prized by the perfume industry as well as aromatherapy practitioners.

floral wax

lightly floral scented solid by-product of the solvent extraction process, used in lotions, creams, and candle making

Carbon Dioxide Extraction

supercritical CO_2 extraction

processing of essential oils through the use of carbon dioxide under pressure; involves multiple distillation steps, first producing a total, then a select essential oil

Also called **supercritical CO_2 extraction**, this technique involves the use of carbon dioxide under pressure as a solvent to extract aromatic molecules and other compounds from plant material. The key to this process lies in compressing the carbon dioxide, which turns it from a gas into a semi-liquid, semi-gaseous state, called a *supercritical fluid*, which is then used to extract the compounds. The resulting extracted matter contains waxes, essential oils, and other compounds, which are then subjected to a secondary carbon dioxide processing at a lower temperature to separate the waxes from the essential oils. After extraction, the pressure is returned to normal, and the CO_2 simply evaporates into a gas once again. This means that CO_2 extraction leaves no chemical residues in the essential oils. In addition, the plant material does not need to be heated as much as during steam distillation, which means that almost all of the plant's compounds are preserved. Some practitioners feel that this produces oils with a richer, more intense scent, because more of the plant's compounds are released through this method.

As botanist and aromatherapy expert Nicholas James notes in his profile in this chapter, "This method of extraction has only been in commercial use relatively recently. It costs more because the equipment needed is more technical and expensive, and only a small percentage of commercially available essential oils are extracted in this manner." He also goes on to point out that there are two kinds of CO_2 extracts: **totals** and **selects**. "The totals contain all the oily components of the plant, not just the volatile aromatic oils. Totals can be extracted from many kinds of plants, both aromatic and non-aromatic, but these are not actually essential oils. Selects are totals that have been redistilled so that only the aromatic oils are captured." James and other aromatherapy experts view selects as bona fide essential oils, though some practitioners claim that only those oils extracted with traditional steam distillation should be considered true essential oils.

totals

a solid blend of waxes and essential oils that result from the first phase of CO_2 extraction

selects

essential oils that result after redistilling a total in the process of CO_2 extraction

Hydrodiffusion

hydrodiffusion

a distillation method of essential oil extraction where the steam is produced above the botanical material and then percolates down

Hydrodiffusion, also called *percolation*, is a relatively new method of essential oil extraction. In this technique, steam is sprayed through plant material suspended on a rack. The steam then condenses and cools, and the essential oils and hydrosol are separated. This process differs from regular steam distillation primarily in its positioning of the plant material below the steam source, rather

the essential oil drops are blended into the carrier oil in the presence of the client directly prior to beginning the treatment.

It is necessary to add the essential oils to the carrier oil drop by drop in order to achieve the correct **dilution**. See Table 11–3 for a list of common carrier oils and their properties. The dilution process is facilitated by aromatherapy bottles themselves, most of which are outfitted with tops that allow one drop at a time to escape when upturned (Figure 11–4). The correct number of drops is 12 to 15 for each ounce of carrier oil. Thus, for a pre-blended mixture, a therapist could use approximately 100 to 120 drops for an eight-ounce bottle of carrier oil.

dilution

a diluted solution; in the case of aromatherapy this refers to essential oils diluted in a base of a carrier oil

sebum

natural oily secretion of the skin, secreted through sebaceous glands

CARRIER OIL	PROPERTIES
Almond, sweet	One of the favorite carrier oils for aromatherapy blends, sweet almond oil is light, non-greasy, and beneficial for all skin types. A favorite with aromatherapists, it blends well with essential oils and has good absorption properties. Contains both oleic and linoleic acid, vitamins A and B, copper, and iron.
Apricot kernel	A smooth, light, soothing oil containing natural vitamin E for all skin types, this oil is especially beneficial for sensitive, dry, inflamed, or mature skin.
Avocado	Often used as an addition to other carrier oils at 10% to 25% strength, this oil moisturizes the skin and so is particularly suited for clients with dry dehydrated skin.
Borage	This oil is a rich source of essential fatty acids.
Calendula	This oil has healing and soothing properties and so is recommended for skin infections, wounds, rashes, bites and inflammations, and scars.
Camellia	Used by Asian women for many years, this oil moisturizes and nourishes skin and hair.
Evening Primrose	Never used as the only carrier oil but rather mixed with others, evening primrose is rich in vitamins and minerals to nourish dry, devitalized skin.
Grapeseed	Light, slightly astringent, odorless, and thinner than almond oil, grapeseed oil absorbs more quickly into the skin and leaves no greasy residue. Appropriate for all skin types.
Hazelnut	Rich in oleic and linoleic acid, hazelnut is particularly recommended for oily skin because it regulates **sebum**.
Jojoba	A liquid wax rather than an oil, usually added to other carrier oils, jojoba is non-greasy and nourishes skin, scalp, hair, and nails as it closely resembles the body's skin oils.
Olive	Olive oil has a strong aroma of its own and may overpower a blend if it is not diluted with other carrier oils, often at 10% strength. It helps retain the skin's own moisture and is an excellent natural skin softener.
Rosehip Seed	Rich in natural plant fatty acids, rosehip seed oil nourishes damaged skin such as scars and burns.
Safflower	Particularly appropriate for sensitive skin and a favorite of many aromatherapists, safflower is light, nearly clear, and does not feel greasy. It absorbs well and washes out of sheets easily. It is good for aromatherapy baby massage.
Sesame	A rich, softening oil for all skin types, sesame oil is also used extensively in Ayurvedic treatments.
Sunflower	Supplying more vitamin E than any other vegetable oil, in addition to vitamins A and D, sunflower oil is easily absorbed into the skin, softening and moisturizing it.
Wheat Germ	Thick and rich in natural vitamins A, B, D, and especially E, as well as proteins and lecithin, wheat germ oil is an antioxidant that is sometimes added to other carrier oils at 15% strength in order to extend their shelf life naturally.

TABLE 11–3 Carrier Oils for Aromatherapy Massage.

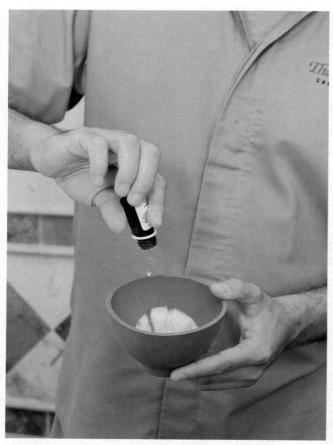

FIGURE 11–4 Essential oils are added to a carrier oil drop by drop.

The use of carrier oils is extremely common in aromatherapy because it is a general rule not to apply essential oils to the skin **neat**, or undiluted. Essential oils may be used undiluted in a diffuser or for other inhalation purposes, but for topical use they are seldom at full strength. Though several oils are safe to use neat on the skin under certain circumstances, it is recommended that only highly trained aromatherapy specialists attempt to do so. Note: The aromatherapy wrap protocol in this chapter calls for very small dabs of neat oils to be applied to the skin on a few specific spots only, which is safe when using the essential oils found in spas. Some aromatherapy practitioners believe it is better to treat clients first with a weaker dilution of essential oils and work up to a total of approximately 2 percent essential oil to 98 percent carrier oils. When treating smaller targeted areas of greater muscle tension, a slightly stronger dilution may be used. Weaker dilutions approximately one-third the strength used for adults should be used for children under twelve. The younger the child is, the more diluted the essential oils should be. Also, older people with delicate skin should use oils at approximately half the strength of the normal adult dilution. Simply inhaling a single essential oil or a blend of oils, rather than applying them topically, is safe in all cases. However, prolonged inhalation of certain oils such as clary sage, jasmine, patchouli, and ylang ylang can be overpowering and lead to headaches. Also, oregano, thyme, pine, spruce, and clover need to be used with care as they are quite strong.

neat

by itself, at full strength; said of 100 percent pure essential oils that have not been blended with a carrier oil or diluted in any other way

The choice of carrier oil can be equally as important as the essential oils used in a blend. As you can see in Table 11–3, each oil has properties that make it appropriate for specific purposes. Some are especially beneficial for revitalizing dry or weathered skin. Some have a lightness that makes them glide especially smoothly over the skin during massage. Others have a slight aroma of their own, which must be taken into account when using them to create blends. No

SPA TIP

Measuring essential oil blends can be tricky because they are sometimes counted in milliliters, other times in drops, and still other times in ounces. We sometimes confuse the three measurement systems. In order to translate most directions from drops to mL to ounces, it is usually sufficient to simply remember the following two basic facts.

- 1 mL of essential oil is between 20 and 25 drops.
- There are 29.5 mL in 1 ounce.

matter which oil is used, it is important to ensure freshness. Carrier oils can go rancid over time, especially if they are not stored in a cool, dry place. In addition to carrier oils, essentials can also be blended into lotions and creams. Certain of these do not readily absorb the oils and must be warmed appropriately to create an **emulsion** that will work for massage. In all cases, stir or gently swirl the drops of essential oil into the medium rather than shaking.

When blending them, essential oils are customarily placed into one of three categories for easy description. **Top notes** are stimulating and uplifting, and their fragrance is strong but lasts just a few hours once it is out of the bottle. **Middle notes** last longer and are potent in their therapeutic effects on the body. They add body and balance to the blend but do not have as strong a fragrance as the **base notes**, which last the longest and are often heavy, sweet-smelling, and calming. The rich fragrance from base notes lasts a long time and can help slow down evaporation of the top and middle note oils. Table 11–2 lists which note is predominant for many common essential oils used in spas. Note that some essential oils could be considered on the border between top and middle, or middle and base. Quantifying the note of a particular essential oil is a subjective business, and as such should be left open to some artistic license.

Certain oils, when blended, augment and refine the effects of aromatherapy treatments. In this sense, a blend of oils is more than the sum of its parts, and to reflect that, a therapeutic mixture of essential oils is given a special name. Aromatherapists call it a **synergy**. An aromatherapy oil that is used alone, unblended, is called a **single note**. As a general rule, oils from the same botanical family that share certain chemical constituents blend well, but it is not necessary to know the makeup of each oil in order to blend them effectively and create an effective synergy. Those oils that smell good when blended are usually a good match. Therapists and clients alike have created therapeutic blends using their noses and intuition alone. Certain essentials, especially jasmine, rose, and lavender, seem to blend easily with most other oils to create pleasant fragrances. Other combinations are not so pleasant, and this is immediately noticeable when they are blended.

emulsion

a mixture of two liquids that do not blend together well, such as oil and water; essential oils and massage creams/lotions, when mixed together, form emulsions, often requiring the application of additional heat in order to blend successfully

top note

an essential oil used in a blend, usually quite volatile, that dissipates quickly and is stimulating and uplifting in effect

middle note

an essential oil aroma that lasts longer than a top note, offering body to oil blends; aromas are usually warm and soft rather than strong

base notes

an essential oil used in a blend; fragrance lasts longer than middle or top notes and is heavy, sweet-smelling and calming

synergy

a therapeutic blend of essential oils

single note

one essential oil, unblended with any other essentials, used in an aromatherapy application

EFFECTS OF AROMATHERAPY

Essential oils add a sense of pleasure to the spa atmosphere with their delightful, exotic, and sometimes sensual aromas, but they also provide real therapeutic benefits. The effects created by essential oils can be broken down into two main categories: emotional and physiological. The emotional effects are created mainly through the process of inhalation, while the physiological effects are created through absorption of the oils through the skin, mucous membranes, and the digestive tract when the oils are ingested, though ingestion seldom if ever occurs in spas. Inhalation also creates some physiological effects when molecules of oil are absorbed into the lungs and enter the bloodstream through this route. The physiological effects most commonly reported for essential oils are diuretic, moistening, analgesic, antibacterial, anti-microbial, antiseptic, anti-viral, anti-inflammatory, antispasmodic, astringent, decongesting, and detoxifying.

SPA TIP

A Royal Oil

In the late 1600s, Anne Marie Orsini, the princess of Nerola, began to scent her gloves and her bath with the essential oil of the bitter orange tree. This soon became a popular fashion, and since that time the name of *Neroli* has been used to describe this oil.

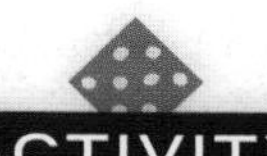

ACTIVITY

Blending Therapeutic Oils

Using essential oils and carrier oils supplied by your instructor, work with a partner to create a blend for aromatherapy massage. Remember the formula of approximately 100 to 120 total drops for an eight-ounce bottle, and adjust your recipe accordingly.

After you have created your blend, give it a name and share it with other classmates. Trade aromatherapy massage with your partner, using the oil you have created. Blend a synergy using small amounts of the essentials you have chosen, with no carrier oil, and place this in a diffuser to fill the massage room with the scent. Note: Only one synergy at a time should be used in a single classroom to avoid commingling of too many aromas.

After you have created the oil and used it in practice, write a one-page paper that lists the recipe, the properties of the oils you chose, and the intended effects of the blend you created, along with its name. Describe your initial reaction and overall impression to the blend. What was your partner's reaction? Was it similar? Different? Conclude with any tips you may have learned regarding the blending of essential oils.

limbic system

area of the brain consisting of the olfactory bulb, hippocampus, amygdala, hypothalamus, and related structures that support emotion, behavior, and memory; strongly affected by aroma and thus aromatherapy

olfactory system

the body's system of smell, including all the structures and processes through which that happens

olfactory epithelia

area of tissue inside the nasal cavity, approximately one inch by two inches in size, located on the roof of the nasal cavity and connecting to the olfactory bulb; directly responsible for detecting odors (singular **olfactory epithelium**)

olfactory bulb

the most forward structure of the brain, transmits smell information from the nose into the brain's limbic system; necessary for the perception of smell

Essential oils have such a profound impact because the sense of smell has a more direct connection to the emotions than any of the other senses. Most people have experienced this personally, when a single whiff of a particular scent brings a memory or an entire series of memories tumbling back into consciousness. This happens because the area of the brain associated with smell is the same one associated with memory. This area is known as the **limbic system** (Figure 11–5). In addition to stimulating the memory centers of the brain, essential oils can engender or enhance moods. Some of the mood words most commonly used by people to describe their experience during exposure to aromatherapy are *stimulating, uplifting, calming, soothing, relaxing, grounding, balancing*, and *centering*.

The physical structures through which essential oils actually enter and affect the body are quite fascinating. They are processed through the **olfactory system**, which detects molecules of essential oil floating in the air (Figure 11–6). When these molecules are breathed in through the nose, they reach a structure called the **olfactory epithelia**, which contains tiny hair-like cilia that are actually the ends of neurons protruding directly from the limbic system in the deepest memory recesses of the brain. These neurons translate the contact of aromatic molecules into nerve impulses that proceed straight into the limbic system via the **olfactory bulb** that sits above the epithelia. Humans have between 10 and 20 million olfactory receptors covering the epithelia, comprised of 300 to 400 different types of receptors that perceive different smells. Mice, on the other hand, have about a thousand types of receptors, and some dogs have over 200 million total receptors, giving them an olfactory sensitivity up to 100 times greater than our own.

The brain's limbic system and associated structures control such basic functions of the body as heart rate, blood pressure, breathing, memory, stress level, and hormone balance. The limbic system is also closely associated with the hormonal system, which can trigger chemical actions within the body, including pain

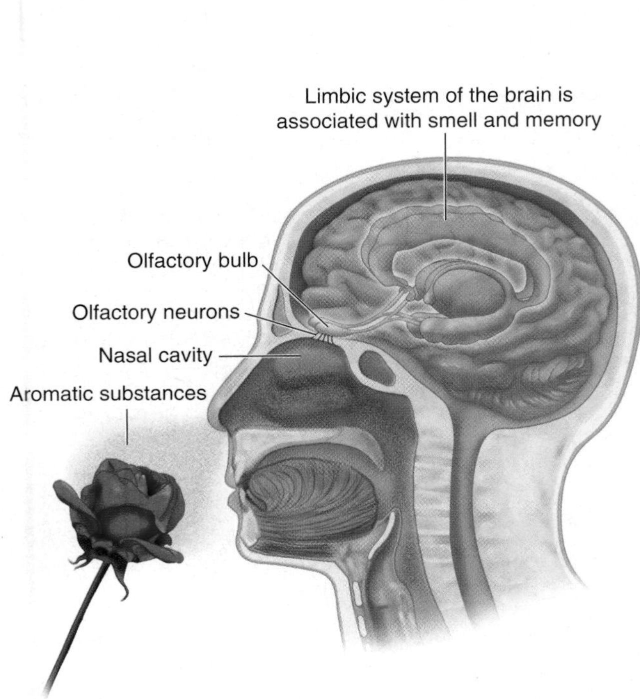

FIGURE 11-5 Aromatherapy triggers emotions because the sense of smell is processed in the same area of the brain as memory.

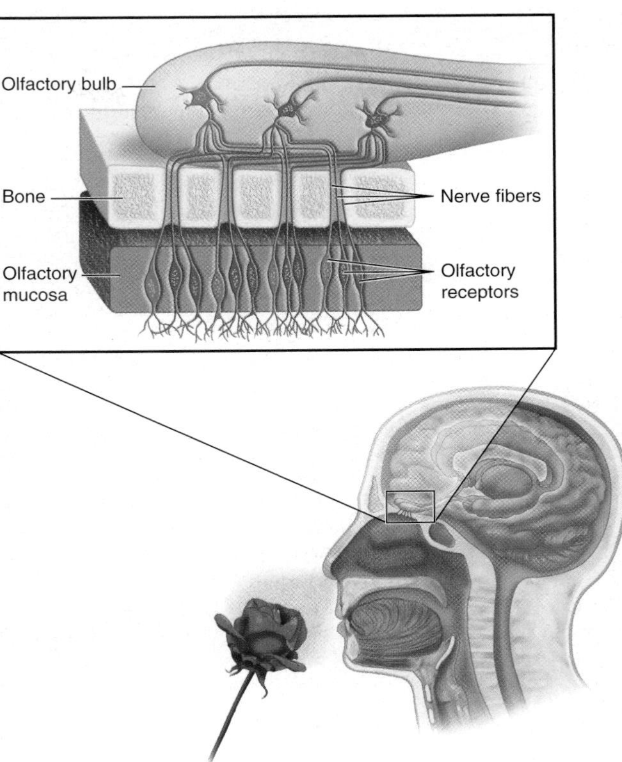

FIGURE 11-6 Specialized nerve cells carry information about aromas directly from our noses to the deepest centers of the brain along nerve pathways.

reduction, sexual stimulation, and relaxation. It is easy to see, then, why essential oils produce such amazing effects on mood, state of mind, and physiology. Practically speaking, when a molecule of essential oil is inhaled, it lands squarely on the tip of a nerve cell that has its roots in the deepest parts of the brain.

Dr. Tiffany Field at the Touch Research Institute in Miami, Florida, specializes in exploring the many benefits of massage and allied therapies. She and her team have undertaken and documented thousands of clinical studies, and over 30 of them were designed to assess the effectiveness of aromatherapy on a wide range of conditions ranging from anxiety to wrinkles. The results from some of these studies are outlined in Table 11–4.

SPA TIP

Colds and viral infections can cause people to lose their sense of smell and thus lower the effectiveness of essential oils. It is usually wise, then, to counsel clients to rebook aromatherapy appointments for another time if they are sick, unless a specific aromatherapy treatment is being administered to try and improve the condition.

STUDY	INTENT	RESULTS
Anxiety	investigate the effects of aromatherapy massage on the anxiety and self-esteem issues experienced by elderly Korean women	The intervention produced significantly lower anxiety and higher self-esteem.
Arthritis	investigate the effect of aromatherapy on pain, depression, and feelings of dissatisfaction in life of arthritis patients	Aromatherapy significantly decreased both the pain and depression scores.
Blood Pressure	evaluate the effects of aromatherapy on blood pressure and pulse using measurements of serum cortisol levels, catecholamine levels, subjective stress, and state anxiety	The use of essential oils can be considered an effective nursing intervention that reduces psychological stress responses and serum cortisol levels, as well as the blood pressure of clients with essential hypertension.

TABLE 11-4 Touch Therapy Institute aromatherapy studies. *(Continued)*

STUDY	INTENT	RESULTS
Cognition	assess the impact of lavender and rosemary on cognitive performance and mood in healthy volunteers	Lavender lowered performance reaction times. Rosemary enhanced memory but also impaired speed of memory. Both rosemary and lavender groups were more content than control group.
Cancer	assess effectiveness of aromatherapy massage on cancer patients with clinical anxiety and/or depression	Patients who received aromatherapy massage had lower anxiety and depression compared with those receiving usual care.
Cortisol	measure the total salivary free radical scavenging activity (FRSA) induced after the smelling of lavender and rosemary essential oils	Lavender and rosemary enhance FRSA and decrease the stress hormone, cortisol, which protects the body from oxidative stress.
Dental Pain	investigate the impact of orange and lavender on anxiety, mood, alertness, and calmness in dental patients	Ambient odors of orange and lavender reduced anxiety and improved mood in patients waiting for dental treatment.
Depression	investigate whether exposure to rosemary oil or lavender oil would change electroencephalographic (EEG) activity in infants of depressed and non-depressed mothers	The two odors did not differentially affect the EEG.
Dialysis	investigate effects of aromatherapy oil on mood and anxiety in patients who were being treated with chronic dialysis	Lavender aroma significantly decreased the mean scores of the Hamilton rating scale for depression (HAMD).
Insomnia	evaluate the efficacy of lavender on insomnia	Lavender created an improvement of −2.5 points in Pittsburgh Sleep Quality Index (PSQI).
Mood	explore the effects of lavender, Neroli, or placebo and suggestions related to the effects of said odors (relaxing, stimulating, or none) on mood	Relaxing odors yielded decreases in heart rate and skin conductance, with stimulating odors yielding the reverse effects under equivalent conditions.
Obesity	compare weight, abdominal circumference and appetite in obese patients given aromatherapy massage	The apparent effectiveness of aromatherapy massage in reducing weight, abdominal circumference, and appetite was noted.
Postpartum	examine the effect of aromatherapy massage in healthy postpartum mothers	Aromatherapy massage may be an effective intervention for postpartum mothers to improve physical and mental status and to facilitate mother–infant interaction.
Stress	measure anxiety and perceived stress when inhaling lavender, peppermint, rosemary, and clary sage essential oils	Physical symptoms decreased, anxiety scores were low, and perceived stress scores were low, showing that aroma inhalation could be a very effective stress management method.
Wrinkles	assess the inhibition of wrinkle-forming elastase activity by various essential oils in aromatherapy massage	Elastase activity was inhibited by essential oils, especially lemon, juniper, and grapefruit. These studies demonstrate a possible rationale for the use of essential oil massage as a preventive treatment for cutaneous wrinkling and aging.

TABLE 11–4 Touch Therapy Institute Aromatherapy Studies.

Contraindications for Aromatherapy

myristicin

a pharmacologically active compound found in various essential oils such as nutmeg

When using essential oils, it is important to remember that they are powerfully concentrated substances and as such should be treated with caution. Several aromatic oils are pharmacologically active, and when used improperly they can overstimulate the body or perhaps even harm a client. The oils of nutmeg, parsley seed, and star anise, for example, contain **myristicin**, a compound that can cause hallucinations and more serious complications if taken internally. Certain other oils are considered toxic as well and should never be used in a spa, including mugwort, pennyroyal, sage, sassafras, and wormwood. Because just a few drops are needed to create an effect, it is better to err on the side of caution and use smaller amounts of any oils you may be uncertain of, especially when treating a client for the first time. In general, it is good advice to read up about each essential oil before applying it on a client. The more information you have, the better. Though aromatherapy is benign and safe for most people, essential oil providers and educators advise caution when treating anybody with specific conditions.

- Stimulating oils of peppermint and spearmint or any other menthol-type plant should not be used on clients with heart disease.
- Health care practitioners should be consulted before applying aromatherapy to clients with certain diagnoses such as epilepsy, skin cancer, kidney disease, or liver conditions.
- Some practitioners suggest that asthmatics should avoid exposure to essential oils as they may provoke asthmatic attacks.
- Be careful not to get essential oils in the eyes. In case this does happen, flush thoroughly with water. The best option is to use an eye-wash station outfitted with sterile saline solution. If this is not available, flush the eye under running water for 15 minutes, keeping it open. For someone with contact lenses, flush the eye initially, then remove the lens and continue flushing. Seek medical attention immediately if the irritation persists.
- Essential oils should never be taken internally in spas unless under medical supervision.
- Certain oils should be avoided altogether because of their potential toxicity or negative effects, including bitter almond, camphor, horseradish, mugwort, mustard, parsley seed, pennyroyal, sassafras, wintergreen, and wormwood, among others. It should be noted, however, that these oils are rarely if ever found in spas.
- The use of essential oils is not a replacement for proper health care. Clients under medical supervision should consult with their health care provider before using essential oils.

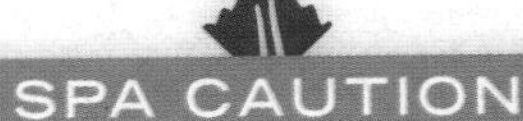

SPA CAUTION

Some essential oils will actually remove the finish from wooden furniture. Painted surfaces and plastic can be affected, too. It is important to quickly wipe up any spills.

Photosensitivity

Certain essential oils, including several citrus peel varieties extracted through cold pressing, cause a heightened degree of sensitivity to sunlight. Any oil that induces this reaction is said to be a **photosensitizer**. Bergamot oil is the most widely cited photosensitizer, along with grapefruit, orange, Neroli, and other citrus. In addition, lavender oil is mildly photosensitizing, and even though it is considered one of the mildest essential oils, is can be **cytotoxic** to human skin cells. Normally, it is recommended that none of these oils should be applied if the client is going to experience direct exposure to the sun within the following four to six hours. However, studies have shown that application of UV protection in conjunction with the oils provides safety.

photosensitizer

any substance that creates sensitivity to the influence of radiant energy, especially light

cytotoxic

the quality of being toxic to cells

Sensitization

Certain essential oils can cause skin and mucous membrane irritations. Included in this group are allspice, cassia, cinnamon bark or leaf, clove bud, oregano, and thyme, none of which are likely to be found on a spa menu. Just in case they do find their way into the treatment room and end up on a client's skin, do not try to rub them off with water, as this will only cause the oil to spread. Instead,

sensitization

a state or condition in which a previously encountered foreign substance, such as a particular essential oil, triggers an immune reaction

haptens

a small molecule, such as those found in certain essential oil components, which can elicit an immune response; see sensitization

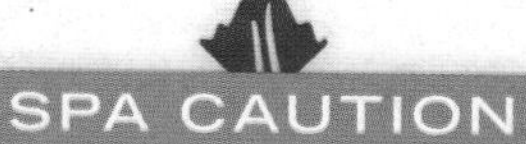

SPA CAUTION

You can use the patch test in order to determine sensitization levels to a particular oil. Using a dilution that is twice as strong as typical massage oil, apply a few drops to the soft skin on the inside of the client's elbow and wait 24 hours, watching for any swelling, redness, or itchiness. If you notice any reaction, do not use the oil on that particular person. People who exhibit irritation to one essential oil may be more susceptible to irritation from others as well. Proceed with caution and test other oils first before performing aromatherapy services.

emmenagogues

any agent that promotes menstrual discharge

apply some pure carrier oil to the area, which will absorb the essential oils and help ease the irritation.

When using any essential oil, it is advisable to proceed with caution, especially when dealing with sensitive skin and clients with skin conditions such as eczema. Avoid rashes and skin breakouts of any kind. If an irritation or allergic reaction develops while using any oil, discontinue use immediately. Remember that these oils are processed through the body in four to six hours, and therefore any reaction should be short-lived. If the irritation persists, seek medical attention.

The process of the body's developing an allergic reaction when exposed to certain essential oils is called **sensitization**. This word does not refer to *people* with sensitive skin or temperaments. It refers to a *condition* that is potentially more serious than irritation. Sensitization is an immune system response that occurs in reaction to foreign molecules called **haptens**, among which are certain essential oil components. Essential oils may become sensitizers because they have become oxidized inside the bottle. Older oils or oils that have been stored improperly may therefore be more likely to cause sensitization. Reactions range from rashes, to difficulty in breathing, to anaphylactic shock in rare individuals who are highly susceptible. Any oil, if overused, can potentially cause sensitization. Though never used in spas, costus oil and saussurea lappa oils definitely cause sensitization and should never be applied to the skin under any circumstances.

In addition to essential oils themselves, the carrier oils used in aromatherapy massage blends can also cause allergic reactions. It is especially important for therapists to be cautious when using nut oils, as many people have nut allergies, some with quite serious implications.

Pregnancy

Pregnant women should be cautious when approaching various essential oils. They should, of course, avoid any of the oils listed above as toxic, and in addition they need to stay away from a class of oils known as **emmenagogues**, as these promote menstrual flow and may be disadvantageous during pregnancy. These oils include chamomile, clary sage, ginger, jasmine, juniper, marjoram, myrrh, rose, rosemary, and peppermint. Note: There are other oils that may be proscribed during pregnancy, but because they are seldom if ever used in typical aromatherapy spa services, they are not listed here.

The first three months of pregnancy are especially delicate. In order to be as safe as possible and err on the side of extreme caution, some spas rule out aromatherapy and all other spa treatments entirely in the first trimester. Others rule out spa services entirely, at any stage of pregnancy. This, however, is generally viewed as overly precautious and ultimately detrimental because it denies women spa treatments at a time when they could most benefit from them. Each spa will have its own policies regarding pregnancy and essential oils. If you ever feel uncomfortable because you believe a spa's policies are too lax and may endanger clients, bring this issue up with spa management rather than speaking about it with clients. Some spas do offer aromatherapy services to pregnant clients but with diluted recipes, offering aromatherapy massages and aromatherapy baths with one-half the normal concentration of essential oils.

There is very little detailed evidence of the toxicological effects of essential oils on the female reproductive system. However, it is known that fetuses have underdeveloped detoxification mechanisms and as such should be treated with extreme care. When in doubt about any risks that may be posed, it is recommended that each client should obtain approval from a physician prior to receiving any type of aromatherapy treatment when pregnant or while breast feeding.

Children and Infants

Keep essential oils out of the reach of children and infants. When applying aromatherapy on children, use strongly diluted versions of the oils—one drop in a bath and two drops per ounce of carrier oil for massage. Inhaling the aromas from essential oils commonly found in spas is fine for children, although they may become overwhelmed by smelling the same scent all day long. In general, small amounts of well-diluted oils used only occasionally pose no problem for children. A good rule of thumb to follow is: the smaller the body, the more diluted the oils should be. It is sometimes recommended not to use essential oils at all with infants. Because of their small size and undeveloped immune systems, they may be more susceptible to the oils' powerful effects. Peppermint and eucalyptus oils are especially intense and should be avoided on children as well as infants. Safer oils such as chamomile, geranium, jasmine, lavender, Neroli, patchouli, sandalwood, and ylang ylang, well-diluted, are extremely unlikely to cause any adverse effects.

RESEARCH

Choose an essential oil that you particularly enjoy and write a one-page report about it. Include harvesting method, area where it is most popularly cultivated, part of plant used, extraction method, major effects, contraindications, and use in history and in modern spas, as well as any anecdotes about its use or background that you find interesting.

AROMATHERAPY SPA TREATMENTS

Aromatherapy is used in a variety of spa treatments. The most popular aromatherapy modality and certainly the one with which therapists will be most familiar is aromatherapy massage. However, stone massage, aromatherapy-infused exfoliations, hydro baths, and seaweed wraps, as well as other types of body wraps, also quite commonly incorporate essential oils. Spas also use essentials for a large number of signature services featuring various components, such as an exfoliation, stone massage, and wrap. Many different manufacturers supply the spa industry with oils, some of them offering training and menu development along with their products. Massage therapists have a tendency to form close attachments to particular brands of essential oils, but it is important to stay open to oils from other companies as well because spas often leave their employees with no choice regarding the brand of oils to use.

Many, if not all, spa treatments can be enhanced through the addition of aromatherapy. As you study and experiment with a variety of spa modalities, you will encounter many opportunities to use essential oils, as outlined in Table 11–5. The possibilities are unlimited. In this chapter you will practice two specific treatments: an aromatherapy massage and an aromatherapy wrap.

SPA TREATMENT	HOW AROMATHERAPY IS USED	BENEFITS
Aromatherapy Bath	drops of essential oils are added to hot water in a bathtub or hydrotherapy tub	the body is warm and pores open to absorb more benefits; inhalation maximized as oils mix with warm water
Aromatherapy Wrap	oils mixed with emollient creams or lotions, applied to skin before wrapping, often includes massage	imparts sense of warmth and security in cocoon, allowing essential oils ample time to soak into pores to benefit body while moistening and healing skin

TABLE 11–5 Uses of Aromatherapy in Spa Treatments. *(Continued)*

SPA TREATMENT	HOW AROMATHERAPY IS USED	BENEFITS
Compress	essentials added to water in which compresses are soaked; sometimes incorporated into other treatments such as cool compress to the head during heat treatment	imparts benefits of essential oils to localized area and adds to intended effects of heat or cold compress application; can add inhalation benefits if used near face
Cooling Wrap	many spas have cooling wraps for clients with sunburn or chapped skin; essential oils are added to the product blend before applying to the body	essentials can help soothe and heal dry, burned skin, often in combination with natural plant materials such as aloe vera
Exfoliation	essentials are added to exfoliant mix, salt, sugar, etc. prior to use; sometimes with client's input at beginning of treatment	can add stimulating, calming, moistening, analgesic, antiseptic, anti-inflammatory, and astringent benefits for the skin; improves aroma of bland exfoliant blends
Face Treatment	essential oils are blended with oils, creams, or lotions and applied to the face during head/neck/face-specific treatment; can also be spritzed on in hydrosol form or used in compresses	essential oils have a dramatic stimulating and regenerating effect on the skin; they can bring oxygen to the cells, soothe irritations, remove excess oils, and more
Massage	essentials are blended directly into massage oil prior to use	essential oils soak into skin along with massage medium, adding physiological effects as well as emotional effects via inhalation
Mud/Clay Wrap	essential oils are added to muds or clay and often warmed prior to application to the skin	the effects of the clay and mud in body wraps can be enhanced by the oils, especially when stimulating or detoxifying effects are sought
Seaweed Wrap	essential oils are added to seaweed prior to application	helps mellow strong seaweed odors while adding benefits of particular oils
Steam Room	essential oil, usually eucalyptus, is mixed with water, then sprayed into the vapor of a steam room	respiratory benefits include healing properties for the lungs, opening of bronchial passages, useful for coughs and colds, antiseptic
Stone Massage	essentials are added to the massage oil applied during the treatment; occasionally essentials applied separately in conjunction with chakra stones	adds pleasurable aromas to stone treatment as well as physiological benefits of particular essential oils as they soak into the skin and are inhaled

TABLE 11-5 Uses of Aromatherapy in Spa Treatments.

Aromatherapy Massage

Some spas hire highly trained practitioners who have undergone hundreds of hours of aromatherapy-specific study to administer aromatherapy massages. This, however, is an exception to the rule. The majority of spas require that all the massage therapists on staff, or at least a significant number of them, perform aromatherapy massage, and they usually offer these therapists a minimum of training on-site to go along with this requirement. It is important for you to feel comfortable and confident when performing these treatments, and it is reassuring to know that the step-by-step procedure for an aromatherapy massage is very similar to that for a typical Swedish spa massage, with a few notable distinctions.

- Before the treatment, the therapist must check the guest's intake form for sensitivities to aromas or, if no form is used, ask the guest verbally.
- Before the treatment, the therapist should explain to the client the therapeutic outcomes desired through the choice of essential oils.
- The massage strokes are predominantly light and flowing rather than deep-tissue oriented.

- Time is allowed for the client to experience the aromas. For example, at the beginning of a sequence over the face, the therapist cups her hands a few inches away from the client's face and asks the client to inhale the oil for its therapeutic benefits. This can be done through the face cradle when the client is prone.
- It is especially important to make sure that blankets and/or an infrared heating lamp are in place if necessary to keep the client warm because spa guests often experience a chill during this treatment, either as an effect of certain oils or because the overall treatment is so calming and sedating.

ACTIVITY

Giving and Receiving a Full-Body Aromatherapy Massage

You have already learned how to perform a full-body massage in school. Now it is time to add the aspect of aromatherapy to the procedure and learn firsthand about the pleasures and benefits of this modality. This will be a three-step procedure.

First, you and a partner choose which single essential oils or blends you would prefer to experience. Using 2 ounces of carrier oil, mix in 24 to 30 total drops of essential oils. So, with a blend of three essentials, you would use 8 to 10 drops of each or some other combination that would equal a total of 24 to 30. Some blends call for one oil to predominate and others to lend just a hint of aroma or effect in the background. You can choose any oil or combination that you desire or ask your instructor for a suggestion. Also, you may try one of the following three blends.

- *Uplifting Blend*: bergamot, lavender, and ylang ylang
- *Grounding Blend*: cypress, frankincense, and sandalwood
- *Anti-Stress Blend*: clary sage, patchouli, and vetiver

Second, start the massage by rubbing a small amount of the blended oil into your hands and cupping them over your partner's face for several moments, instructing him to breathe deeply in order to appreciate the aromas and absorb their properties into his body. Then, when you begin the massage, concentrate primarily on soothing effleurage and petrissage strokes. Also, if you are familiar with lymphatic drainage techniques, you can apply some during the treatment, as several essential oils such as rosemary aid in detox and drainage of the body. See Chapter 12 for more information on lymphatic drainage. After the massage, switch roles so the receiver now gives the massage. At this time, if it is allowed by the instructor, you can create another two-ounce blend to be experienced by the second recipient.

Third, on separate pages, each of you provide written responses to the following:

1. Did the essential oil blend provide the experience you expected as far as aroma? Was the aroma strongly detectable throughout the massage? Only at the beginning? Was it too strong?
2. Do you think you experienced any detectable effects from the oils above and beyond what you would experience during a massage without essentials added?
3. How was your experience giving a treatment with essential oils? Was it completely positive, or did the oils become overwhelming after a time to you as a therapist?
4. What would you do differently next time you give or receive an aromatherapy massage? Would you choose different oils? Strengthen the concentration slightly? Dilute further? Would you choose a different carrier oil or lotion?
5. Write a two- or three-sentence paragraph describing the experience of receiving an aromatherapy massage with this blend. Craft the sentences so they could be used as a treatment description on a spa menu to entice clients. Call this paragraph "Aromatherapy Massage Menu Description."

Aromatherapy Wrap

An aromatherapy wrap uses essential oils, a carrier medium which is usually an emollient lotion, and wrapping layers such as muslin sheets and blankets to create a cocoon experience for the client. Some spas prefer to use pre-blended products, while others customize the treatment, blending oils according to the client's preference. The treatment is quite gentle and meditative, focusing more on the client's mood and state of mind than any musculoskeletal problems. In fact, at some spas, the therapist forgoes massage entirely during the aromatherapy wrap and instead simply applies the product with long, gliding, superficial strokes over the entire body. Some spas offer a choice between this simple application and a more comprehensive aromatherapy wrap with massage included.

To start the treatment, the therapist places a drop of essential oil blend on her fingertip, then touches it to several energy points along the body. After this, the lotion/oil blend is applied to the body in long strokes, and the client is covered immediately afterward to assure warmth. The client turns over and the procedure is repeated on the front of the body before wrapping the client in layers of muslin and blankets. A bolster is placed beneath the knees, the lights turned low, and the client is left wrapped for 20 minutes on average in most spas. During this time, the therapist often applies a light, non-invasive therapy such as craniosacral therapy to the head and neck area.

Performed with a strong therapeutic intention, the aromatherapy wrap can be a profound experience for spa guests, even though it is quite simple to perform and not taxing on therapists' hands or bodies. It is an excellent way to take advantage of the power of essential oils.

TREATMENT: AROMATHERAPY WRAP	
Wet Room/Dry Room	Dry room
Table Setup	blanket, sheet for wrapping, draping towels or sheet
Treatment Duration	30 minutes, 60 minutes if a more extensive massage is applied
Needed Supplies	1 to 2 tablespoons emollient body lotion, 20 to 25 drops essential oil(s), heating unit to warm product, spa bowl, blanket, 2 sheets, draping towels or sheets, bolster
Contraindications	skin conditions, rashes, caution during first three months of pregnancy and avoid emmenagogic oils, avoid sunlight after application of photosensitizing oils, avoid contact with eyes, caution for asthmatics, stimulating menthol-type plant oils should not be used on clients with heart disease, clients with epilepsy, skin cancer, kidney disease, or liver conditions should consult physician prior to treatment
Draping	Same draping as massage therapy during application. Wrapping sheet can be used as additional drape during wrap itself.
Treatment Order	Aromatherapy wraps can be given after exfoliation and before massage.
Safety, Sanitation Issues, & Clean-Up	Discard unused emulsion as it can become rancid rather quickly. Lotion usually soaks into client's skin, so it is not necessary for client to shower after treatment.
Body Mechanics & Self-Care	Same body mechanic concerns as massage therapy. Oils can be powerful and therapists should take care to avoid exposure to pure, undiluted essentials. Their scent may become overwhelming over a period of many treatments. Get fresh air between services. Keep oils away from eyes.

(*Continued*)

TREATMENT: AROMATHERAPY WRAP	
Product Cost	less than $1 for lotion and drops of essential oils
Treatment Price	Add $10 to $20 on top of massage price for equal time frame.
Physiological Effects	Depending upon the oils chosen, the aromatherapy wrap can be diuretic, moistening, analgesic, antibacterial, anti-microbial, antiseptic, anti-viral, anti-inflammatory, antispasmodic, astringent, decongesting, or detoxifying. In addition, emotional effects and mood enhancement are often reported.
Pregnancy Issues (information provided by Elaine Stillerman, LMT, author and developer of MotherMassage)	Wraps should be comfortable and not binding. Avoid during the first trimester and only if the second/third trimester client is not too hot. All aromatherapy should be avoided during the first trimester, and scents with emmenagogic oils or those with hormonal influences must be avoided at all times. Be sure that the oils are 100% pure, essential oils and not degraded with preservatives that may be contraindicated during pregnancy.

Aromatherapy Wrap Preparation

1. Prepare the treatment table with a blanket, sheet, and draping (Figure 11–7). Muslin sheets are often chosen for comfort.
2. Use a pre-blended synergy or a single-note, or choose oils to blend. With a total of 20 to 25 drops, set aside ¼ in a small receptacle and place the rest in a spa bowl. Add lotion to the spa bowl and mix thoroughly. Note: When blending oils in certain lotions or creams, it may be necessary to warm the lotion first in order for the essential oils to mix in and form an emulsion.
3. Warm the mixture by floating it in hot water or nestling it between hot towels.

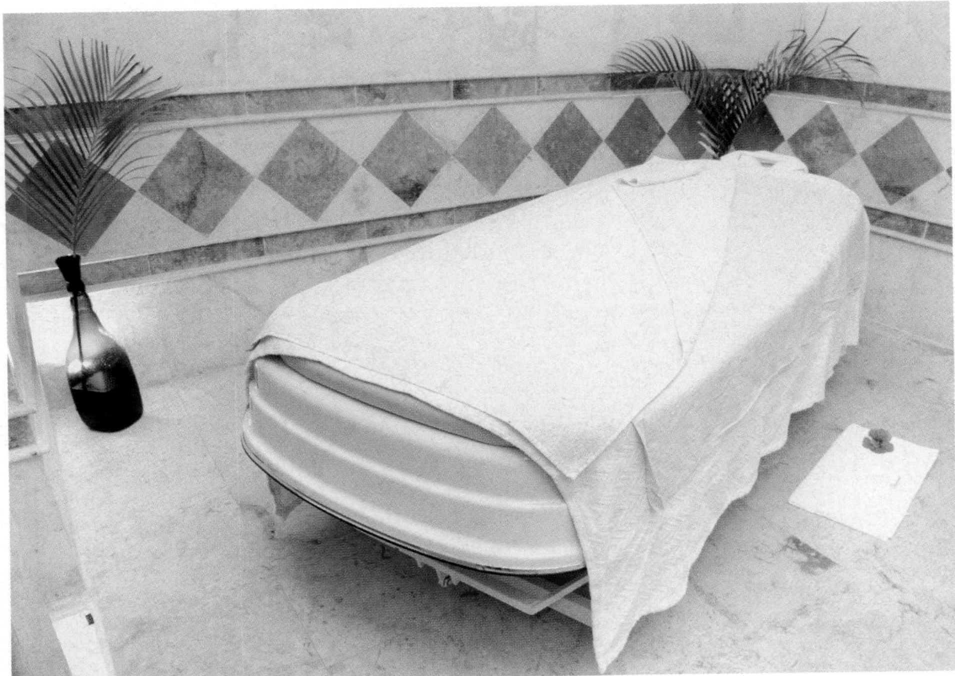

FIGURE 11–7

Aromatherapy Wrap Procedure

1. Ask the client to lie prone beneath a drape sheet or towel and atop a muslin sheet while you step out of the room.
2. Hold the small receptacle of essential oils beneath the face cradle and allow the client to breath in the aroma for several moments (Figure 11–8).

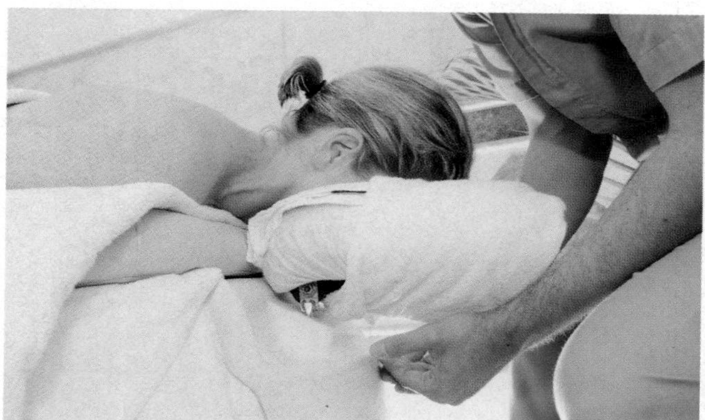

FIGURE 11-8

3. Dab one finger into the pure oils and then touch the finger to each energy point along the left leg, starting at the center of the bottom of the foot (Figure 11–9). Hold each point for five seconds with light pressure, then move up the leg (Figure 11–10). Repeat on the other leg, then apply to five points up the spine, beginning at the sacrum (Figure 11–11). Refer to Figure 11–25 for point locations.

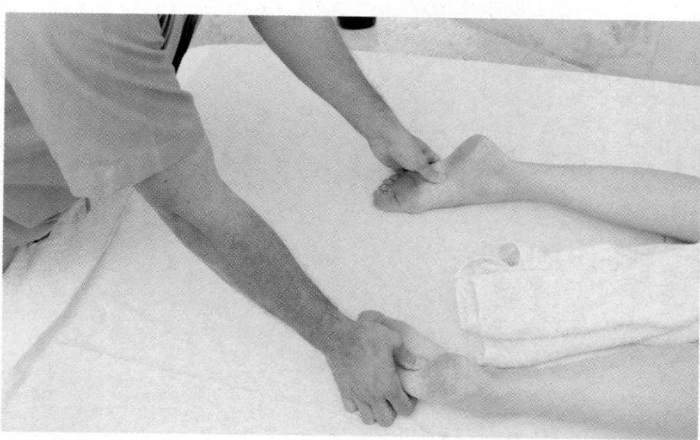

FIGURE 11-9

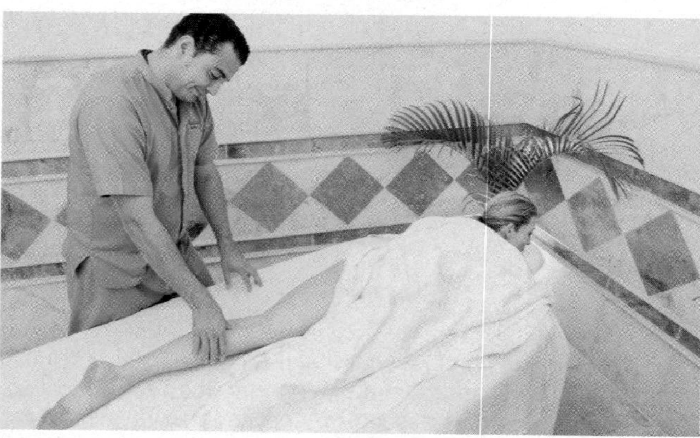

FIGURE 11-10

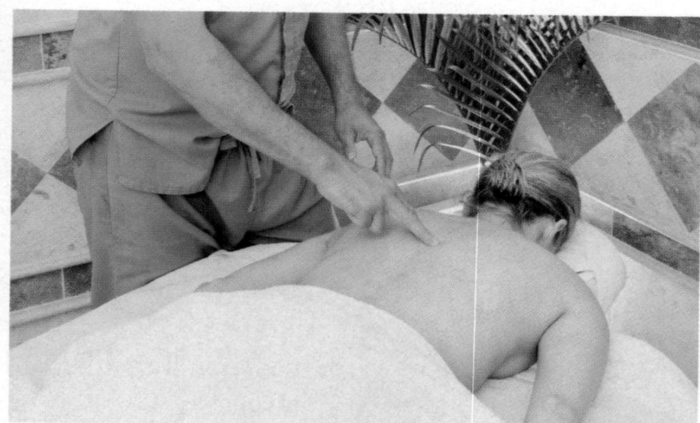

FIGURE 11-11

4. Apply lotion and the essential oil mixture to the back of the left leg using light effleurage and petrissage movements (Figure 11–12). Repeat on the other leg. Then apply the mixture to the back (Figure 11–13). The application to the entire back and legs should last only five minutes. When applying a longer one-hour version of the treatment, this massage segment can be extended to 15 minutes.

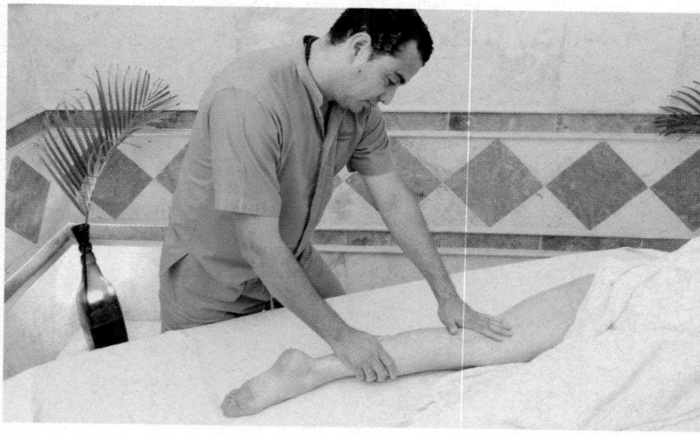

FIGURE 11-12

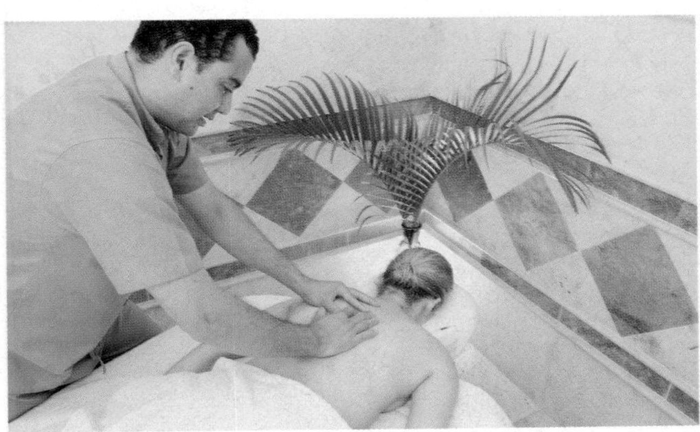

FIGURE 11–13

5. Maintaining proper draping, instruct the client to turn over into a supine position.
6. Beginning on the left foot (Figure 11–14), dab the essential oil mix to energy points on the front of the body as outlined in Figure 11–25. Continue up the left leg (Figure 11–15), then the left leg and torso (Figure 11–16), to the head (Figure 11–17). For female clients, insert a breast drape to expose the abdomen.

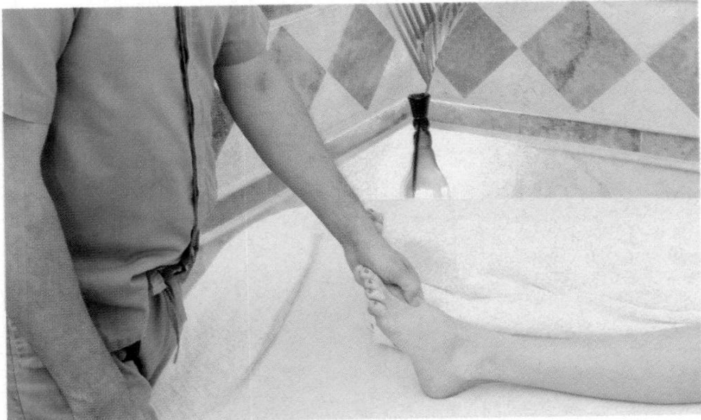

FIGURE 11–14

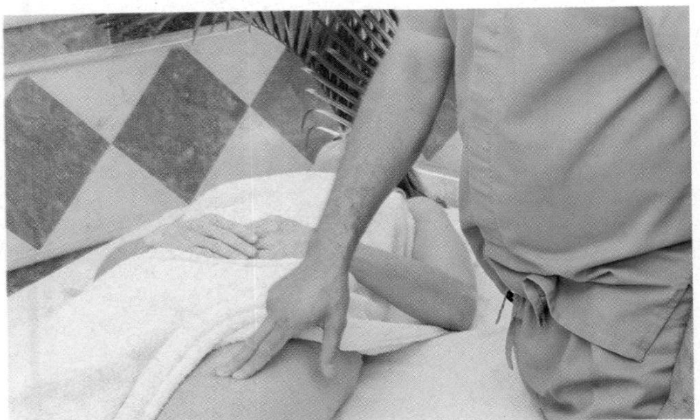

FIGURE 11–15

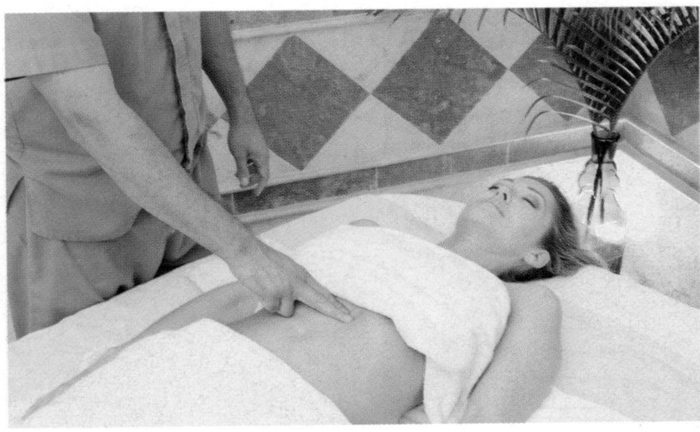

FIGURE 11–16

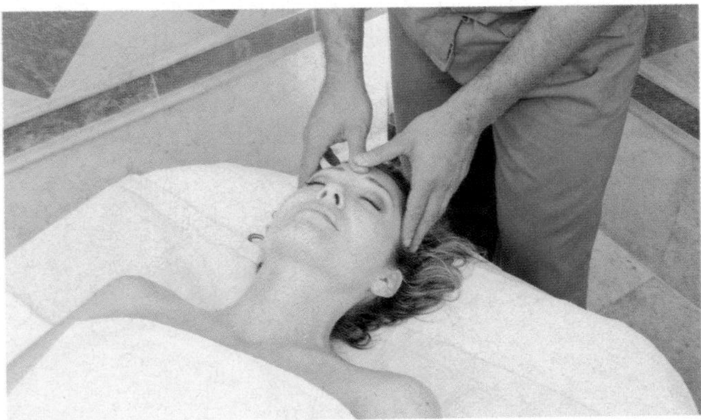

FIGURE 11–17

7. Apply the lotion and oil mixture to the left foot and leg using effleurage and petrissage techniques (Figure 11–18). Cover the area with a muslin sheet as you complete the application (Figure 11–19).
8. Repeat the application on the right leg and cover with a sheet.
9. Apply the mixture to the torso (Figure 11–20). Steps 7 through 9 should last 5 minutes for a short aromatherapy wrap or 15 minutes for a one-hour treatment.

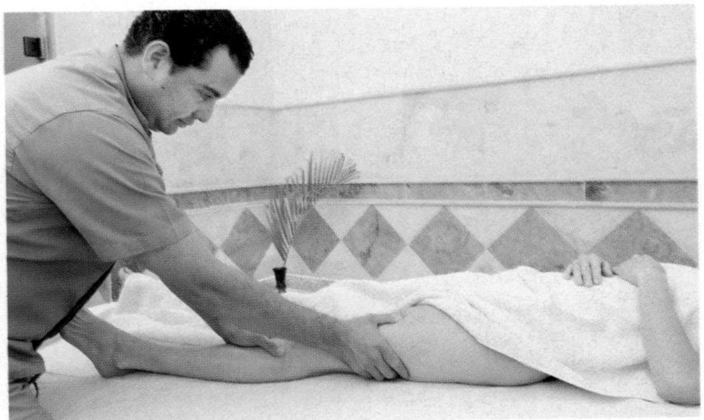

FIGURE 11–18

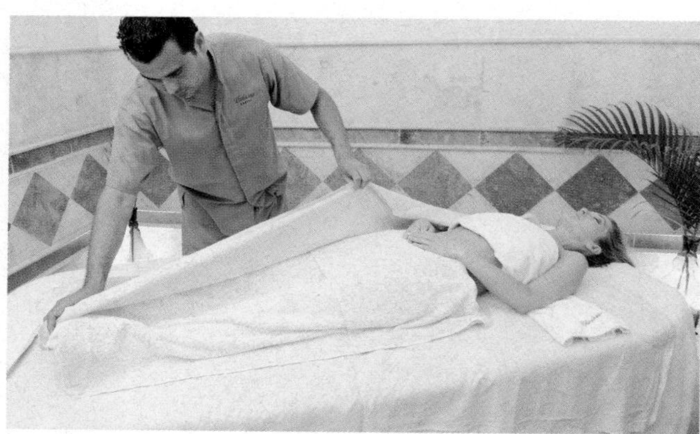
FIGURE 11–19

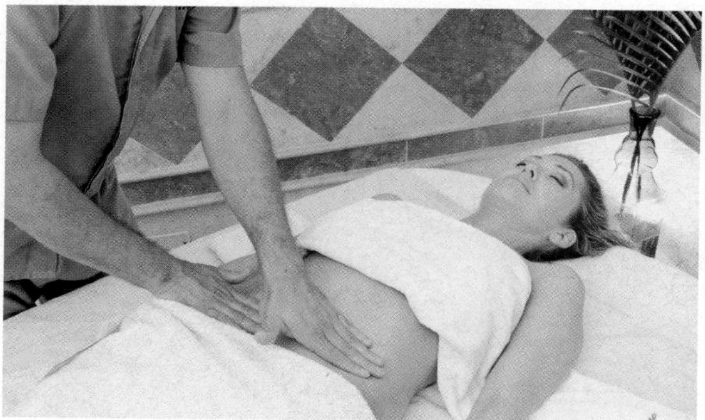
FIGURE 11–20

10. Sit at the head of the table and apply the mixture to the shoulders, neck, and face (Figure 11–21).

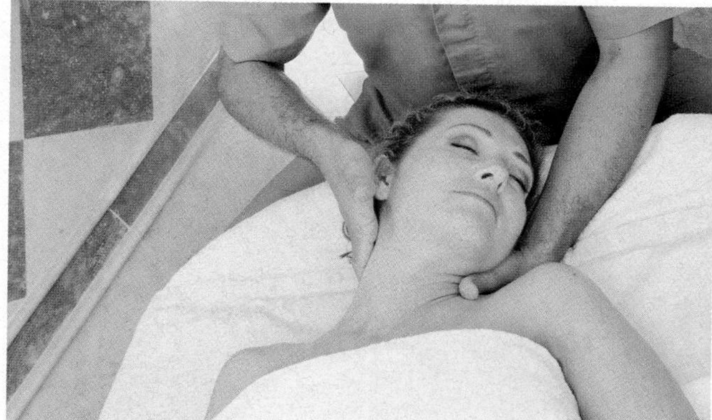
FIGURE 11–21

11. Wrap the muslin sheet and underlying blanket around the entire body.
12. Place a bolster beneath the knees.
13. Ensure that the client is comfortable. While the client remains wrapped for 20 minutes, move to the head of the table and apply light massage to the face and head (Figure 11–22). If you are familiar with them, you can use Reiki, craniosacral, or similar light techniques at this time.

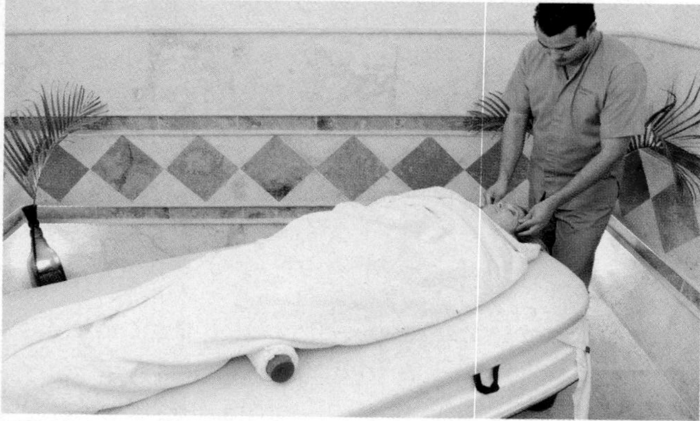
FIGURE 11–22

14. Unwrap the client one side at a time, starting with the right side (Figure 11–23). Assist the client in sitting up, then standing, maintaining modest draping at all times. A robe can be offered (Figure 11–24). The lotion and oils can be left on to soak further into the skin.

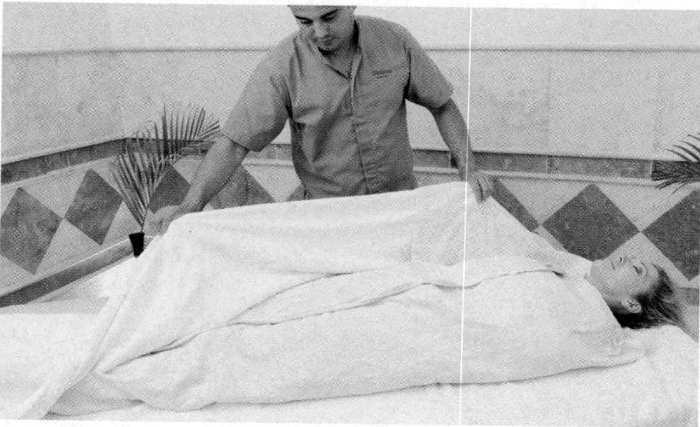
FIGURE 11–23

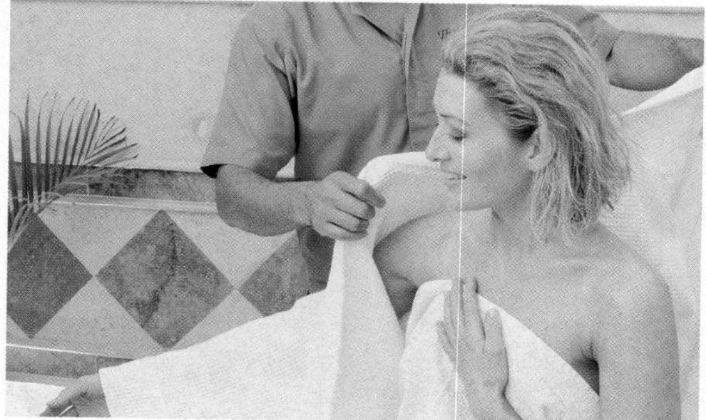
FIGURE 11–24

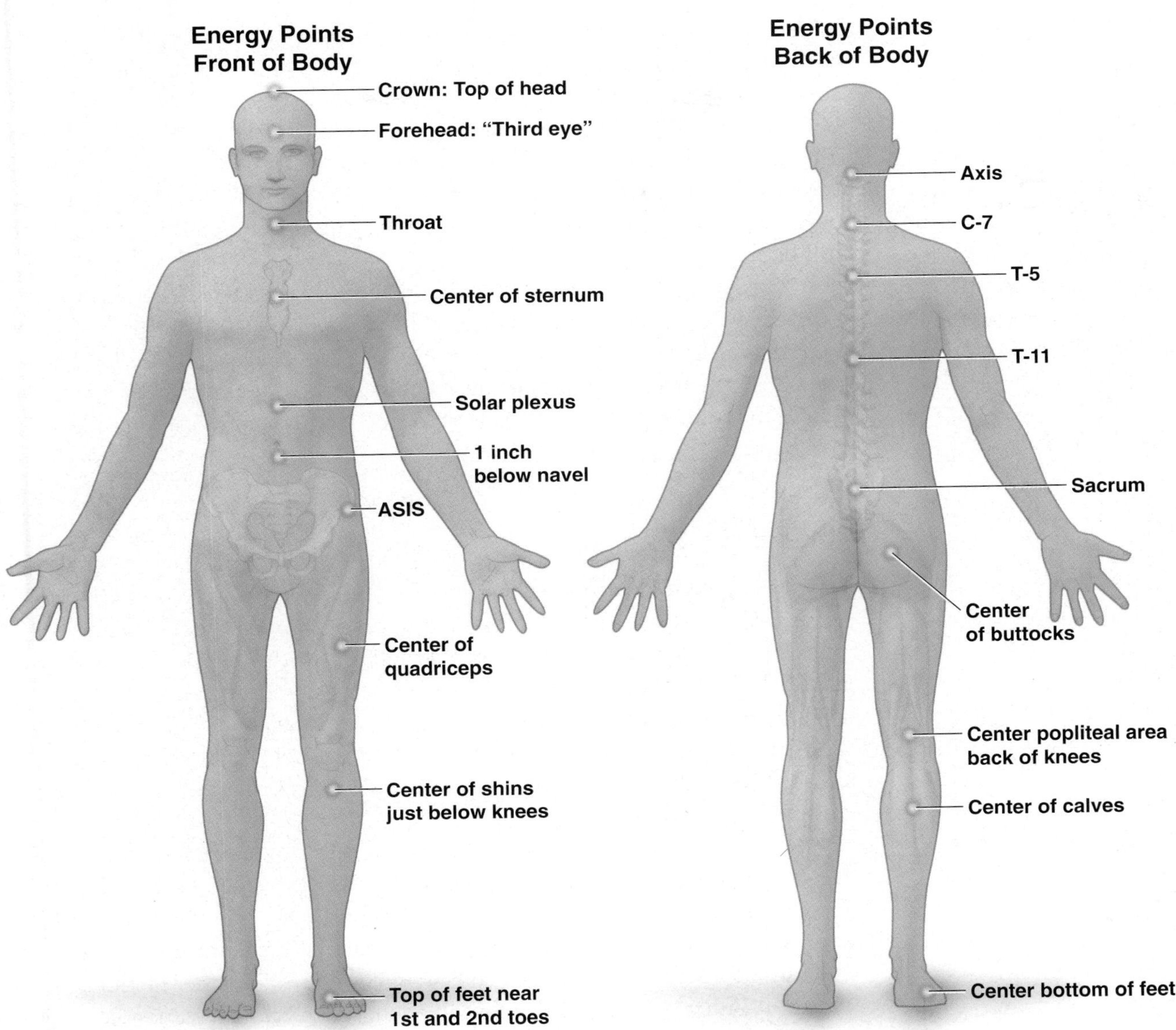

FIGURE 11–25 Dab a small amount of essential oils to each of the points at the beginning of the aromatherapy wrap.

Aromatherapy Wrap Cleanup

1. Discard unused emulsion.
2. Clean the spa bowl thoroughly so future treatments are not affected by residual aromas.
3. Launder the sheets and towels.

Aromatherapy Baths

Aromatherapy baths are popular in many spas. They can be defined as any bath that incorporates the use of aromatherapy essential oils. In this sense, many hydrotherapy baths on a spa's menu may in fact be aromatherapy baths, although they are not labeled as such, as essential oils are routinely added to hydrotherapy tubs to enhance the client's experience. Popular essential oil choices for aromatherapy baths include chamomile, lavender, rose, and rosemary. The material used to dilute essential oils in a bath is, of course, water, and in this sense, water can be considered a "carrier." These oils, however, are not soluble in water and should be dispersed as much as possible by stirring or agitating the bath. Some therapists thoroughly disperse the oils first in a pitcher or other container before adding them to the full bath.

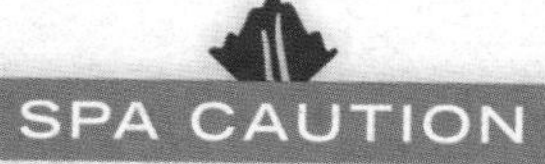

SPA CAUTION

Certain oils, especially cooling or highly stimulating ones such as peppermint, ginger, or juniper, should be avoided in aromatherapy baths, especially for children.

Typically, 4 to 6 drops of essential oil are added as the bath is filling. These drops may be blended with a carrier oil beforehand if a silkier texture is desired for the bath. The warm water, usually 100°F to 104°F, helps release the aroma of the oil, so the benefits of inhalation are increased. To perform an aromatherapy bath, follow Therapeutic Bath Protocol or the Hydrotherapy Tub Protocol found in Chapter 4.

Inhalation

Much of the benefit from essential oils comes from simply breathing them in, regardless of what type of treatment is being applied. Receiving molecules of essential oils onto the olfactory epithelium, in this sense, can be considered a kind of therapy in itself, even when no wrap or massage or exfoliation accompanies the inhalation. Spas take advantage of this through the use of diffusers that spread these molecules around. There are four main processes for diffusing essential oils: nebulization, ventilation, humidification, and heat.

Nebulization breaks essential oils down into tiny particles, which is why it is also called atomization. This requires a pressurized stream of air moving through a specially designed jet nozzle at high velocity (Figure 11–26). It is the most effective manner for providing both maximum aroma and maximum therapeutic value without altering the oils in any way. Unlike other methods of diffusion, nebulizers create particles small enough to reach the deepest layer of the lungs and thus be absorbed most thoroughly into the blood stream. This is why physicians and respiratory therapists prescribe the use of nebulizers to administer medicines. Unfortunately, nebulizers are more expensive when compared to other forms of diffusers.

Ventilation uses a small fan to make air flow over a cotton pad or other absorbent layer containing essential oils. This evaporates the oil and sends molecules into the air. This type of device is often referred to as a *fan diffuser* (Figure 11–27). It is simple and economical, and since there is no heat involved, the chemical composition of the oils is not changed. The particles produced are too large to penetrate deeply into the lungs, however.

In humidification, water and essential oils are mixed together, and then a fan, heat, or ultrasonic energy forms a mist from this mixture, which then fills the air. This adds moisture to the inhalant, but at the same time it dilutes the oil.

When using heat, several different methods are effective at dispersing the scent of essential oils. Candles are often used, as well as electric heaters, clay

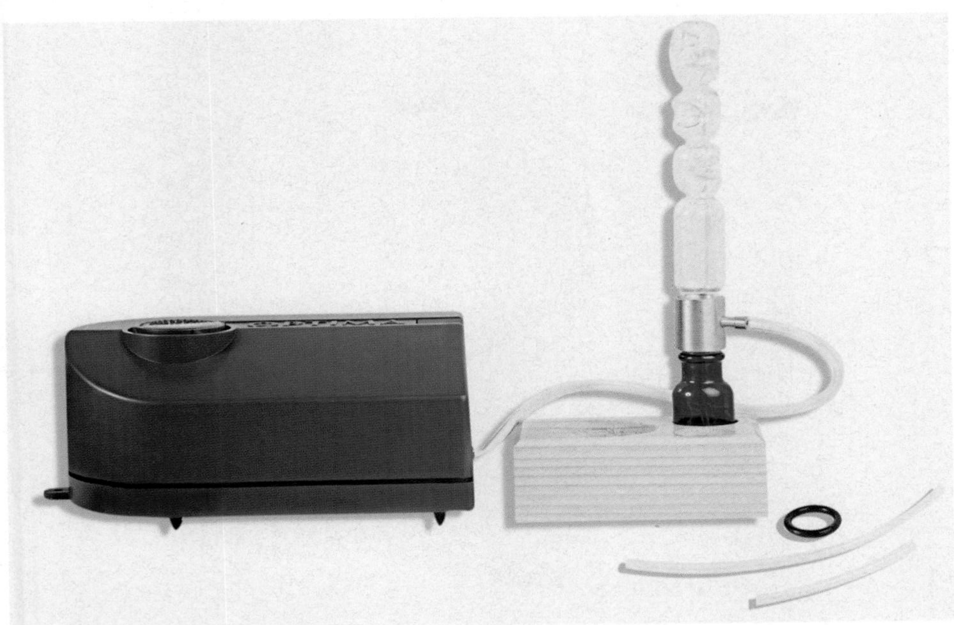

FIGURE 11-26 Nebulizers are the most effective way to diffuse essential oils.

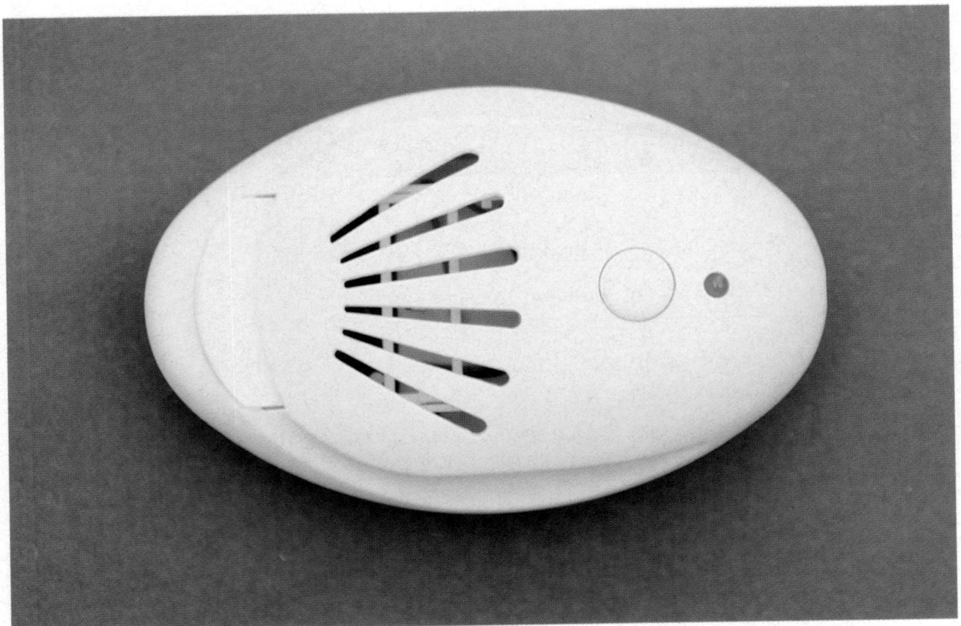

FIGURE 11-27 Fan diffusers are simple devices that make use of ventilation to spread aromas through the air.

pots, and even light bulbs. This method works well enough to disperse aroma into a room, but the heat can alter the chemical balance of the oils and diminish their therapeutic value. Sometimes oils are placed in a receptacle and left to simply evaporate with no heat applied (Figure 11-28).

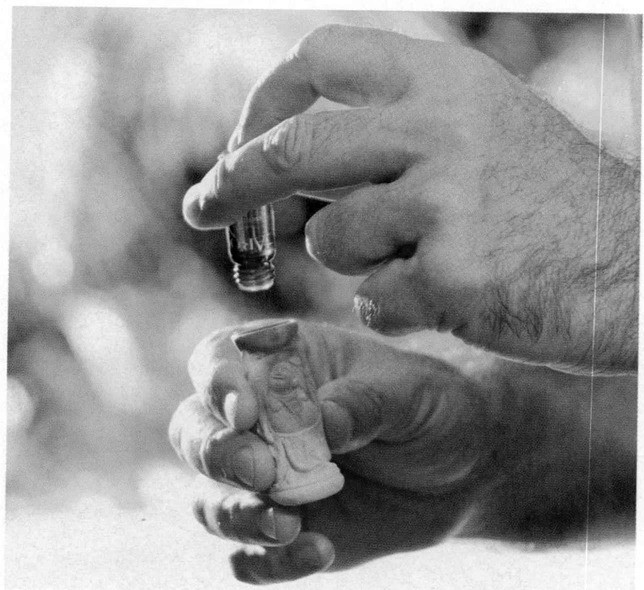

FIGURE 11–28 A small clay pot can be used to diffuse essential oils into a space.

Particle Size Matters

Did You Know?

There is an inverse relationship between the size of essential oil particles in the air and the depth of penetration into the respiratory tract. In other words, the larger the particle, the less depth, as shown in this little table.

PARTICLE SIZE	DEPTH OF PENETRATION
5 to 20 microns	nose, larynx, trachea
2 to 5 microns	shallow part of the lungs
1 to 3 microns	deep part of the lungs: alveolar region

Therefore, to achieve maximum penetration, the diffusing technique that creates the smallest particles of essential oil will be the most effective. Nebulization fits the bill in this regard. Any diffuser will create a pleasant aroma and improve the atmosphere of a room, but nebulizers offer maximum therapeutic benefit and are therefore highly recommended for therapeutically oriented spas.

Diffuser Confusion

Did You Know?

In spas, when people want to use a device that spreads the scent of aromatherapy throughout a room, they often use the word *nebulizer* interchangeably with *diffuser*. This is a mistake. Once again, we have a squares-and-rectangles problem. Every nebulizer is a diffuser, but not every diffuser is a nebulizer. A diffuser is any device that imparts scent via evaporation. A nebulizer is a very specific kind of diffuser that uses high-pressure air through a nozzle to disperse particles of essential oil of a particularly small size.

SPA PROFILE

Nicholas James, owner Body Bliss, Sedona, Arizona

Nicholas James is an Oxford University–trained botanist who has followed his bliss into the career path of aromatherapy. He now owns a company called Body Bliss, based in Sedona, Arizona, and he spends much of his time creating custom products for an ever-expanding list of spas. He notes that, as the industry becomes more saturated, spas are finding it important to distinguish themselves from each other, and an increasing number of them are turning to indigenous ingredients and plants to create aromatherapy-based products that uniquely reflect each particular spa and its environment. To achieve this goal for his clients, James finds himself engaged in pursuits that he perhaps never imagined while an undergrad at Oxford, such as keeping track of the destructive path of hurricanes in Florida. "Much of the grapefruit crop in Florida was destroyed due to hurricane activity," he explains, "and that created a shortage of organic grapefruit oil, causing prices to rise dramatically. When you're using hundreds of different natural raw materials, not a week goes by without facing shortages, price fluctuations and so on. Aromatherapy is an interesting industry that is actually woven quite tightly into the fabric of our economies and cultures worldwide."

James spends a lot of time interfacing with spa owners, spa directors, and spa therapists. "Spas are my main customers," he says, "and my most important point of contact is with the spa director, but I spend a lot of time talking with the therapists, training them on aromatherapy and product knowledge."

James says that the most important idea he tries to communicate to therapists during his trainings is regarding quality. "You can actually get profound and dramatic results in a spa setting, or any setting," says James, "but that only happens when you use oils of a sufficiently high standard. This is the gist of what I teach therapists. Quality is paramount. In nature, the sun shines energy on plants, and these plants manufacture a great variety of compounds. Essential oils consist of a vast array of aromatic compounds, and the more we can preserve the full spectrum of those compounds, the more optimally effective and powerful the oil will be."

According to James, the preservation of plants' integrity during processing varies depending upon the method used. "When you remove lesser compounds of a plant," he states, "you remove some of its effectiveness, because every compound has a purpose. At Body Bliss, one technique our distillers use is called *supercritical carbon dioxide extraction*, which is perhaps the best method for retaining all of a plant's compounds. In a nutshell, when you apply pressure to carbon dioxide just above room temperature, it becomes a supercritical fluid, somewhere between a liquid and a gas, which can be used to extract the oil-soluble components of the plant. Using this process, you don't have to heat the plants up very much, as you do with steam distillation, and therefore practically all of the compounds are preserved. This method of extraction has only been in commercial use relatively recently. It costs more because the equipment needed is more technical and expensive, and only a small percentage of commercially available essential oils are extracted in this manner. We don't use this technique with every oil, though, and we still produce some fabulous oils using steam distillation with low pressure over an extended time. Many companies, unfortunately, produce oils which are steam-distilled at too high a temperature, too quickly.

"People are not used to smelling the complete range of aromas that come from a plant. They can be incredibly complex, containing 300 to 400 compounds, but many commercial processes take that complexity away. Eucalyptus and peppermint oil, for instance, are deliberately distilled and redistilled for consistency in commercial applications

(Continued)

SPA PROFILE

Nicholas James, owner Body Bliss, Sedona, Arizona *continued*

because people would become disturbed if their toothpaste or other everyday products smelled different each time."

James finds himself doing some highly creative work with the high-quality oils he produces. "Each oil has its own frequency," he says, "a blueprint of sorts, that can be sensed. I spent two or three weeks studying each oil, and I wrote profiles of them from an energetic point of view, pairing them all with different human archetypes. Vetiver corresponds to the monk, for example, as it inspires meditation and centering. Frankincense is the father. Each oil has its own type. Eventually I began doing readings for people. They would choose an essential oil and it would reveal parts of their personality to me. Coming from a scientific background, in the beginning, I tended to be skeptical about my own claims in this arena, but the more readings I did with people, the more confident I became in the process. Many therapists have expressed a lot of interest in the technique."

According to James, aromatherapy is one of the key pillars of spa work. "Aromatherapy can and should be used in almost any type of spa modality," he says, "as it increases the pleasure and effectiveness of them all. It is perfectly suited to being used with massage, energy work, water treatments, body wraps, and face treatments. And now we're noticing a trend of aromatherapy moving into nontraditional areas of spa and hospitality, such as the in-room amenities. People want these products to be made in sustainable ways with natural ingredients, and essential oils fit the bill."

When it comes to obtaining the best aromatherapy education, James advises therapists to find somebody they trust and to learn from them, but at the same time he says they need to trust themselves. "You've got to compare oils and decide for yourself," he says. "It's not at all difficult to do so. I often take along some mediocre oils and some very good oils to my trainings and ask therapists to compare. They never have any problem distinguishing them. The nose is a fantastically sensitive instrument, and the world of essential oils is a fantastically rich one to explore."

CONCLUSION

Many massage therapists are attracted to using aromatherapy oils, and aromatherapy has become a major part of the spa landscape in recent years. No spa is complete without some component of aromatherapy playing a part on the treatment menu in one manner or another. Though a wide range of advanced training courses are available for therapists interested in honing their skills in this area, it is not necessary to become a highly trained expert in order to offer spa clients many of the benefits of aromatherapy. Through a moderate amount of study and practice, any spa therapist can become proficient in the blending and application of common essential oils, offering clients a wide range of therapeutic and mood-enhancing benefits, in addition to the sheer pleasure the aromas provide. You owe it to your future clients to make aromatherapy a basic part of your spa repertoire.

ACTIVITY

Determining Doshas

Several different techniques are used to determine which dosha is predominant in an individual. Experienced practitioners and Ayurvedic physicians can tell much about a patient through discussion and close observation alone. In addition, they use three main techniques to assess conditions and provide a diagnosis. These techniques include taking the pulse, testing urine samples, and examining the condition of the tongue, nails, and skin.

In spas, however, the most typical method of determining a client's dosha is through a simple questionnaire or "constitutional analysis." Figure 12–1 shows a popular constitutional analysis card used by Ayurvedic

TARA SPA THERAPY INC. TRAINING PROGRAM

TARA™
AYURVEDA

CONSTITUTIONAL ANALYSIS

In each of us resides the elements Ether, Air, Fire, Water and Earth.
To discover which elements predominate in your constitution,
mark the characteristics which pertain to you most.

	Vata (Ether & Air)	Pitta (Fire & Water)	Kapha (Water & Earth)
PHYSICAL FRAME	m thin, tall or short, small boned	m medium, well proportioned	m thick, stout, stocky, well developed, large boned
BODY WEIGHT	m light, prominent joints, under developed muscles	m moderate, good muscles, athletic physique	m overweight, heavy
SKIN	m dry, rough, cool, cracked, prominent veins, thin, fine pores	m soft, oily, warm, fair, sensitive, red, moles, skin eruptions, yellowish	m thick, oily, prone to acne, cool, pale
HAIR	m dry, curly, frizzy, kinky, coarse,	m fine, oily, baldness, early graying, reddish or blonde	m thick, shiny, oily, lustrous, wavy
EYES	m small, dry, dark, few eyelashes	m medium, sharp, pene-trating, green, yellowish, light sensitive	m large, round, blue or brown, thick eyelashes
LIPS	m thin, dry, chapped	m soft, medium	m large, smooth, full
TEETH	m can be crooked or protruded	m yellowish, sensitive gums	m strong, white, large, even
NAILS	m brittle, ridged, cracked	m soft, flexible	m strong, thick
STRENGTH	m low, poor endurance	m medium	m strong, good endurance
APPETITE	m variable, erratic, small amounts frequently	m strong, unbearable at times, persistent	m slow but steady
PHYSICAL ACTIVITY	m very active	m moderate	m less active, can be lethargic
MIND	m active, restless	m intelligent, sharp, focused	m calm, slow
EMOTIONAL TEMPERAMENT	m changeable, fearful, unpredictable, insecure, anxious, nervous	m assertive, aggressive, easily irritated, hot tempered, angry	m waves of emotions, tearful, attached, calm, passive

FIGURE 12–1 Constitutional analysis card. *(Continued)*

(Continued)

TARA SPA THERAPY INC. TRAINING PROGRAM

TARA™ AYURVEDA

CONSTITUTIONAL ANALYSIS (CONTINUED)

	Vata (Ether & Air)	*Pitta* (Fire & Water)	*Kapha* (Water & Earth)
MEMORY	m recent memory good, remote memory poor	m excellent	m slow but sustaining
SPEECH	m fast, talkative, breathy	m sharp, precise	m slow, melodic
SLEEP	m scanty, interrupted	m little but sound	m deep and prolonged
DREAMS	m fearful, flying, movement	m fiery, angry, violence, passionate	m watery, ocean, river, peaceful, romantic
ELIMINATION	m dry, hard, constipation	m soft, oily loose	m thick, oily, heavy, slow
IMBALANCE TENDENCY	m constipation, nervousness, anxiety, insomnia, cracking, popping joints	m inflammatory disease, hypertension, rash, skin disorder, hypersensitive, aggressive behavior	m respiratory congestion, water retention, obesity, lethargy, cystic acne, lymphatic congestion

TOTAL

Constitutional Analysis: ______________________________

____

____

____

NAME: ____________________

DATE: ____________

Reference: ***Ayurveda, The Science of Self Healing*** **by Dr. Vasant Lad**

FIGURE 12–1 Constitutional analysis card.

spa product provider and trainer Tara Spa Therapy and originally sourced from Dr. Vasant Lad's book, *The Science of Self Healing*. Answer the questions to determine your own predominant dosha type. In spas, once a client's dosha is determined, specific products that are most beneficial for that type are then applied to the skin.

Deep Cleaning

Did You Know?

True traditional pancha karma includes elements that many spa clients would most likely find unpleasant. Self-induced vomiting and enemas, for example, are not usually on the list of preferred treatments for someone on her way to a spa getaway with a group of girlfriends. However, for those people seeking true deep cleaning and renewal, nothing beats the full pancha karma program, which includes the following five cleansing procedures:

1. *nasya*: cleansing of the nasal and sinus passages
2. *basti*: cleansing of the colon
3. *verechena*: cleansing of the small intestines
4. *vamana*: cleansing of the stomach and lungs
5. *rakta moksha*: cleansing of the blood

Each day during this cleansing process includes an oil massage and steam treatment to help circulate and eliminate any toxins released in the body.

or kapha and to leave the body in a state of balance. Traditionally, in Ayurvedic spas, pancha karma is given over the course of seven days, but in most other spas, the treatments are modified and can be given one at a time.

Ayurvedic practitioners believe that the right food is the best medicine, and they use specific types of food to treat disease. Pancha karma includes a regimen of fresh nutritious foods prepared daily during a program. Medical doctors and highly trained experts administer pancha karma in spas such as the Chopra Center in California, and people report feeling lighter and healthier after undergoing the full program. Sometimes, chronic conditions and diseases are improved or eliminated. Most spas, however, do not offer such intensive programs and instead feature just a few Ayurvedic-inspired treatments on their menus.

Although the cleansing therapies used in pancha karma may vary from one person to another, depending upon dosha and particular goals, two elements remain consistent for almost everybody undergoing a pancha karma program. These are the oil massage known as **abhyanga** and the full-body steam immersion called *swedana*. Other Ayurvedic therapies are also used, several of which are offered in all types of spas. They are listed below.

abhyanga

four-handed Ayurvedic oil massage

Abhyanga

This full-body massage is normally two hours long and is usually given by two experienced therapists who are familiar with Ayurvedic protocols, though a single therapist can administer the massage as well. The therapists synchronize their movements and apply massage to specific circulatory channels and **marma points**, 107 of which are located on the body. In Sanskrit, *marma* means *hidden* or *secret*, and the points can be found at the junction of different types of tissues, such as muscles, ligaments, bones, joints, or veins. Practitioners also point out that they are the meeting points of mind and matter. As in acupressure point massage, the idea behind marma massage is to unblock energy, or **chi**.

marma points

a total of 107 specific points on the body that are stimulated as part of an Ayurvedic massage

chi

life force energy in the body stimulated by massaging marma points in Ayurvedic treatments

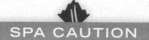

SPA CAUTION

Because of the relatively large amount of oil used in abhyanga massage, it is especially important to wipe the client's feet off at the end of the treatment with a moist towel so she does not slip when rising from the table.

Each marma point is said to have three receptors, one for each dosha, and the points are massaged in specific ways with particular oils depending upon which dosha is being affected. In general, a very light stimulation is applied over these points. It is a subtle technique using direct pressure or circular movements, either clockwise or counterclockwise, depending upon the desired result.

Sesame oil—or an oil chosen according to one's body type, or dosha—is typically used, and the massage is often followed by the swedana steam treatment, which is meant to help the oils penetrate the skin and lubricate body tissues. Much more of this oil is used than in a normal spa massage, and clients should be told about this beforehand so they are not overwhelmed by the amount of lubricant.

Shirodhara

shirodhara

Ayurvedic treatment featuring the pouring of oil over the "third eye" area

Shiro means "head," and *dhara* signifies the flow of liquid. In **shirodhara**, the client lies on the massage table with her head just slightly over the top, and experiences a continuous flow of warm oil pouring over the forehead from a special container held in place in a support stand (Figure 12–2). This process lasts approximately 30 minutes. Though the oil is often poured over the "third eye" area of the forehead by itself, a variety of herbs and medicated milks may be added to it as well. The treatment is quite relaxing, and some Ayurvedic practitioners claim it can help open energies in the "third eye" area and stimulate psychic strength. It is used in cases of memory loss, headaches, tension, and insomnia. Shirodhara is always administered in conjunction with an abhyanga full-body massage.

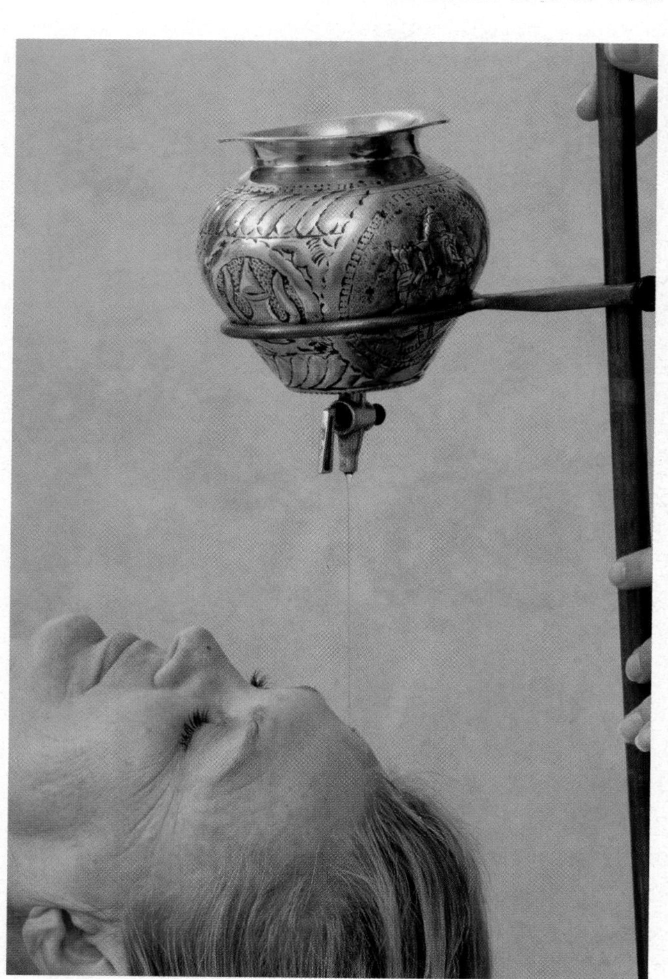

FIGURE 12–2 A shirodhara treatment.

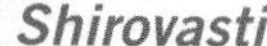

Shirovasti

Shirovasti is an Ayurvedic head bath featuring special herbal oils. Traditional Indian leaves and flowers are soaked in oil, which is then poured into a cap and placed on the head. With this treatment, practitioners seek to reduce eye strain, sinus congestion, and headaches.

Garshana

Garshana is the Ayurvedic version of exfoliation, a dry lymphatic skin brushing performed with a silk glove. This creates all the benefits of exfoliation explained in Chapter 6, increasing circulation and cleansing the skin so that other spa products and oils can penetrate deeply. It is usually offered in combination with other treatments, especially the abhyanga massage and shirodhara.

Pinda Sweda

In *pinda sweda*, hot herbal poultices are applied, similar to the Thai herbal balls described in the "Herbal Compress Therapy" section of Chapter 8. The hot poultices are pressed into the skin all over the body, especially in areas such as the joints where pain or stiffness may be felt.

Udvarthanam

This treatment is known as "flower petal massage" or "Ayurvedic powder massage." The powder derives from dried and finely ground tropical flowers which are applied to the skin by one or two therapists.

Lepana

In the *lepana* treatment a paste of Ayurvedic herbs is applied over the whole body. The paste is left to dry and is then removed using deep tissue massage techniques.

CRANIOSACRAL THERAPY

As its reputation for being both effective and gentle has grown, craniosacral therapy (CST) has proven increasingly popular in many spas. Spa clients seeking a lighter touch than typical massage find that craniosacral fits the bill perfectly. While it could be considered "energy work," the modality has also built a solid therapeutic reputation. People have read about it in newspapers and magazines, or they have heard anecdotal stories from friends and relatives. The technique has helped many people, even some seriously ill ones. Therapists who spend the time and money to pursue further training in this modality stand a good chance at being able to use their skills at top spas, many of which seek out qualified craniosacral therapists.

The technique is called *craniosacral* because it deals with the movement of **cerebrospinal fluid** (CSF) through the spine, from the *cranium* to the *sacrum* (Figure 12–3). In this technique, therapists place their hands gently on the client's spine, skull, and other areas of the body, and tune into the natural pulse of CSF, facilitating subtle releases and realigning bones to their proper positions. This is said to treat many kinds of mental and physical stress, from back pain to migraines, from fibromyalgia to posttraumatic stress.

cerebrospinal fluid

the fluid in the ventricles of the brain, between the arachnoid and pia mater, and surrounding the spinal cord

The pulse felt by practitioners is known as the **craniosacral rhythm (CSR)**, and there is some controversy as to whether this pulse actually exists. The technique of manipulating the craniosacral system was developed originally by osteopathic doctor William Sutherland, who first posited that cranial bones might move slightly at their sutures, facilitating the CSR. This pulse was synchronous all the way down to the sacrum. Sutherland instituted a new field known as *cranial osteopathy* to disseminate his findings, training others to teach the technique.

craniosacral rhythm (CSR)

a naturally occurring pulsation of cerebrospinal fluid through the ventricles of the brain and around the spinal cord; its existence is questioned by some authorities

Osteopathic physician John E. Upledger continued this work at Michigan State University, where he set up a team of medical professionals to study Sutherland's theories. His studies led him to believe that the craniosacral rhythm indeed exists, and he claims to have observed it during an operation when a patient's spinal cord was visible. Upledger then developed his own treatment style, naming it *craniosacral therapy* and teaching it to thousands of hands-on practitioners around the world through his Upledger Institute. This is the main therapy that many spa clients seek out today, and it has inspired several subspecialties such as emotionally based work and lymphatic drainage techniques.

THE CRANIOSACRAL SYSTEM

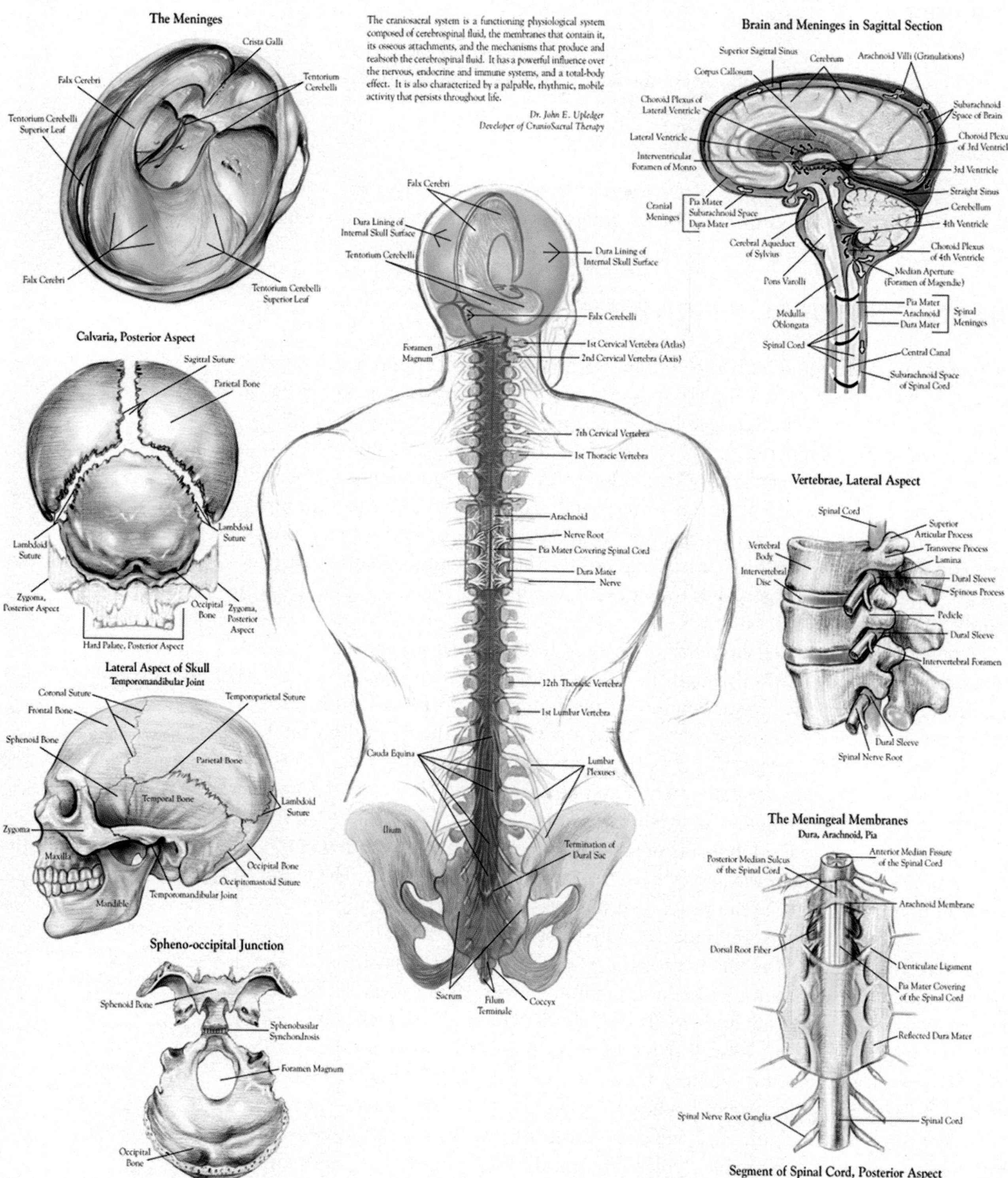

FIGURE 12–3 The structures of the Craniosacral System. Courtesy of The Upledger Institute.

Some spas offer craniosacral therapy as a stand-alone selection on their menus, while others incorporate it into another treatment. Some therapists use aspects of craniosacral when they are performing a massage, especially one that requires light touch, as when working with elderly or frail clients. In general, the modality is a good non-invasive adjunct therapy. While there is some continuing controversy regarding the scientific verifiability of craniosacral therapy, many highly positive results have been achieved, and spa clients continue to book the treatment on a consistent basis.

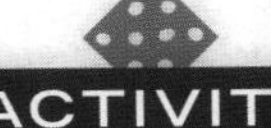

SPA TIP

Craniosacral therapy has been known to positively impact the lives of people living with a variety of serious medical conditions. If you are working in a spa where CST is not available, consider referring out to a qualified CST therapist for clients who present with any of the following complaints:

- Migraines and headaches
- Chronic neck and back pain
- Stress and tension-related disorders
- Motor-coordination impairments
- Infant and childhood disorders
- Brain and spinal cord injuries
- Chronic fatigue
- TMJ syndrome
- Scoliosis
- Central nervous system disorders
- Learning disabilities
- ADD
- Posttraumatic stress disorder
- Orthopedic problems

ACTIVITY

Feeling the Craniosacral Pulse

The problem most therapists run into when they first attempt to detect the craniosacral rhythm (CSR) is that they are unable to feel anything because they are applying too much pressure. The Upledger Institute recommends applying "pressure equaling the weight of a nickel" on the client's skin in order to most effectively access the pulse.

Try it.

1. Find a partner and take turns lying supine on a massage table.
2. Sitting at the head of the table, place a nickel on your partner's upper chest and watch it move up and down with his or her breath.
3. Now, place a fingertip or thumb alongside the nickel and try to match the pressure of its weight into your partner's body. Chances are it will be quite difficult to remain so superficial. Hold this light touch for a few minutes.
4. Then change hand locations, placing your fingertips gently along the temporal bones behind the eyes and just in front of and above the ears.
5. Maintaining light contact, feel for the craniosacral rhythm, which will be a slow, steady inward and outward movement of the bones.
6. Be aware that the CSR is not the heartbeat, which you may detect in the superficial temporal arteries, nor the breath, which you will experience as a slow rising and falling. This is a separate pulse, slower and subtler than the other two, usually experienced by the practitioner as slight expansion and contraction.
7. Trade partners. When you have both practiced nickel pressure and tried to feel the CSR, discuss your experience.

INDONESIAN TREATMENTS

Geographically specific spa treatments from a number of countries are popular, as already noted in the Ayurvedic offerings from India. You will also discover lomilomi from Hawaii and Thai treatments from Thailand. Spas are constantly seeking new, exotic locales on which to base their treatment offerings, to entice clients who have already sampled the mainstream spa offerings of Swedish massage and hydrotherapy applications. One of the lesser-known up-and-coming location-oriented therapy traditions has its origins in Indonesia, especially Bali and Java. The Indonesian-inspired treatments focus on ingredients found on the lush jungle islands of the region, including frangipani, ginger, jasmine, coconut, and aloe vera. Natural rice bran and fresh yogurt are often used for exfoliation, and an abundance of fresh tropical blossoms is typically strewn throughout the treatment area to recreate an island feeling. The most popular Indonesian offering is a service called the **Lulur**, which is described below.

Lulur

type of spa service that recreates an Indonesian pre-nuptial ritual, including exfoliation, massage, yogurt application, and bath

Javanese Lulur Procedure

The Lulur spa experience was originally inspired by a seventeenth-century ritual from the royal palaces of Central Java, in Indonesia. During this ancient tradition, every day for 40 days prior to a marriage celebration, the bride-to-be would receive "Lulur" from the other women in the family, as a way of passing on wisdom and nurturing. In modern times, the complete Lulur is now a popular spa treatment suggested for both men and women, and not only on wedding days. It is often promoted as a romance ritual, a celebration of love. Jasmine and frangipani are the two main ingredients incorporated into every authentic product for the Lulur.

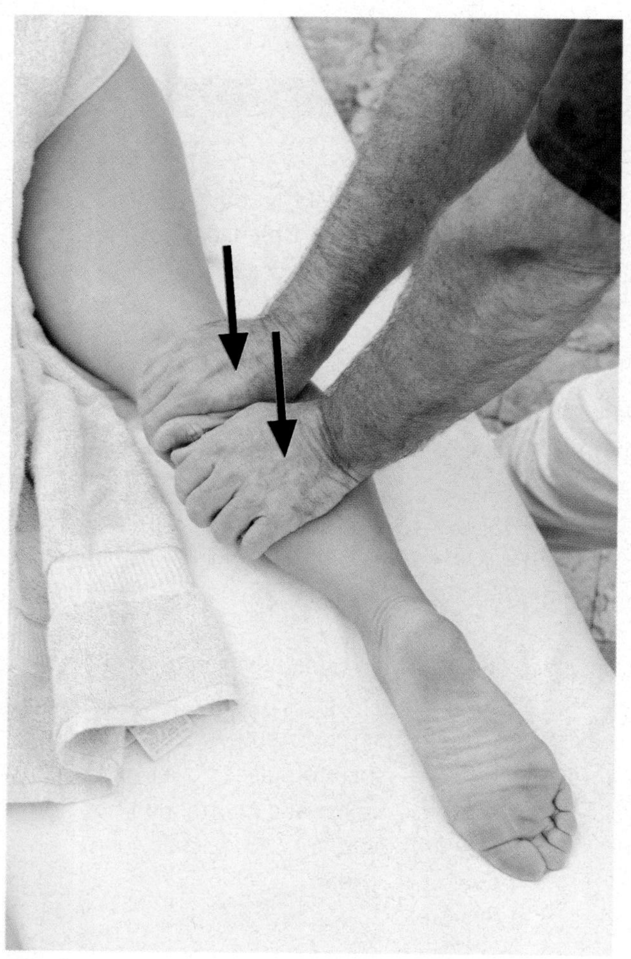

FIGURE 12–4

Notes on procedure: Several aspects of this protocol can be altered to suit the situations found in massage school classrooms. Authentic Lulur ingredients are usually sourced from Indonesia, but generic products may be substituted for the massage oil, exfoliant, bath gel, and body butter. At one point during the treatment, fresh yogurt is traditionally applied to the skin as a natural exfoliant. This can be substituted with a hydrating lotion in your classroom if desired, for practice purposes, as will be noted in the procedure. Also, a bath is normally part of the treatment, but if none is available in your practice area, hot, wet towels can be substituted.

There are nine Indonesian-inspired massage strokes and techniques used in this treatment, as explained below. For the first five movements, only the hands are used. Jasmine and frangipani massage oil is incorporated into the last four techniques.

1. *Compression*: Palm pressure using both hands at the same time (Figure 12–4).
2. *Thumb Walk*: Thumbs "walk" continuously over each other (Figure 12–5).

3. *Crab Walk*: Gently grasp and lift the muscle, then "walk" one hand over the other to the next area (Figure 12–6).
4. *Wringing*: Using cupped hands, alternate compression inward (Figure 12–7).

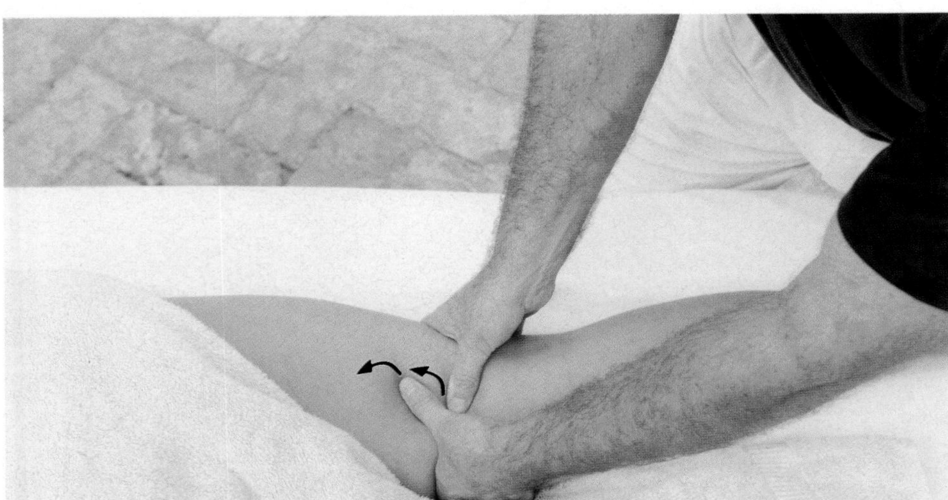

FIGURE 12-5

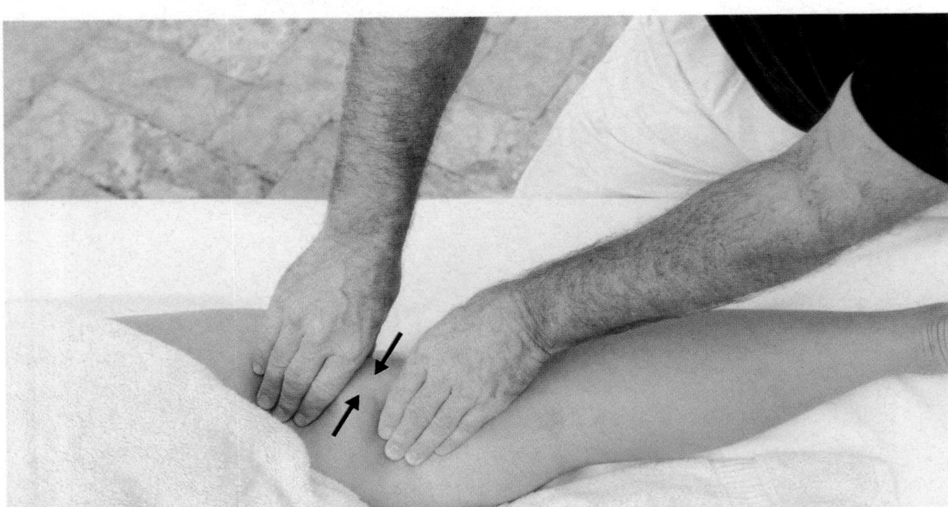

FIGURE 12-6

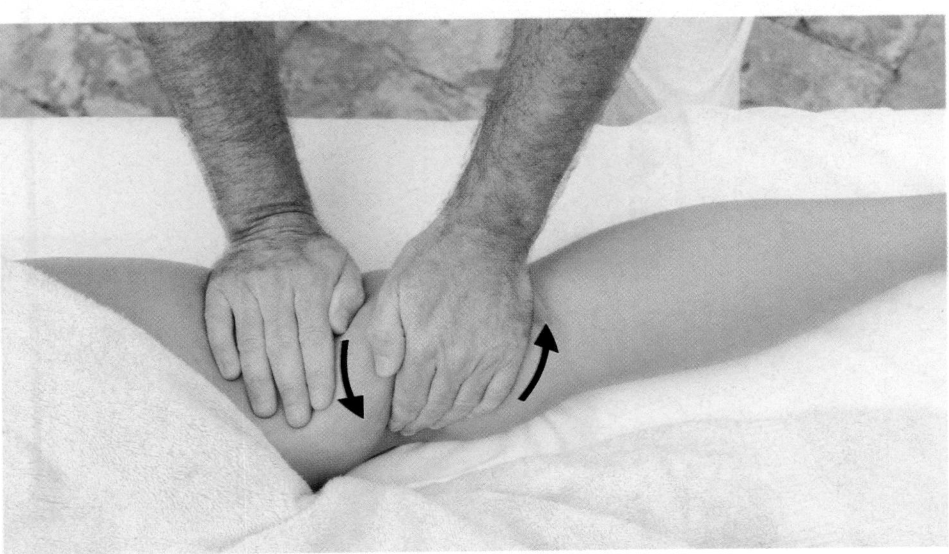

FIGURE 12-7

5. *Skin Rolling*: Gently lift and roll the skin using thumbs and forefingers in a forward motion, then use light nerve stroked back (Figure 12–8).
6. *Oil Application*: Use effleurage to apply Jamu massage oil (Figure 12–9).
7. *Knuckling*: Apply muscle stripping with thumbs together and knuckles moving away from you (Figure 12–10).

FIGURE 12-8

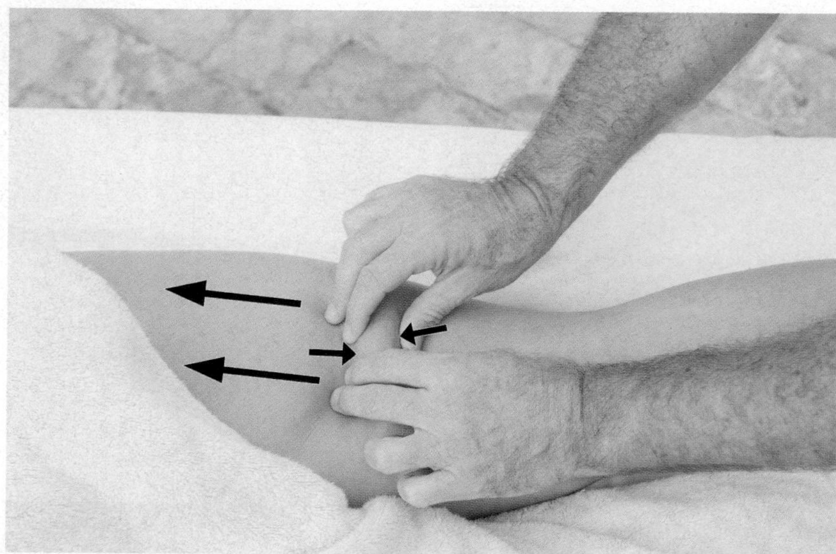

FIGURE 12-9

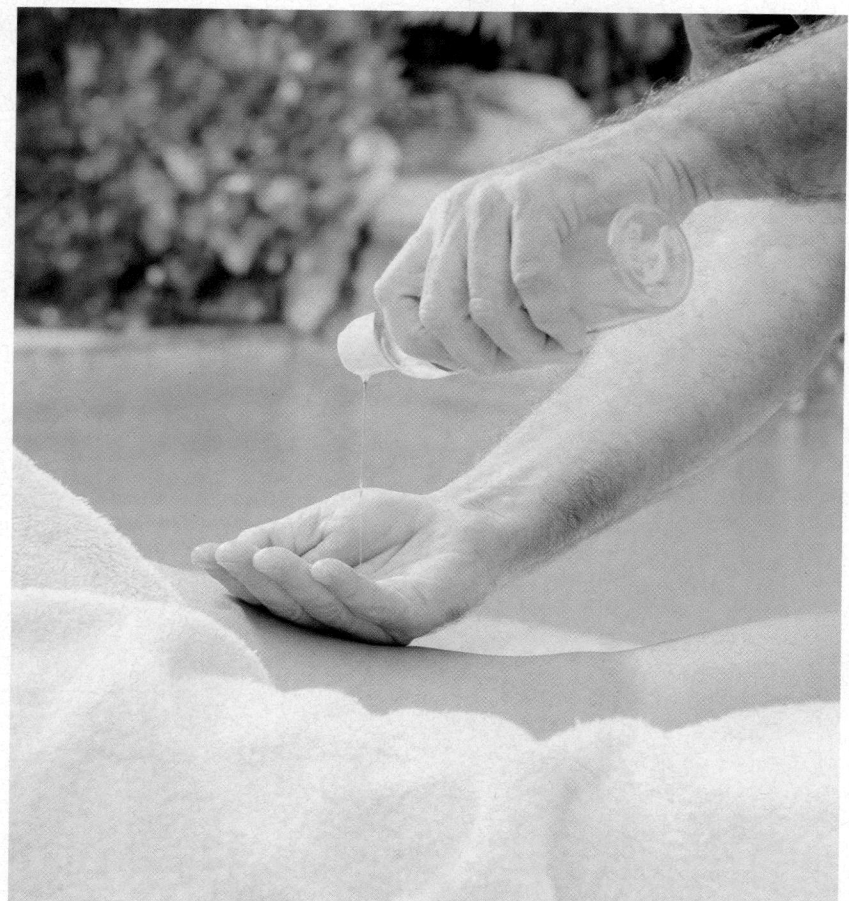

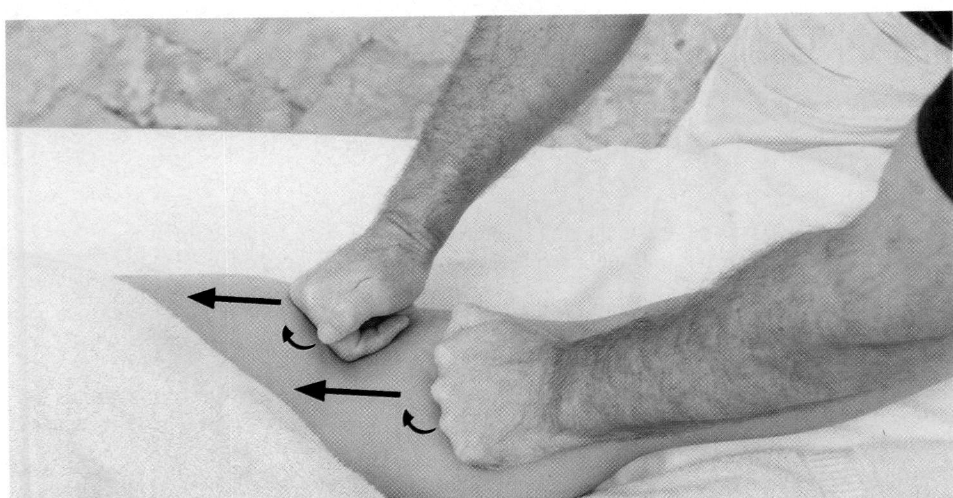

FIGURE 12–10

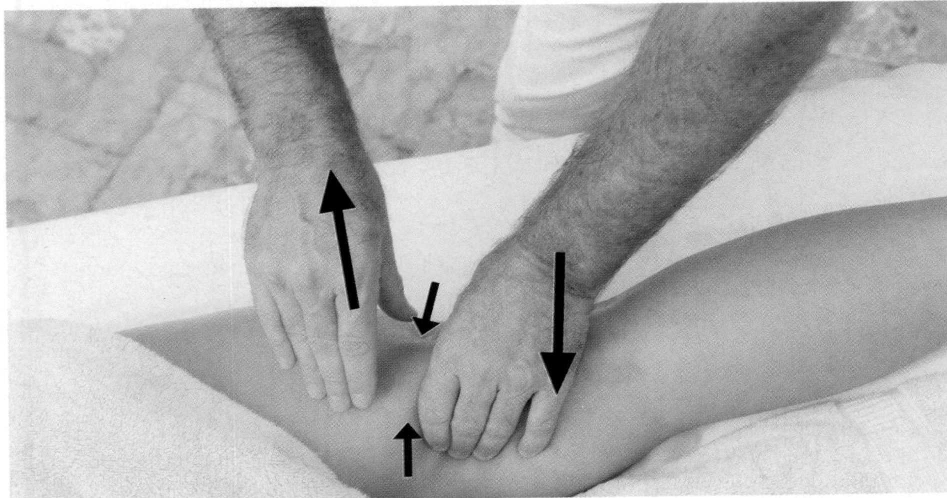

FIGURE 12–11

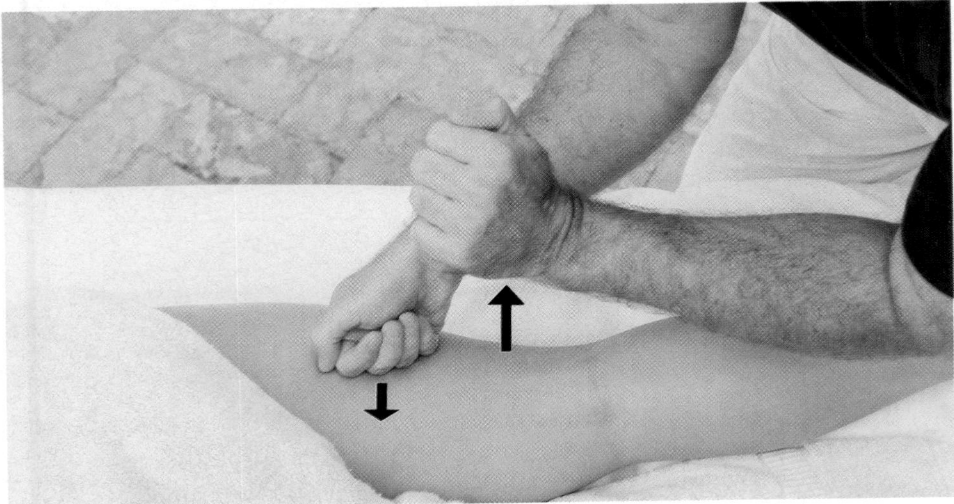

FIGURE 12–12

8. *Bumbu*: **Bumbu** means to add "spice" with this alternative skin-rolling technique that incorporates all four fingers opposite the thumb instead of just the forefinger (Figure 12–11).
9. *Percussion*: Use soft fist pounding, "bird's beak pecking," and light chopping in a rhythmic and energizing tempo (Figure 12–12).

Bumbu

meaning to add "spice," a skin-rolling massage technique incorporating all four fingers opposite the thumb, used in Javanese Lulur treatments

TREATMENT: JAVANESE LULUR	
Wet Room/Dry Room	wet room
Table Setup	fitted table sheet, blanket, lower sheet, upper sheet, towel drape
Treatment Duration	90 minutes
Needed Supplies	hot towel cabbie, towels, Lulur massage oil, Lulur body scrub, hydrating lotion or body butter; optional: yogurt, Lulur bath gel, bath salts
Contraindications	Caution is advised for pregnant clients as the bath water temperature could possible raise core body temperature. Also, the blend of many aromas may be too much for sensitive individuals, including pregnant clients. Also contraindicated: sunburn, cuts, abrasions, sores, eczema, thin/delicate skin, allergies to exfoliants, and recent shaving. Untreated hypertension is contraindicated for the massage and heated bath portions of this treatment with a physician's approval. Note: The yellow coloring of the scrub is due to turmeric, and may remain on the skin for several hours. Suggest that clients not wear white clothing directly after treatment.
Draping	Employ normal draping as for massage; see Bath Entry Draping Protocol in Chapter 4 for details on draping prior to the bath that is a part of this treatment.
Treatment Order	Lulur contains a scrub, a bath, and a massage, and can be considered a type of package consisting of several different treatments. It can be given before a facial.
Safety, Sanitation Issues, & Clean-Up	Floors may become slippery after the bath. Always use a bath mat. Take care to maintain bath water at proper temperature, near 100°F. Flowers, oils, and scrubs need to be cleaned up after every service.
Body Mechanics & Self-Care	Take care when bending over bath. Use normal massage therapy body mechanics during massage and scrub.
Product Cost	$2 per treatment, more if fresh yogurt is used
Treatment Price	$125 to $200
Physiological Effects	Exfoliation removes dead skin cells, improving appearance and preparing body for absorption of therapeutic products. Massage benefits circulation, relieves minor aches and pains, stretches soft tissues, initiates relaxation response. Warm/hot bath opens pores, relaxes muscles. Ingredients in the oil and exfoliant include antibacterial, antiseptic, anti-inflammatory and antioxidant effects, while lotions and body butter provide emollient action.
Pregnancy Issues (information provided by Elaine Stillerman, LMT, author and developer of MotherMassage)	Not advised during pregnancy if water temperature is too warm, aromatics contraindicated, or scrubbing too aggressive on the lower extremities. Employ lymphatic drainage on the legs during pregnancy and up to three months postpartum.

Javanese Lulur Preparation

1. Place a flower bowl under the face cradle with floating blossoms and essential oils.
2. Place a bath mat at the entrance side of table, with flower blossoms/petals on it.
3. Prepare a minimum of five hot, moist towels in a towel cabbie.
4. Create a presentation tray with the Lulur, body butter, bath salts, and scrub. Top spas also include freshly shredded ginger root, sprigs of fresh rosemary, and fresh blossoms to beautify the experience.
5. Prepare the massage table with linens (dark linens are best), a strip of accent fabric, and blossoms/petals.

Javanese Lulur Procedure

1. Present the tray of products to the client and briefly explain the treatment, inviting any questions.
2. Place Lulur scrub, enzyme lotion, and body butter in a hot towel cabbie to be kept warm.
3. Invite the client to lie supine on the massage table while you leave the room. Return when she is under the drapes on the table.
4. Touch your palms to the lower legs above the ankles slowly and consciously, and offer a silent blessing for the treatment.
5. Begin compression atop the draping towel on the left leg at the ankles with both palms, and move this compression up the leg, up the left arm, across the upper chest, then down the right arm and back down the right leg, all atop the drape (Figure 12–13).

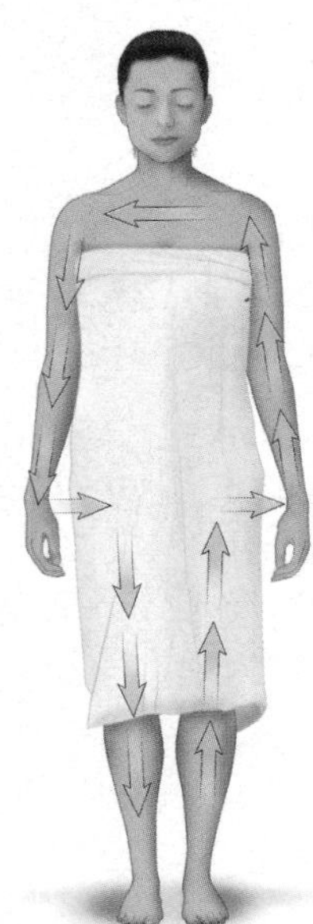

FIGURE 12–13 All maneuvers follow the same circular pattern over the body during the Lulur treatment.

6. Do the first five "dry" techniques up the left leg, up the left arm, then on the right arm and back down the right leg.
7. Follow with oil and the remaining techniques over the same areas in the opposite order—up the right leg, up the right arm, then on the left arm and back down the left leg.
8. Ask the client if she would like abdominal massage, and follow the breast draping procedure for women if so, using only the last four techniques, with oil.
9. Sit at the head of the table and apply the last four techniques, with oil, on the head, neck, and shoulders.
10. The client turns over to repeat this procedure, applying the first five techniques, without oil, on the back of the right leg, up over the back, and down the left leg.
11. Reverse the direction using oil for the last four techniques. If the client is comfortable, the back and leg can be undraped at the same time.
12. Start the bath. If no bath is available, skip this step.
13. Apply warm, pre-blended Lulur scrub to the back of the body, beginning at the right foot, one section at a time: up the right leg, over the back, and down the left leg.
14. Lightly remove the Lulur scrub with warm, moist towels, one towel for the legs and feet, one towel for the back.
15. Apply a thin layer of fresh, plain, organic yogurt to the back of the body—*only* if including the bath step later. If no bath is available, skip this step and apply finishing lotion to the back of the body.
16. Ask the client to roll over, rolling the top sheet out from underneath. First, have the client roll to the far side of the table, roll the sheet toward the middle of the back, then have the client roll back to the near side of the table and pull the sheet completely off the table before having the client lie down on her back atop the clean second sheet.
17. Apply warm, pre-blended Lulur scrub to the front of the body, beginning at the right foot, one section at a time: right leg, right arm, left arm, left leg, torso, and décolleté.
18. Lightly remove the Lulur scrub with warm, moist towels, one towel for the legs and feet, one towel for the arms and hands, and one towel for the torso, décolleté, and shoulders.
19. Apply a thin layer of fresh, plain, organic yogurt to the front of the body—*only* if including the bath step later. If no bath is available, skip this step and apply finishing lotion to the front of the body.

20. Optional: Shut off the bath and add bath gel and sea salts, then spread the flower petals on the water.
21. The client is wrapped for 12 to 15 minutes—wrapped in yogurt if the bathtub is being used, or wrapped in hydrating lotion when no bath is being used.

PERFORM STEPS 22 THROUGH 25 ONLY IF USING THE BATH

22. Unwrap and escort the client to the bath, keeping her covered in the second sheet. Follow the Bath Entry Draping Protocol from Chapter 4.
23. The client bathes for 10 minutes with Lulur bath gel and bath salts (Figure 12–14).
24. After the bath experience, invite the client back to the treatment table to lie down prone, first under the drape, and apply body butter for five minutes on the back of the body.
25. Ask the client to turn over, and apply body butter for five minutes on the front of the body.

TAKE UP TREATMENT AGAIN HERE IF NO BATH IS USED

26. Assist the client in sitting up and getting into a robe.
27. Offer a cup of warm jasmine/orange tea.
28. Optional: Place a flower behind the client's ear.

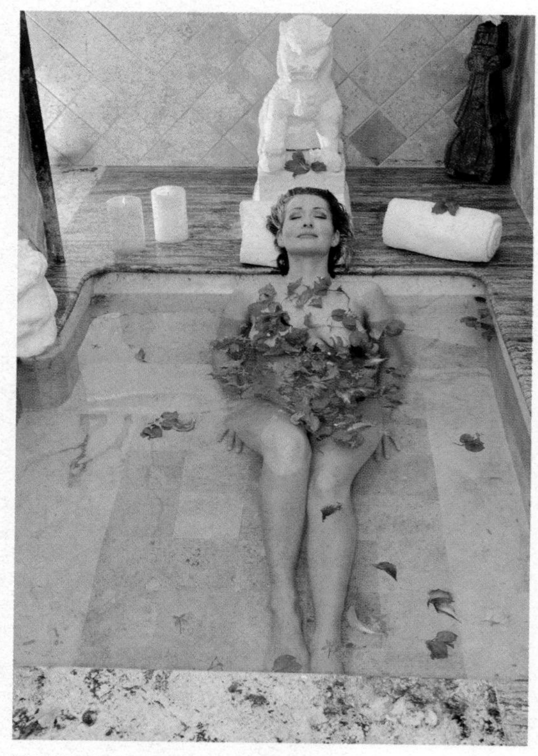

FIGURE 12–14

29. Finish by placing hands together in front of the heart and offering the traditional Indonesian blessing called **Terimakasih**:

    "Lulur treatments in Indonesia are traditionally given with a spirit of kindness and peacefulness. We acknowledge this with a special word—terimakasih. This means, 'I have received your love.' Thank you for giving me the opportunity to work with you today."

Terimakasih

Indonesian blessing word uttered at end of Lulur and other spa services there, meaning "I have received your love"

kahunas

Hawaiian healer skilled in the full spectrum of lomilomi techniques that extend beyond massage, including diet, herbal medicine, counseling, elements of chiropractic, and more

Javanese Lulur Cleanup

1. Change table and launder the linens.
2. Empty and wash the bathtub with disinfectant.
3. Dispose of flower petals or save for the next treatment.

LOMILOMI

Lomilomi massage has become a mainstay on many spa menus, especially in Japan and Europe, and its popularity is increasing in the United States as well. What clients in a modern spa experience as lomilomi is a refined and abbreviated adaptation of a much broader and more comprehensive healing tradition that had its roots in Polynesia hundreds of years ago as Polynesian settlers on Hawaii adapted ancient hands-on healing techniques into a unique system all their own. As it evolved over time in separate valleys on different islands, lomilomi branched into several distinct styles with varied techniques.

In the past, before Western influences became all-pervasive, the practice of lomilomi was not restricted to Hawaiian healers, known as **kahunas**. Rather, everyone in the family massaged each other on various occasions, and the techniques were known to all. In addition, everyone knew about healing herbs for various ailments. Natural healing and massage were part of the culture. Special lomilomi sessions were reserved for tribal chiefs, who basked in luxury, eating rich foods and receiving massages meant to relax them and aid in the digestion of their vast meals. In fact, one of the earliest uses of the word "lomilomi" by a native Hawaiian was in reference to the "person who took care of the chief's excrement."

Beyond massage, traditional lomilomi healing sessions are likely to include chiropractic manipulation, physical therapy, stone therapy, bone setting, hydrotherapy, herbal medicine, and dietary advice. And beyond these physical techniques, an element of prayer—**Pule** in Hawaiian—and spiritual counseling is also involved. Practitioners often help resolve disputes and heal crises by having the parties involved open new lines of heartfelt communication, a method with the Hawaiian name of **ho'oponopono**.

Pule
Hawaiian for *prayer*, traditionally part of lomilomi healing sessions

ho'oponopono
method of resolving disputes and clashes within families and tribes; part of traditional Hawaiian lomilomi

La'au
sticks used as therapeutic massage tools in lomilomi treatments

Na'au
the word for large intestine or colon in Hawaiian; also means *soul* or *heart*

Did You Know?

Real Lomilomi

Although most lomilomi work experienced by spa clients today is a somewhat watered-down version, it is still possible to taste the original flavor of the technique by traveling to Hawaii or other locales and visiting a practitioner versed in traditional lomilomi healing techniques. People who do so may be quite surprised by what they find. For instance, many lomilomi practitioners employ the aid of a very large stick, a ten-foot pole, actually, when plying their trade. They use it to balance themselves while walking all over their clients, cracking bones and affecting myriad chiropractic adjustments. Practitioners might also make use of smaller sticks called **La'au** as powerful massage tools, as shown in Figure 12–15. Then, there may be several minutes of Hawaiian prayer incantation, which lends an exotic island feeling to the proceedings. And clients should not be surprised if the practitioner spends a lot of time working on the belly. Traditional lomilomi always features extensive work on the gastrointestinal area; the word for *colon* in Hawaiian is **Na'au**, which also means "soul" or "heart."

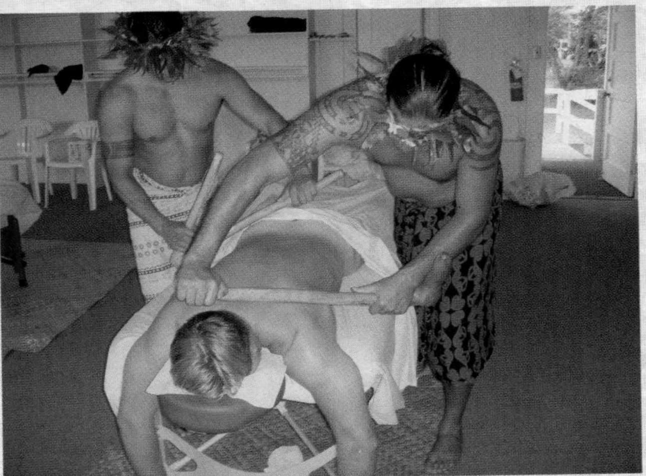

FIGURE 12–15 Traditional practitioners performing La'au lomilomi.

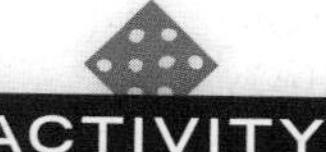

ACTIVITY

Simplified Lomilomi

Although traditional lomilomi is a rich and complex system of healing, some of the pleasure and therapeutic effects created by the technique can be experienced through simple maneuvers that are typically practiced by massage therapists in spas. Therapists who take weeklong retreats or seminars become familiar with these techniques, the most familiar of which is assuredly the forearm effleurage stroke, which has become symbolic of the overall modality. Practitioners may also use the palms, fingers, knuckles, elbows, knees, feet, and stones, but the forearm stroke epitomizes the technique for most people. You can practice the basic technique yourself with a partner using the following simple steps.

1. Have your partner lay prone on the massage table and undrape one leg (Figure 12–16).
2. Apply a liberal amount of massage oil, slightly more than you would normally use, with normal effleurage strokes at first (Figure 12–17).

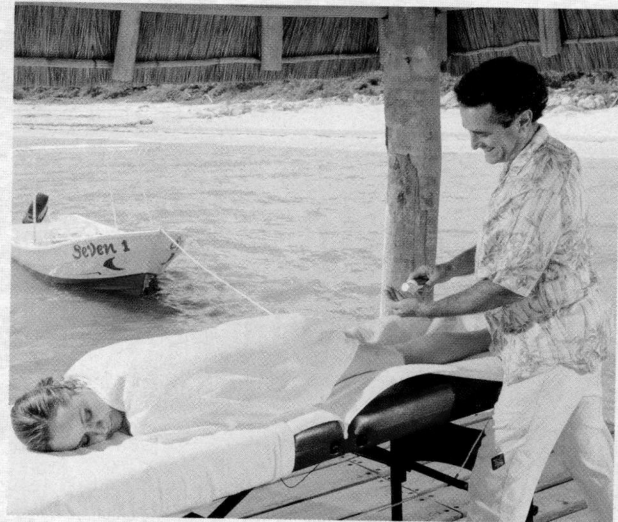

FIGURE 12–16

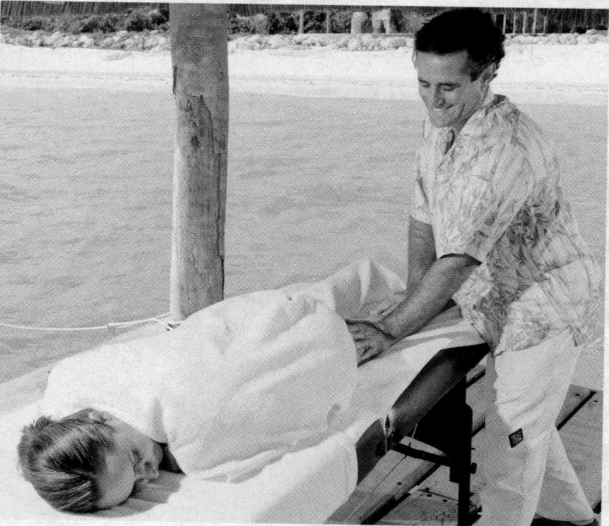

FIGURE 12–17

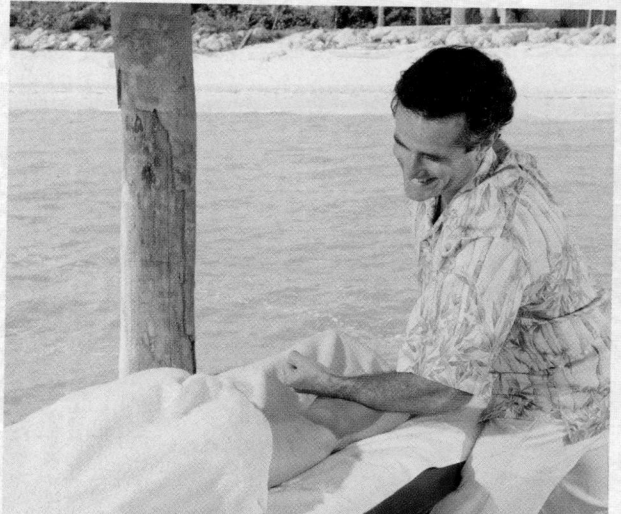

FIGURE 12–18

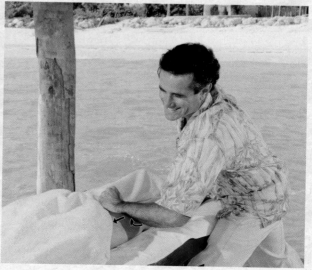

FIGURE 12–19

3. Bending your knees, get your hips down at table level and lean onto your partner's lower hamstrings with your forearm (Figure 12–18).
4. Slide your forearm up the hamstring, pronating it as you go (Figure 12–19).
5. Slide the forearm back down the hamstring with lighter pressure and repeat several times without supinating the forearm (Figure 12–20).
6. Repeat on the other hamstring and experiment on other areas of the body such as the calves and the back, being gentle and careful (Figure 12–21).
7. On the front of the body, you can practice these forearm strokes on the quadriceps (Figure 12–22).

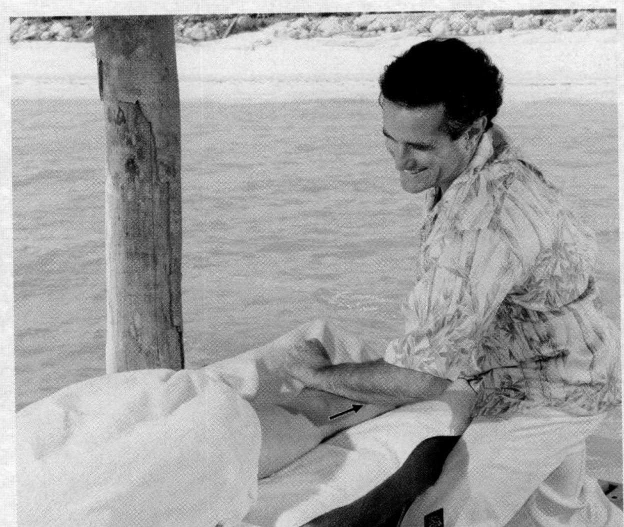

FIGURE 12-20

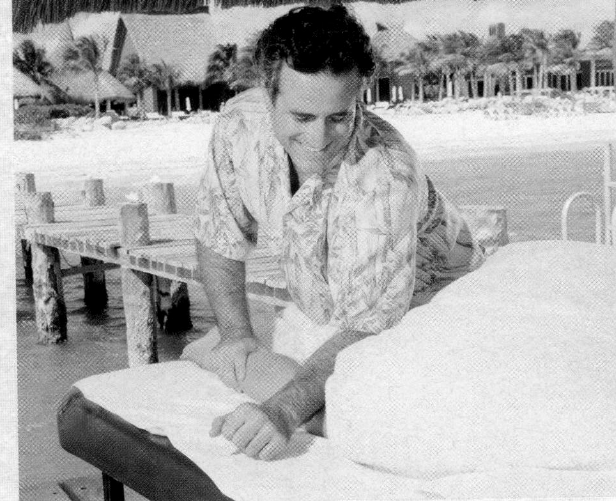

FIGURE 12-21

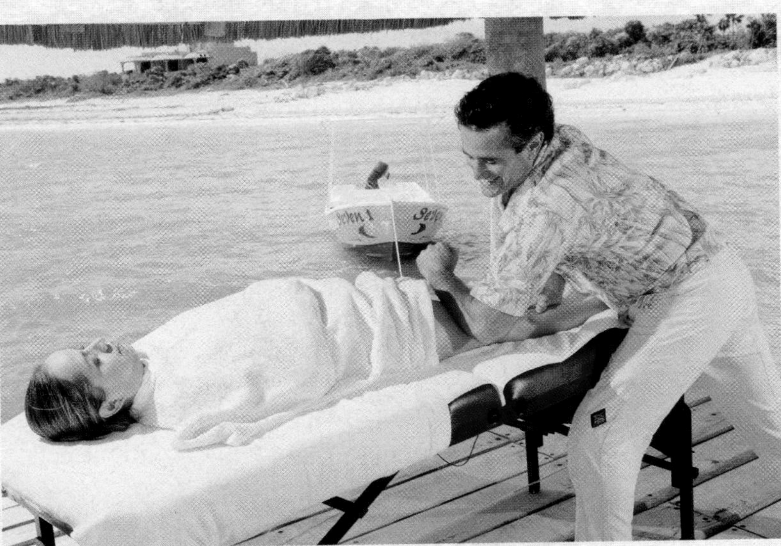

FIGURE 12-22

The traditional practice of the art of lomilomi gradually gave way to more modern influences after the arrival of foreigners, especially missionaries, who decried the practice as heathen or primitive. As modern Western medical techniques began to hold sway, the lomilomi healing tradition went underground, being practiced by individuals in private homes and out-of-the-way sites. The massage aspect of lomilomi remained popular, however, even among foreigners who came to the islands, and its popularity spread.

The state of Hawaii legitimized the practice of lomilomi massage in 1947 when the Board of Massage was established, and a law was passed requiring the successful completion of an exam prior to working as a massage therapist. Several "old school" traditional healers did not wish to undergo such examinations, and they held their healing practices and teaching sessions outside legally recognized channels. This did not keep their work from becoming extensively sought after, though, and several individuals attained near-mythical status as teachers and healers, foremost among them being "Auntie" Margaret Machado and "Uncle" Freddie Tira. It was not until 2001 that an act was passed that allowed trained native practitioners to work without needing to take the exam.

MANUAL LYMPHATIC DRAINAGE

Manual lymphatic drainage (MLD) is a gentle, superficial massage which helps move lymphatic fluids through the body and promote better elimination. Because the lymph system depends mostly on muscular activity to drain properly, some people experience difficulties associated with improper drainage, which can lead to complications such as **lymphedema**. People who are bedridden or immobilized due to injury or sickness are especially vulnerable to this condition. Manual lymphatic drainage has been shown to improve the flow of lymph and thus help the body in one of its important natural processes of elimination.

lymphedema

swelling caused by lymph accumulating in the tissues; often treated with manual lymphatic drainage (MLD), which complements many spa therapies

The lymph system is a network of vessels and bodily tissues that carry lymph through the body (Figure 12–23). The spleen, tonsils, thymus, and bone marrow are also considered part of the lymph system because they produce and circulate **lymphocytes** in the body. Lymph is formed when interstitial fluids enter the lymph system: it is composed of clear fluid, lymphocytes, and **chyle**.

lymphocytes

a leukocyte that normally makes up a quarter of the white blood cell count but increases in the presence of infection

chyle

a milky fluid in the lymph formed of emulsified fats; formed in the small intestine

The lymph system has three main duties:

1. removing interstitial fluid from tissues
2. absorbing fatty acids and fats from the digestive system in the form of chyle and moving them to the circulatory system
3. producing lymphocytes and other immune cells

The lymphatic system is extremely important, as it helps filter unwanted materials, even cancer cells, from the body. It can also help improve appearance when it efficiently transports fats out of tissues. When they apply manual lymphatic drainage in spas, massage therapists are usually aiming to improve appearance and help clients in their quest to feel revitalized and reenergized. In medical spa settings, these intentions may be more remedial or curative, as when clients exhibit signs of swelling or infection.

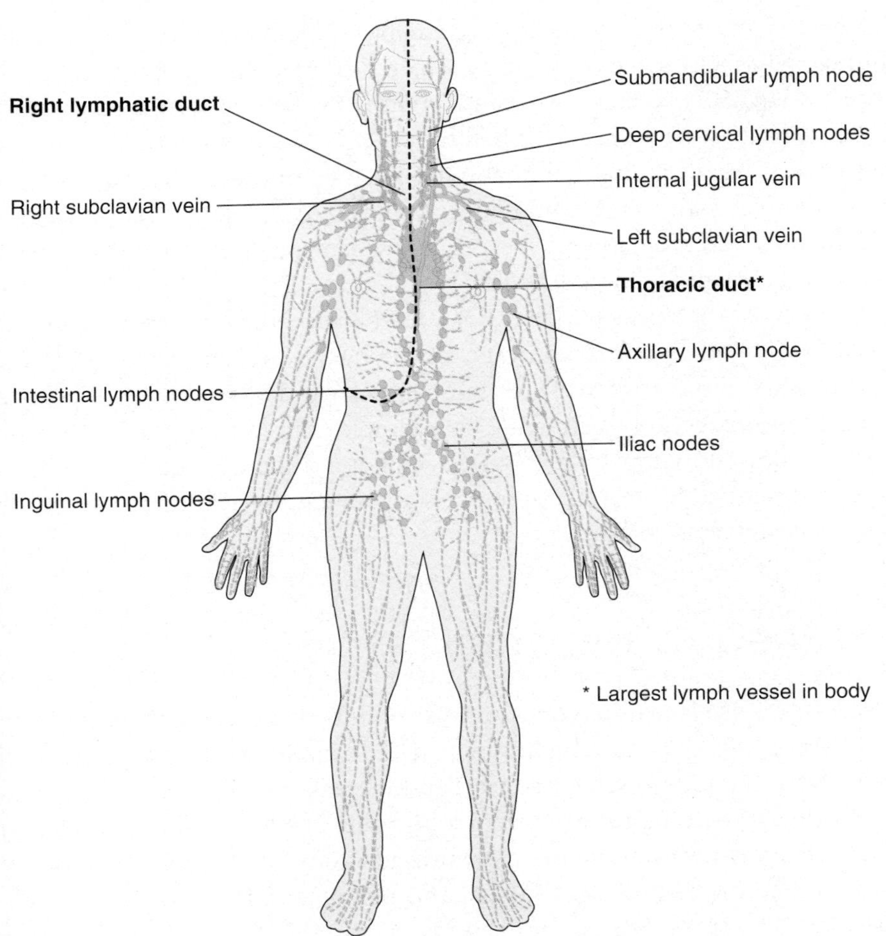

FIGURE 12–23 The lymph system.

The technique of manual lymphatic drainage was developed in France by Dr. Emil Vodder in the 1930s. He worked on patients with chronic colds and other infections, noticing that they had swollen lymph nodes. Vodder studied the lymph system thoroughly and developed specific gentle manual techniques that could effectively move the lymph. This massage technique is now accepted as a viable therapy in the management of lymphedema, and many certification courses are offered for massage therapists, physicians, and others.

Manual lymphatic drainage techniques are typically quite superficial and aim to move lymphatic fluid toward lymph nodes, the main ones being located in the axillary region and groin area, as shown in Figure 12–23. Three types of spa services most frequently call for manual lymphatic drainage techniques:

1. revitalizing treatments
2. cellulite treatments
3. detoxifying treatments

Revitalizing treatments are meant to improve appearance and well-being. They use MLD to drain excess fluid from the body and face, which can create the appearance of slimming and more youthful skin. Cellulite treatments in spas attempt to improve the appearance of affected areas through a number of methods, including the use of MLD techniques, which helps to lessen the inflammation that can exacerbate this condition. See Chapter 7 for more information on anti-cellulite spa services. Detoxifying treatments such as the herbal wrap are enhanced when MLD is offered in conjunction with them. For instance, a typical spa detoxification package might include an exfoliation, an herbal wrap, and a massage featuring manual lymphatic drainage techniques. The two main adjunct therapies paired with manual lymphatic drainage in spa services are hydrotherapy and aromatherapy, especially when applied with detoxifying oils or oil blends meant to aid in drainage.

In order for therapists to offer full manual lymphatic drainage sessions, they need to be trained and certified in the techniques. However, some spa protocols use a minimal number of MLD techniques as part of a larger overall program, as in cellulite-reduction treatments, for example, and in these cases, therapists are often allowed to apply a few basic lymphatic drainage techniques that are precisely described in treatment protocols and taught by lead therapists or other qualified individuals at the spa.

MYOFASCIAL RELEASE

Myofascial release is featured on a number of spas menus, especially those spas that focus on therapy and rehabilitation. The modality works primarily on the **fascia**, with the intention to ease pain and increase range of motion by releasing tension and holding patterns often found between fascia, skin, muscles, and bones. Fascia is the web of connective tissues found throughout the body. It covers and connects muscles, organs, and bones, and it connects the skin to underlying structures. Muscle (*myo*) and fascia together form the myofascial system. Work done on one area of this system can be felt in distant areas and can have effects far removed from the treatment site itself. Tightness or restrictions in the myofascial system can be caused by stress, injuries, chronically poor posture, and other problems. A release of the fascia in one area can bring relief to the entire person.

fascia

a sheet or band of fibrous connective tissue separating or binding together muscles and organs

A typical myofascial release session might include structural assessment, massage and stretching. Therapists use fingers, knuckles, elbows, or forearms to manipulate the fascia in order to reorganize layers of connective tissue that may have become tight or entrapped in some way. Some myofascial sessions require the client to stretch and move in ways not typical to a Swedish massage session, and the therapist will often suggest deep breathing accompany these movements, which can be quite deep and intense. Myofascial work often begins with a lighter massage to palpate tissues and warm up the area to be treated, especially the underlying fascia.

The roots of myofascial work extend back to the 1940s, when Janet G. Travell, M.D., used the term "myofascial" to refer to musculoskeletal pain and trigger points. Her book, *Myofascial Pain and Dysfunction: The Trigger Point Manual*, published in 1983, has become a well-used reference on the topic. The modality rose in popularity during the 1990s, with many therapists opting to become certified in the method. Two main methods of myofascial release techniques are taught: direct and indirect. The direct method works directly on restricted fascial tissue, with practitioners applying deep pressure through progressively deeper layers of fascia to gradually stretch this tissue and achieve release. This type of work is in the same therapeutic family as structural integration, which includes such specialties as **Rolfing** and **Bindegewebsmassage**. Its practice is usually restricted to therapists with credentials in these specialties. The indirect method of myofascial release is by far the most popular type used in spas. It involves a more gentle stretch, with very light pressure which is meant to "unwind" the fascia. Therapists practicing this technique use a light touch with relaxed hands to slowly stretch the fascia until it reaches a point of restriction. The stretch is held for several minutes until the tissue softens and releases. This technique increases blood flow and warmth in the area, aiding the body in self-healing and proper alignment. Physical therapist John F. Barnes has popularized the technique and taught it to thousands of therapists through his seminars, books, and DVDs.

Spa clients in search of relief from specific conditions are often drawn to the indirect method of myofascial release. It has been shown to be especially good for people who suffer from fibromyalgia, back pain, and other muscle-specific problems. Regular use of the therapy can provide clients with improved posture, greater freedom in movement, emotional resolution, and a reduction in pain. Because it is usually more effective when applied in successive sessions over time, day spas with local repeat clientele are more apt to list this modality on their menus.

Rolfing

type of deep structural alignment body work developed by Ida Rolf in the 1950s, not often offered in spas because of its intensity and the need for several consecutive sessions in order to be optimally effective

Bindegewebsmassage

a type of myofascial release massage that uses light strokes to affect the superficial fascia, rarely offered in spas

NEUROMUSCULAR THERAPY

Neuromuscular therapy (NMT) is a specific type of massage in which static pressure is applied to myofascial trigger points with the intention of relieving pain. The technique manipulates the soft tissues of the body to balance nerve impulses in the central nervous system. Neuromuscular therapists undergo extensive post-massage-school training to become certified, focusing their studies on kinesiology, biomechanics, and the physiology of the nervous system, specifically on the nervous system's effects on the musculoskeletal system. Spa clients who are suffering from back pain, neck pain, sciatica, or similar complaints often turn to NMT to provide relief. The modality addresses five main causes of pain:

1. *Ischemia*: lack of local blood supply to soft tissues
2. *Myofascial Trigger Points*: irritated points in the muscles which cause pain in other parts of the body
3. *Nerve Compression*: pressure on a nerve caused by soft tissue, cartilage, or bone
4. *Postural Distortion*: imbalance of the muscular system caused by stress or trauma
5. *Biomechanical Dysfunction*: improper repetitive movement patterns such as typing, tennis strokes, golf swings, and lifting objects

Neuromuscular therapy was developed almost simultaneously in both Europe and North America. Osteopaths, naturopaths, physical therapists, and physicians use the technique, and it has become widely practiced by massage therapists, though more frequently in clinics and doctors' offices rather than spas. Paul St. John and Judith Walker DeLany have been the two foremost proponents and instructors of the technique in the U.S.

Because neuromuscular therapy is often used to treat referred pain, spa clients are sometimes confused when their NMT therapist begins working on a distant area after they have requested work on the painful site. Therapists who perform NMT in spas therefore need to become especially skilled at communication, and they need to share their knowledge of the modality with co-workers such as front desk staff and spa technicians so that everyone can adequately answer clients' questions about the technique.

REIKI

Reiki is a type of energy work, and practitioners of the technique say that they can transmit healing to other people through the gentle application of their palms or sometimes with no contact at all (Figure 12–24). Advanced practitioners even claim they can transmit this energy over the phone, at a distance. While no substantial scientific evidence has ever been produced that would prove the existence of this energy or its effectiveness in the promotion of healing, many people claim to have been helped by the technique, and it has become quite popular on a number of spa menus. Perhaps the quality of a Reiki treatment that spa clients most appreciate is its gentleness. While there are many skeptics who dispute claims that Reiki helps people, the technique has never been shown to cause any harm to people, either.

Reiki was the spiritual brainchild of a Japanese man, Mikao Usui. In 1922, he fasted and meditated for three weeks on Mount Kurama in Japan, and the result of this introspection was a personal revelation in which he claims to have received the ability to transmit universal healing energy. One part of this transmission process, called **tenohira**, is similar to the laying on of hands in other healing traditions. The word *reiki* itself has a colorful origin, roughly

tenohira

the "palm healing" aspect of the Reiki modality, in which the practitioner comes into physical contact with the client

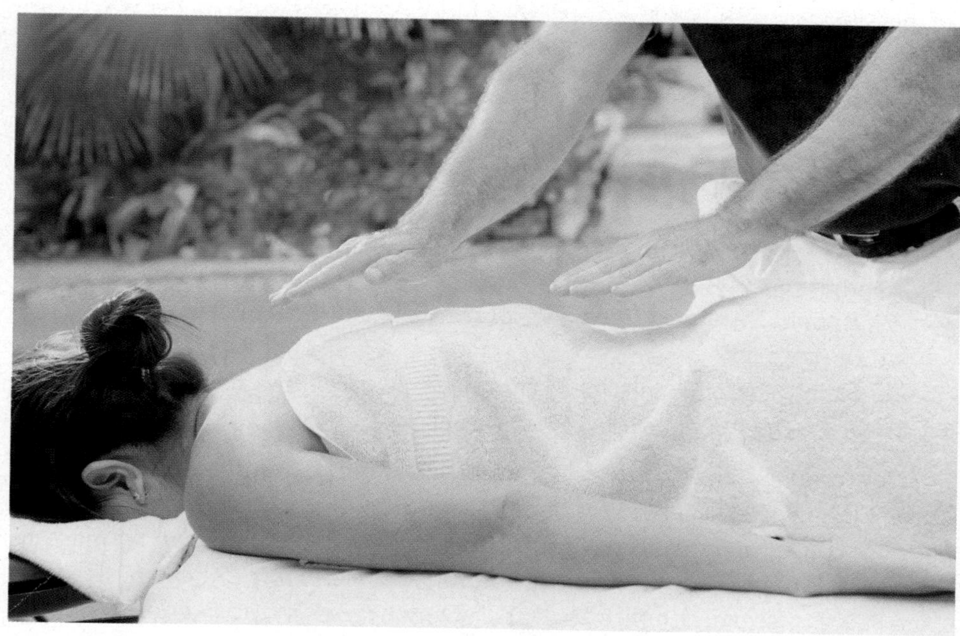

FIGURE 12–24 Reiki treatments include the lightest of touch or no touch at all.

translated from the original Japanese as "mysterious atmosphere," "spiritual power," or "feeling of mystery." The more popular modern translation, however, is "universal life energy," though this is not technically correct. *Ki* does mean "life energy," but *rei* does not mean "universal." Rather, it means "ghost, spirit, soul; supernatural, miraculous or divine." The word *reiki* can be used as a noun, a verb, or an adjective, as in: I perform *reiki*; I *reiki* my clients; and I perform *reiki* treatments.

People wishing to become trained in Reiki do so by studying with someone who has had the technique passed down to them through the lineage of teachers that started with Usui. Such teachers are known as Reiki masters. In order to be able to access the spiritual healing power, one needs to go through a process known as attunement, in which the Reiki master passes along the ability to the student. Anybody can go through the attunement process, not just massage therapists or other hands-on professionals. Courses, usually two days long, are offered in three levels; first-degree, second-degree, and third-degree. Successful completion of all three leads to designation as a Reiki master. Many different teaching methods, time frames, and costs are used by various Reiki teachers, and no single organization is responsible for regulation or accreditation.

Reiki has enjoyed increasing acceptance in recent years as people become more receptive to the concepts of energy work. In spas, Reiki is offered either as a stand-alone treatment, as a series of treatments, or in some cases to treat specific problems. Sometimes Reiki is combined with other modalities; it may be added to a body wrap or a massage, for example. Stemming from the origin of one man's spiritual insights, the modality has helped thousands of spa clients tune into subtler energies. This universal life energy they experience while having a Reiki session may actually be nothing more than a closer focus on their own life energy that pulses through them with every heartbeat and every breath, but if Reiki can help spa clients tune into that, it is performing a valuable service.

SHIATSU

Shiatsu is a popular modality offered at many spas. Some spas offer a modified version that can be performed on a massage table and incorporates several aspects of Swedish massage as well. Other spas offer a more traditional version which is performed on a mat on the floor (Figures 12–25A and 12–25B). The root of the word comes from the Japanese *shi*, meaning *finger*, and *atsu*, meaning *pressure*. The founder of Shiatsu was a Japanese man, Tokujiro Namikoshi. He is said to have discovered his healing touch at the age of seven when treating his mother for rheumatoid arthritis. After establishing the Japan Shiatsu College in 1940, he trained many students, some of whom went on to develop their own forms of his technique. These forms, known as derivative styles, are the ones primarily practiced in U.S. spas, the most popular being the one taught by Wataru Ohashi, known as **Ohashiatsu**. All of these styles incorporate traditional Japanese massage, influences from Chinese medicine, and a modern understanding of anatomy and physiology.

Ohashiatsu

derivative style of shiatsu developed by Wataru Ohashi in the U.S.

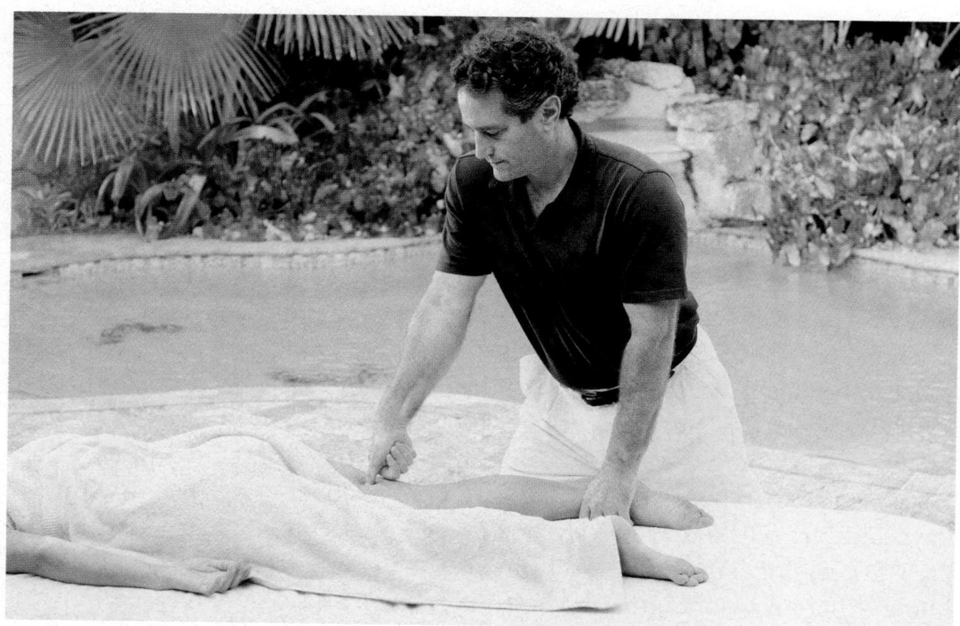

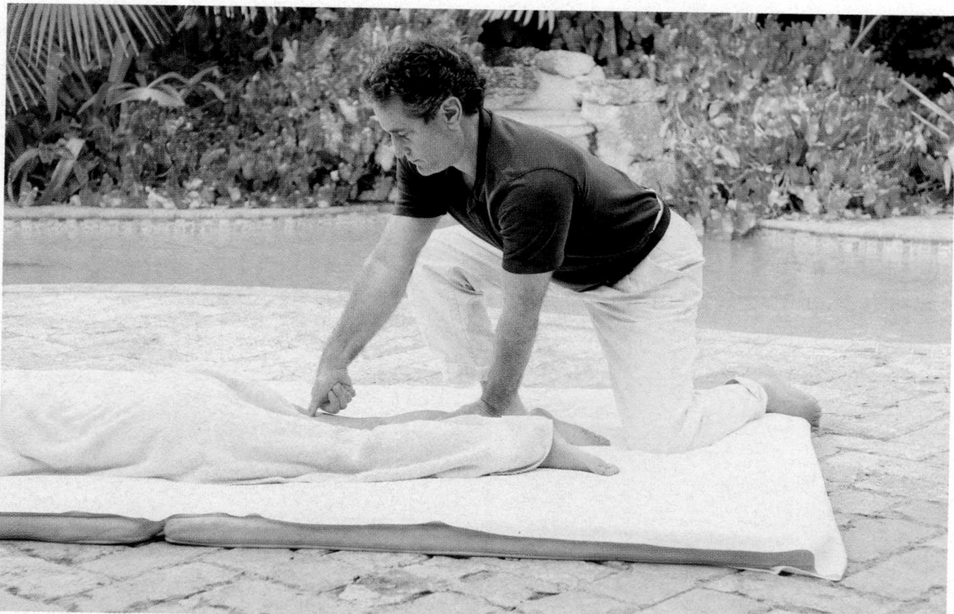

FIGURE 12–25A, B Shiatsu can be performed on a table or on the floor in the spa setting.

During a shiatsu session, practitioners put pressure on specific points (Figure 12–26), typically holding the pressure for 5 to 7 seconds. Most points are stimulated with the thumbs, but fingers and palms are used as well. An important aspect of the original Japanese therapy combined a type of diagnosis with this palpation, and extremely experienced practitioners are said to be able to give sessions that are both diagnosis and therapy combined. This, of course, is almost always inappropriate in spas. While spa clients may be seeking relief from specific complaints, therapists should never offer a diagnosis of specific conditions, as this is outside their scope of practice.

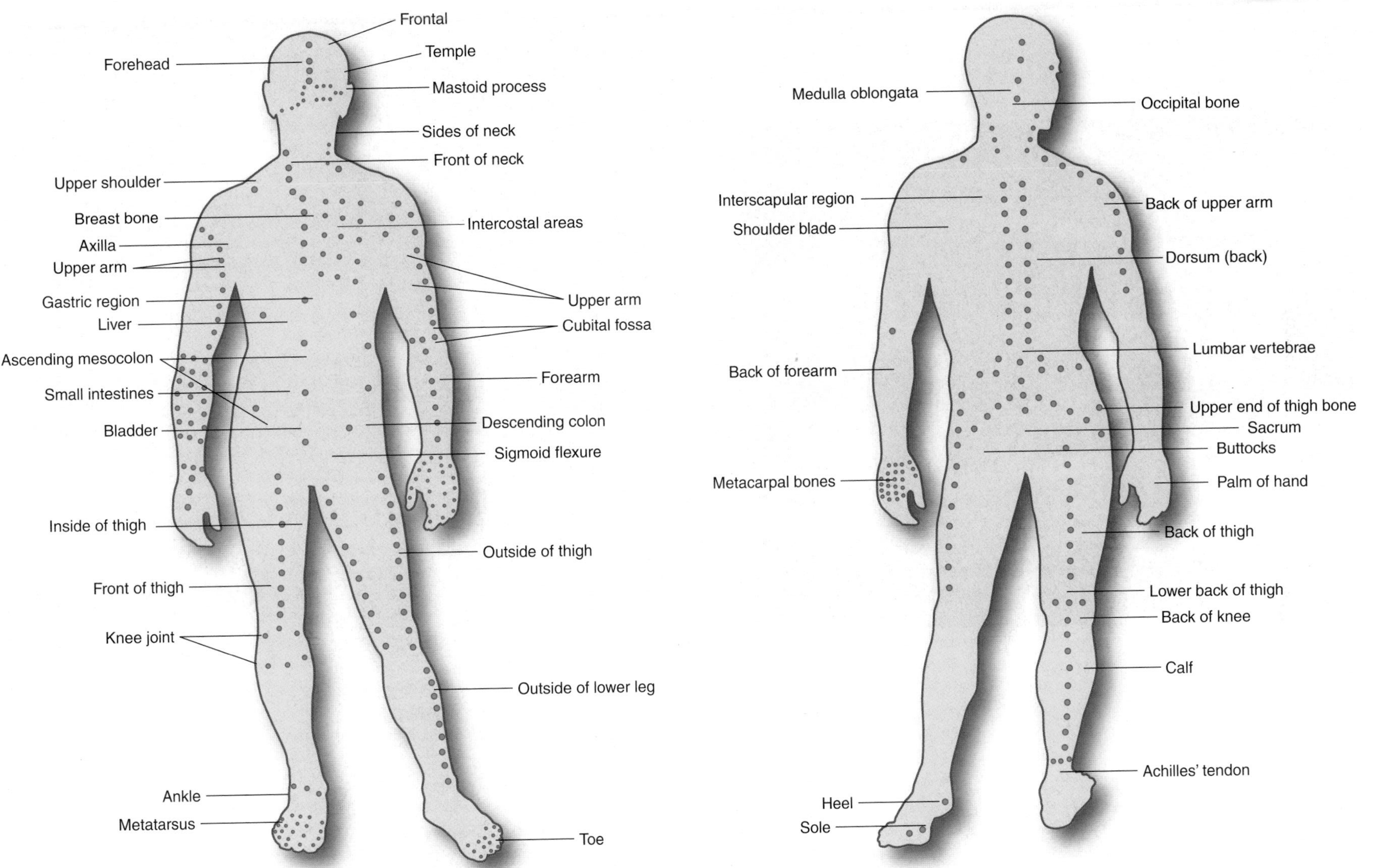

FIGURE 12-26 Shiatsu points.

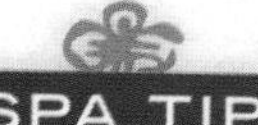

SPA TIP

Shiatsu is usually offered as a stand-alone treatment in spas, not given as part of a treatment package, although some spas specializing in Asian modalities will include it in a package featuring other Asian products or services. One example would be a "Zen" package featuring a hot tub soak, a scrub with dried herbs from Asia, and a shiatsu massage.

SPA CAUTION

It is important to be properly trained before attempting to press forcefully on shiatsu points. Some points are located near endangerment sites, and therapists who are not trained could potentially injure a spa client. This is especially important when using the feet to apply pressure. Lawsuits have been filed by spa clients who claim they were hurt during such a massage. Spas and spa therapists need to protect themselves through proper education, proper insurance coverage, and proper application of this technique.

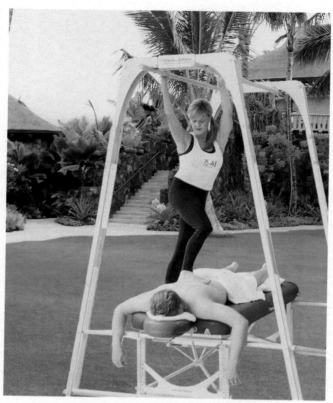

FIGURE 12–27 Ashiatsu is performed with the feet while the practitioner grasps bars overhead.

A recent development in shiatsu offered in many spas is called Ashiatsu Oriental Bar Therapy®. *Ashiatsu* comes from a Japanese root similar to *shiatsu*'s, but in this case, the Japanese word *ashi* is used. *Ashi* means *foot*, and *atsu*, of course, means *pressure*. This modality is performed standing on top of the table grasping bars overhead, with most of the work being done with the practitioner's feet (Figure 12–27). Ashiatsu is included on the menu at many top spas. Although the use of overhead bars and foot pressure has been a part of traditional Japanese therapy for many years, this particular modality, with its use of lubricant and its emphasis on centrifugal and centripetal pumping motions that practitioners claim can create structural improvements in soft tissue problems, was developed in the U.S. in the 1990s. Many therapists appreciate using their feet, thus saving the wear and tear on their hands and upper bodies normally experienced while doing deep tissue work.

THAI MASSAGE

Thai massage is growing in popularity in spas for a number of reasons. It is exotic, effective, and pleasurable, but perhaps most attractive to many spa clients is the fact that recipients do not need to undress. Thus, draping and modesty are not an issue. Unlike Swedish and many other Western style massage modalities, which require a lubricant to be applied to bare skin to be optimally effective, Thai massage is done through clothing. Typically, recipients recline on a mat, futon, or hard mattress, wearing loose-fitting garments. Often, pajama-like

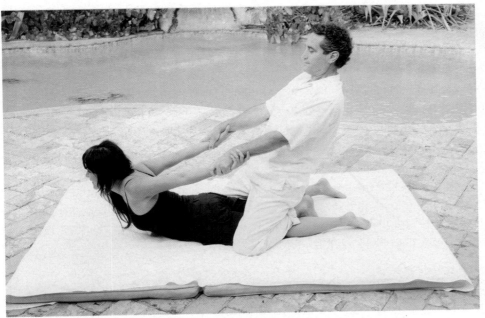

FIGURE 12–28 Thai massage includes stretches similar to yoga.

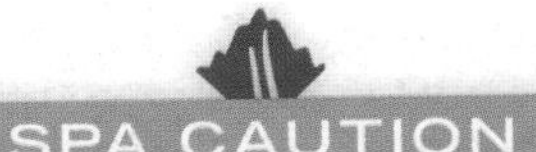

SPA CAUTION

Therapists always need to exercise caution when applying Thai massage movements, especially stretches. Many spa clients may be unprepared for such intense maneuvers and could potentially be injured. Communication and gentleness are key. All therapists need to be properly trained by a Thai massage instructor prior to applying these techniques.

clothes are supplied by the spa or massage establishment, which the client dons prior to the treatment. The treatment itself consists of acupressure-like movements and a good deal of stretching (Figure 12–28). In fact, so much stretching is involved in Thai massage that it is often referred to as *Thai yoga massage*, *passive yoga*, or *assisted yoga*.

In Thailand, massage is ubiquitous and inexpensive. It is a part of daily life for millions of Thais and many foreigners as well. Thais refer to it as "Nuat," which translates as simply "massage," though the full name for the technique in Thai is *Nuat phaen boran*, which translates as "massage, ancient, manner" or "old style massage." It is also referred to as the Northern style or Old Medicine Hospital Style, since the most popular form experienced by Westerners is taught and promoted in the northern Thai city of Chiang Mai. This style, in turn, was developed from the teachings at Wat Po, the main temple in Bangkok, which has a Thai massage school and clinic right on the temple grounds. Thai massage originated in India, based on yoga and Ayurveda. It is believed that the style was brought to Thailand by Shivago Komarpaj over 2500 years ago, around the same time that Buddha was teaching.

Thai massage theory focuses on an invisible energy in the body that is said to flow along *sen sib*, which are similar in concept to meridians in Chinese medicine. Practitioners seek to unblock the energy flow along these pathways, helping the body regain balance and well-being. The pressure point applications and stretches are all meant to free up this energy. Heat and herbs are often applied as well, using special herbal compresses called *luk pra kob* (see Chapter 8 for more information on this technique).

In Thailand, massage is given on a mat or futon on the floor, or a raised platform, and some spas recreate this type of atmosphere for their clients. Other spas offer a modified form of Thai massage on a massage table. Spas sometimes have a particular Thai massage protocol which they choose to provide for their

SPA TIP

Creative individuals in the spa industry have developed advanced modalities that are actually combinations of two or more existing modalities. One example of this trend is **Swe-Thai**, which is a melding of Swedish massage and Thai massage. You can look for this trend on spa menus yourself. Wherever you see the words "fusion" or "synergy" or an invented word you have never heard of before on a spa menu, there is a chance the "modality" has actually been around for a very short period of time.

Swe-Thai

combination treatment featuring elements of Swedish and Thai massage

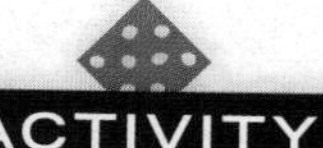

ACTIVITY

Thai Style Stretches

The following three stretches are included in many Thai massage routines. They are quite gentle, yet offer a taste of the relaxation and increased range of motion offered by this modality. Choose a partner and have the recipient lay supine on either a massage table or a mat. The giver starts sitting at his partner's feet.

1. Cross one foot over the other and pull toward you, applying plantar flexion to both feet. Switch the top and bottom foot and then repeat three times (Figure 12–29).
2. Move to your partner's side and gently slide the knee up and out while the foot moves toward the body, allowing the leg to open to the side, supporting it if necessary. Then apply gentle pressure with one palm up the inner thigh on several points for a few seconds each, while the other hand anchors the lower leg (Figure 12–30). Repeat three times, then move to other leg.

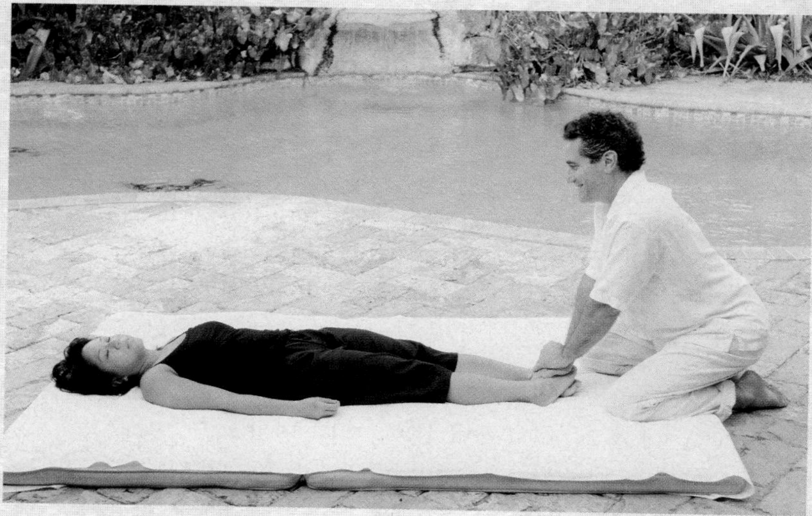

FIGURE 12–29

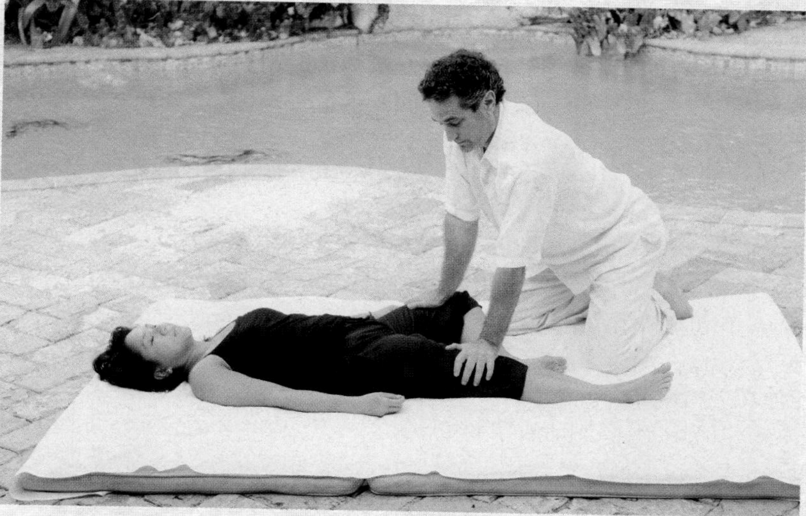

FIGURE 12–30

(Continued)

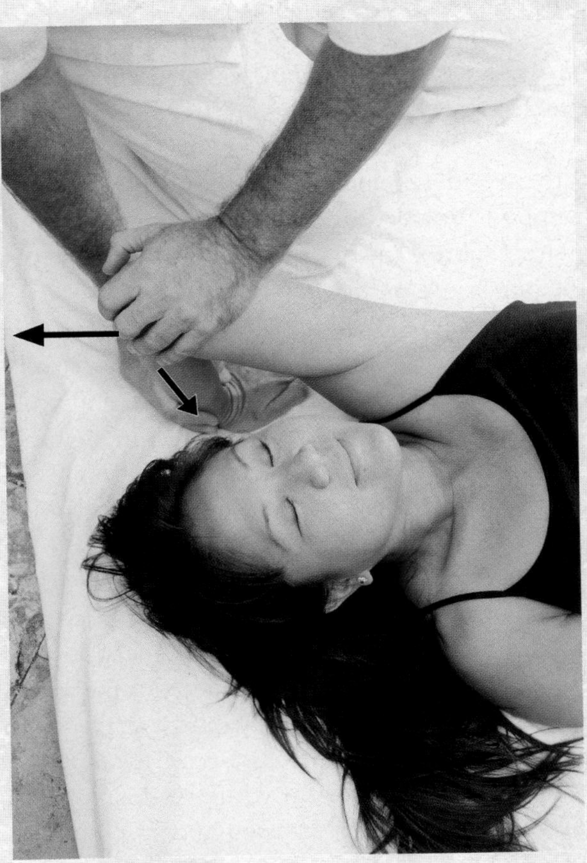

FIGURE 12–31

3. Moving to sit near your partner's head, take one arm over and place the palm flat on the surface directly above the shoulder, fingers pointing down toward the feet while applying an upward stretch to the elbow (Figure 12–31). Hold for five seconds. Repeat on the other arm.

Remember, you must receive proper training before applying these or any other Thai moves on an actual client.

guests, training therapists in the specifics, or they may allow therapists to apply the modality as they have learned it in a workshop. And, increasingly, spa therapists are making the trek to Thailand to study the form at its origin. Gaining mastery of this modality, in any manner, will make any therapist more attractive to employers at many spas.

WATSU

Watsu is an advanced modality developed by Harold Dull at Harbin Hot Springs in northern California. He founded a school there to teach the technique, and he instituted the Worldwide Aquatic Bodywork Association (WABA) to further the goals and principles of this modality. The technique itself is performed in a pool, with the practitioner standing in chest-deep warm water. The water at

Harbin comes from natural underground springs, which is preferred for treatments, but Watsu can be performed in normal swimming pools also, as long as the water is warm enough, the recommended temperature being approximately 94°F. The therapist assists the client in floating atop the water, sometimes with the aid of flotation devices (Figure 12–32). Gentle body movements and stretches are applied, helping to bring the client into a meditative state. The buoyancy and support provided by the water creates an extra opening for the client's body to release, and it enables the therapist to perform maneuvers that would otherwise be impossible on dry land.

The name *Watsu* is derived from *water* and *shiatsu*, which can be somewhat misleading, because the technique itself bears little resemblance to shiatsu. Harold Dull studied Zen meditation and shiatsu in Japan, however, and he believed his new water-based technique brought about similar states of mind to those created by the Japanese traditions. Although Watsu is the most well-known, other forms of water-based bodywork have been developed, including **Wassertanzen**, from Germany, which is often performed in combination with Watsu. Like Watsu, Wassertanzen, which means "water dance" in German, begins with the client being cradled, stretched, and relaxed on the surface, but then the therapist takes the client beneath the water for a few moments at a time while the client wears a nose clip to keep water from entering air passages. A certain form of craniosacral therapy, described earlier in this chapter, can be done in the water also. Known as Ocean Therapy™, the technique involves multiple therapists aiding a client while he floats in calm water. As the name implies, ocean water is preferred, though a pool can also be used. Several other aquatic techniques are practiced in spas, including Hydroholistics, Jahara, Aqua Wellness, Aqua Bliss, and Multi-Dimensional Movement Arts.

Wassertanzen

a form of aquatic bodywork similar to Watsu but featuring full submersion of the client under water

Watsu is a wonderful addition to any spa menu, and an increasing number of spas are offering it. The modality requires a large investment in infrastructure, however, because the technique is usually offered in a purpose-built pool with

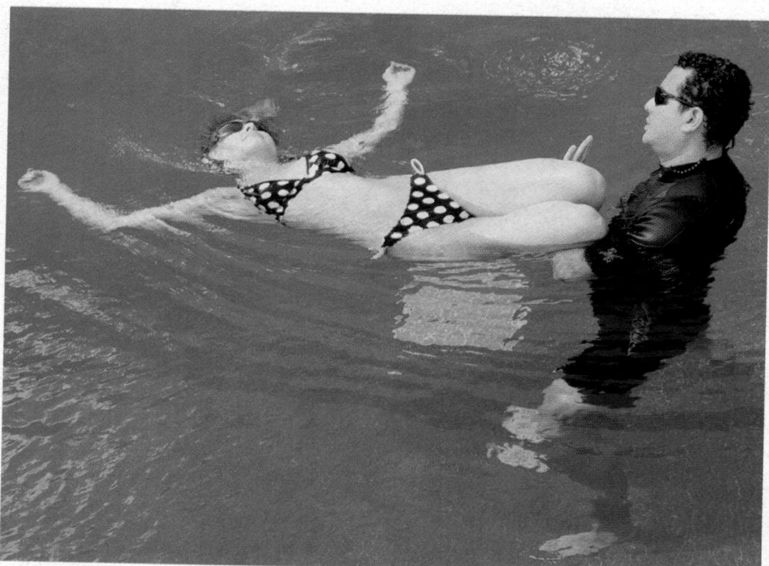

FIGURE 12–32 Watsu® is performed in a pool of warm water.

a separate temperature control. This means that only larger, well-funded spas or smaller Watsu-specific spas are likely to offer it. Therapists usually love performing the modality, as it is deeply therapeutic and meditative, and it offers a break from massage work on the table. Therapists trained in the technique are highly sought after by spas, and some spas offer their staff therapists on-site training.

SPA ETIQUETTE

Because the therapist and client come into close contact during a session, some people consider Watsu to be sensual in nature. Therefore, because of its intimacy, Watsu needs to be performed with exceptional professionalism. Communication, respect for boundaries and a discrete awareness of how the client's body is being touched and held are extremely important. Therapists who are adept at making this advanced modality both comforting and therapeutic are highly prized by spa owners and directors.

Did You Know?

Exotic Modalities

A number of spas feature one-of-a-kind treatments that are one part showmanship, one part creativity, and one part therapy. The Liquid Sound facility at the Toskana Therme in Bad Sulza, Germany, is an example of one such exotic spa offering. Built on natural salt-water springs, the entire town of Bad Sulza has been a center for health seekers since the mid-1800s. Today, the Liquid Sound project features six swimming pools under glass domes where spa goers float in body-temperature salt water while experiencing rhythmic light shows projected onto the ceiling and listening to underwater music that vibrates their bones (Figure 12–33). The signature spa treatment, called *Aqua Wellness,* is an underwater massage similar to Watsu performed in the Liquid Sound chamber. This exotic treatment has become a multimedia social event, but it is also quite therapeutic and has become popular with people suffering from respiratory, rheumatic, and chronic conditions. Each year, Professor Jonathan Paul De Vierville, who was profiled in Chapter 4, leads a group of spa professionals to the site for his "Avant-Garde Spa Culture Seminar: Dream Spa Course, Liquid Sound Workshop & Kur Tour Course®."

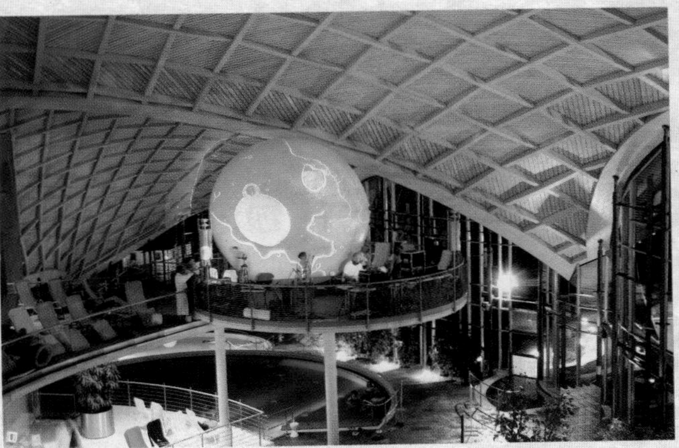

FIGURE 12–33 The Liquid Sound® Chamber in Bad Sulza, Germany.

Another exotic treatment features the use of many people's favorite food—chocolate. At the Spa at the Hershey Hotel, also known as the Chocolate Spa, clients can experience a number of treatments based on the cocoa bean. Examples include the Whipped Cocoa Bath, in which clients settle into a foaming chocolate milk bath, the Chocolate Bean Polish, which combines the exfoliating properties of cocoa bean husks with a softening cocoa body moisturizer, and the Chocolate Fondue Wrap, which features the application of chocolate "fondue" made of warmed moor mud and essence of cocoa.

RESEARCH

Do some Internet research to find an exotic service listed on a spa menu anywhere in the world and describe it in one page. In which country did it originate? Does it involve the blending of two or more modalities? What treatment building blocks does it include: hydrotherapy? massage? exfoliation? thermal therapy? Using the knowledge you have been gathering while studying spa therapies, explain the main therapeutic benefits such a treatment would offer clients. What physiological effects would the treatment create on the body? What contraindications might be involved?

SIGNATURE SERVICES

Spas often distinguish a special treatment or combination of treatments as particularly representative of their business. These signature services are usually quite unique and differ widely from spa to spa, yet they share certain common characteristics, including:

- *Singularity*: Spas strive to set themselves apart from the competition in several ways, and developing a one-of-a-kind signature service helps in this regard.
- *Elaborateness*: Most signature services combine more than one element, such as a hydrotherapy bath and massage, or hot stones and exfoliation, in order to further differentiate the treatment.
- *Expense*: The signature service is typically billed as something to experience on special occasions and is seldom among the cheaper items on the menu.
- *Exotic Ingredients*: If, for instance, a spa's signature service features Swedish massage, the oil used for the massage might be special oil reserved only for this treatment. If hot stones are used, the stones themselves may be from a special source, or the manner of applying them may be different from that used in other spas.
- *Location Specificity*: If the spa is located near a particular landmark or natural feature, the signature service may reflect that. Many spas located at hot springs, for instance, include the spring's water in their signature service.

While some signature services include an advanced modality, others focus on core treatments such as massage or exfoliation and add a twist of some kind, such as a foot treatment to go along with a wrap. Many spas combine two of their core treatments together to make a signature service. In that sense, the line between signature services and spa packages can become quite blurred. Sometimes the two are indistinguishable, in fact, and spas have been known to recognize this by listing a number of "signature packages" on their menus. Many spas offer more than one signature service—the larger the spa, the more apt it is to offer a number of special treatments targeted to various demographics among their guests. Depending on the type of spa and the particular clientele it serves, signature services can be customized to attract certain people. For instance, a golf resort spa might create a "Get Back in the Swing" signature service targeting muscles used on the course. A spa attached to a yoga ashram might offer a "Spiritual Quest" service featuring energy work and deep breathing exercises combined with massage and a wrap. A detoxification clinic might offer purging herbal therapies and an intense sweat inside an infrared sauna. Also, a meal is sometimes included in the signature service, in those spas where food is available.

The following list of signature services is inspired by actual offerings on the menus of top spas. Details have been changed to protect their exclusivity.

1. Natural Relaxation (at a small, owner-driven spa)
   This experience features homemade herbal remedies developed by the spa owner, including massage oils, essential oils, and lotions. These custom-made botanicals are introduced with a combination of massage modalities, including Swedish, deep tissue, trigger point therapy, and Reiki energy work.
2. Deep De-Stress Hydro Massage (at a hot springs spa)
   This signature treatment begins with a therapeutic soak in warm spring water, followed by a Swiss shower and Scotch hose treatment targeted to tight back and shoulder muscles. Heat packs are applied to further relax the back before the final phase of the treatment—a deep tissue massage for the back, neck, and shoulders.
3. Beautiful Dreaming (at a salon-oriented day spa)
   This treatment begins with an individual steam shower treatment plus stress-relieving hydrotherapy soak, putting you in the mood for our relaxing Jasmine Facial, full manicure and pedicure, and delicious spa cuisine lunch.
4. Acu-Lomi Relaxation Treatment (specific to a medical spa)
   This treatment combines acupuncture needling specific to relaxation points interspersed with a soothing lomilomi massage. If you have ever wanted to experience the benefits of acupuncture but were uncertain you would enjoy it, try this guaranteed-to-please experience.
5. Cooling Ti-Leaf Sun Relief (at a resort spa on the beach)
   A calming aromatherapy wrap that features lavender-infused aloe vera gel which is spread luxuriously on the body then covered with fresh, cooled Hawaiian Ti leaves. The body is then wrapped to optimize hydration while your therapist applies gentle, therapeutic face and scalp massage.
6. The Zen Face Treatment (at an Asian-themed day spa)
   Warmed Chakra stones are placed gently on the face to begin this treatment. Soft meditation music plays in the background, the lights are dimmed, and natural, organic products are applied in luxurious succession: an anti-aging mask, vitamin infusion, and sea extract. Stress melts away as your feet and hands are encased in warmed paraffin. After your skin is gently cleansed at the end, the sound of Tibetan bowls will follow you into the rest of your day.
7. Golfer's Delight (at a sports-oriented destination spa)
   This treatment begins with a soak in our hydrotherapy tub. Afterward, you will receive a vigorous massage with Biofreeze pain-relieving gel targeted especially to lower back, shoulders, and arms. Twenty minutes of golf-specific stretches round out your treatment.

8. Spring Cleanse (at a spa specializing in fasting and detox)
   First, you will enjoy our private herbal steam chamber to open your pores and begin the internal cleansing; then a wrap with detoxifying herbs pulls impurities from your entire body. A vigorous two-therapist abhyanga massage follows, meant to stimulate lymph flow, soften joints, and improve circulation. Afterward, your therapist will give you a cup of warm tea that will stimulate healthy digestion. You will leave with our exclusive five-day detox-in-a-box program to continue your journey of healing and renewal at home.
9. Avocado Wrap (at a country spa in an avocado grove)
   A dry brush massage thoroughly sloughs dead cells from your skin before an application of just-picked avocados mixed with rosemary and jojoba oils. You are wrapped in a warm cocoon to let the natural vitamin-rich avocados work their magic while your therapist treats your feet to relaxing reflexology. A warm towel wrap and nourishing scalp treatment finish the treatment.
10. All About You (at a full-service day spa)
    This treatment is truly "All About You"! You meet with your therapist prior to the treatment to discuss your needs and desires; then you co-create an entirely customized program lasting two and a half hours and spanning the gamut of all our spa has to offer. Your therapist will recommend appropriate combinations and add a personal therapeutic touch to your experience. Afterward, you will receive a special gift from our spa shop reserved exclusively for those customers who have received our signature service.

SIGNATURE SERVICE NAME	
MENU DESCRIPTION	
Wet Room/Dry Room	
Table Setup	
Treatment Duration	
Needed Supplies	
Contraindications	
Draping	
Treatment Order	
Safety, Sanitation Issues, & Clean-Up	
Body Mechanics & Self-Care	
Product Cost	
Treatment Price	
Physiological Effects	

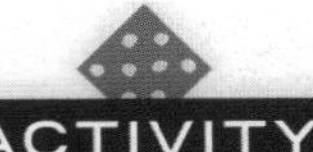

ACTIVITY

Create a Signature Service

Now is time for you to put together the information and experiences you have gathered during your spa studies and create your own signature service. Keep in mind proper treatment order, body mechanics, safety issues, contraindications, and all other relevant issues by filling in the treatment matrix table on the previous page. Give your signature service a unique name and an imaginative description such as one you would find on the menu at a top-notch spa. List steps for preparation, procedure, and cleanup. Mention any special music, lighting, or other additions that might create the optimal ambience for the treatment.

Preparation

1. ______
2. ______
3. ______
4. ______
5. ______

Procedure

1. ______
2. ______
3. ______
4. ______
5. ______
6. ______
7. ______
8. ______
9. ______
10. ______
11. ______
12. ______
13. ______
14. ______
15. ______
16. ______
17. ______
18. ______
19. ______
20. ______

Cleanup

1. ______
2. ______
3. ______

Beyond Modalities

Did You Know?

Larger spas, especially destination spas, offer their clients a wide assortment of activities outside the realm of traditional spa services. These activities can broaden and deepen a client's experience while at the spa and even afterwards upon returning home. They include such pursuits as Native American healing rituals, nature walks, rock climbing, archeology, painting, and sculpting. Some spas have purpose-built rooms in which to hold classes on these topics. Other spas can be found in natural settings, surrounded by opportunities for outdoor exploration. One spa in the southwest U.S., for example, features guided hikes into the surrounding mountains, where guests can view ancient Indian petroglyphs etched onto the stones. Spas offer their clients these activities in order to help them get in touch with themselves, with nature, and with the world around them. Spa therapists who work in spas that offer these activities can play an important supporting role in the client's experience. For example, a client who undertakes an art therapy course while at the spa will likely be accessing the artistic/creative right side of her brain more consistently than in daily life back home. Therapists can facilitate this process by providing a deeply relaxing massage, flotation in a hydrotherapy tub infused with brain-stimulating aromatherapy oils, and verbal visualization techniques to help the client tune into her subconscious.

Some spas also offer lifestyle programs that deal with issues such as weight loss, sexuality, grief, heart health, and more. Physicians, psychologists, and other professionals are on staff to lead group sessions, individual counseling, and workshops on these topics and more. In addition, some spas also offer team building, ropes courses, and other self-empowerment challenges. The Miraval spa in Arizona, for example, bills itself as the spa to go for "Life in Balance." It features an obstacle course in which guests climb all the way up a telephone pole, balancing on its tiny round top in order to conquer their fears and self-doubts.

SPA ETIQUETTE

Does This Spa Bathrobe Make Me Look Fat?

A spa client will sometimes ask the therapist for an honest assessment of her body, especially if she is undergoing a weight-loss program at the spa. This is dangerous ground, and therapists need to be especially sensitive to clients when answering such questions. It is reasonable for the client to seek an informed opinion from the therapist, who, after all, has extended opportunities for close observation of the client's body. However, weight-loss advice and dietary recommendations are not advanced massage modalities and are definitely outside the massage therapist's scope of practice. The correct and most sensitive way to respond to such questions is to compliment the client on her desire to improve her body and then refer her to the spa's exercise physiologist or nutritionist. Therapists may also suggest that the client undergo a body analysis of some kind to objectively determine her current condition and formulate realistic weight-loss goals. There are a number of body composition tests available, including skin fold measurement, bioelectric impedance, and hydrostatic weighing, the most accurate being **DEXA**, which is available at top spa resorts and medical spas.

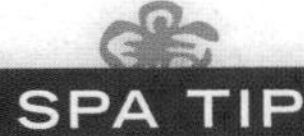

SPA TIP

Spas Can Change Lives

More than simply offering massages and other treatments, spas can give clients the opportunity to make profound changes in their lives. As a service provider in the spa setting, you should remember that you are part of a potentially life-altering enterprise. People have quit smoking, lost weight, weaned themselves from drugs, improved personal relationships, gotten back into shape, and retooled the way they live in their own bodies, all because of spas. Some people have literally saved their own lives through the experiences they have had and the lessons they have learned in spas. When you are working in the spa setting, your interaction with the clients is about more than simply massaging, exfoliating, or wrapping. It is about supporting people on a journey of transformation. Knowing this can help keep you inspired on your own journey as well while you go through the inevitable ups and downs in your career.

SPA PROFILE

Angela Keen, ESPA

Angela Keen is ESPA's National Training Manager for America, a position that entails intimate knowledge of advanced spa treatment protocols as well as the psychological makeup of massage therapists. In addition, over the past several years, her job has included a good bit of international travel. ESPA is a world leader in spa training and management, having formed strategic relationships with many top properties, including the Four Seasons and Mandarin hotel chains. So, what exactly does a globetrotting national spa training manager actually do? How does one prepare for this position? And how can her experiences training so many therapists on advanced modalities help you as you prepare for a career in the spa field?

"Well," explains Angela in her lovely British accent, "where I come from, things are done a bit differently as far as training goes. Back in England, I was dual-qualified as both a therapist and an esthetician, a practice that is quite common there. My primary studies in the field lasted three years and included work in reflexology, sports therapy, aromatherapy, massage, esthetics, retailing, and spa management, as well as some additional courses. So, in a sense, my basic training included certain things that would be considered advanced training here in the U.S. Since graduation, I have always worked within the spa industry, starting out as a therapist then eventually joining ESPA as a retail manager. I then went to open two ESPA properties, in London and Portugal, acting as spa director in charge of recruitment, hiring, training, and operations. It was a very scary responsibility, an amazing process I'm glad I went through. After finishing my stint at the spa in Portugal, I decided I wanted to get back into doing treatments, so I became an ESPA trainer."

Though it has a worldwide presence, only two hundred or so people work directly with ESPA. Launched in 1993 by Susan Harmsworth, the company employs various methods of operation depending on the spa property, and their services include design, management, product sales, treatment development, recruitment, training, and more. Some spas are ESPA-branded, while others retain their own brand and are served behind the scenes by the company. In all cases, the focus is on the therapies and the therapists.

"We're truly a treatment-led spa company," says Angela. "Although we offer full support for all stages of the spa business, our primary goal is to develop holistic versatile treatments that really work and can help to counteract the stress we're all subject to these days. In order to achieve this, typically the therapists in our spas will undergo a full eight-week training program in order to get up to speed with the full menu. Afterwards, we try for a week of training time per quarter."

(Continued)

SPA PROFILE

Angela Keen, ESPA *continued*

When asked what one lesson she feels is most important for all the therapists she trains, Angela's answer is not so much about hands-on technique as it is about attitude. "It all comes back to their initial training," she says. "Massage schooling is based on techniques, as it should be, but now more than ever, therapists within the spa industry need to focus on client service, client expectation, personal presentation, communication, customer care, and body language. I believe a truly holistic spa treatment extends out from the treatment room to encompass the entire experience at the spa and even outside of the spa if we can encourage them to take home some therapeutic products for self-care. In our trainings, therapists are made aware from the very beginning that, even though their massage skills are valued, we are very much a holistic company. Everything about their work at the spa, including the customer service and retailing aspects, needs to have the same therapeutic intention as their massage therapy.

"As far as the actual treatments go, what we focus on and are very passionate about are philosophy-based treatments, such as Ayurveda, ones during which therapists can truly nurture the client. We call these in-depth, philosophy-based treatments 'journeys.' The most popular is the Ayurvedic journey, designed around marma points, which is our signature treatment. Thai-inspired and Balinese-inspired journeys are also well-liked. Journeys might include a welcoming foot soak, a body brush, and a specialized scalp treatment in addition to the main modality, creating a full experience for the client. Many therapists appreciate this because they get to know the client a little better, to spend more time with them and discover what they truly need, which is, in the end, what therapy is all about.

"The *E* in 'ESPA' stands for *education*, which is at the core of the success of ESPA in its therapist training and treatments. Once a therapist goes through our training, they are truly educated about the value and impact of spa therapies. If therapists subsequently want to take further continuing education classes for their own knowledge, we encourage them to do so, and many of the hotels where we operate will offer support to subsidize this training. There are loads of opportunities out there. My best advice to therapists or therapists in training is really just to keep an open mind. And remember to research the spa industry prior to going into it. I even suggest to work in a spa over a holiday season when they need extra help, just to find out what it is really like. Find out as much as you can about the specific spa you are interested in working in. Are you suitable for the spa and is the spa suitable for you? And, even if you're an amazing body therapist, consider going for a dual license in esthetics as well, because an increasing number of spas are looking for that flexibility. Keep yourself open, have fun and enjoy everything this industry has to offer!"

DEXA

acronym for dual energy X-ray absorptiometry, a full-body scan used in some spas to measure bone density and body fat percentage and location, offering a very high degree of accuracy

CONCLUSION

Advanced modalities add something special to spa menus, giving spa clients the opportunity to expand their experience of life with luxurious ingredients and exotic treatments. Spas can also help clients heal themselves with the aid of highly trained therapists applying advanced skills. You will benefit yourself and your future clients in the spa by learning one or more advanced modalities yourself. This will increase your pride in what you do, enable you to help more people, and improve your earning potential in the spa industry. Spa directors and owners are constantly in search of therapists who are skilled in multiple modalities. If you have your sights set on working at a particular spa, do some

FACE TREATMENTS

Massage therapists working in spas, or even in their own private practices, can offer effective and pleasurable face treatments to clients. These treatments create some, but by no means all, of the benefits experienced during facials performed by a licensed esthetician. The benefits that massage therapists can offer include increased localized circulation, cleansed pores, relaxed facial muscles, and drainage of excess fluids from the area, all of which support improved appearance and well-being. Some of the many skin conditions that massage therapists should never attempt to diagnose, treat or improve, however, include **acne**, **rosacea**, **comedones**, **milia**, **seborrhea**, and **asteatosis**. In fact, when any excess redness, inflammation, or other abnormality is at all present on the skin, therapists should not provide treatment to the face but rather should refer the client to an esthetician or physician.

A large number of products can be used in spa face treatments, and their application is well within the boundaries of a massage therapist's job description. Some examples of such products include vitamin E, aloe vera, fresh herb powders, essential oils, and moisturizing creams and lotions (Figure 13–1). The physical techniques that massage therapists can ethically and professionally apply include, of course, massage, and also exfoliation, heat application and cold application, and cleansing. When these techniques are combined with natural products, a wide range of pleasant and effective treatments can be created, as is evidenced by the many offerings on massage therapists' menus in spas and private practices.

There are two primary methods of application for these face-oriented therapies in the spa setting: stand-alone face treatments, and mini face treatments that are administered as part of a longer spa service such as a body wrap. Face treatments can be combined with hand, foot, scalp, or back treatments to create an esthetically oriented package or signature service. In addition, many massage

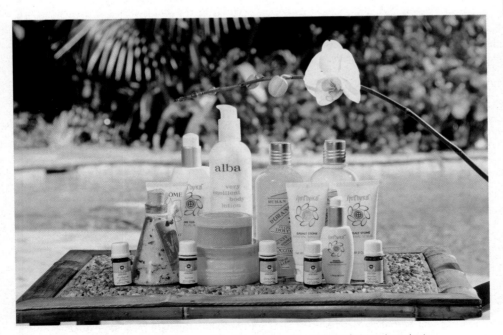

FIGURE 13–1 Massage therapists can ethically apply a wide variety of natural products to the face.

extractions

the squeezing out of blackheads or whiteheads from skin pores performed by estheticians using a variety of techniques, some of which include the use of instruments or steam

acne

chronic inflammation of the sebaceous glands caused by retained secretions; in severe cases cysts and nodules can form, resulting in scarring

rosacea

a skin disease in which blood vessels of the face enlarge, resulting in a flushed appearance and sometimes pustules

comedones

also called a *blackhead*, this is a hardened mass of sebum that has become lodged in a hair follicle

milia

small white or yellowish nodules resembling millet seeds, produced in the skin by the retention of sebaceous secretion

seborrhea

oily or shiny skin caused by abnormal excess secretion of sebum

asteatosis

diminished or arrested action of the sebaceous glands caused by advanced age and exposure to cold, resulting in dry, scaly skin services that focus primarily on the body can feature a face-specific component. Stone massage treatments are ideal for this, as therapists can modify the service to focus more time on the face, or they can create a face-only stone service that in essence miniaturizes the full-body stone massage, repurposing it for the face, neck, shoulders, and scalp alone, using both hot and cold stones. See Table 13–2 for a partial list of possible face treatments that can readily be performed by massage therapists.

TREATMENT	DESCRIPTION	SCOPE OF PRACTICE ISSUES
Face Stone Massage	Using the smallest stones in a stone kit, therapists apply heat and cold combined with oils, moisturizers, and exfoliating products to create a treatment that deeply tones and stimulates the muscles and integument of the face. The neck and shoulders are also relaxed with stones and manual massage.	Therapists who have not been trained in the use of massage stones should not apply them, especially to the delicate face and neck areas, even though it is within their scope of practice. Obtain proper training beforehand.
Ayurvedic Face Treatment	Packaged products featuring herbs, oils, floral waters, moisturizers, and cleansers created with Ayurvedic ingredients and applied in accordance with Ayurvedic principles are well within the boundaries of massage therapists' domain. Simple questionnaires to determine clients' body type or "dosha" can help therapists apply the most appropriate products. See Chapter 12 for more information.	These treatments should be restricted solely to product applications and not involve any type of diagnosis, which can happen if therapists use information about clients' doshas to prescribe certain protocols. Dosha information should only be used to choose appropriate products.
Seaweed Face Treatment	Seaweed preparations are applied to the face, typically to form a mask that is then either peeled or washed away. Other steps may include cleansing, exfoliation, massage, and moisturizing.	Seaweed application is often performed by estheticians, and therapists need to take care not to diagnose any type of skin condition that might benefit by seaweed. Rather, a general application good for all skin types should be used.
De-Stressing Spa Face Treatment	This treatment uses hot towels to cleanse and pressure points to massage, thus relaxing facial muscles and rejuvenating the client. Afterward, soothing Swedish strokes and a rich moisturizer lock in the benefits.	This treatment is straightforward massage, but therapists need to be careful not to overly cleanse during towel application and cleaning, avoiding any trace of extractions.
Aromatherapy Mini Face Treatment	Given while the client is cocooned in an aromatherapy wrap, this face treatment complements the chosen oil that was mixed with the emollient lotion and applied to the body. It lasts only 15 minutes while the client rests in the wrap.	Simple, straightforward protocols as provided by the spa should be followed, and therapists need to resist prescribing certain essential oils if they have not been trained in their use.
Head-to-Toe Treatment	This treatment features spa reflexology and a mini face treatment combined into one. Clients can remain dressed while their face, hands, and feet are treated with simple natural products and plenty of massage.	Therapists must remember not to perform any extractions or diagnose any skin conditions.
All-Natural Herbal Face Massage	This treatment features an herbal exfoliation, mask, and moisturizer. It should be applied by those therapists who have been properly trained and are comfortable working with natural herbs and herbal formulations, many of which have been adapted for use on the face.	As long as the products used are consumer-grade and readily available to the public, their use should present no problem in these treatments. Therapists need to remember only to cleanse, exfoliate, and massage. No other techniques are appropriate.

TABLE 13–2 Examples of Face Treatments Massage Therapists can Perform in the Spa Setting.

SPA TIP

When referring to face treatments performed by a massage therapist, it is best to refrain from using the word "facial," which is used by estheticians. It is more descriptive and less confusing to use terms such as "face massage," "face treatment," and "head, neck, and face treatment" when referring to these services when they are performed by massage therapists. The use of these terms implies that esthetician-specific protocols such as skin-type diagnosis and extractions are not to be performed.

RESEARCH

Go receive a professional facial treatment by a licensed esthetician at a local spa. Afterward, write a one-page paper about your experience, noting specifically which parts of the procedure you, as a massage therapist, would not be allowed to perform.

Mini Face Treatment

The relatively short face treatment protocol featured here, at only 20 minutes, can be slightly expanded to be a stand-alone half-hour treatment, or it can be applied as-is during another spa service such as the body wrap described in Chapter 7.

upcharge

an additional charge added to the stated price of a commodity or service, as for a face treatment given during a longer service such as a body wrap

TREATMENT: MINI FACE TREATMENT	
Wet Room/Dry Room	dry room
Table Setup	The table can be set as for a massage, with a blanket, bottom sheet and top draping sheet. If the mini face treatment is administered as part of a longer service such as a wrap, follow the table setup for that service.
Treatment Duration	20 to 25 minutes
Needed Supplies	2 cotton pads, astringent cleanser spray, ¼ cup reconstituted sea clay (other chosen product can be substituted for application, such as moor mud, rose clay, herbs, etc.), 4 drops lavender essential oil, 1 tablespoon moisturizing face lotion, warmer such as a hot towel cabbie, 2 hand towels, optional natural bristle brush for product application
Contraindications	skin conditions in the face and neck area, including severe acne, rashes, skin viruses, cuts, bruises, abrasions, recent surgeries, recent skin peels, sunburn, cold sores, extremely sensitive or delicate skin
Draping	For a stand-alone treatment, clients can remain dressed if so desired, lying atop table linens or even on a reclining chair. Alternatively, a top sheet can be used for draping.
Treatment Order	The mini face treatment is either given during another spa body treatment or by itself, in which case it should be scheduled after an exfoliation, massage, or wrap. When administered after other services, the client's cleansed skin and improved appearance can be more easily maintained.
Safety, Sanitation Issues, & Cleanup	Keep products out of client's eyes, using cotton pads to cover the eyes if necessary. If paraffin is used, monitor temperature often to maintain a safe operating environment.
Body Mechanics & Self-Care	It is recommended to sit at the head of the table on a comfortable stool or chair while applying the face treatment in order to avoid stress on the lower back.
Product Cost	less than $1
Treatment Price	sometimes given as an add-on for other services at no extra charge, or for an **upcharge**, typically in the $20 range; as a stand-alone treatment, $40 to $80
Physiological Effects	The mini face treatment helps remove dead cells from the skin, unblocking pores; products nourish skin; lotions and creams moisturize; massage stimulates circulation, moves lymph and relaxes muscles, creating a relaxation response and improving appearance.
Pregnancy Issues (information provided by Elaine Stillerman, LMT, author and developer of MotherMassage)	Safe during pregnancy. In the latter stages of pregnancy, positioning modifications must be implemented since pressure from the heavy uterus on the inferior vena cava (from lying supine or insufficiently bolstered) may cause impaired venous return and supine hypotensive syndrome.

Mini Face Preparation

1. Set the table and prepare the room.
2. Moisten and warm two hand towels.
3. Warm the products to be used in a spa bowl.
4. Have all products close at hand for easy access.

Mini Face Procedure

1. For stand-alone treatment, instruct the client to lie supine on the table or recline on a chair. Drape as appropriate. If the client is already on the table as part of a longer service, make sure that she is comfortable. In either case, use a bolster under the knees for support while the client is lying supine for an extended period.
2. To protect the hair, fold a hand towel diagonally and wrap around the hairline, tucking the ends behind the head (Figure 13–2).

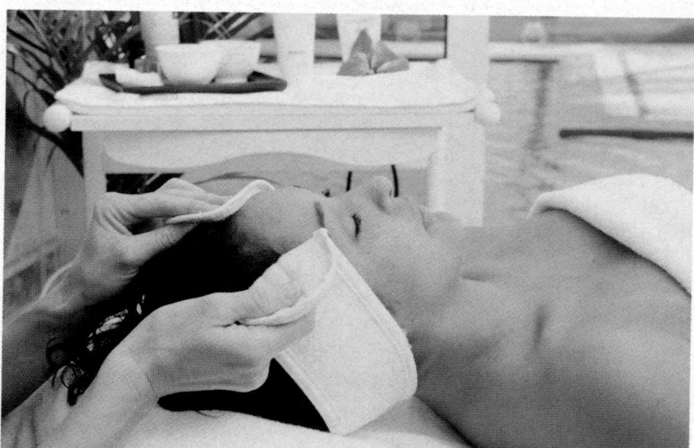

FIGURE 13–2

3. Spray cleanser onto two cotton pads and wipe the client's face, using upward motions starting at the chin (Figure 13–3).

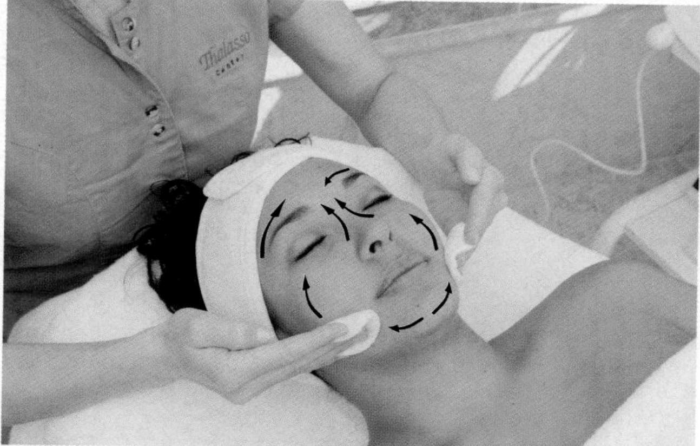

FIGURE 13–3

4. Apply the first hot towel to the face and hold it in place using slight pressure over the eyes for 30 seconds (Figure 13–4).

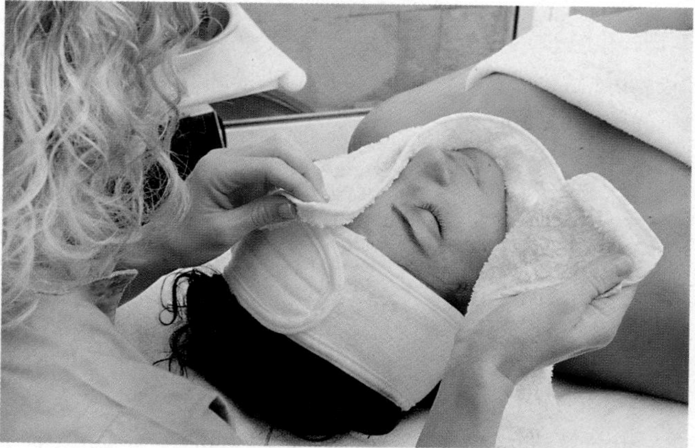

FIGURE 13–4

5. Drip two drops of lavender essential oil into each hand and apply pressure point massage along the chin, jaw, and cheeks, around the eyes, and on the forehead and scalp (Figure 13–5).

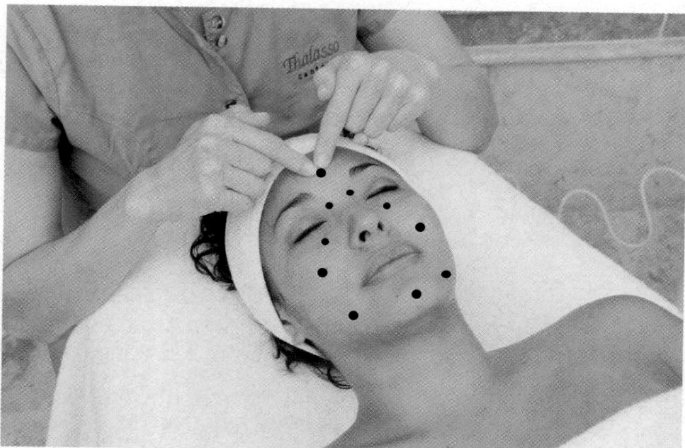

FIGURE 13–5

6. Apply warmed sea clay (or other chosen natural product) to the skin of the face in a thin layer using your hands or a natural bristle brush (Figure 13–6).

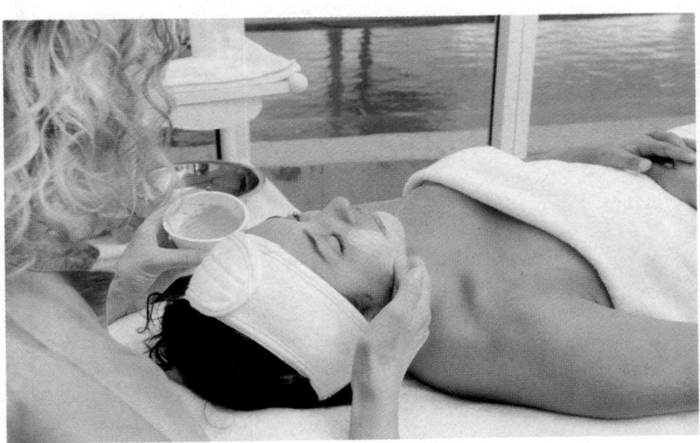

FIGURE 13–6

7. Once application is complete, wipe your hands on the used hot towel. If the client is chilled, wrap her in a blanket if she is not already wrapped as part of another service (Figure 13–7).

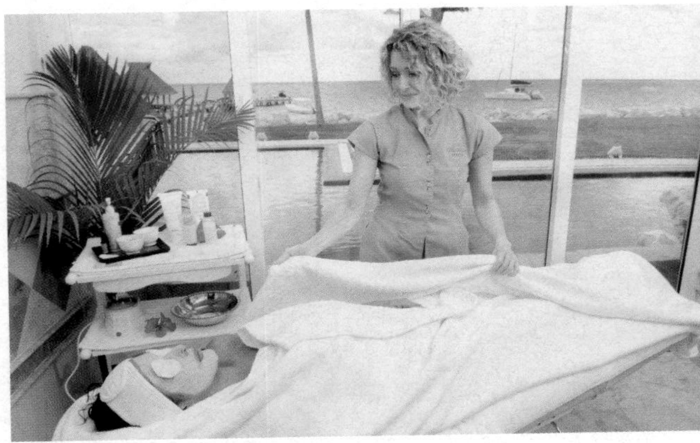

FIGURE 13–7

8. Apply scalp massage (Figure 13–8).

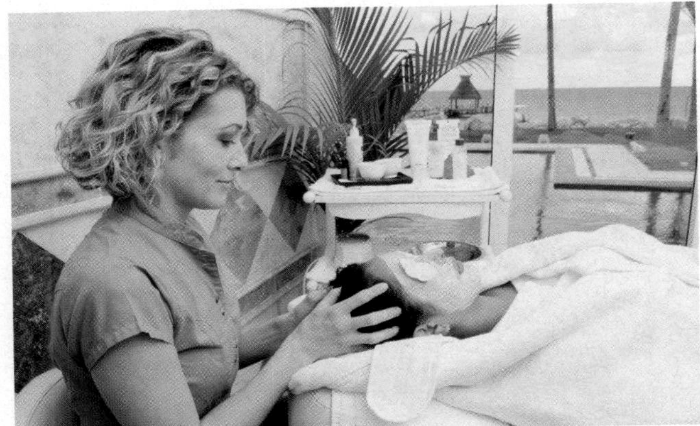

FIGURE 13–8

9. If the client's hands are accessible, offer hand massage (Figure 13–9).

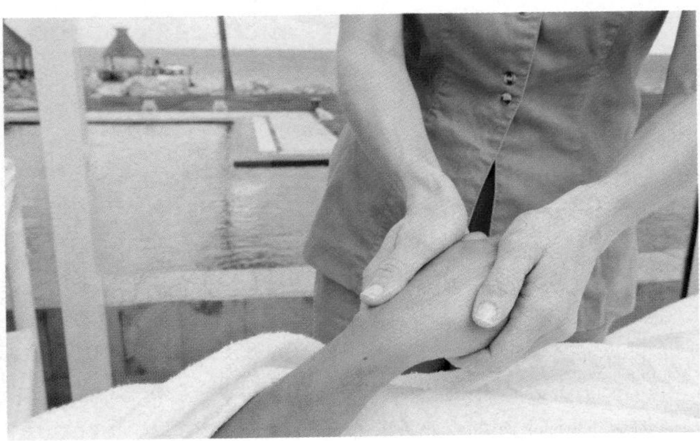

FIGURE 13–9

10. Use a second hot towel to cleanse the product from the client's face (Figure 13–10).

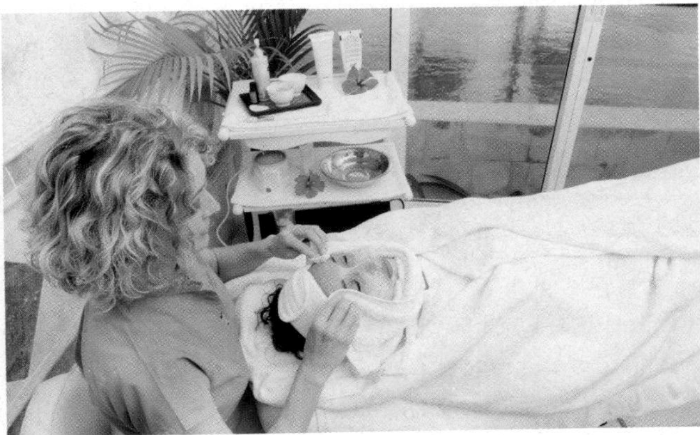

FIGURE 13–10

11. Apply emollient lotion using massage strokes in an upward motion (Figure 13–11). Make the massage longer for a stand-alone treatment.

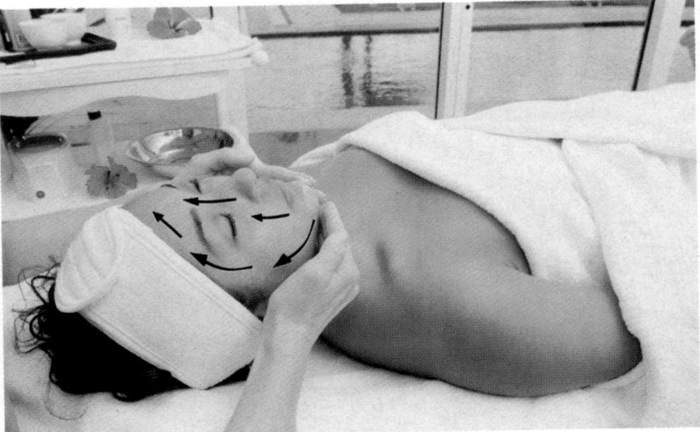

FIGURE 13–11

12. Unwrap and assist the client in getting off the table.

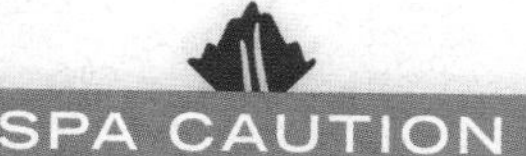

SPA CAUTION

Be careful when applying hot towels to the face. Always check the temperature on your hands first, and then place the towel over the client's face, being sure to leave an opening for the mouth and nose so that the client can breathe freely. Even though caution is rightfully advised, however, you should also be aware that the towel will feel hotter to your hands than it will to the client's face. It takes a little practice with this technique before you will feel completely comfortable applying hot towels to the face and getting the temperature just right for each client.

Mini Face Cleanup

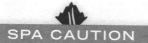

1. Launder the sheets and towels.
2. Change the linens on the table.
3. Wash out the spa bowls.
4. Discard the cotton pads.

Face Treatments with Paraffin

Because it is a substance that can heat and relax the muscles, paraffin can be used by massage therapists for many types of therapeutic applications. When meant for application to the face and neck, paraffin is typically spread atop a layer of gauze, keeping it in place and providing texture into which the wax can harden over the contours of the skin. Details about paraffin and its application in spas have already been described in Chapter 5. Therapists often take advantage of the penetrating heat and occlusive barrier created by paraffin to treat not only their clients but also their own aching hands after extended periods of work. See the activity sidebar for step-by-step protocols for using paraffin on the face.

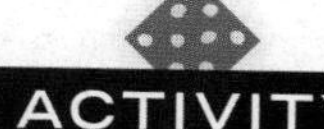

ACTIVITY

Paraffin Application to the Face

Paraffin application to the face feels great and has immediate therapeutic effects, sealing in rejuvenating moisture while heat penetrates into muscles and connective tissues. Try exchanging this simple paraffin face application with a classmate. You will need, in addition to the supplies for the face treatment explained in this chapter, three additional items: a pre-cut gauze face cloth, heated paraffin, and a brush.

Step by Step:

1. Warm the paraffin. The facial paraffin often comes in a small container that can be warmed in a special unit, bringing it to the proper temperature for application.
2. Cleanse the face with cotton pads and an astringent.
3. Apply a small amount of moisturizer and massage it into the skin.
4. Lay the facial gauze on the face, making sure to match up the mouth and nose openings over the proper area (Figure 13–12).

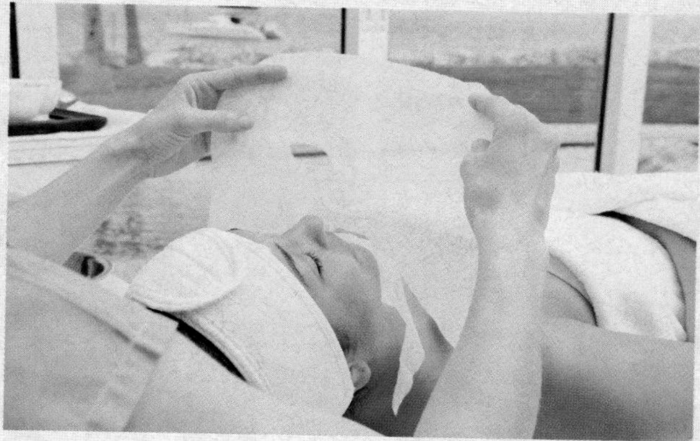

FIGURE 13–12

(Continued)

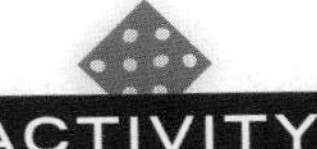

ACTIVITY

5. Dip the brush into the paraffin, let excess drip off, then paint the paraffin over the gauze, starting at the neck and working up to the forehead, avoiding the eyes (Figure 13–13).
6. Repeat the painting application until it is three layers deep (Figure 13–14).
7. Let your partner relax for 10 to 15 minutes, applying hand massage. If it is available, you can also dip your partner's hands in paraffin and wrap them in plastic.
8. Remove the gauze and paraffin together, peeling it away from the face, starting at the neck and moving upward (Figure 13–15).
9. Dab the balled-up paraffin on the face to attract any leftover pieces (Figure 13–16).
10. Apply a moisturizing lotion and massage into the face.

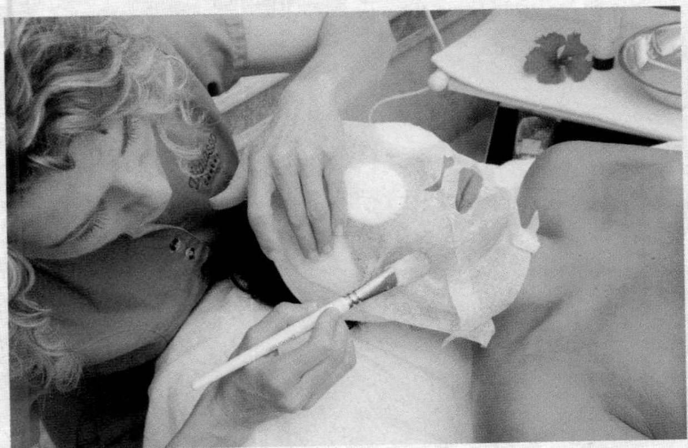

FIGURE 13–13

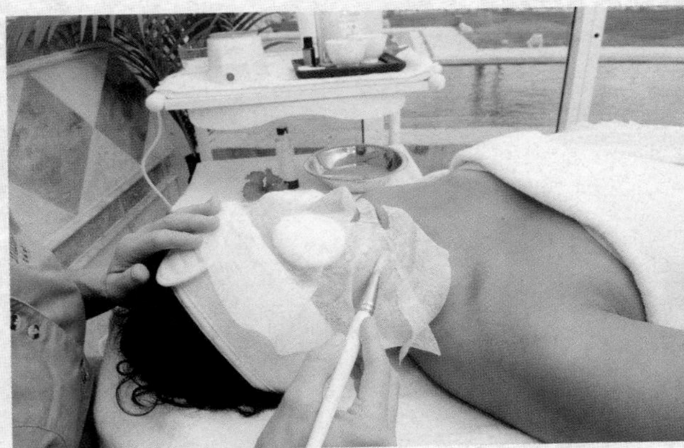

FIGURE 13–14

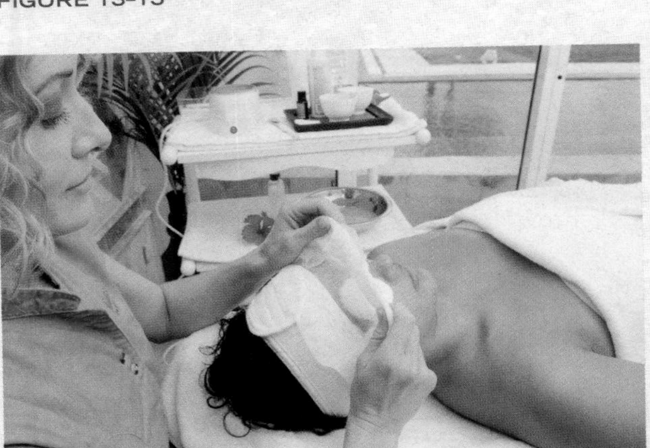

FIGURE 13–15

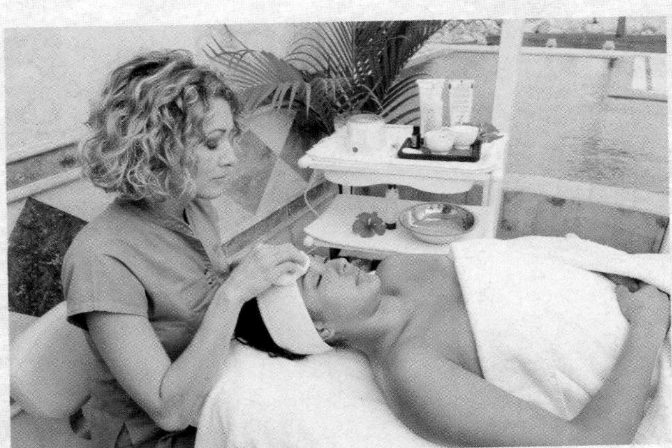

FIGURE 13–16

Face Treatments with Natural Chemical Exfoliants

It should be repeated here that massage therapists, unless they are trained and licensed otherwise, are not estheticians. Nor are they physicians, physicians' assistants, nurses, or certified laser technicians. Therefore, even when these therapists are working within the confines of a spa where the rules are "bent" at times regarding the application of products and services that have a profound effect on the skin, such as physician-strength alpha hydroxy acids and hair-removal laser machines, it is up to each individual therapist to decline to work outside his or her scope of practice.

However, in spite of these caveats, it is also important to remember that massage therapists can apply certain products that do have an effect on the skin, as long as that effect is within their scope of practice. One example of this type of product is a natural enzyme exfoliant, the most popular being papaya enzyme. At low doses, this enzyme can chemically dissolve dead skin cells and assist the therapist as he cleanses, exfoliates, massages, and moisturizes the face, all of which contributes significantly to improved appearance and well-being. There is a simple, reasonable rule of thumb to follow when determining which strength of product is appropriate for use by massage therapists, and that consists of a single question: Is the product available for purchase by the general public? If the answer is yes, then therapists can use it without trepidation. If, on the other hand, it is necessary to first obtain a particular license or other qualification to purchase the product, it may be too concentrated for use by untrained personnel and should not be used by therapists, even if they are familiar with the product and confident in their ability to use it.

SPA TIP

Men in Esthetics

Desiree Collazo, Education Manager at the Florida College of Natural Health, has noticed a new trend: many male therapists who graduate and work in the field for a few years are coming back to study skin care. By becoming dually licensed, they can find better employment opportunities. They do not necessarily work as practicing estheticians, but they find that more doors are opened to them in the spa industry just because they have the extra credential. They are also more qualified to perform body treatments such as wraps and exfoliation, as they have a greater knowledge of the skin.

Ayurvedic Face Treatments

The Ayurvedic tradition offers several face treatments which massage therapists can perform quite readily because they do not involve extractions or other advanced esthetic techniques. Cleansers, herbal exfoliants, herbal masks, and moisturizers made with Ayurvedic ingredients are simple to apply, and several variations on Ayurvedic face treatments are used by therapists in spas large and small. One specialized version of an Ayurvedic face treatment is called **Soundaryam Vardhini**, which is not so much a traditional facial but rather an application of fresh fruit- and vegetable-based creams, astringents, and ointments, combined with massage to marma points, which creates a relaxing and beautifying treatment. As in all face treatments performed by therapists, this service features no extractions or trauma to the skin. The marma-point massage focuses on the face, neck, and shoulders, toning local tissues and reinvigorating the client.

Soundaryam Vardhini
Ayurvedic face treatment using fresh fruit and vegetable preparations and marma-point massage

BACK TREATMENTS

Some spas offer their clients the opportunity to experience a treatment that focuses exclusively on the back area. More than just purely massage, these services usually focus on some kind of cleansing and skin rejuvenation featuring products that are sometimes applied to the face. For this reason, these services are sometimes called "back facials," even though no extractions or diagnoses are being performed. This term can sometimes be confusing, though, as clients might rightfully assume that any kind of a "facial" treatment would be performed by an esthetician. The types of products applied range from mud to seaweed to clay to paraffin. Modalities used can include exfoliation, Swedish massage, stone massage, lymphatic drainage, heat therapy, and others. These treatments are especially enjoyable for clients who are not accustomed to disrobing completely for spa treatments. The back is usually a non-threatening area of the body on which to work, and clients can remain dressed below the waist if they so choose.

Estheticians who perform back treatment can, of course, use extractions and other techniques meant to benefit certain skin conditions. For this reason, clients with acne and other skin problems are best advised to receive back treatments from estheticians. However, for a majority of clients—those who are seeking spa services for relaxation and wellness—back treatments given by massage therapists are enjoyable and effective.

The following protocol is typical of back treatments performed in many spas. It does not require a wet room, though a spa that has a wet room available would most likely make it available to their clients, as showering simplifies the cleansing of products from the skin, especially when drying clays are used. When paraffin is applied during a back treatment (and also for a full-body treatment), large strips of gauze are laid over the skin and the melted paraffin is applied over the gauze with a brush.

TREATMENT: BACK TREATMENT	
Wet Room/Dry Room	dry room
Table Setup	table cover, sheet, draping sheet
Treatment Duration	45 minutes
Needed Supplies	4 hot wet towels, sheet of plastic cut to the size of client's back, exfoliating body scrub, product (mud, clay, seaweed) to apply to back, emollient lotion, 2 spa bowls, optional infrared heating unit
Contraindications	cuts, abrasions, sores or bruises on the back, recent surgery on the back area, severe or aggravated acne or other skin conditions, difficulty in lying prone such as during pregnancy
Draping	The client remains prone throughout this entire treatment. Draping is performed with a sheet, uncovering and covering the back from the sacrum up to the neck.
Treatment Order	The back treatment is typically given as a stand-alone treatment, though a full-body massage can be incorporated at the end, or an exfoliation beforehand.
Safety, Sanitation Issues, & Cleanup	Excess product may be washed down the drain. Soiled towels should be laundered soon after treatment to prevent mold. Take care if using infrared lights for warming purposes, as these can burn if touched directly.
Body Mechanics & Self-Care	Therapists should use the same body mechanics as they do during massage.
Product Cost	$2 or less for product and plastic wrap for back
Treatment Price	$70 to $100
Physiological Effects	The back treatment opens the pores through exfoliation, cleansing the skin and making the penetration of therapeutic products easier. Products applied can draw impurities from the skin. Heat from the hot towels and products relaxes muscles and connective tissues. Massage releases tension from the back and shoulders, and emollient lotions lock moisture into the skin.
Pregnancy Issues (information provided by Elaine Stillerman, LMT, author and developer of MotherMassage)	Safe during pregnancy if the client is safely and comfortably positioned on the body support system or sitting upright.

Back Treatment Preparation

1. Place 1 tablespoon exfoliating scrub in one spa bowl and ½ cup body mud, clay, or seaweed in the other spa bowl, and warm.
2. Moisten and heat the four hand towels.
3. Prepare the table and room, noting that clients often feel chilled after having their backs wrapped, then exposed, so it is important to keep the room warm or to have an infrared heating unit that can be placed near the client's back.

Back Treatment Procedure

1. Apply the first hot towel to the back and allow the heat to penetrate for a minute while applying steady pressure over the entire back area (Figure 13–17).

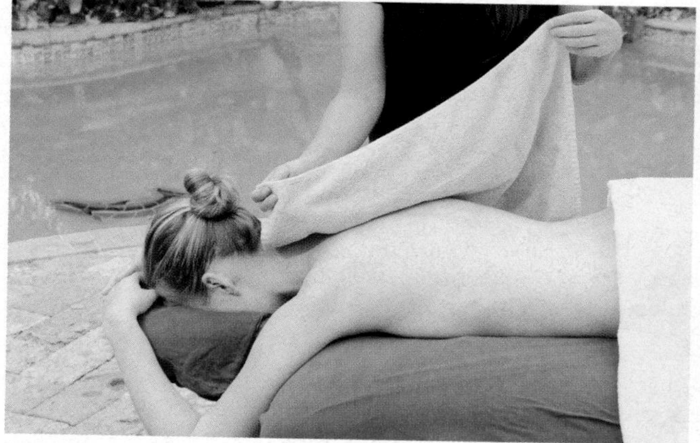

FIGURE 13–17

2. Apply exfoliating body scrub over the entire back, sprinkling a little water over the area if needed, though the back may already be moist enough from the hot towel application (Figure 13–18). Use the exfoliation techniques learned in Chapter 6.

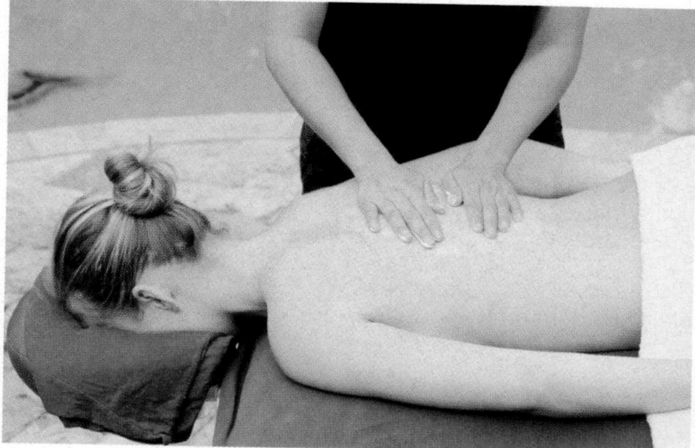

FIGURE 13–18

3. Wipe exfoliant from the back with the second hot towel (Figure 13–19).

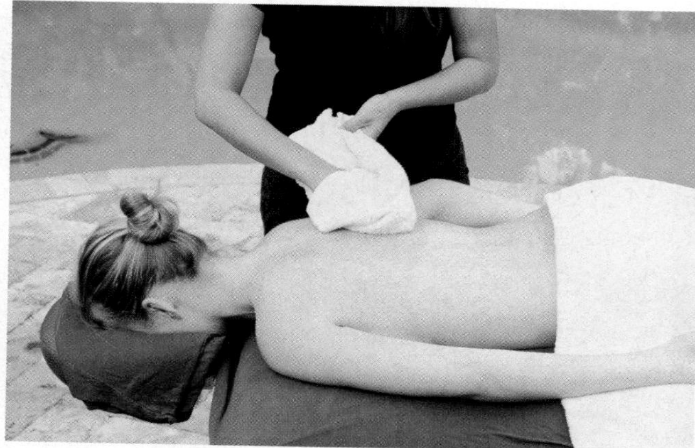

FIGURE 13–19

4. Using your hands or a natural bristle brush, apply seaweed, mud, or clay to the back (Figure 13–20). Specific benefits and contraindications for these products are found in Chapters 7 and 8.

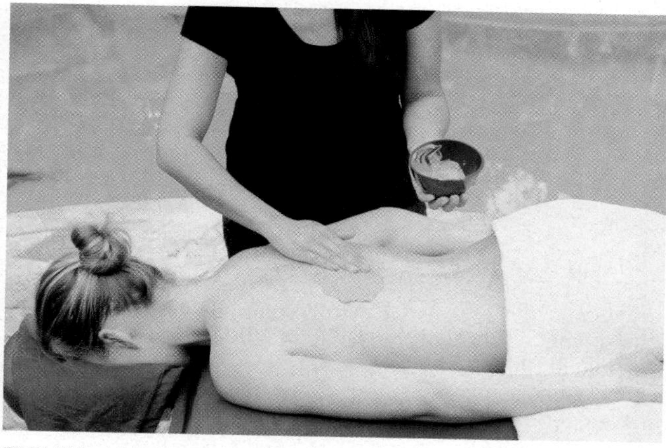

FIGURE 13–20

5. Cover the client's back with piece of plastic wrap, then cover with a bath towel and the top sheet drape (Figure 13–21).

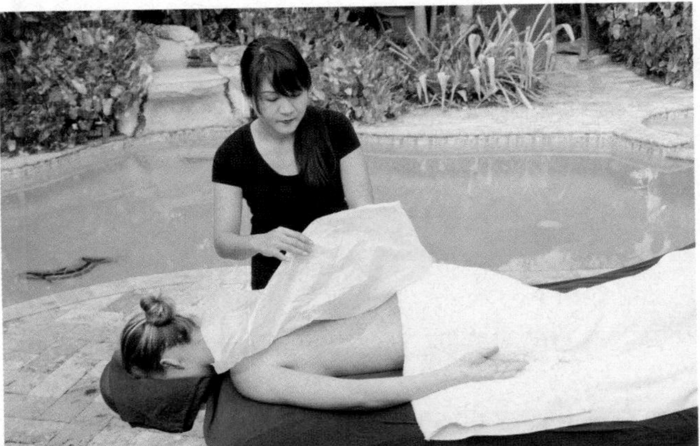

FIGURE 13–21

6. The client rests, remaining in the prone position for 10 to 15 minutes, during which you can apply light massage to the hands, feet, or scalp (Figure 13–22).

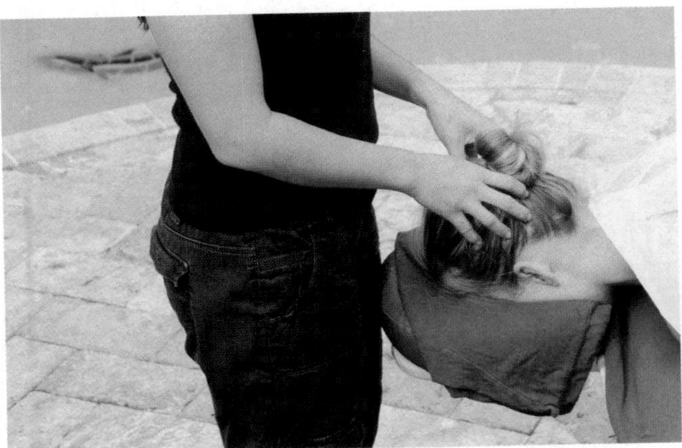

FIGURE 13–22

7. Use the remaining two hot towels to wipe the product from the back, patting dry with a clean towel if necessary (Figure 13–23).

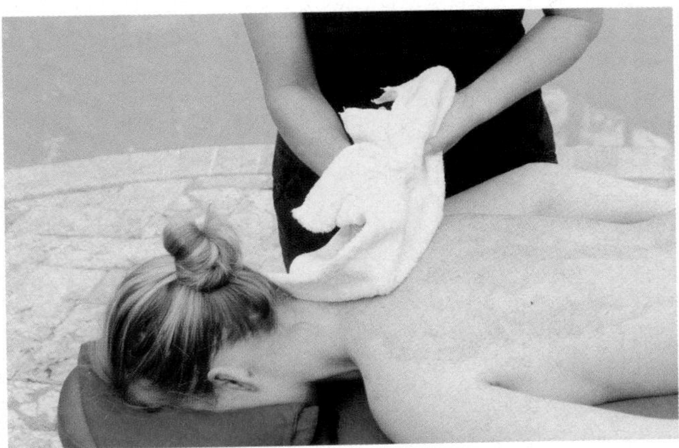

FIGURE 13–23

8. Massage emollient lotion into the skin of the back, shoulders, and back of the neck (Figure 13–24).

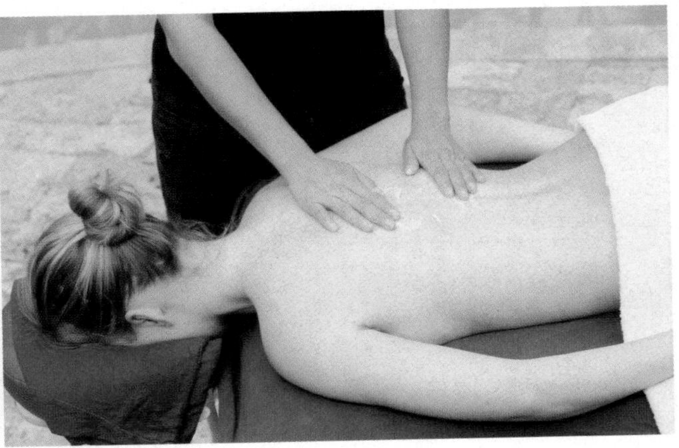

FIGURE 13–24

Back Treatment Cleanup

1. Launder the towels and sheets.
2. Clean the spa bowls.
3. Discard the plastic wrap.

SCALP TREATMENTS

Scalp treatments are a simple, delightful addition to massage therapists' repertoire of spa services. Though not as therapeutic as certain other services—such as the herbal wrap or hydrotherapy bath, for example—these treatments

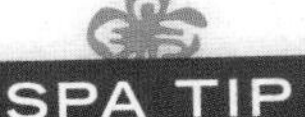

SPA TIP

To make the back treatment longer or shorter (for a 60-minute or 30-minute treatment), increase or decrease the length of time the client rests with the product applied, and also the massage application at the end.

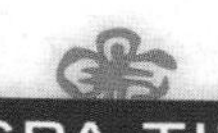

SPA TIP

For added enjoyment and therapeutic effect, 4 to 6 drops of essential oil may be added to both the exfoliant and the product applied in the back treatment. Good choices for this include bergamot, geranium, orange, tea tree, and vetiver. See Chapter 11 for more details about these oils' effects.

trichology

the branch of medical and cosmetic study and practice concerned with the hair and scalp

follicle

the sheath of cells and connective tissue that surrounds the root of a hair

keratinization

the process of changing into keratin, the hardened protein substance that makes up hair, nails, claws, etc.

sebaceous glands

a small gland in the skin which secretes a lubricating oily matter called *sebum* into hair follicles to lubricate skin and hair

can be quite beneficial for the hair and scalp, adding moisture and a natural sheen. In the same way in which full facials and esthetics services must be left to those estheticians who are licensed to perform them, hair services must be left to cosmetologists, who have been trained in the physiology of hair and its proper maintenance and beautification. Massage therapists may apply products and techniques with the intent to therapeutically benefit bodily tissues, but they may not choose specific protocols for particular hair types or scalp conditions. However, it is important for therapists to have a basic understanding of the hair and scalp in order to be aware of contraindications. The branch of science that deals with the scalp and hair, and which cosmetologists must study, is called **trichology**.

Human hair can be divided into two main parts, the hair root and the hair shaft, the root being located beneath the skin and the shaft above (Figure 13–25). Hair begins its growth process beneath the skin in the **follicle**, gradually turning from living material into hardened, dead cells in a process called **keratinization**. Although it may look luxurious and vibrant, visible hair is actually dead. Hair comes in many thicknesses and lengths, with different individuals displaying a wide range of hair types. Some people may even have different types of hair on different areas of their scalp, such as coarse, thick hair in most areas but thinning, brittle hair in one patch. The scalp treatments that spa therapists can perform are beneficial for all hair types.

One of the primary benefits of spa scalp treatments is increased moisture for dry and damaged hair. The culprit behind dry hair and scalp is inactive **sebaceous glands**, and it can be made worse by a dry environment. Scalp treatments ameliorate this condition by introducing natural products and increasing localized circulation. The scalp and hair need a certain amount of natural oils to remain healthy, and without these oils, the skin can become dry, itchy, or irritated. Overuse of synthetic soaps and shampoos can cause unnaturally low oil levels that lead to these conditions. Spa scalp treatments reintroduce natural oils to the hair and restore balance.

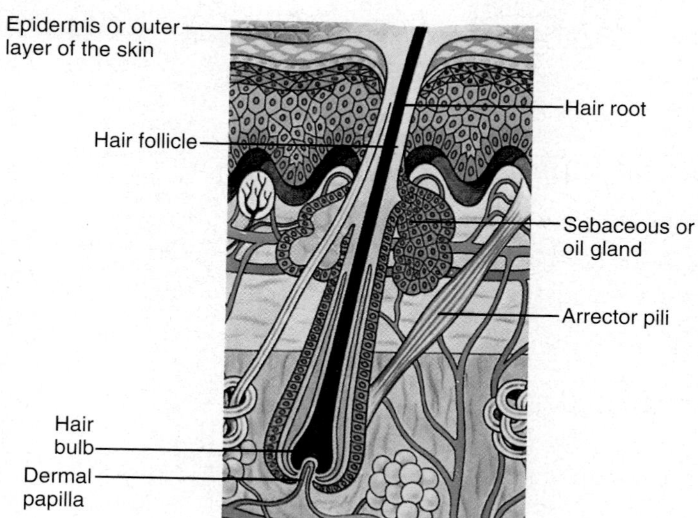

FIGURE 13–25 Cross section of human hair and skin.

Did You Know?

Can Spa Scalp Treatments Stimulate Hair Growth?

The average person has about 100,000 strands of hair on his or her head, and although some therapists have been known to suggest that vigorous scalp massage can help ward off hair loss, this has not been proven. The average rate of hair loss for most people is 35 to 40 strands per day, and no amount of massage will prevent that. However, there have been studies suggesting that the massaging of certain essential oils into the scalp does stimulate new hair growth. As noted in *Prevention* magazine, dermatologists in Scotland conducting a randomized, double-blind study over a seven-month period found some promising results. Participants suffering from **alopecia areata** were each given daily scalp massage, with an essential oil blend of thyme, rosemary, lavender, and cedarwood in jojoba and grapeseed carrier oils for half of the group, and with only the carrier oils for the other half. The study showed that 44 percent of the group exposed to essential oils experienced improvement and hair growth, compared with 15 percent of the other group. Overall, study results showed the use of essential oils to be a safe and effective treatment to stimulate hair growth in individuals suffering from hair loss.

Aromatherapists believe that many essential oils have benefits for the scalp and hair, including:

- Basil: benefits oily hair
- Cedarwood: stimulates scalp and hair follicles; used in treating hair loss
- Chamomile: gives golden highlights
- Clary sage: dandruff treatment
- Eucalyptus: antiseptic, anti-dandruff
- Lavender: used for itchiness, dandruff, and even lice
- Lemon: adds gold highlights to hair; benefits dry scalp, dandruff, and underactive sebaceous glands
- Lemongrass: useful for oily hair, slows down scalp's oil production
- Patchouli: used to treat dandruff
- Rose: soothes scalp, pleasant aroma
- Rosemary: good for dandruff; promotes hair growth (contraindicated for pregnancy)
- Sandalwood: good for dry or damaged hair
- Tea tree: good for dry scalp, dandruff, and underactive sebaceous glands; stimulates hair follicles
- Thyme: promotes hair growth
- Ylang ylang: antiseptic, helps control sebum production, good for oily hair

In addition, jojoba is a good choice of carrier oil because it effectively moisturizes the scalp and helps balance natural sebum levels in the skin. Some therapists also use unrefined coconut oil, as it has a soothing effect on dry, itchy scalps and dandruff.

Scalp treatments can easily be performed in a typical massage room, as the protocol below will show. If, on the other hand, the treatment is given in a wet room, the use of a sink, floor drain, or shower can be helpful. Wherever it is experienced, the scalp treatment is deeply relaxing. Some call it meditative. And it can be pleasurable as well, like a luxurious shampooing at a first-rate salon, but performed by a massage therapist instead of an attendant.

alopecia areata

a condition in which hair is lost, usually from the scalp, creating bald spots, especially in the first stages; certain essential oils have been shown to have a positive impact on the condition

Macassar Oil

Did You Know?

Although modern spa scalp and hair treatments are enjoyed primarily by women, men have traditionally used these very same products and techniques on their hair as well. Gentlemen in the Victorian and Edwardian eras, for example, applied a compound known as *macassar oil* to their hair to keep it fragrant, neat, and sleek. Macassar oil is comprised of coconut oil or palm oil blended with essential oil of ylang ylang, and sometimes other essentials as well. This concoction was called *macassar oil* because it was said to have been made from ingredients originally sourced in the port of Makassar in Indonesia.

Because this rich, fragrant macassar oil often transferred from a gentleman's hair to the backs of chairs and couches that he happened to sit upon, a special piece of crocheted or embroidered fabric was developed, called the *antimacassar*, that was placed over the back of furniture to protect it. Perhaps the most famous example of this in American history can be found at Ford's Theatre in Washington, D.C., the site of Lincoln's assassination. Dark stains on the back of the chair are sometimes purported to be Lincoln's blood, but they are actually macassar oil.

TREATMENT: SCALP TREATMENT	
Wet Room/Dry Room	dry room or wet room
Table Setup	waterproof table cover, sheet
Treatment Duration	30 minutes for *à la carte* service
Needed Supplies	shower cap, pitcher to pour warm water, basin to catch water, chair or stool on which to place basin, spa bowl, 1 to 2 tablespoons jojoba oil, 2 drops each of essential oils (thyme, rosemary, lavender, and cedarwood), massage lotion for hands, shower cap or plastic wrap, natural shampoo, waterproof covering to protect massage table
Contraindications	skin conditions or inflammation of the scalp, recent surgery in the scalp area, certain essential oils such as rosemary contraindicated for pregnancy
Draping	a bath towel for the upper body for protection from water and oils, as clients can remain clothed, or a top sheet can be used for draping if the client is disrobed
Treatment Order	The scalp treatment is typically offered after other spa services or as part of a longer service that includes a body wrap.
Safety, Sanitation Issues, & Cleanup	Oils should be thoroughly washed from hair after application. Take care not to overheat the oil, as it may scald.
Body Mechanics & Self-Care	Therapists should use a chair or stool at the head of the table to avoid excessive bending at the waist, which may injure the lower back.
Product Cost	under $1
Treatment Price	sometimes given as an add-on for other services at no extra charge, or for an upcharge, typically in the $20 range; as a stand-alone treatment, $40 to $80
Physiological Effects	exfoliates and cleanses scalp, adds moisture to hair, in addition to having a relaxing and calming effect overall; essential oils can positively affect mood
Pregnancy Issues (information provided by Elaine Stillerman, LMT, author and developer of MotherMassage)	The position of the pregnant client may be of concern in this treatment; her upper torso should be elevated between 45 and 70 degrees; 30 minutes in a position that puts too much pressure on the inferior vena cava is never recommended.

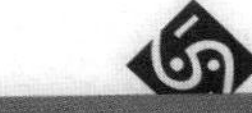

SPA ETIQUETTE

Always ask before applying oil to a client's hair. Some clients prefer never to have oil in their hair, though they may enjoy a modified scalp treatment without the oil.

Scalp Treatment Preparation

1. Mix jojoba oil and essential oils in a spa bowl and warm.
2. Moisten and heat one hand towel; place in a hot towel cabbie or insulated container.
3. Place the empty basin atop a stool or chair to be used to catch water and oils.
4. Position plastic wrap or a thermal blanket over the head of the table to protect it from water and oils.

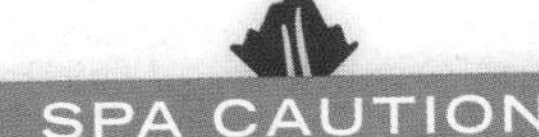

SPA CAUTION

During scalp treatments, water or oil can be spilled on the floor, making the area slick and causing a slipping hazard. Always be prepared with extra towels to place on the floor in case of spills.

Scalp Treatment Procedure

1. Position the client so that the top of her head extends slightly off the end of the table.
2. Rinse the client's hair with warm water (Figure 13–26).

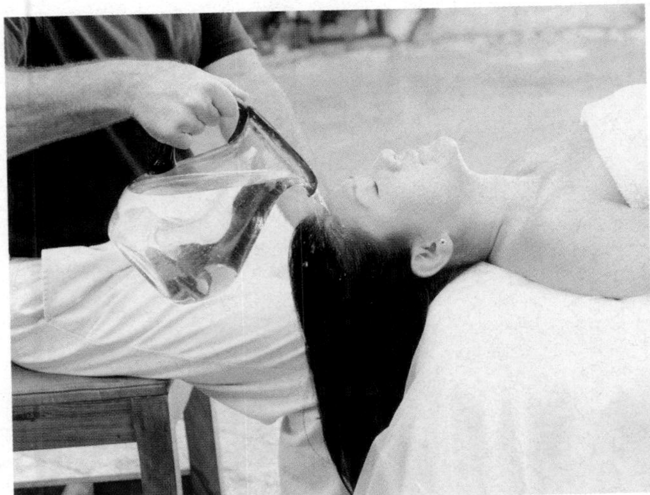

FIGURE 13–26

3. Cover the top of the head and forehead with a hot, moist towel to warm tissues for treatment and remove excess water from hair (Figure 13–27).

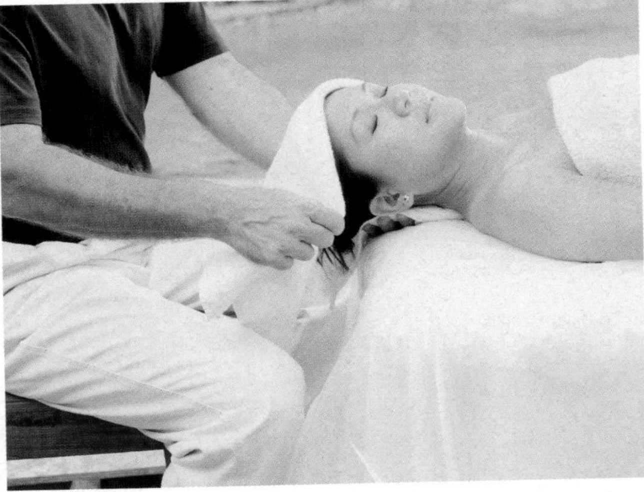

FIGURE 13–27

4. Massage jojoba and essential oil mixture thoroughly into the hair and scalp using firm, circular strokes with the fingertips (Figure 13–28). Begin massaging at the hairline above the forehead, and work back over the top of the scalp and down toward the occipital region. Lift your fingers away from the scalp slightly while moving from one spot to the next. Once you have reached the client's neck, move in circular movements up over the sides of the head toward the temples. Repeat this

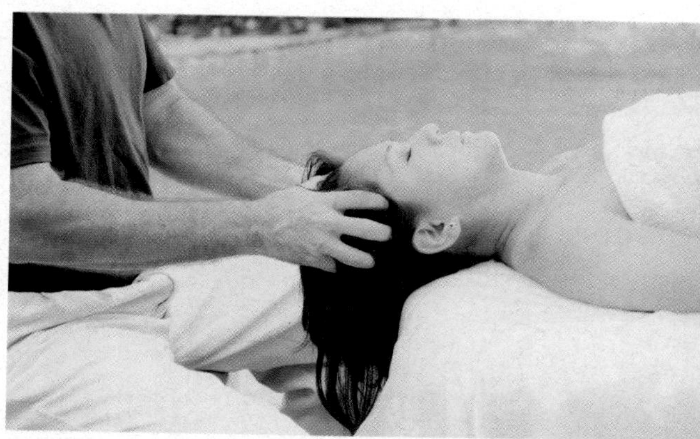

FIGURE 13–28

sequence several times until the oils are thoroughly massaged into the scalp.

5. Cover hair with a shower cap or piece of plastic wrap (Figure 13–29).

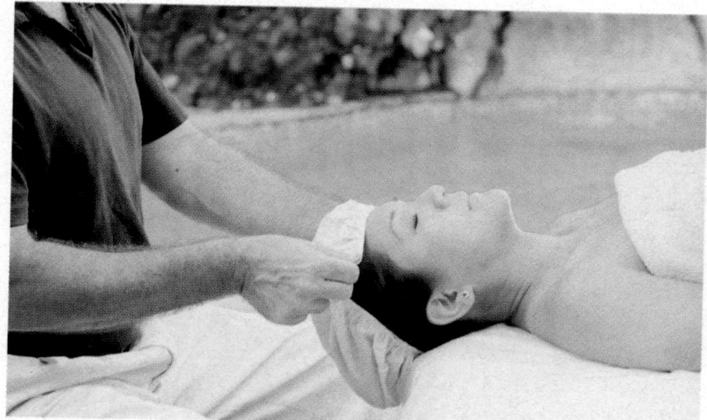

FIGURE 13–29

6. Massage the client's hands using emollient lotion, leaving oils in the hair for as long as possible for optimum effect (Figure 13–30).

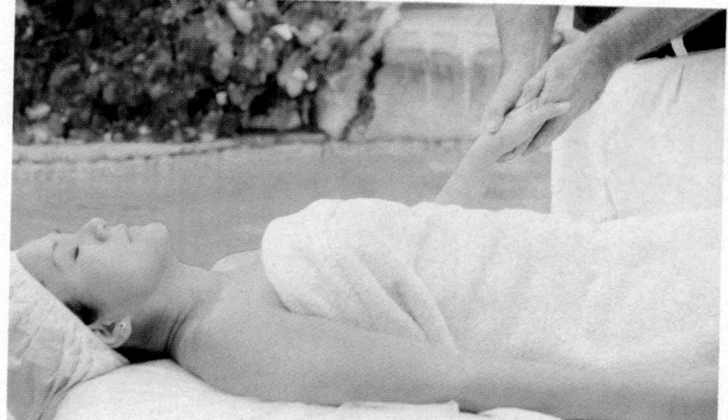

FIGURE 13–30

7. Remove the shower cap and rinse the oil from the hair with fresh water.
8. Apply a small amount of shampoo to the hair, massaging in and rinsing out (Figure 13–31).

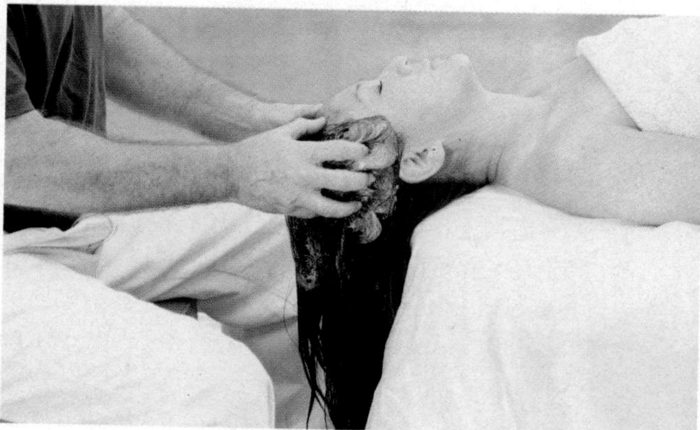

FIGURE 13–31

9. Gently towel-dry the hair (Figure 13–32).

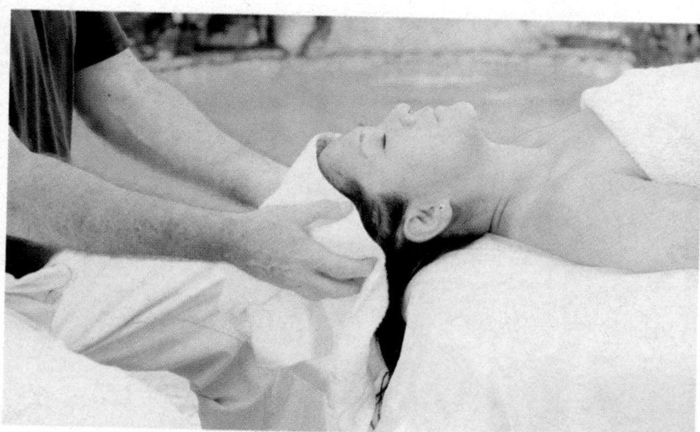

FIGURE 13–32

10. Brush hair until smooth (Figure 13–33).

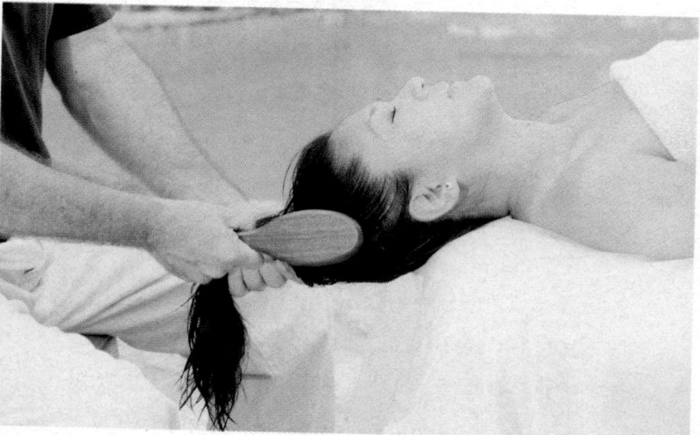

FIGURE 13–33

Scalp Treatment Cleanup

1. Discard the plastic or wash out the shower cap.
2. Launder the sheets and towels
3. Make sure that all oil and water spills are wiped from the floor.

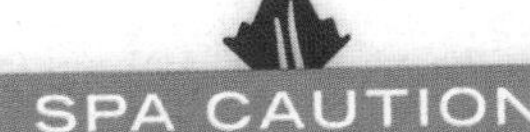

SPA CAUTION

Be cautious about introducing excessive oil into the hair, as it may become difficult to wash out, causing a greasy or sticky sensation for the client. When it comes to oil, a little goes a long way.

HAND AND FOOT TREATMENTS

Massage therapists can use their skills to add therapeutic benefits and deep enjoyment to spa hand and foot treatments. When cosmetologists administer manicures and pedicures, they often include some massage procedures, but since their expertise is not in massage therapy (unless they are dual licensed), clients are sometimes left wishing for a more thorough hand or foot massage experience. Therapists can offer this, as long as they remember not to overstep their bounds and perform any of the procedures reserved for cosmetologists. The procedures that are not allowed include cutting, filing, shaping, or buffing the nails, applying or removing nail polish, and trimming or shaping **cuticles**. Therapists, however, can massage the hands and feet, exfoliate the hands and feet, and apply therapeutic heat and cold to the hands and feet, in addition to moisturizing and nourishing the skin in these areas. Hand and foot treatments also provide an ideal occasion to offer the benefits of reflexology to clients, and the spa reflexology protocols outlined in Chapter 9 can be incorporated into any of these services.

One positive aspect of hand and foot treatments is that they can be performed in public spaces within the spa, such as waiting rooms and relaxation areas. Performing hand and foot treatments in these areas creates a tranquil mood and also inspires other spa clients to inquire about the services they see being offered. Some spas turn the offering of foot treatments into a ritual and perform it before every service in one of the spa's waiting areas. Attractive receptacles are used to wash the feet, such as ceramic basins or carved wooden bowls. Flower petals and essential oils can be added to the water to make these public services even more appealing. Services performed in public spaces do not take up valuable treatment room time, which can then be booked for other revenue-generating services.

Hand and foot treatments can be offered while the client is sitting fully clothed in a chair, which makes them especially attractive to modest people. Reclining chairs are optimal for this purpose, but the standard straight-backed chairs found in most waiting rooms can be used as well. The therapist generally sits in front of the client, either on a cushion, stool, ottoman, or another chair, taking the client's feet in her hands and holding them on a pillow or towel on her lap. If the client is scheduled for another spa service and has already changed into a robe, it is important, for modesty reasons, to keep the front of the robe tucked securely around the client's legs. A bath towel can be draped over the front of the robe for extra modesty in this circumstance.

Special care must be taken to ensure that all foot treatments are performed in a sanitary manner. Some clients are particularly sensitive to hygiene issues when their feet are being touched, and so therapists need to take this into account. It is important to always wash your hands prior to and after working on the feet, especially if you are going to be working on the face area afterward. For this reason, a cleansing step is usually incorporated into each foot treatment

SPA TIP

Additional spa products, such as mud, clay, and seaweed, may be massaged into the hair as part of the scalp treatment, and some therapists incorporate fresh, natural products such as ground avocadoes to add natural oil to the hair. These products are added after the oils have been rinsed out; they are then left on for another 10 to 15 minutes to provide extra benefit while additional hand or foot massage is provided to the client. In order for these products to be washed out easily, the hair must be thoroughly moistened beforehand, and it is recommended to have a sink available to completely clean the hair and scalp afterward. These products are sometimes too messy for use in dry rooms.

cuticles

nonliving epidermis surrounding the edges of the fingernails and toenails; therapists are not licensed to work on this area with implements during hand and foot treatments

SPA CAUTION

Massage therapists are not licensed to use any cosmetologists' tools to perform hand and foot treatments, including cuticle nippers, cuticle pushers, emery boards, nail brushes, nail buffers, nail clippers, nail files, and tweezers.

onychosis

any disease or disorder of the nails

at the very beginning. While some spas use a basin or pedicure station, others choose hot towels for this first step. It is permissible to request that clients wash their feet and hands before arriving for these treatments.

Cosmetologists and nail specialists need to be aware of certain contraindications and disease conditions that may affect their ability to perform a pedicure or manicure. **Onychosis** refers to any condition that adversely affects nails. These conditions can be quite severe, such as blue nails, in which nails can turn a variety of colors, indicating a deeper systemic problem. In addition, certain fungal conditions can affect the skin of the feet, including athlete's foot and ringworm, which can be contagious and are definite contraindications for spa foot treatments. Therapists, of course, are not in a position to diagnose specific diseases or conditions of the hands or feet, but they can and should report any irregularities they observe to the client to potentially be checked by a physician.

TREATMENT: HAND AND FOOT TREATMENT	
Wet Room/Dry Room	dry room
Table Setup	A chair can be used. For massage tables, only a sheet is necessary, with massage draping if client is disrobed. A blanket may be placed beneath for wrapping if the service is given as an add-on to a longer treatment.
Treatment Duration	30 minutes
Needed Supplies	ottoman or stool for therapist to sit on, footstool for client's feet, emollient lotion, essential oils of lavender, peppermint, and chamomile, 2 hand towels, 2 bath towels, 2 spa bowls, large receptacle for foot soaking (optional), ¼ cup body mud, 1 tablespoon exfoliating sea salts, liquid body bath, 2-foot square piece of plastic wrap
Contraindications	nail diseases, fungi such as athlete's foot, cuts, abrasions, or sores on the foot, hand, lower arm, or lower leg; caution urged with ovarian and uterine reflex points on feet and hands during pregnancy
Draping	No need to drape if client is clothed; if client is disrobed, use normal massage draping. Take care to maintain modesty if client is wearing a spa robe during treatment.
Treatment Order	often given before other treatments as a prelude to spa visit, or included as part of a longer treatment such as a body wrap
Safety, Sanitation Issues, & Cleanup	Sanitize hands after performing a foot treatment and before working on client's face.
Body Mechanics & Self-Care	Keep spine straightened when leaning over client's feet in order to avoid sore lower back.
Product Cost	less than $1
Treatment Price	typically $50 to $75 as a stand-alone treatment; given free as an incentive as part of longer services; sold as an upcharge to other services for an average of $25
Physiological Effects	stimulates local circulation, providing relief to muscle soreness and joint complaints such as arthritis; improves appearance of hands and feet through exfoliation; products moisturize and nourish skin
Pregnancy Issues (information provided by Elaine Stillerman, LMT, author and developer of MotherMassage)	Safe during pregnancy. Caution must be taken to avoid Large Intestine 4 on the hands, and the ovary/uterus reflexes, Liver 3, Bladder 67, Kidney 1, and Spleen 6 on the feet and legs. The temperature of the foot bath must not be too hot. Therapists are advised to have the client stand up and walk around after 20 to 25 minutes of sedentary sitting. Essentials oils cannot be used during the first trimester.

SPA PROFILE

Desiree Collazo – Education Manager, Florida College of Natural Health, a Steiner Leisure company *continued*

the spa need to follow certain precautions. "I know when to draw the line when it comes to teaching the hands-on portion of facial massage for therapists," she says. "For example, I always tell the students not to remove makeup from the face, as that is off-limits. It is possible a client may get an eye infection and blame the therapist for not knowing proper makeup removal technique. You have to think about what could go wrong. However, therapists can definitely ask clients if they want a face massage, in which case I recommend using upward, firming strokes, just like estheticians do. Clients can remove their own makeup if necessary, and therapists can apply a warm, moist towel afterward to open the pores and prepare the area for massage. Spas can charge more for this additional service. It's not really a facial, but the therapist is treating the face."

Collazo offers further advice for massage therapists who wish to work alongside estheticians in a professional manner. "Therapists need to learn the difference between fungal and viral infections," she says. "They need to be aware of the most frequently seen skin conditions. Sometimes, just recognizing something, and knowing who you have to refer the client to, is a life saver. There have been occasions where therapists have found cancerous lesions on the back where the client could not see them. Therapists are not supposed to diagnose, but it is important to identify certain skin conditions and know who to refer to, whether it be a physician or an esthetician. And always remember to document every observation and referral!"

Collazo believes that therapists can definitely have an esthetic impact on spa clients. "Just the massage itself increases circulation, firming and toning the tissues," she says. "The mere fact of bringing in circulation will enhance the person's appearance. All the same benefits derived by massaging the body are created by massaging the face. In fact, perhaps there's a little extra benefit for the face. The massage rejuvenates tissues, accelerating the cell renewal process. No products are needed for that.

"If massage is your passion, stay true to what you're doing, "Collazo counsels." Continue to educate yourself about spa services, but stay within your scope of practice. By knowing what your boundaries are, you can serve the client completely. But I definitely have to encourage you to think about dual licensing! It is the future, and it will open doors for you that you cannot even imagine now. Without a doubt, it is a smart move."

CONCLUSION

Uplifting, rejuvenating spa treatments that improve clients' mood and appearance are well within the bounds of what massage therapists can offer, and if you expand your professional capacities to include these services, you will increase your value as a spa employee. A good number of spa clients will appreciate your efforts at making them feel cared for through these esthetically based treatments. If you find that you enjoy performing them, you may consider seeking dual licensing by attending a professional esthetics school, as have many other successful therapists before you. Spas are blurring the line between esthetics and therapy, and there is no need to feel you are underusing your massage skills by performing treatments that help clients feel better about their appearance.

Remember, you will be offering your clients the profound benefits of massage therapy at the same time. Your intention is what counts the most, and performing esthetically oriented spa services with an attitude of dedication and service will bring you and your clients a high level of fulfillment.

REVIEW QUESTIONS

1. Instead of diagnosing skin conditions and using skin-specific products, what can massage therapists apply to the skin during face treatments?
2. How is paraffin typically applied to the face by massage therapists?
3. What is the most popular natural enzyme exfoliant used by massage therapists in spas?
4. What is a common term for the back treatments offered in spas? Why are they called this?
5. When performing scalp treatments in the spa, therapists are not allowed to choose specific protocols for particular hair types or scalp conditions. Why not?
6. What is the condition most commonly benefited by spa scalp treatments? What causes this condition? How do spa scalp treatments help?
7. What procedures are massage therapists not allowed to perform when giving a hand or foot treatment?
8. What are some of the benefits of performing foot treatments in a spa's waiting area?

PART 4

SPA CAREERS

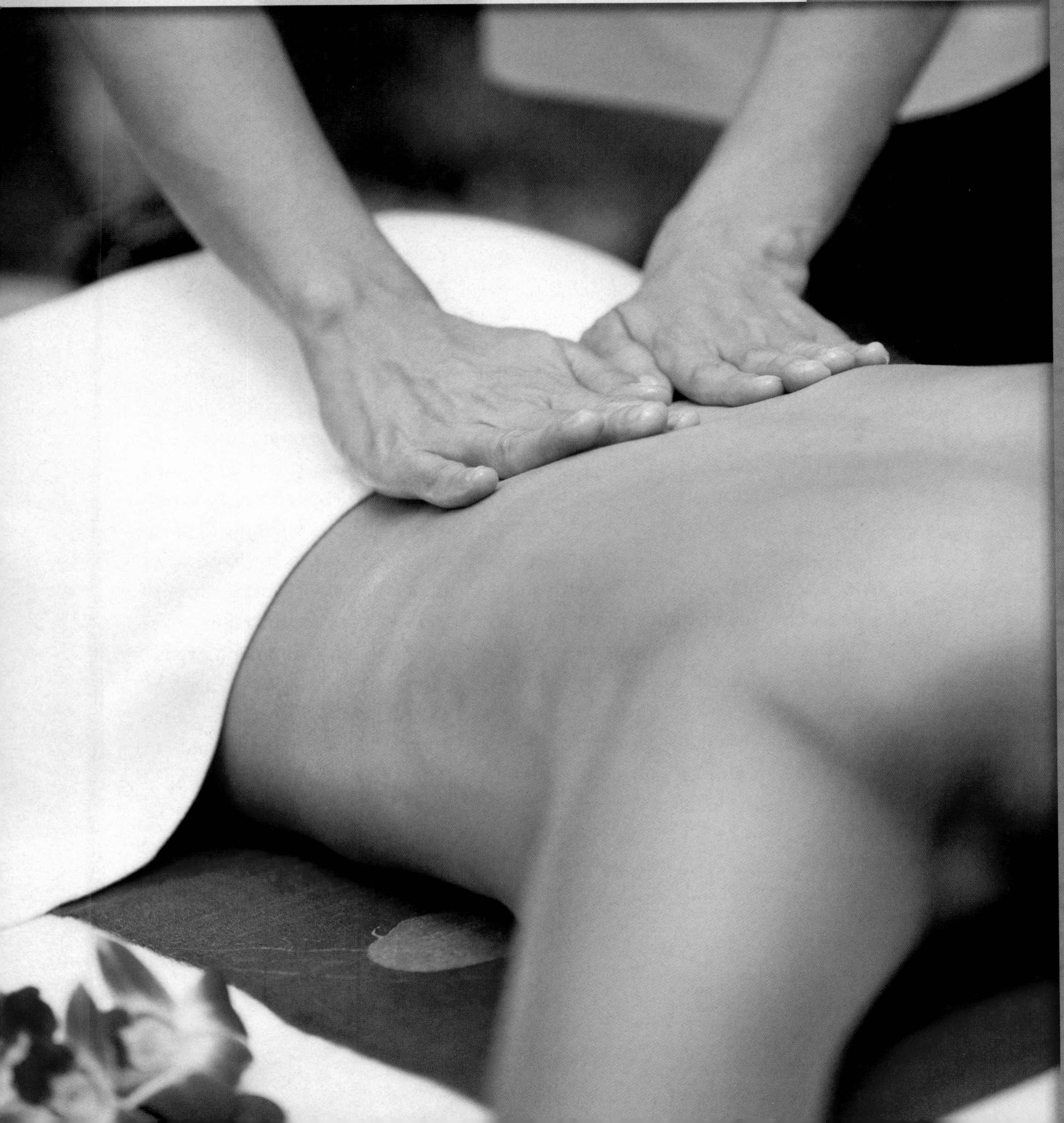

"I've failed over and over and over again in my life. And that is why I succeed."

Michael Jordan

If you pursue a career in the spa industry, you will no doubt encounter some challenges and maybe even a few setbacks, but this field is so filled with opportunities and possibilities that you will certainly find your place, as long as you remain persistent and positive. A spa career means different things to different people. For some, it may mean the security of a job at a large company, with health benefits and abundant prospects for camaraderie. For others, it may mean a chance to hone an entrepreneurial spirit, to build something new from the ground up and succeed with a thriving business of one's own. And for many, spa modalities are simply one more path to heal, to touch, and to connect with the people we call clients.

This section of the book will give you some guidance as you lift your head from your hands-on lessons and begin to look out toward the world of employment. Chapter 14 will help you as you prepare to seek your first spa job, giving practical advice regarding how to present yourself to prospective employers and create the best chances for a successful start. Once you have found a job, the learning and the growth will not suddenly stop. In fact, you may be faced with the greatest tests once you've already passed the hurdle of securing work. Chapter 15 shows you how to pass those tests by becoming the most valuable spa employee possible. One test you will likely encounter is when a spa director or owner calls upon you to sell products, even though it may not come naturally to you. Chapter 16 will help you feel comfortable with this necessary part of the spa industry. Many therapists dream of opening spas of their own one day, which is a big undertaking that will require much thought and the help of many other people. Chapter 17 will help you get thinking along the right track if you are considering this option yourself, and it will introduce you to some of the professionals who can be your helpers along the journey toward spa ownership. Once a therapist has made the leap to spa ownership, even if it is in a small one-room spa of her own, an entirely new set of responsibilities will be encountered, such as marketing, motivating employees, payroll, scheduling, and planning for expansion. Chapter 18 covers these topics and more.

CHAPTER 14

Finding Spa Work

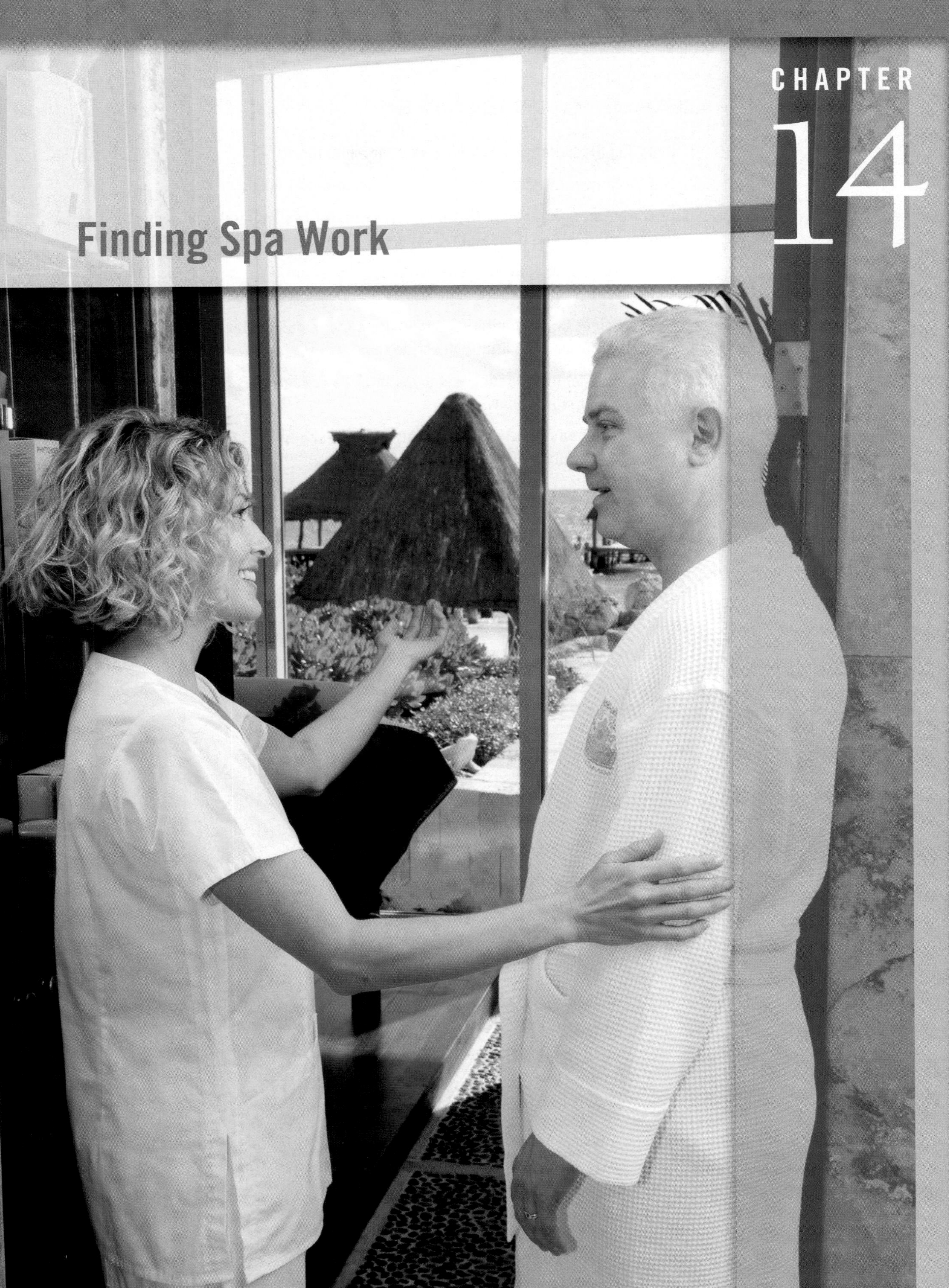

LEARNING OBJECTIVES

1. **Describe the benefits of working as a therapist for a spa.**
2. **List three key traits spas are looking for in potential employees.**
3. **Describe the main components of a successful résumé and name five ways to enhance the information on the résumé.**
4. **Describe the properties spa directors are looking for on résumés and "deal-breaker" items on résumés that may decrease the chance of being hired.**
5. **List the eight components involved with successfully filling out a spa employment application, and briefly describe them.**
6. **List four guidelines for successful spa interviews regardless of which staff member is doing the interview.**
7. **Explain the concept of Social Styles and how it applies to the personality of a massage therapist applying for a spa position.**
8. **Describe "interview massage" and provide four techniques for giving a successful massage as part of the interview process at a spa.**
9. **Define "provisionary employment" and give examples of the procedures involved at two spas.**
10. **Explain why lower wages for therapists (as compared to private practice) are necessary and beneficial in the spa.**
11. **List and explain three factors influencing therapist compensation in spas.**
12. **Explain the pros and cons of a *salaried spa therapist* position versus a *contracted labor* position.**

INTRODUCTION

When you walk out the door of massage school on that last day, along with thousands of other graduates across the continent, you will be searching for a way to put your newfound skills to work. Statistically, you stand a better chance of putting these skills to work in a spa than in any other workplace environment. According to *Massage Magazine*, spas hire more massage therapists than any other single industry—more than chiropractors, doctors, and private massage clinics. The spa industry, as discussed in Chapter 2, is large, employing tens of thousands of people, and a good percentage of those employees are massage therapists. In addition to all the positions that must be filled for the new spas that continue to open, many existing positions are left vacant each year by therapists who move on to other jobs or move up into management. Many spas are seasonal enterprises, with much heavier guest loads at certain times of the year, and they continually need new therapists to take the places of others who have left at the end of one season and do not return at the beginning of the next. This chapter focuses on how you can find your place in this large and growing industry.

SEEKING SPA EMPLOYMENT

Even though you are studying the spa industry and spa modalities, you still may secretly not be convinced that working in the spa industry is desirable. You may feel, as many therapists do, that starting your own private practice and including spa modalities is better than working for somebody else. Or you may be planning to open a spa of your own one day. In this case, Chapter 17 will cover the information you need in detail.

There are benefits to working for a larger spa as outlined in Table 14–1 (see Figure 14–1).

SPA TIP

Do not underestimate the benefits of working as an employee in a spa. Too many therapists judge spas solely on compensation levels compared to compensation in a private practice; 30 percent or 40 percent sounds like a bad deal versus 100 percent until you factor in all the hidden benefits (see Table 14–1).

WHAT EMPLOYERS ARE LOOKING FOR

While it is true that many spas are actively seeking massage therapists to hire, the pool of available therapists continues to grow, and as a result, competition to find and secure the best spa jobs can be intense. This does not mean that you cannot find a position, even if you are fresh out of school. You may encounter spas that prefer seasoned veterans with several years of practice and some advanced training; however, don't be discouraged if you do not have much or any relevant work history when seeking your first spa position.

SPA EMPLOYMENT BENEFIT	EXPLANATION
Proving Grounds	Spas provide a proving ground for your skills. Many bodies will pass beneath your fingers in a relatively short period of time while working in a spa. You'll "log" many bodies in the same way in which a pilot needs to log many hours in the air in order to reach expert status.
Low Barriers to Entry	Many spas are eager to hire therapists fresh out of school. They want to be able to mold the therapist's actions, attitudes, and skills according to their own practices. The barriers to entry in the industry are lower than in some clinical settings. You will not usually need to know advanced modalities, which may cost hundreds or thousands of dollars to learn.
Camaraderie	It can be lonely working as a private practitioner. Although many therapists dream of working alone in their own practice, when they achieve this goal, they often miss the camaraderie of working with other therapists.
Experience	Experience makes you a better boss if you one day run your own spa. There is no better way to grasp the unique challenges and typical complaints faced by spa owners than by working as a therapist in a spa. The biggest complaint against spa owners by therapists is that they do not understand the therapists' point of view. Working in a spa as a therapist before opening your own spa will eliminate this complaint.
Training	Spas often allow therapists the opportunity to learn new modalities at the spa's expense. Many spas cover the cost of training for therapists who demonstrate loyalty.
Automatic Clientele	New therapists tend to overlook the difficulties of finding new clients and building a thriving private practice, which can be time-consuming and challenging. Spa jobs offer an automatic clientele, leaving you free to focus on therapy.

TABLE 14–1 The Benefits of Working for a Spa.

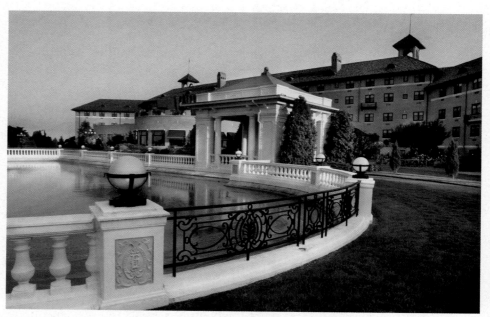

FIGURE 14–1 Many large hotels and resorts around the country, such as The Hotel Hershey in Hershey, Pennsylvania pictured here, feature spas and offer job opportunities with great benefits.

Spas will be looking for three key traits in all of the therapists they hire. These include:

1. **A positive attitude and pleasant appearance:** The law states that employers cannot discriminate on the basis of race, color, religion, political affiliation, national origin, disability, marital status, sex, or age, but you do have to realize that you will be judged by your appearance when you interview for a job. Employers will assume that the way you look during an interview will predict your appearance in the future. Show up for any application, interview, or testing looking your best. You do not have to be a movie star to work in a spa. However, spas are places people go in order to feel and look their best. If they are greeted by slovenly personnel with a negative attitude, they will probably go elsewhere. It is up to you to display a positive attitude and to look your best as you apply for spa jobs.
2. **A history of success/longevity in positions:** If you've never worked at a spa before, or even if you have never worked at any job before, your potential employers are still going to look for something in your history that signals success and longevity. Have you joined an organization or volunteered your time and stuck with that commitment over months or years? Have you built something of value, whether a business, an organization, or a family? Have you completed a course of study on your own, outside of school? Accomplishments such as these should be highlighted and documented on a résumé. This is one criteria your potential employer will use to determine whether to invite you for an interview.
3. **A well-put-together résumé:** The process of putting together your own résumé will help you reflect upon who you are and develop your

positive qualities more fully so that you can broadcast them loud and clear to potential employers. Your résumé is more than just a piece of paper. In a way, having a strong résumé is a way to boost your own confidence. Self-confidence is a crucial factor in getting the job you desire.

CREATING YOUR RÉSUMÉ

Spas owners, directors, and managers want to know who they are hiring, and one of the best ways to let them know who you are is by creating an informative résumé. Your résumé is a potent tool to let employers know who you are, what your attitude is, and what you are capable of. The main components of a résumé are objectives, experience, education, references, and skills (Figure 14–2). You can look upon the creation of your résumé as a way to elaborate upon and refine your self-definition as an employee. Putting time and care into the creation of a superior résumé may even emphasize those areas where you could use improvement, thus leading you to upgrade your abilities and improve your chances for future success. The following five suggestions will help you to enhance the information on your résumé.

Customize the Résumé

If possible, customize the résumé with information that will be particularly relevant to the specific spa where you are applying. It is not always necessary or appropriate to place the actual name of each spa where you apply on the résumé. However, there are other ways you can customize the information to the spa industry. For example, you can emphasize the fact that you learned retailing at a popular clothing outlet and then relate that experience to how it will help you sell products in the spa.

Call Yourself a Therapist

Call yourself a massage therapist, even if you have only recently graduated from school and have not truly begun your career yet. As long as you have a license or certificate to legally practice in your municipality, it is permissible to use this terminology.

Emphasize Your Strengths

Don't be afraid to "toot your own horn" and play up all of the positive qualities, useful experiences, and particular strengths you possess that could make you a more valuable employee. Dig into your past and be creative about where you've gained experience and knowledge. For example, you can showcase the strengths you've built up through healthy lifestyle choices, sports activities, hobbies, reading, and self-directed study.

Remember, when employers review your résumé, they are hoping to find a positive individual who will fulfill all their requirements. Fill your résumé with information that will make spa owners and spa directors curious to know more

Deborah Thompson
123 Main Street
Any Town, NY 12345

have a website set up that tells more about you

555.555.2008 home
555.333.2008 mobile
deborah@thomsonmassage.net
www.thomsonmassage.net

customize the résumé and name the specific place where you are applying if possible

Deborah Thomson, LMT, NCTMB

Objective

Challenging position as massage therapist treating varied clientele with excellent body therapies and supporting overall business success through retail sales in the Therapeutic Day Spa

Experience

2008–Present Self Employed Any Town, NY

Massage Therapist

Currently treating 8-10 clients per week in the greater Favoritown area.

Specialize in impeccable customer service.

Generate 15% of revenue through retail product sales to clientele.

call yourself a therapist, even if you've just begun

2006–2008 Bally Fitness Any Town, NY

Fitness Club Associate

Sold memberships

don't be afraid to "toot your own horn"

Assisted members with exercise routines

Responsible for safety of members in use of equipment and proper exercise techniques

mention customer service skills

2005–2006 The Gap Clothing Store Any Town, NY

Sales Associate

Trained with the major retail leaders in the Favoritown area to become proficient at customer service and sales techniques.

Responsible for opening and closing facility.

Extensive cash register and computer use.

2003–2004 Interact Club Any Town, NY

Head of Planning Committee

Organized charity events to benefit the homeless and women's shelter system of Favoritown, New York

Education

2007 Favoritown School of Massage Any Town NY

Certificate in Therapeutic Massage

Advanced trainings in Thai Massage, CranioSacral Technique

stress skills applicable to your new position

2004–2006 Favoritown Community College Any Town, NY

A.A., Business Administration

Graduated with honors.

choose references wisely

References

- John Smith [past employer], Anytown, Vermont (323) 288-1234
- Alicia Great [college professor], Somewhere, New York (212)123-4567

Avocations/Skills

- Nationally Certified in Massage & Bodywork
- Sculpting, Art, Weight Lifting, Tennis, Reading
- Fluent in Spanish.

show strengths through life-style choices

FIGURE 14–2 Your résumé is a potent tool to let employers know who you are.

about you. Then, if you are hired, follow up all that positive information with on-the-job reality. Live up to the image you have created for yourself.

Emphasize Customer-Service Skills

A massage therapist's customer-service skills are a crucial factor in the hiring decisions of most spa directors and owners (see Chapter 15 for more information about customer service). They look at you and at your résumé, and they think to themselves, "Does this person have the skills and background to give my customers the level of service they expect? If not, can he or she be trained?" Take every opportunity in your résumé to highlight any customer-service experience you may have.

If you don't yet have any experience in customer service, consider getting some. Before you graduate from your spa program or immediately afterward, work for a time in a restaurant, hotel, or resort—as a busboy, waiter, hostess, or desk clerk—and focus on building your customer service abilities while there.

Choose References Wisely

While it may be more comfortable to list your mother or your best friend as a reference, spas will place more weight behind a reference from a massage instructor, college professor, a well-known person in the community, or a spa industry professional. If possible, choose a reference from a past job experience. Future employers are going to be interested in speaking with past employers whether they are listed as references or not, so it is a good idea to list them here, showing a willingness to have the spa contact people for whom you have worked in the past.

Did You Know?

Spa Directors Speak

When asked what they were looking for on therapists' résumés, a panel of spa directors from top properties said there were four minimum requirements:

- correct spelling
- full dates for all employment and education
- full disclosure of past history, including different jobs held with each employer
- massage school attended

The spa directors also pointed out four "deal-breakers" on résumés that greatly lessened the chances of a therapist getting hired:

- "job junkies" who jump from one job to the next without demonstrating loyalty or stability
- a history of multiple past injuries that would hamper ability to perform massage
- attendance at a poorly run or unaccredited massage school
- leaving prior jobs because of poor relationships with management

Note: Data gathered at East West College's spa directors symposium in Portland, Oregon.

Always check with people beforehand to make sure they are willing to provide a reference for you. Pick these people carefully. The most common references are past employers, teachers, and family friends. If you have not held any other jobs previously, it is perfectly acceptable to provide **character references**. Later, you will have professional references who can attest to your performance on the job.

character references

people used as references on jobs applications (usually family and friends) who cannot attest to job performance but can vouch for attitudes and qualities such as "responsibility" and "maturity"

Keep in mind that past employers are often constrained by law from saying anything other than, "I can only confirm that [massage therapist name] worked here from [begin date] to [end date]." That's it. So, by including a previous supervisor or boss as a personal reference that includes private contact information, you will allow that person to speak on your behalf without constraint.

SPA EMPLOYMENT APPLICATIONS

The prospect of filling out employment applications as you seek your first spa job may not fill you with enthusiasm and joy. However, there is no need to turn this necessary process into a stressful one. At first, an employment application may seem complicated, but once you have created your résumé, you will already have most, if not all, of the information necessary to complete this or any other application you will encounter. At larger destination spas, resort spas, or at day spas with several locations, you may have to fill out your application in the **human resources** department. At smaller spas, you will deal directly with management. Regardless of to whom you turn over your application, you should adhere to the following guidelines while actually filling it out.

human resources

in larger spas, a separate department in charge of recruiting and hiring new personnel and overseeing the employment application processes

Arrive Prepared with Everything You Need

When you head out to complete spa applications, make sure to bring these key items: your résumé, social security card, driver's license, massage license, names and addresses of previous employers, starting and ending dates at previous jobs, and pay for each job. Having too much information is better than not having enough.

Follow the Instructions on the Application Carefully

Each employer is different. Although application forms may appear boringly similar to you, if you read between the lines, you may discover certain points that are important to the particular spa where you are applying. For example, if the application asks you for the name of a massage school teacher or administrator who may be contacted, you will know that education is a high priority at that spa. You can therefore stress the high quality of your own massage school experience.

Be Neat and Thorough

If you display messiness and a lack of organization on the job application, employers will assume you will display the same qualities on the job. Consider bringing an erasable pen to fill out the application or some correction fluid/tape to fix any mistakes. Spas want the same information from all of their applicants, so make sure not to leave any blanks on the application. If certain questions do not apply to you, write "not applicable" or "n/a" in the space provided. Do not write "see résumé."

Provide Plentiful Information

Just as you do with your résumé, you want the information you provide to create the biggest positive impact possible on the spa where you are applying. When you are provided blank lines to write in more information, use them. Let the spa know about any awards, experiences, schooling, volunteer work, plus any general skills and qualities that will make you an especially good choice and set you apart from other applicants.

Be Truthful but Not Negative

Always provide truthful information on the application. Although most spas will not go to the trouble of checking every fact, just one falsehood could lead to dismissal when it is discovered, even if that happens months after you've been hired. At the same time, however, you do not want to dwell on negative information. If you have been "downsized" out of a past job, for instance, try to be as positive as possible, leaving a longer explanation as to why the job ended.

Do Not Mention Specific Salary Requirements

In most negotiations, it is said, the first person to mention a number loses. Let the spa tell you what they are willing to pay for the therapist position. Employers often use this question to screen out inappropriate applicants, and you can be eliminated from consideration if you give the wrong answer. If the application asks you to quote your "salary requirements" or "expected pay level," it is better to put "open" or "negotiable" in the blank and let them tell you what the pay scale is like at their spa.

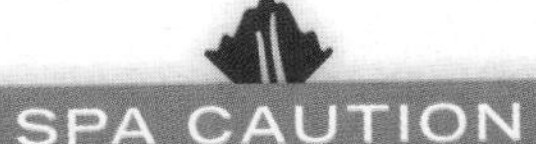

SPA CAUTION

An exclusive day spa in Los Angles was hit with a lawsuit after one of their male therapists confessed to sexually molesting a female guest. The guest was paraplegic. The therapist had excellent references that included work at a Ritz-Carlton spa. In spite of this, and in spite of the fact that the day spa checked these references thoroughly, doing everything possible to hire a good, upstanding therapist and train him appropriately, they were faced with staggering court costs and the possible closing of their business. Due to occurrences such as this, you can expect to have your references and past employment history thoroughly checked. Therefore, it is in your best interest to have all your paperwork in order. If possible, obtain letters from previous employers and clients to use as part of the application process if necessary.

Check Your Application Before Turning It In

After completing the application, go back over it slowly and carefully, scanning for any errors, misspellings, or other mistakes. Make it as neat and complete as possible. You will be judged partially on how the document looks as well as what it contains. Also, check to make sure that the information you've provided is the same as that on your résumé. Inconsistencies will raise eyebrows and perhaps trigger questions that could lead to your not being hired.

INTERVIEWS

Going out on a job interview for a massage therapist position can be especially nerve-racking. You will be judged not only on your past history, your education, your attitude, and your knowledge, but also on something much more personal than most job applicants have to worry about—your touch. If you have just recently graduated from school and your massage skills are still untested, the prospect of being judged like this can be daunting. This section will help guide you through the process of successfully interviewing for the position of spa therapist.

At smaller spas, you will probably interview with the spa manager, director, or owner. Some larger spas require applicants to speak with several different people, on different days, and a few even require a **staff review** during which new therapists are interviewed by the therapists already on staff to make sure they are a good fit for the team. Regardless of which person you are speaking with, keep the following guidelines in mind.

staff review

process by which potential new therapists at a spa are interviewed by the therapists already on staff to make sure they are a good fit for the team

Be Flexible

One of the first questions many spa interviewers will ask is, "How flexible is your schedule?" They want to know if you have many other obligations that would keep you from working at peak operational hours. Be prepared to be as flexible as possible with your hours. Spas require some unconventional working hours of their therapists, especially weekends and early evenings, when massage and spa treatments are most popular. If you have certain commitments that make it impossible to work at certain times, try to show flexibility in other ways. For instance, you could say, "I usually pick up my son at day care around 5:00 p.m., but the school has extended after-school care until 7:30 p.m., and I would be happy to stay until 7:00 on those nights you need me."

Part-time employees do not need to be quite as flexible, but remember that peak hours (late afternoons, early evenings, and weekends) are usually when the most part-time employees are called upon to work. If you do not have any of these hours available, it may be harder to secure a position.

Speak Up

You are your own best advocate when it comes to getting that job you dream of. Sometimes, you will be your only advocate. It is up to you to speak up for yourself in the interview. Even if your hands-on skills are impeccable and you have a résumé that speaks for itself, there will still come a time during the job-getting process when spoken words are absolutely necessary. You're going to need to talk. If you are shy or uncomfortable when it comes to speaking with others in formal situations, keep these few tips in mind:

Slow down: Many therapists get nervous and rush through the interview process. They feel what they have to say is not that important and so they gloss over their observations, rushing through sentences to finish the interview as quickly as possible. This may lead the interviewer to conclude that the therapist does not truly wish to be offered the position. Take your time.

Be concise: On the other end of the spectrum are those therapists who tend to use a chatty, talkative tone in an interview. When you are asked a question, provide a thorough answer, but then finish your statement after making it. Do not digress too far from the point you are making, and don't ramble.

Be confident but humble: Do not brag about being a great therapist, but do not shy away from plainly stating a healthy belief in your own talents and skills. Employers want to know that you are a great believer in your own abilities as a therapist. This will come across in just a few confident words.

Be Prepared to Answer Questions

You will definitely be peppered with questions from your interviewers, and it is best to be prepared by knowing the general type and tone of question before they are asked. The following are examples of questions asked by an assortment of spa directors from top resort spas and day spas:

1. "Can you give me an example of an unhappy guest and how you would turn the situation around?"
2. "Give me an example of what you've done to encourage teamwork in your previous jobs."
3. "How would you deal with a guest who exhibits sexually inappropriate behavior?"
4. "Can you give me an instance of something you felt was unfair in your past work life or personal life?"
5. "How much do you know about our facility, and why do you want to work for this spa in particular?" (Directors and owners in particular want their therapists to be raving fans of the spa, and they only want to hire therapists who really want to be part of the team.)
6. "Why did you get into massage?"
7. "What do you enjoy most about giving massage?"

Watch Out for Negativity

You may have noticed that a couple of the questions listed above are actually traps that can lead you into speaking negatively. Number four in particular may lead you in that direction. Spa directors use such questions purposefully in order to weed out those therapists who are prone to complaining and putting blame on other people. Try to be aware of this type of question, and avoid slipping into negativity whenever possible. Also, during the interview, watch yourself and be wary of using specific "deal-breaker" words and phrases that spa directors have noted often in negative therapists (see the Deal-Breaker Words sidebar).

Deal-Breaker Words

Did You Know?

Spa directors have noted that the following words and phrases heard during the interview processes denote a possible negative attitude on the part of potential new employees. Known as "deal-breakers," they send up immediate red flags that could halt the interview in its tracks. Some of them include:

"Backstabbing" – When this word is uttered about past employers or co-workers, it often turns out to be true of the therapist/interviewee.

"Unfair" – This word usually signals a victim mentality in the therapist/interviewee and is often used by people who do not take responsibility for their own feelings and experiences.

"In my last spa . . ." – Therapist/interviewees who constantly refer to a former employer may be looking into the past too much and feel that the way things were done at their previous place of employment is the only way they can be done, thus making it harder to learn in a new job environment.

"It would be so relaxing to work here." – Saying something like this shows that the potential therapist/interviewee does not have a true appreciation for the amount of work required in spas.

Remember: While avoiding these deal-breaker words may improve your chances at making a positive impression, you will need to present a positive attitude and actions, not just words, in order to find and keep the best spa jobs.

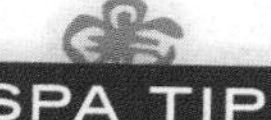

SPA TIP

Your entire background, education, attitude, and skill set will come into play when you apply for a spa position, and people in different positions within the spa each have a distinct set of qualities they're looking for in the massage therapists they interview. Keep this in mind and you'll fare better when you're face-to-face with those who have the power to hire you. Following along with the information in Table 14–2 will help you understand each person's point of view and what in particular they are looking for from an interviewee, giving you a better of idea of which of your qualities to stress.

Of course, you should stress these traits not only during the interview but also once you are employed, honestly striving to uphold your end of the bargain in exchange for being given a chance at employment.

THE PERSON IN AUTHORITY...	IS LOOKING FOR THIS IN PARTICULAR, SO...	YOU SHOULD STRESS...
Spa Owner	loyalty	that you are honestly looking for a stable position and plan on dedicating yourself to your job at the spa
Spa Director	responsibility/reliability	that you will be on time, be familiar with required conduct, and never give reason for disciplinary action
Spa Manager	ability to work with others	that you are a team player who believes in pulling your weight and making life easier for co-workers
Human Resources Manager	willingness to adhere to company policy	that you are aware that massage therapists working in a spa environment need to understand the company's overall hierarchy, chain of command, proper procedures, and mission

TABLE 14–2 Traits Prized in Massage Therapists by Different Interviewers.

PERSONALITY TESTING FOR SPA THERAPISTS

You should be aware that you may be given a "personality test" to determine whether you are a good candidate to work in a particular spa. This is not a test to measure your ability in massage therapy or any other task you may need to perform while on the job. Rather, it is a test to find out whether your basic personality traits will be a good fit for the spa's **corporate culture**.

corporate culture

the shared values, traditions, customs, philosophy, and policies of a corporation; also, the professional atmosphere that grows from this and affects behavior and performance

You cannot cheat on these tests. Although you may be tempted to check the boxes you think the spa wants you to check, these tests are devised in such a way that you will most likely not be able to figure out what your answers ultimately mean, and it is therefore difficult if not impossible to craft a response that will make you look like a better candidate for the job. It is best just to answer honestly, following your intuition when replying. The test is meant to give employers insight into your basic "type," allowing them to determine if your presence on board their team will hinder or enhance the spa's overall success. Several companies administer these tests, and each has its own take on what makes a person a better choice to hire. In essence, they seek to categorize people so that spas can understand them in order to better use their innate strengths while minimizing the adverse impact of their weaknesses.

The Five-Factor Model of Personality as taught at the Center for Applied Cognitive Studies, for example, focuses on the following attributes: need for stability, extraversion, originality, accommodation, and consolidation. The Keirsey Temperament Sorter offers four basic personality types: *artisans, guardians, idealists*, and *rationalists*. The most widely used traditional personality profile test is the Myers Briggs Type Indicator® Career Assessment Test (MBTI®). Personality profiling tests such as these are used by a few spas, but the one that has turned out to be the most widely applicable to the spa industry in general has been the **Social Styles** model that was developed by David W. Merrill and Roger H. Reid. This model consists of four primary archetypes—*analytical, amiable, driver*, and *expressive*—as seen in Table 14–3. The traits of the "amiable" type have been modified slightly here to more accurately reflect the specific strengths and weaknesses of massage therapists in the spa setting.

Social Styles

a personality profiling model that was developed by David W. Merrill and Roger H. Reid, consisting of four primary archetypes—*analytical, amiable, driver*, and *expressive*—that many spas use to categorize potential employees

Massage therapists, not surprisingly, tend to fall squarely under the "amiable" personality type, with all of the good and all of the bad that comes with that category. Spa directors, managers, and supervisors constantly have to

PERSONALITY TYPE	POSITIVE TRAITS	NEGATIVE TRAITS
Analytical	precise, methodical, organized, rational, detail-oriented	critical, formal, uncertain, judgmental, picky
Amiable (massage therapists)	cooperative, compassionate, warm, listener, negotiator	undisciplined, independent, rebellious, overly creative
Expressive	enthusiastic, persuasive, outgoing, positive, communicator	ego-centered, emotional, exploitive, opinionated
Driver	persistent, independent, decision-maker, effective, strong-willed	overly aggressive, strict, intense, relentless, rigid

TABLE 14–3 Social Styles Personality Types.

keep reminding therapists to be more disciplined, proactive, and self-directed, while at the same time becoming just a little bit more of a team player and less independent.

Tips for Cultivating Your Positive Social Styles for Job Interviews

You can use this knowledge to your advantage as you approach spas for a job. The people who are hiring will already know that you probably fall into the "amiable" category and will be on the lookout for the weaknesses that come with this Social Style. Starting right now during your schooling, if you can begin to cultivate the positive traits of the amiable style while weeding out some of the negative aspects, you'll be on your way toward creating better chances at successful job interviews and subsequent employment. You can accomplish this by taking a look at some of the positive traits of the other Social Styles and beginning to cultivate those yourself, even if at first it does not seem natural (see "Practice Cultivating Your Positive Social Styles for Job Interviews" activity).

Your Analytical Side

Your analytical side is precise, methodical, organized, rational, and detail-oriented. To reveal these aspects of your personality during the interview, you can say, "I plan on being successful in my spa career by carefully analyzing situations I run into and making well-thought-out decisions. I will approach problems logically, and I will follow the appropriate procedures to help the spa run smoothly."

Your Expressive Side

Your expressive side is persuasive, outgoing, positive, and communicative. To reveal these aspects of your personality during the interview, you can say, "I understand that every interaction in the spa should be focused on customer service, and that we should concentrate on sales because what spas sell is health and well-being. Your spa guests need this, and this is what they come to you for. I look forward to helping you increase sales and customer satisfaction in any way possible."

Your Driver Side

Your driver side is persistent, independent, decisive, effective, and strong-willed. To reveal these aspects of your personality during the interview, you can say, "As a member of your spa team, I will seek out innovative solutions to any problems that I am faced with regarding customer service, spa operations, sales, or anything else. I will always focus on maximizing profitability for your business. Regardless of the task or challenge, I will try to establish standards of excellence to guide myself by in order to help you grow your business and achieve the spa's ultimate goals."

Your Negative Amiable Side

The negative side of the typical amiable personality is perhaps the most bothersome aspect of massage therapists for most spa directors. This is the undisciplined, independent, rebellious, and overly creative side. To downplay these characteristics during the interview, you can say, "Although I value the creative healing nature of my work as a massage therapist, I also understand the realities of business and the need for professionalism at all times. As an employee of your spa, I will never let my own independent nature and artistic vision supersede your need to maintain a disciplined team that offers a consistent standard of service over time. My goal is to help you maintain the best spa possible by fulfilling your goals and visions for the business."

Of course, once these words have been spoken in a job interview, you have to follow them up with on-the-job performance, as already mentioned. By striving to become a more well-rounded individual who prizes the many diverse qualities of your own personality, you will become a more valuable spa employee.

ACTIVITY

Practice Cultivating Your Positive Social Styles for Job Interviews

Spa owners, directors, and managers appreciate therapists who are able to rise above their own limitations and display some of the positive characteristics of differing personality types. When they interview you as a prospective new therapist for their staffs, they are hoping beyond hope that you will be someone who breaks the stereotypical mold of the "amiable" therapist to become a high-quality all-around employee. You can help make it easy for them to choose you as their next employee by revealing the analytical, expressive, and driver sides of your personality. We all have these aspects in our personalities to some degree, but in massage therapists they are often undervalued and thus not cultivated.

Practice exchanging job interviews with classmates, and see if you can discover your hidden strengths by emphasizing some of your own positive social styles.

THE INTERVIEW MASSAGE

Therapists who apply for positions at spas are usually called upon to give at least one full massage session to somebody on staff to test the quality of the massage and determine if the style is compatible with the spa's overall bodywork methods. This step in the interview process is called the **interview massage**. The interview massage recipient on staff at the spa has to be in a critiquing mode in order to hire the best staff for the business, which makes it difficult to simply relax and enjoy the massage. Tension is inherent in this situation, as the applicant tries his best to relax someone who is being critical and cannot relax. You can adhere to the following guidelines in order to make this paradoxical and sometimes difficult experience as painless as possible and help you secure the job you are seeking.

interview massage
massage given to staff personnel to determine eligibility for employment as judged by hands-on techniques, customer-service skills, and other qualities

Tips for Giving an Interview Massage

- Forget that it's an interview massage, if at all possible.
- Remember all the basics—wash your hands beforehand, use proper draping, inquire about sore areas or physical problems, respect boundaries, be polite.

- Dress similarly to the therapists who work at the establishment where you're applying.
- Give an entire massage, if it's requested. Do not say, "Well, it's been five minutes. You must know if you like me by now. Do I have the job or not?"
- Use conversation sparingly. After the first couple minutes, only respond to the interviewer's remarks instead of initiating exchanges.
- Only give an interview massage if you're already confident and comfortable with your technique. This is not a time for practice.
- At the end of the massage, step quietly out of the room and wait. Do not ask how you did.
- When you say good-bye, shake hands firmly. Looking your interviewer straight in the eye, smile, and say, "Thank you for this opportunity."
- Remember that if this the first interview massage you've given, the next one will be much easier.

Therapists can overcome some of the anxiety that attends these interview massages by practicing on as many people as possible before applying for the position, ideally with several of these practice treatments given back-to-back, as this is the way in which many spas are now conducting interview massages. In order to simulate the real-world conditions of a spa, applicants are often asked to give two or three massages in a row to see how well they hold up under the pressure and the strain.

It must be remembered that the interview massage is not just about massage. Applicants are also being screened for certain invisible—yet still crucial—attributes which can make or break a therapist's chances at getting a

SPA CAUTION

Interview Massage Disasters

A spa manager who has received over 100 interview massages from job applicants offers some words of advice for you when you head out to give your own interview massages. "I've encountered some unbelievable situations," he comments. "I can't believe that applicants continue to make the same basic mistakes. If you watch out for these problems yourself when performing an interview massage, you'll at least avoid the most common disasters and give yourself a better chance at getting the job. The following all really happened to me when receiving interview massages.

- One man who gave me an interview massage kept banging my own hand into my head really hard over and over again while I was supine and he was working on my triceps with my arm raised up over my head. When I asked him to stop, he kept doing it!
- One man was sweating so profusely during his interview massage that he got my body all slicked up with his own moisture. If this is a problem for you, I suggest wearing an undershirt and using a heavy-duty antiperspirant.
- Suggesting that the client take a few deep breaths during massage is fine, but one woman had me breathing so deeply and so intensely during an interview massage that I almost passed out from hyperventilation.
- During one interview massage, a woman intoned some Polynesian-sounding prayers over my body before beginning the session, and then proceeded to "clear the room" of negative energies with a bundle of dried sage that she took from her bag and swept about the room in large sweeping movements. Afterwards, out came the chakra stones. These personal touches to a massage treatment are fine in private practice or during specific exotic treatments at the spa, but what owners and managers are looking for during an interview massage is a straightforward display of the therapist's skills. Save the creative flourishes for the appropriate time.
- Once an applicant came to give an interview massage immediately after eating a big plate of Mexican food featuring plenty of beans (he admitted this to me afterwards). The flatulence that ensued during the massage was embarrassing for both of us."

job. Although newly graduated therapists are rightfully proud of their technical skills, it is not massage talent alone that can get them that coveted position at an exciting spa, but rather character, personality, presence, and attitude.

SPA TIP

How to Get Hired at Any Spa

If you are one of those people who have become fixated on working at a certain spa and refuse to take no for an answer, try this suggestion: Become a locker-room attendant or spa attendant first. Swallow your pride and agree to begin work at a lower-paying job in the spa of your dreams. Some of the best spas are staffed by therapists with long experience and advanced training. Spend time with them. Learn all the operating procedures of the spa. Be as helpful as you possibly can. If you continue to hone your therapeutic skills at the same time, chances are good that you will eventually be asked to join the ranks of the therapists there. Sometimes, the best jobs need to be earned.

WHAT HAPPENS AFTER THE INTERVIEW

After you turn in your application, go through one or more interviews, and give an interview massage, the hiring decision is then left up to the spa. It is best for you to concentrate on other matters after that, as you have no way of improving your chances at getting hired once the interview process is finished. During the period immediately after the interview, the spa will quite likely run a background check on you, contact references, and speak with previous employers when possible. Afterward, the spa's decision makers will discuss the plusses and minuses of taking you on as a team member. You may be hired. Or you may not.

If you are not hired, this does not necessarily point to some fault or deficiency on your part. The spa may be going through their slow season. They may be looking for someone with more experience—or less experience. They may want to hire female therapists only at this time, and if you are a male, there is nothing you can do to help your chances. Do not take it personally if you are not hired. Simply continue to improve your skills, hone your customer service knowledge, and increase your relevant experience as you seek employment elsewhere.

PROBATIONARY PERIODS

If you are hired at a spa, you may have to undergo a **provisionary employment** period during which the spa can terminate the employment at any time. This may seem unreasonable to you, but spas have found through hard experience that some therapists who look good during the interview process turn out to be deficient employees. These probationary periods range from a few days to a few months. During this time, it is of course advisable to be on your best behavior and to focus diligently on learning all the policies and procedures of the spa. Each spa has its own version of this provisionary period, and it is often not as stressful as it sounds. For example, some therapists are treated to spa services to familiarize them with the spa's procedures. The following are comments from spa directors at top properties regarding their procedures immediately after hiring therapists:

provisionary employment

period immediately after hiring during which the spa monitors performance and can terminate the therapist's employment at will with no need for an explanation

- "We go over all of our protocols, procedures, and employee guidelines. Then we spend time training therapists in safety and health, specifically regarding bloodborne pathogens and AIDS awareness."
- "We give our new hires the employee handbook, then give them a set period of time in which to study it and become familiar with all aspects of their responsibility in the spa. Then we give them a 'Spa Q' test, and depending on the results we keep them on or suggest they seek employment elsewhere."
- "The first 21 days of employment is known as *certification training* for our therapists. If they can achieve the level of knowledge and skill necessary for us to certify them, they get to keep their job."

SPA CAUTION

The first day on any job can be an intimidating experience, but the first day at your first spa job can be particularly daunting. You will not only be faced with a new boss and new co-workers, but also a whole lineup of new customers, each one of whom you sincerely want to impress. Your hands-on skills as well as your personality and your customer-service abilities will be put to the test many times over on that first day. It can be a taxing experience. How you handle it will set the stage for the rest of your tenure at the spa.

One piece of advice: Do not judge yourself too harshly on this first day. Many spa owners and directors will go out of their way to make your first impressions positive ones on this first day because they know how challenging it can be. Let them take care of you. Relax into the position, focusing on what you do best, one person at a time. If you make any mistakes or commit a faux pas with a guest, quickly forgive yourself. For at least this one day, after all the work you've done in school and in preparing for the job, you've earned the right to go easy on yourself. So go easy.

- "We simply spend time talking about the flow of massage, and we have therapists spend time with supervisors, their fellow therapists, and other employees. It's low-pressure."
- "We have instituted a 'buddy system' for the initial phase of employment during which new therapists shadow a current employee in order to learn proper procedures."
- "Our spa offers new employees hours of classroom training, and then we have them give three test services on long-term employees to determine whether they've reached the appropriate skill level."
- "Our new therapists receive a spa treatment first thing. Their very first day on the job should be as low-stress as possible in order to imprint positive memories and associations about the spa in the new employee's mind. They should receive at least one service that day, preferably more."
- "Our new hires get to stay at the resort one night to see what it feels like for the guests."

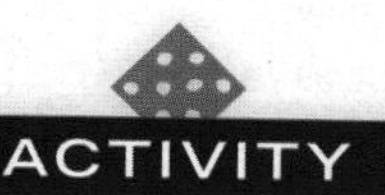

ACTIVITY

Your Ideal Spa Job

Write down the answers to the questions in the Finding the Right Spa section. Then, fashion all the details into a one-page narrative about the ideal spa in which you hope to work (or which you hope to own) one day. This exercise will enable you to recognize your ideal spa job when it comes along and help you weed out those jobs that are not so ideal.

FINDING THE RIGHT SPA

Numerous types of spas offer job possibilities for a wide range of therapists with diverse skill sets and personality types. How will you know where to look and how to determine in which type of spa you are best suited to work? There are several questions you should ask yourself when you first start your search for a spa position, including:

- What is the spa's ambience? What type of spa is it? Medical? Resort? Weight-loss? Esthetic?
- Is the spa seasonal, busier one time of the year and slower another?
- What are the spa's staffing needs (part-time/full-time/on-call)?
- What, if any, benefits are offered to therapists at this spa?
- Does the spa follow a seniority system regarding pay, benefits, promotions, and scheduling? If so, how long have senior therapists already been there, and what are my chances to advance?
- What compensation model does the spa follow? Commission? Straight salary?
- Is this spa a good fit for my own personality and massage style?

amenity spa

located within a larger resort setting that caters to guests on vacation and business travel, these spas are often looked upon as secondary to the guest experience and are therefore not expected to make much profit or offer superlative therapies

Spa Ambience

You will want to consider which type of spa is most suitable for your level of massage skill, your personal preferences, and your ultimate goals (Table 14–4). Some therapists are more comfortable in a clinical spa setting, while others prefer the

TYPE OF SPA	REASONS FOR SEEKING EMPLOYMENT
Medical Spa	The medical spa setting is ideal for those therapists who want to work with doctors, move into the medical field, and perhaps eventually become a physical therapist, chiropractor, or physician. Therapists in this setting may be exposed to invasive procedures and should be comfortable around needles, prescription medications, and medical terminology. Therapists are sometimes called upon to add their expertise to the overall treatment of patients' conditions, so advanced "medical massage" training may be necessary.
Club Spa	The club spa environment is fitness-focused and part of a larger business geared toward exercise. Therapists who work in this environment are usually physically fit themselves, as this gives them firsthand knowledge of the conditions presented by the clients. They are often versed in the specifics of sports massage because so many of the clients need work tailored to performance, flexibility, and strength.
Salon Spa	The salon environment is often social and relaxed. At times, in fact, it is too relaxed for many therapists, who prefer a more tranquil and focused atmosphere in which to practice. Salon Spas can be chatty places, and the salon aspect of the business often overshadows the spa aspect. Therapists who work in salon spas should be comfortable with this sociable aspect of the job and be willing to promote their own offerings to the salon's customers.
Day Spa	Many different types of spas could be categorized as day spas, but the pure version is one that is dedicated first and foremost to providing spa services to the guest rather than offering these treatments as an adjunct to salon services, fitness options, and so on. Therapists who work in a true day spa need to be serious about the industry and actively involve themselves with the clientele. Loyal repeat clients are the mainstay of day spas, and it is up to the therapist to consistently keep these clients satisfied. This builds success for the individual therapist as well. In day spas, therapists who are requested the most by repeat clients make the most money.
Urban Spa	Urban spas have a distinctively modern feeling, with sleek furniture and design, set in a big city downtown area. They are usually housed in larger buildings or lofts. Therapists who work in urban spas should be comfortable with modern fashion trends and be willing to project a chic, trendy image as well as offer good therapy.
Retreat Spa	Retreat spas often have a greater educational purpose, such as yoga programs, wilderness trekking, spiritual or meditative disciplines, and more. Therapists who work at these spas need to be comfortable living in rural areas and working closely with guests as they experience the transformational programs offered at the retreat spa.
Destination Spa	Destination spas are dedicated solely to the spa experience, so they bring focused and dedicated clientele, but this clientele is transitory. It is difficult, therefore, to develop a rapport with the guests unless they become repeat visitors. Therapists who work at destination spas should be comfortable supporting guests' overall goals at the destination spa, which usually include increased well-being, weight loss, improved diet, detoxification, and physical fitness.
Hot Springs Spa	Hot springs spas are built directly on the site of natural hot waters fed from underground springs. Therapists who work in these spas should be especially conversant in the effects, benefits, and contraindications of hydrotherapy in general and its thermal effects in particular.
Resort Spa	Resort spas are located inside the larger confines of a resort environment, often in large hotels in vacation areas. Spa guests at these resorts are usually on vacation, and they may look upon the spa as an **amenity spa** rather than a crucial part of their experience. Therapists who work at these spas should be comfortable as part of a larger team of employees at a big company, and they should be willing to support the guests in their quest for relaxation and escape from everyday stress.
Cruise Ship Spa	Every cruise ship has some form of spa on board, many of them as elaborate as those found on land. The clientele is transitory, of course, and the cruise lines have strict rules that keep therapists from socializing with passengers. Therapists who work in cruise ship spas need to be comfortable in the regimented environment on board and be prepared to work several hours a day straight through in sometimes cramped quarters. They also need to be willing to sell the spa's branded products and maintain professional customer-service standards. Perks include extensive travel and low expenses.

TABLE 14–4 Types of Spas and Reasons for Working in Them.

more relaxed atmosphere of a resort. High-quality massage work is performed in all spa environments, but the modalities, the mood of the clientele, and the general ambience are often quite different.

At times, you may need to compromise when it comes to choosing the type of spa in which to work. You may have to take a spa job that is available and convenient, rather than ideal. However, chances are good that you will find more than one option because of the large and growing number of spas. Remember, if you concentrate on developing and improving those skills that make you attractive to spa employers (see the next two chapters for information on those skills), you will create more job options for yourself and have more spas to choose from.

Seasonality Concerns

seasonality

the tendency for a business to be more popular in certain times of the year than others, which especially affects spas in summer resort and winter resort areas

Many spas are extremely affected by the **seasonality** of their respective locations. Therefore, it is important to time your application with the upswing in business that accompanies the beginning of the busy season for the spa. For example, the best time to apply at a spa at a beach resort that is fully booked all summer is in April and May as the spa is trying to fill all the therapist positions it needs. Likewise, the best time to apply at a ski resort is in October and November. Some spas transcend the seasonality factor of their location and build a strong year-round clientele, but they are still usually looking for more employees during their traditional busy season.

Staffing Needs

on-call therapist

a contracted worker (usually receiving no benefits) who is not guaranteed a particular number of work hours per week but rather called only when the spa is busy and in need of extra therapists

Most spas where you apply will have specific staffing structures in place and expect you to fit into them. If you cannot work full-time, but that is the only option available at the spa, no amount of skill or enthusiasm on your part will make you a more attractive employee. Many spas offer the option of becoming an **on-call therapist**. This gives you much greater flexibility in scheduling your hours, but it diminishes some of the benefits such as insurance and job security. You should know beforehand what your needs and desires are regarding part-time, full-time, or on-call work and be up-front about them with the spa. This should be the first item you discuss with prospective employers, as it can be a waste of time to determine your eligibility for the job only to find that you cannot satisfy the spa's staffing needs.

Benefits

For some people, receiving employment benefits such as insurance, child care, and 401K plans is an extremely important consideration. It is, of course, expensive for spas to offer these benefits to their employees, and so they usually reserve the benefits for full-time personnel. Some spas only offer benefits to those employees who demonstrate their loyalty by first maintaining their employment at the spa for a prescribed period of time. These benefits should be factored into the equation when you are considering the compensation level at the spa. Your hourly per-treatment wage may be lower, but the trade-off in benefits makes it worthwhile for many therapists.

Seniority Systems—Pros and Cons

The seniority system in place at the spa is another important factor to consider when applying for a job. Many spas have a strict system that rewards longtime therapists with priority in scheduling, choice of treatments, higher pay, and more hours. The only way to achieve this yourself is to stay at the spa for a long time. While a strict seniority policy encourages loyalty among the therapists, it can also have the opposite unwanted effect of encouraging complacency. Senior staff members sometimes do just enough to get by and retain their senior status, while more eager, ambitious, and hardworking therapists below them strive fruitlessly for advancement because the best positions are already filled and will remain so for some time. This situation has been called the "**seniority syndrome**," and it has frustrated many new therapists seeking to advance their careers.

seniority syndrome

the practice at many spas of according priority in scheduling, choice of treatments, higher pay, and more hours to those therapists who have been on staff the longest, sometimes causing frustration on the part of ambitious therapists hired more recently

To counteract the initial frustration that many therapists feel when confronted by an impenetrable seniority system, it is helpful to take a step back and consider how you might feel if you find yourself in a senior position one day. If that were to happen, you might resent the energy and enthusiasm of an upstart such as the person you are right now.

The problem is not so much with individual therapists, but with the system itself. Given sufficient motivation and opportunity, most spa therapists will want to continue to improve themselves and their work.

One alternative to the seniority system that has worked at some spas can be called the "merit system." Rather than awarding therapists solely for sticking around, this system is based on monthly guest comment cards, plus longevity on the job, which does count for something, after all. If the therapists who garner the most favorable comments also receive the most prized shifts and optimal number of hours, it will work for the benefit of the spa, the guests, and the therapists as well, who will be motivated to do their best work.

SPA TIP

If possible, when applying for a position at a spa, ask a therapist on staff how the other therapists feel about the compensation offered. You will find that one spa may have a primarily happy team of therapists, while another has a staff that constantly complains about compensation issues. Ironically, the pay may be the same at these two spas. The key is strong leadership and good communication on the part of the spa director/owner. Set your sights at working for a spa with a happy team, and you'll end up being happy with your compensation too, regardless of the exact dollar amount you are paid.

It is appropriate and permissible for you to inquire about the seniority system or the merit system in place at the spa where you are applying. It is not appropriate, however, to criticize the spa's procedures. Simply learn what type of system would await you were you to accept a position at each spa, and use that knowledge in your final decision regarding where to work.

Compensation Models

Of course, the big question on your mind as you apply for a spa job may be: How much are they going to pay me? While therapists learn in school that they can expect $50 to $100 per hour for their massage work, this is not the pay scale you will find in spas. Spas cannot afford to pay therapists that much, no matter what the cost of the treatment. Typically, pay ranges from $15 to $30 per hour, or 30 to 40 percent of the cost of the massage or spa treatment. However, those numbers may be deceiving, because several other factors come into play when determining the actual pay you will receive, as explained in Table 14–5.

When you are thinking about accepting a position on a spa staff, it is important to consider the various forms that compensation can take. Some therapists are more comfortable with a straight percentage of the cost of each treatment they perform. Others prefer to work for an hourly wage, regardless of how many treatments they perform in a given day. Each compensation model has

FACTORS INFLUENCING THERAPIST COMPENSATION	EXPLANATION
spa's overhead expenses	The high overhead expenses of running a spa make it impossible to offer therapists what they are accustomed to receiving for doing massage in a private practice.
locale	Spas in some rural locations or where the local economy is depressed cannot charge high prices and therefore cannot afford to pay therapists high wages.
therapist seniority	Wherever you apply, there will be other therapists working there already, unless the spa is a startup. These therapists may already be receiving higher wages, making it difficult for the spa to offer high wages to beginning therapists on staff. Often, beginning therapists will start at lower wages.
benefits offered	Full-time therapists and other employees may be receiving benefits such as insurance and paid vacations, which takes a percentage of the proceeds from each treatment.
seasonality	During the spa's off-season, therapists perform fewer treatments, often coming into work for just a few hours per day, thus lowering overall wages.
spa policy	Some spas just plain pay low wages, compared to the average in the area. That is their policy, and nothing will change it. At times this fosters a "revolving-door" atmosphere at the spa, with many therapists coming and going on a frequent basis, resulting in lower quality for the guests. Spas in resort locations with few return clients sometimes have this policy. After a time, these spas develop poor reputations among therapists.

TABLE 14–5 Factors Influencing Therapist Compensation.

its positive and negative aspects, depending upon your needs and desires, as explained below.

Salaried Positions

Many spas offer salaried positions to massage therapists, but the number of salaried positions compared to part-time and on-call positions is usually small. This is because spas need to pay their full-time salaried people extra in the form of benefits. Consider yourself quite lucky if you can land a full-time salaried therapist position at a spa straight out of school. This is the exception rather than the rule. Usually, spas will start new therapists as part-timers, especially during any probationary period required at the beginning of employment.

If you do receive a salaried position, be prepared to accept a lower hourly wage to start with than you would perhaps have hoped for. Sometimes, this wage is lower than that paid to part-time therapists. Remember, salaried positions carry the extra compensation of stability, a guaranteed minimum income, and benefits. If these factors are important to you, you should inquire about how realistic a chance you would have of attaining a salaried position at the spas where you apply. Also, it is important to learn the time frame for attaining this status. At many spas, therapists have to wait several years before they achieve full-time salaried positions.

contracted labor

in spas, therapists hired to perform massage and spa treatments in exchange for an hourly wage with no benefits and without becoming an actual employee of the spa

Contracted Labor

Many spas draw upon a pool of therapists who are not actually employees but rather work as **contracted labor**. These therapists fill in during busier times at the spa and are free to pursue their own clientele on their own time. This situation works out well for therapists who are interested in building up their own practice but who appreciate the added income of a part-time spa position. In some spas, a contracted labor position can be full-time and even include overtime during busy seasons, but there is no guarantee of employment, and the schedule is subject to change from day to day, week to week, and month to month.

Tips and Service Fees

Gratuities constitute a good percentage of the pay for many spa therapists. Some spas have a service charge built into the price of each service, and the bulk of this charge (usually between 10 and 20 percent) goes to the therapist, with the rest divided among support staff. If the spa charges $100 for an hour-long service, for example, and the therapist receives a 15 percent built-in service charge, that is $15 in tips for each service given. The hourly pay is often lower, between $8 and $12 per hour on average, but the combined wage and tip adds up to an average of $25 per hour, which is a respectable wage for a spa employee. In some spas, the gratuity is left up to the individual client. Some clients leave larger tips than others, but the average is still 15 percent. Some therapists believe that it may not be appropriate to receive gratuities for massage therapy. The ethical aspects of accepting tips in the spa are covered in the next chapter.

Renting Space

Some spas offer therapists the opportunity to rent space in their facility and essentially run their own business as independent operators, with the added benefit of marketing and support staff. Often referred to as **booth rental**, a term from the salon industry which has carried over to the day spa industry, this setup can be optimal for self-directed therapists who like the idea of not having to answer to a boss. Booth rental leaves you free to close up shop and leave whenever you want to. It allows you to take as many or as few clients as you can handle. It also requires a good deal of self-promotion and self-motivation, so if you are more comfortable in a structured environment, with other people giving you guidance and assistance on the job, this is probably not the best option for you.

booth rental

(taken from the salon industry where it means renting a hair styling booth from a business owner) the practice of paying a business owner for the right to operate a massage or spa practice within the owner's facility for a set weekly or monthly rental fee, with all other proceeds retained by the practitioner

Personal Factors

When it comes down to deciding which spa is the right "fit" for you, sometimes you need to listen to your intuition. Regardless of whether the spa offers the compensation model you desire, a seniority philosophy you can believe in, or the 401K plan of your dreams, you have to ask yourself one question: "Does it feel right?" Do you like the people you meet there during the interview process? Is the environment attractive? Do you feel you will be able to offer your best work there? The best advice is to weigh carefully all the considerations listed in this chapter, but also to trust your instincts. The spa that is right for you at one stage may not be where you will work for the rest of your career. Choose a job to which you can dedicate yourself 100 percent *because it feels right*. As time goes on, your enthusiasm and dedication will help you move up the ranks at this spa, or move toward work at another spa or perhaps at an allied business.

The Spa Hiring Paradox—A Lower Starting Wage Is Good for You

Did You Know?

Many therapists, eager to get started and make their fortunes in the spa industry, rush out on their first set of interviews, expecting the pay scale to be a starting wage of 40 percent, 50 percent, or even higher. And, strangely enough, they find it to be true! As hundreds of new spas open every month in towns and cities across the land, many spa owners fuel these unrealistic expectations by offering therapists more money than they can actually afford to pay. Because of this mistake, many spas have had to either shut down or completely restructure their compensation model in order to stay in business.

The thinking of these new spa owners goes something like this: "If I pay a really good wage, I'll attract really good therapists. Then I won't have to worry about training them because they'll already be excellent at what they do. My clients will love them, book more repeat business, and I'll be well on my way to opening my second spa, which will be part of a massive chain of franchises I'll roll out across the entire country."

Instead of looking for "really good therapists," these spa owners should look for "really responsible and giving therapists willing to dedicate themselves to my business while they grow and learn in a mutually beneficial give-and-take relationship." In order to attract and hire the second type of therapist, smart spa owners implement a model of incremental compensation increases based on rewards for accomplishment and loyalty. In other words, *they offer a lower starting wage.*

If you seek out those wiser spa owners and spa directors with this attitude, you will end up with steady work that allows you to focus on building your skills and serving clients. This is a solid foundation for a career in the spa industry. Those therapists who insist on seeking out the highest pay right out of the gate regardless of how realistic that pay is are setting themselves up for potential disappointment.

It is your choice.

RESEARCH

Realistic Spa Compensation Expectations

Many beginning therapists in the spa industry experience major disappointment when they head out for their first job, because the pay they are offered is not what they expected. One way to gain some realistic expectations about spa compensation is to do some research and determine the actual compensation model used for the therapist staff at real spas. You can find this information in help-wanted ads, by calling spas and asking the treatment staff supervisor about pay, and by searching on the Internet for spa jobs. Find out what therapists are paid at one day spa and one larger resort or destination spa—the full package including benefits and other types of compensation—and then share this information with the class.

RESOURCES FOR SPA JOBS

When you head out looking for a spa position, the most likely resource for you to use is your local newspaper. While this makes sense and does at times offer leads, spas these days are more apt to advertise online or in trade magazines. You can also find spa jobs by going through the job placement program offered at many massage schools. This can be something as basic as a bulletin board or as extensive as a fully staffed office. Massage schools often have relationships with directors and owners of local spas, so it is important for you to cultivate a positive relationship with school faculty and ownership right from the beginning in order to improve your chances at positive recommendations for spa jobs once you graduate.

You can also check the Web site of the particular spas you are interested in applying to. Some of them, such as The Spa at the Hotel Hershey profiled later in this chapter, post job openings on their sites. Others use job posting sites specific to the spa industry to seek out new employees. One valuable industry resource is the Web site of the International Spa Association, which has a section devoted to job seekers and spas seeking employees (see Figure 14–3). Visit http://www.experienceispa.com and look under the Education & Resources > Job Bank heading for listings of dozens of therapist jobs.

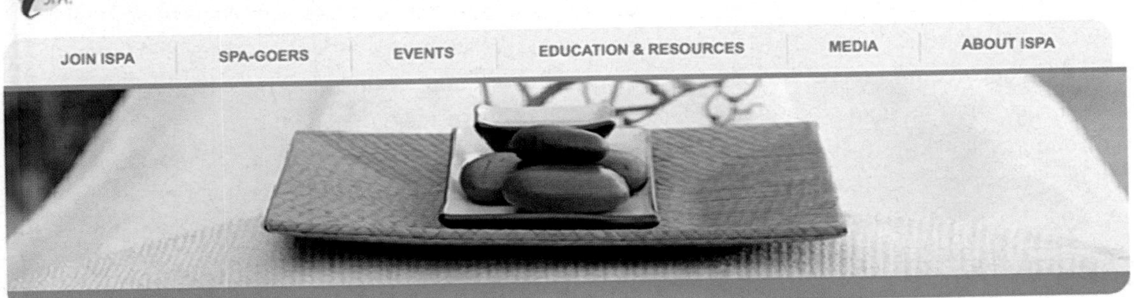

Job Title	Posted	Company	City	State	Country
Massage Therapist	2/21/2009	Glen Ivy Hot Springs Spa	Valencia		United States
Massage Therapist	2/20/2009	moss wellness spa	Scottsdale	AZ	United States
Massage Therapist	2/16/2009	Glen Ivy Hot Springs Spa	Brea	CA	United States
Massage Therapist	2/13/2009	Spa Chakra	San Francisco	CA	United States
Licensed Esthetician for Make-up Artist position	2/12/2009	Daired's Salon & Spa Pangea	Arlington	TX	United States
Massage Therapists	2/12/2009	Daired's Salon & Spa Pangea	Arlington	TX	United States
LMT	2/8/2009		Lake Placid	NY	United States
Massage Therapist	1/29/2009	Hotel Del Coronado	Coronado	CA	United States
Massage Therapists	1/23/2009	Bacara Resort & Spa	Santa Barbara	CA	United States
Massage Therapist	1/12/2009	Westmoor Club	Nantucket Island	MA	United States
Massage therapist	1/12/2009	Sole Spa	Tortola		BRITISH VIRGIN ISLANDS
Massage Therapist	1/7/2009	Spa Chakra	Short Hills	NJ	United States
Experienced Massage Therapist	1/3/2009	Bella Sante The Spa on Newbury	Boston	MA	United States
NYS Licensed Massage Therapist	12/15/2008	Equinox Fitness Clubs	New York	NY	United States

FIGURE 14–3 The International Spa Association (ISPA) has many therapist positions listed on its job bank page.

SPA PROFILE

Jennifer Wayland-Smith, spa director, The Spa at the Hotel Hershey, Hershey, Pennsylvania (Figure 14–4)

With approximately 65 massage therapists on staff, spa director Jennifer Wayland-Smith knows what she's talking about when it comes to seeking out, interviewing, and hiring qualified candidates. So, what exactly does she look for when she posts a job opening on the resort's Web site and begins receiving applications that have been filled out online by eager massage therapists?

"I think the main quality I look for in therapists is the ability to roll with the inevitable changes that happen in the spa," says Wayland-Smith. "They need to demonstrate a certain amount of flexibility in scheduling, in learning new techniques and procedures. They need to show me they are willing to go for it when it comes to trying new things. Most of all, I need to sense confidence in their skills. Also, I'm thinking about whether they are going to fit in with our particular team. You can't be a loner in the spa business. You have to be a team member. You can't work in an isolated world when there's a staff of over 125 people to think about."

Wayland-Smith keeps just 12 therapists on full-time status, and the rest are part-time. Full-time at The Spa at the Hotel Hershey means some serious benefits, including 401K plans, paid holidays, and vacations. All massage therapists at the spa, full- and part-time, start at Level One, with the same wage structure, which is paid regardless of whether the therapist is giving a treatment in a given hour. On top of that, they receive 17 percent of the price of the services they render to the guests. Each year, the wage is increased 3 percent, and there is also the potential of moving up to Level Two after a year on the job, Level Three after six years, and Level Four after nine years. Each step up carries an additional wage increase.

"Yes, we have some happy therapists," notes Wayland-Smith. "For the most part they're happy with their paychecks, and there is very little turnover, especially in the full-time positions. We currently have a full-time position open, but it's the first time that's happened in a couple years."

Understandably, therapists are eager to work at The Spa at the Hotel Hershey, and so Wayland-Smith has her pick when it comes time to hire new personnel. "I am on the advisory board for a local massage school and I stay in close touch with other massage school owners. Often, when therapists apply, I will call the school owner and ask what kind of students they were. Were they attentive? Did they show up on time, display responsibility, and treat their studies seriously? My massage manager and I personally interview every therapist who applies. This usually takes about 45 minutes to an hour. We chat, going over the therapist's background and previous job history, whether it's in the spa industry or not. We also familiarize them with our standard procedures and pay structure. Then after that we have two hands-on auditions, with myself and my massage manager, sometimes on the same day, sometimes different days. Based on the interview, those two auditions, reference checks and the call to the school owner, we have enough information to make a pretty good decision. Just in case, all employees undergo a four-month probationary period. During that time, they can be terminated for poor attendance, poor performance, guest complaints, or any other reason, with no need for the normal disciplinary process. I think that over the past five years or so we've only terminated two or three people during the probationary period."

At some spas, the therapists complain about the pay scale, but that does not seem to be the case at The Spa at the Hotel Hershey. "I think when therapists work here, they understand the guests are not paying over $100 for a massage alone," says Wayland-Smith. "They're paying for an entire spa experience, which includes all the overhead: robes,

(Continued)

CUSTOMER SERVICE ON STEROIDS

Customer service is a big focus in many businesses, especially within the **hospitality industry**. Numerous books have been written on the topic, and hundreds of experts whiz around the world on jets giving presentations to large corporations about upgrading and maximizing the customer-service skills of their employees. It is obviously a big priority for many industries. But when it comes to spas, customer service goes beyond a priority to become a crucial, do-or-die necessity. Spa customers expect the very best customer service on the planet—"customer service on steroids." They expect to be coddled, cared for, remembered by name, and catered to at the drop of a hat. Why? There are several reasons:

hospitality industry

the entire economic sector, including spas, that serves the public through lodging, dining, personal services, and entertainment offerings

- Spas are, in one sense, the womb recreated, and as customers lay enveloped in warm sheets or tended to by loving hands, they allow their natural defenses to relax. In this state, they are especially vulnerable, both physically and emotionally, and need to be handled with extra care.
- For many people, spas epitomize the height of luxury. Customers cannot imagine a destination that would more thoroughly match their idea of a fantasy fulfilled. Any chink in the armor of that fantasy creates grave misgivings about the entire experience.
- Spas set themselves up for these high expectations by giving themselves names such as "Bliss," "Nirvana," and "Heaven."
- Whether it is true or not, the public generally regards spas as palaces of indulgence which charge very high prices for their services. They do not understand the high overhead costs involved with running a spa and therefore think that spas "owe" them extra service for the money they are paying.

For these reasons, it is vital that you as a spa therapist learn those techniques and skills that will add to the spa's ability to provide top-notch customer service. In order to excel in this area, you must first understand precisely what exactly customer service is. Customer service can be defined as "the ability of an organization or individual to take care of the needs, wishes, questions, requests, and complaints of its clientele." Excellent customer service consists of doing these things consistently, to a very high standard of satisfaction, and in a largely transparent manner, which means that the customer often does not even notice the efforts being made on his behalf.

The Seven Main Customer Service Skills for a Spa Therapist

What are the skills and qualities that a spa therapist needs to cultivate in order to provide exceptional customer service? There are several, the most important being *sensitivity, flexibility, positivity, humility, responsibility, maturity,* and *connectivity.* Each of these are explained below in order to help build your awareness of these principles in the spa.

The Seven Habits of Highly Effective Massage Therapists

Did You Know?

Sensitivity—the strength of compassion
Flexibility—the strength of adaptability
Positivity—the strength of hope
Humility—the strength of self-confidence
Responsibility—the strength of respect for others
Maturity—the strength of experience
Connectivity—the strength of communication

Sensitivity

As a massage therapist, you are most likely a sensitive person. Empathy is high on your list of important personality traits. Nonetheless, empathy for a client's pain, tightness, or stress is not the same as empathy for a client's customer-service needs. Just because you know how to release a person's frozen shoulder does not mean you will be able turn her into a completely satisfied spa guest. In fact, your empathetic abilities can sometimes actually get in the way of this process; you are so involved with clients on a therapeutic level that you forget some of their other needs. This often happens in physicians' offices. Many doctors, though certainly not all, are notorious for their brusqueness and insensitivity to patients' needs outside of the treatment or operating room. In fact, the concept of "customer service" might seem laughable to them. You might want to search your own soul a bit and see if you discover any of this attitude within yourself.

When you work in a spa, you are not only a therapist, you are also by default a guest-services expert. This may cause you to bristle somewhat, saying to yourself, "I should not be forced to pander to these people's needs just because they are paying big bucks to be here. That's somebody else's job." In order to be a truly effective spa therapist, you must break through this limiting self-definition, expand the concept of your role, and see yourself in a new light. If you find the strength of character to do this, it will increase your chances of success in the spa industry.

To be the best spa therapist you can be, you need to be sensitive to the guest on many different levels. For example, when working as a spa therapist, you can ask yourself the following questions:

> "Is this guest comfortable with me as a therapist? Perhaps it is his first time receiving a massage and I have to do my best to assure he is at ease, even if that means excusing myself and suggesting a different therapist."
>
> "Does this guest need anything else besides therapy, such as a drink of fresh water, tea, or juice? A clean towel? A new robe or slippers?"
>
> "Is my work area neat and tidy? This will be my guest's living space, for at least one hour, so I have to be aware of how the environment will make her feel."
>
> "Am I providing a uniform image through my attire and attitude that matches the rest of the spa so that the guest will have a smooth overall experience?"

Flexibility

In the spa environment, your ability to accept change is absolutely vital. Without it, you will flounder at crucial moments when you should be steady and strong. If you are too attached to unchanging schedules and routines, you will not be able to accommodate constantly fluctuating guest demands and workplace conditions. Although the work life of a spa therapist might look serene from the outside, and perhaps even boring, the reality is much more fluid, dynamic, and at times even upsetting (see the section on "Spa Stress" and the "Battleground Scenarios" later in this chapter). You must be able to stop on a dime, assess any new situation, and turn in a completely new direction if it is warranted.

One example where flexibility is necessary is in scheduling. Often, spa guests will change their appointments at the last minute, or an appointment will be added or dropped from the schedule without your knowledge. These are moments that can cause you frustration, and you have to be ready for them. Instead of getting upset, which will definitely carry over and influence any guest interaction you have afterward, perhaps even souring a therapeutic session, you can take the opportunity to remind yourself once again that customer service comes first. If you cannot learn to maintain a positive mindset during the inevitable fluctuations in your daily routine, you will not become the most valuable spa therapist you can be. This will cause you to miss opportunities for advancement and perhaps keep you from getting a spa job in the first place.

Positivity

Because spa guests can be so demanding, you may find yourself at times stretched to the limit of your capacity to stay positive when it comes to meeting those demands. However, it is imperative that you find a way to turn their experience into a positive one, to say "yes to the guest" (see Did You Know? Saying "Yes to the Guest").

As part of your massage training, you have learned that during physical contact, we share an invisible energy with our clients. Although we cannot see it, we can measure the electricity and warmth that pass between our bodies when we touch. Some people also believe that negative thoughts and emotions can be felt by clients and thus affect the massage. Negative thoughts and emotions include judgment, regret, anger, and jealousy, among others. At the very least, these emotions will affect your clients when they see the expression on your face and hear the inflection in your voice. Labeling these states "negative" does not make them wrong. However, they are generally not states that spa guests pay a great deal of money to experience. It is part of your job as a professional spa therapist to find a way to give the guest a positive experience, regardless of your personal situation at the time. You may have gotten into a car accident, had your wallet stolen, and broken up with your boyfriend or girlfriend all in the last week, but these issues should not be brought into the treatment room. It is important to note that most guests will be very kind if you bring up personal problems, thus compelling you to share more, creating a cycle of negativity. While it is most appropriate to share concerns and troubles with friends outside of work, spa guests are there for another purpose.

The interactions you have with guests in lounge areas, locker rooms, at the front desk, and on the phone should all be tempered by the same professional

Saying "Yes to the Guest"

Did You Know?

A spa director from one of the Ritz-Carlton properties, which are famous for their attention to customer service and guest satisfaction, has stated that her goal and the goal of all the therapists on her staff is to be able to say "yes to the guest" (Figure 15–1). This means turning any request, complaint, suggestion, or problem into a positive experience. The guest should always walk away feeling that his needs have been met. "We Are Ladies and Gentleman Serving Ladies and Gentlemen," is the Ritz's motto, and they strive to always do so in a positive manner.

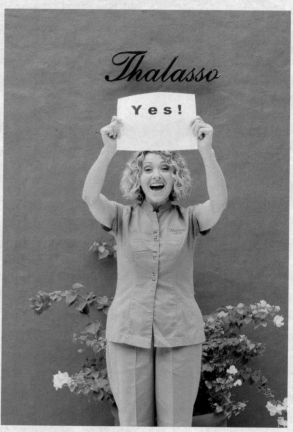

FIGURE 15–1 It is important to turn any request, complaint, suggestion or problem into a positive experience and say "Yes to the guest."

While this goal sounds good, how can you as a spa therapist learn to implement it consistently? Perhaps you can take a lesson here from the world of dramatic arts. One of the fundamental rules of improvisational theater is to always say "yes" to everything that is thrown at you. Thus, if you are an actor on stage during an improv performance and somebody says to you out of the blue, "You are a 10-foot-tall carrot!" your immediate response is, "That's right, and my greatest fear is giant rabbits." Actors who are unable to flow into the unknown impede the performance.

In the same way, the end result to any spa guest's query should always be "yes." Even if the situation seems hopeless, there is usually a way to solve it. Here are some examples:

If a guest on your treatment table asks for a Red Delicious apple, you can say, "Let me go try to find one for you right now." (This actually happened to a spa therapist in Florida.)

A guest signs up for a scalp treatment but arrives with her hair up in ribbons and says, "I'm going to an important affair this evening, so you cannot touch my coiffure." You smile and proceed to give her the best scalp treatment she's ever received, while concentrating on her neck, forehead, temples and upper shoulders, avoiding her hair entirely.

A pregnant guest comes to you for a prenatal massage then requests that you concentrate on her feet because she loves reflexology. It is the spa's policy to avoid reflexology on pregnant guests because of the possibility of stimulating an early birth. Your response? "Yes, of course, I'd love to offer you reflexology. I can't do it right now because of our policy against endangering guests, but I'm going to give you a special certificate for a discount on reflexology the next time you visit the spa, and in the meantime today I'll concentrate on your lower legs and back. I'm sure they're sore from carrying the extra weight."

positivity. If you are passing through a difficult time personally and need time off for truly pressing needs, respectfully request it from the spa director or owner, explaining your situation, rather than risk creating negative situations with guests. Management will appreciate your forthright communication and your concern for the guests' welfare, and this will translate itself into greater success for you in the spa eventually, even if it means missing a day or two of work in the short term.

Humility

It is important to remember that the guest should be the center of attention in the spa, not the therapist. While this may seem obvious, it entails a degree of retraining for some therapists, especially American therapists, who rankle easily at anything that might be termed "subservience." This is why it has traditionally been difficult for American therapists to work aboard cruise ship spas. There is a distinct division between the serving class and the receiving class aboard a cruise ship. Therapists are not allowed to roam all passenger decks freely, for example, and there is a sublimating of the crew's desires and needs and freedoms in order to make the guest's experience more exceptional. While this "class division" is not as overt at most spas as it is on the cruise ships, it is important to remember that there is indeed a division. For those moments of professional interaction in the spa, we are the serving class. If you cannot place yourself even temporarily in this humble stance, you will consistently run into problems.

It is also important to cultivate humility when faced with your own therapeutic limitations. You may find yourself working in a spa one day faced with the temptation to overstep your abilities and knowledge. A guest may ask you to treat a condition or problem for which you are not adequately trained. It is important at that moment to humbly state that you are not certified for that type of work, rather than attempting heroics.

Spa therapists also need humility when it comes to following instructions. At times, our independent natures lead us to shrug off directives from our superiors. This is not a good idea. In order for a spa to work smoothly, a certain amount of hierarchy is necessary. Your pride may not like this, thus making it an excellent opportunity to expand the scope of your humility. Relax and breathe into the reality of your boss.

Responsibility

When you become a spa therapist, not only will you have the typical responsibilities you would expect with such a position, such as punctuality, cleanliness, therapeutic integrity, and so on, but you will also carry the additional responsibility of playing a type of role model for the guests who come to the spa expecting to be instructed (both verbally and non-verbally) in the arts of healthy living and lifestyle. You will, in a sense, be responsible for *being* a certain kind of person. This does not mean that you cannot simply be yourself. But, at least while you are on the job, you will need to maintain an awareness that you are representing the spa, and beyond that, the spa lifestyle.

Any habits, behaviors, or attitudes you display that run counter to this spa lifestyle may cause unease or even confusion amongst the guests. For example, a therapist who arrives for a massage or spa therapy appointment with the smell of cigarettes on his clothes, hair, or breath can completely break the charming spell cast by an attractive facility.

You will also be responsible to your immediate supervisor, and beyond that, to the spa directors, owners, and perhaps even shareholders, if it is a public company. Thus, when you are working in a spa, you are part of a larger structure than you may not have experienced before, unless you have previously worked in a corporate environment.

Maturity

Spa directors and owners love it when their therapists exhibit a mature desire for continuous improvement in their professional lives. They look closely at how many continuing education classes their therapists have taken, the breadth and depth of the work they offer to the spa's clientele, and their overall commitment to their massage therapy careers. Mature therapists are attractive to employers, and *mature* in this sense does not mean old or even well-seasoned. It means someone with a long-term perspective, someone who brings knowledge, commitment, and passion for their work into the spa, for the betterment for the guests and, one would hope, an improvement in the overall business.

There is another type of maturity that is greatly appreciated by spa owners. As you grow in the spa industry and decide that you would like to commit yourself for a number of years, perhaps even carving out a lifelong career within the spa world, you will have to make a mature decision to set aside some of the independence that comes with a private practice and some of the lost revenue that comes with working in someone else's establishment. If you can make this decision without remorse, knowing that along with the drawbacks come many benefits, you will be a pleasure to work with. Too many therapists work in spas, take home a decent paycheck, and then complain bitterly that they could be making more on their own. If that is the case, then perhaps it would be best to go out on your own and make more. (See the discussion on compensation in Chapter 14.) It is a mature therapist who knows better than to spread the sentiments of remorse and regret amongst co-workers and perhaps even the guests.

It is natural to think about bettering yourself, and you may continue to feel a need to explore other options, even while staying committed to the spa where you presently work. That is fine. What matters most is your attitude. If you are grateful for what the spa is offering you, and you strive in a mature way to demonstrate that gratitude by doing the best work you can, in the most positive way, then everyone—spa owners, directors, guests, and fellow therapists—will find you a joy to work with. One way to help you maintain this mature attitude is to look at your work in the spa from a different viewpoint. The spa is actually offering you something very valuable in exchange for the percentage of income you are "losing" by not treating the clients in your own private practice. What the spa offers you, according to noted spa owner and consultant Peggy Wynne Borgman, is **professional career management**. This consists of a number of valuable services that many therapists take for granted, such as scheduling, billing, payroll, medical benefits, marketing, rent, supplies and equipment, and more. A spa can take you fresh out of massage school and turn you into a successful, busy massage therapist at absolutely no cost to you. In fact, you will be paid while your career is being developed by these professionals. That is a good deal, and mature therapists realize it.

professional career management

a number of valuable services that therapists receive as spa employees, including scheduling, billing, payroll, medical benefits, marketing, rent, supplies, and equipment

SPA PROFILE

Peggy Wynn Borgman, Preston-Wynne Day Spa, Saratoga, California

"Professional Career Management" for Spa Therapists

Preston-Wynne Day Spa owner Peggy Wynne Borgman is an expert at keeping employees happy in the workplace. She has devoted an incredible amount of time and effort to devise standards and procedures that allow her dozens of staff members to remain optimally productive and develop successful careers. This effort has paid off, as Preston-Wynne has been ranked the top day spa in the U.S. several times by the Day Spa Association.

One key to her success is something she calls "professional career management" for her staff of therapists and estheticians. "We try to create a situation where the support staff truly provides career management to the hands-on employees," she says. "For that reason, the support team needs to know absolutely everything about the menu, the spa, and the therapists. They also have to be intelligent, well-paid (we pay from $10/hour for a new employee, up to $15 for an accomplished individual) and very well-trained. The training for the support team at Preston-Wynne is actually longer than the training for therapists."

What exactly do therapists receive as part of this professional career management? "To begin," says Borgman, "the spa takes away all those concerns about where the money is going to be coming from. We offer a built-in clientele, marketing, advertising, appointment booking, billing, payroll, supplies, equipment, training, support staff, and a clean facility. Everything down to laundry services is taken care of so the therapist can concentrate on what he or she is best at—therapy.

"Of course, we charge for all this career management. There is a true cost to having a great work environment and to having all those details in place that make it possible for the right therapist to flourish. And by *flourish* I mean not only to do well financially, but also to receive some other meaningful rewards that are important to creative, intuitive, artistic individuals. Above and beyond pay raises, therapists appreciate greater flexibility in their hours, visits to other spas to sample treatments, scholarships for continuing education classes, and public recognition for their input and their worth."

Borgman has found that one of the biggest stumbling blocks to therapists' fulfillment and ultimate happiness with their spa careers is a misunderstanding of one basic principle. "The main problem," she says, "is that we have to cut the connection between the charge-per-service and the wage to the therapists. There is no connection!

"Optimally, therapists should understand that the percentage pay they receive from each service is less important than the 'real dollars' they are making as an employee. Many therapists can't seem to understand that it is the size of the pie—not the size of the slice—that matters as far as pay goes. The bigger the whole pie, the spa's overall income, the more money therapists are going to make over time. While raising the percentage rate on someone's pay from 30 percent to 35 percent, for example, may seem on the surface to be the quickest way to a bigger paycheck, it may not actually make that much difference if the number of clients does not increase. Therapists working in spas everywhere will benefit greatly if they understand this principle. There are a couple little formulas I use that sum this principle up. To arrive at the appropriate pay for the therapist, I use this formula:

skill + knowledge + effort = therapist's treatment rate

And to arrive at the appropriate dollar figure to charge my clients, I use this formula:

therapist's rate + overhead + profit = price of service

(Continued)

SPA PROFILE

Peggy Wynn Borgman, Preston-Wynne Day Spa, Saratoga, California *continued*

"The important thing to notice here is that the 'price of service' is not part of the formula for coming up with the treatment rate, and yet therapists constantly make the error of thinking that their pay should somehow be tied to the rate we charge the client. They feel that the more we charge, the more they should be paid. This is fallacious reasoning.

"No matter how hard I might try to explain the fairness of this and other policies, I as a spa owner might still be discredited by my employees, even though I've been a hands-on esthetician myself, because the employer–therapist relationship can often be a parent–child relationship.

"In general, I find that the best long-term spa employees are not entrepreneurs. The more entrepreneurial type therapists eventually move on to work at their own businesses. We like to work with those therapists who appreciate what it is we're offering them in the way of professional career management and who thrive in these conditions. We help them reach their potential by creating the right environment, offering benefits and stimuli for constant improvement, and then getting out of the way so they can work their magic with the clients. We think this is a pretty good arrangement and an excellent deal for the right kind of therapist.

"In the end, we measure our spa's success through our clients' satisfaction, and one of the best ways to assure that satisfaction is through the professional career management we offer to our therapists. The happier and more well-taken-care-of the therapists feel, the more satisfied customers we'll have. So focusing on the career management of our therapists is, in the end, one of the best ways to assure return clientele and a successful business. It's a win-win-win."

SPA TIP

Spa Therapist Compensation Equations

It is especially important to note that the price of a spa service should not be a factor in determining therapists' pay, as shown in Peggy Wynn Borgman's Spa Therapist Compensation Equations:

skill + knowledge + effort = therapist's treatment rate

therapist's rate + overhead + profit = price of service

Connectivity

Your job as a spa therapist will put you in almost constant physical contact with your customers, but in order to be the best spa therapist you can be, you should also connect with your clients in other ways, opening as many avenues of communication as possible. Good communication skills include:

Verbal: Speak clearly and simply when telling guests about the services they are going to receive. They may be nervous or apprehensive or shy, especially if it is their first experience in a spa. It is up to you to put them at ease.

Visual: Look guests directly in the eye when addressing them. This inspires trust. Direct guests' attention to useful details, such as the location of hooks for hanging robes or clothes, bathrooms, handrails for safely entering tubs, showers, etc.

Tactile: Other moments of shared contact with your guest outside of the treatment room are also important. For example, when you meet your clients, shake hands firmly (Figure 15–2). A reassuring pat on the shoulder can quell nervousness. Direct guests' awareness to comforting tactile sensations in the room such as heating pads and soft linens.

Auditory: Remember that each guest has a unique preference for auditory stimulation during massage or spa treatment sessions. One guest's blissful serenity may be another's dreary boredom. Do not assume that every client will prefer the same music choice or volume. If you have the ability to change either, do so

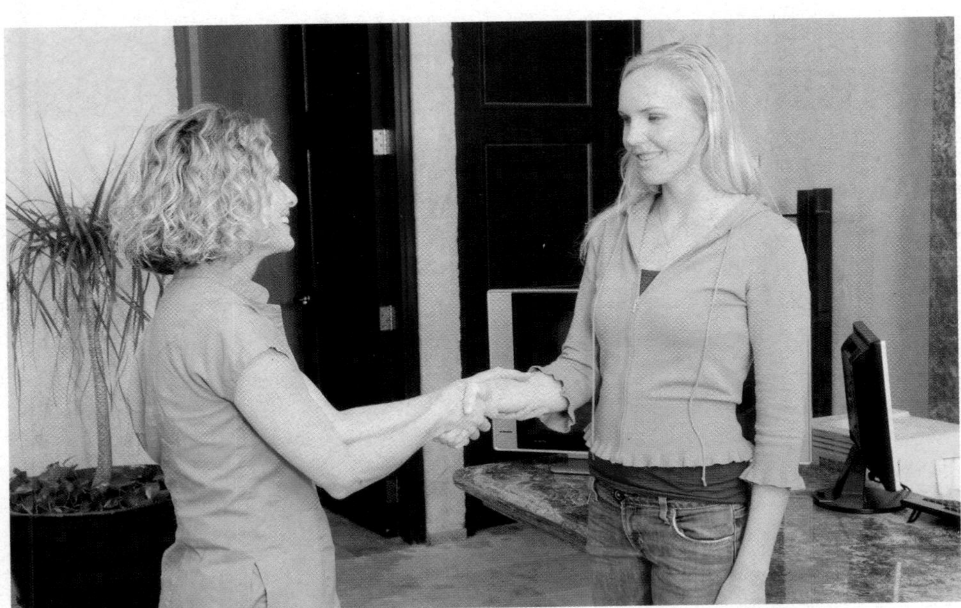

FIGURE 15–2 When you meet your clients, shake hands firmly.

at the guest's request, and also ask him what his preference is at the beginning of the treatment. Also, if you have control over any other auditory influences such as background noises, try to adjust these for the guest's comfort. However, be aware that in many spas, the management has set a uniform environment for all guests, and you may not have control over all the details. In this case, it is better to accept the uniform conditions imposed by management and strive to make the guest as comfortable as possible within those parameters.

Olfactory: In your treatment room, you may have some control over the aromas through the use of candles, essential oils, and incense, but before you use any of these, you must be given permission by spa management. Then, of course, the guest must have her say-so as well. Communicate with the guest directly regarding any preference in aromas. Some guests love a well-scented treatment space, while others find scents distasteful or might even be allergic.

The invisible: It is best to approach the spa's clients with a caring, open heart, treating each one as if she were a client in your own private practice, or even a guest in your home. This creates several benefits: first, your own customer-service skills will improve, and this will serve you well for the rest of your professional life; second, spa management and ownership will look favorably upon you, increasing the likelihood of promotion and pay raise; third, the spa's business and bottom line benefit by increased customer loyalty brought about by your efforts; fourth, and most important, the customer feels deeply cared for, which is the essence of the spa experience. Rubbing people down, scrubbing them off, or wrapping them up are simply the external excuses for the inner connections we make with our guests. The best services and the best interactions occur in an atmosphere of acceptance and heartfelt communication. In many Asian spas, guests are greeted the traditional way, with palms raised in prayer position for "Namasté." This image is good to keep in mind when you greet each of your own spa guests. Though it might not be appropriate to raise your hands, you can open your heart and "bless the divine within" each person who enters your treatment room.

ACTIVITY

Role Playing Customer Service Skills

Engage in a role-playing scenario based on one of the seven qualities and skills listed above. You and a partner choose roles—either guest or spa therapist—and then interact from the moment of first greeting the guest up through the moment the massage begins. Then continue the interaction after the massage up until the moment of parting from the guest. Switch roles with your partner afterward, choosing another of the seven qualities. You can do as many role-playing scenarios as you like. Each will last 3 to 5 minutes.

HOSPITALITY

Here is a quick, one-question "pop quiz" for you: When you work in the hospitality industry, it is extremely important for you to be:

(a) super-intelligent
(b) very good looking
(c) good with math
(d) hospitable

That's right. Though it might seem overly obvious, being hospitable is the most important quality for someone in the hospitality industry. Make no mistake about it: When you work in a spa, you are working in the hospitality industry. This is true regardless of whether the spa has guest rooms, like a hotel. Even the smallest day spa is operating in the hospitality sector of the economy, the same sector as hotels, cruise ships, ski lodges, and golf resorts. Hospitality, in its simplest form, can be defined as "kindness in welcoming guests or strangers." It is the last word in that definition that is most important. Do you have within you what it takes to welcome a stranger and make him feel comfortable (Figure 15–3)?

Some people argue that the quality of hospitality is an inborn personality trait, or perhaps a cultural phenomenon, and that it cannot be taught. Hawaiians, they

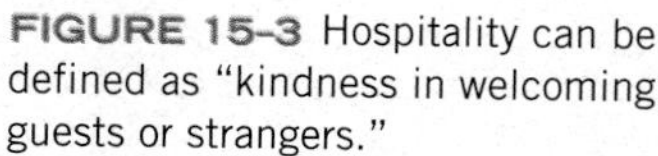

FIGURE 15–3 Hospitality can be defined as "kindness in welcoming guests or strangers."

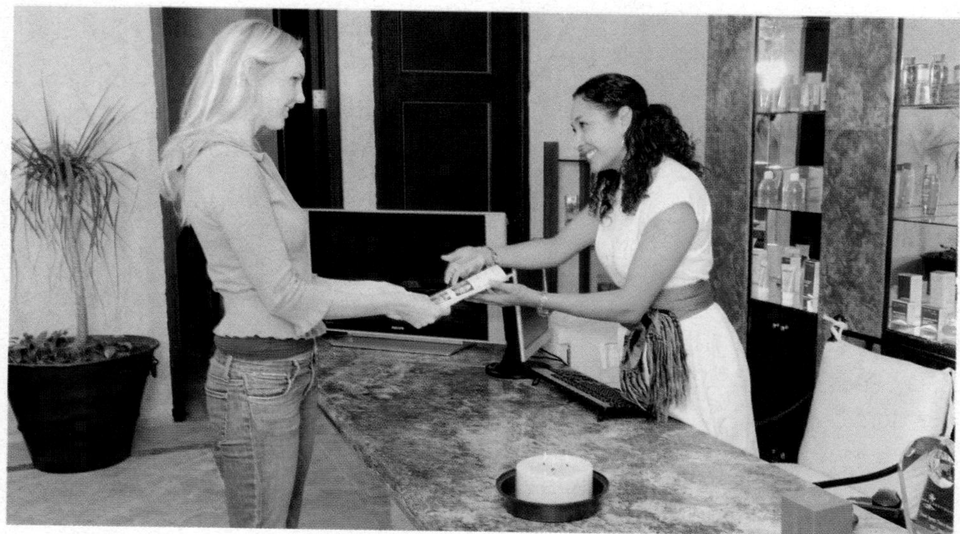

say, are more hospitable by nature than people from North Dakota. People from Thailand are more hospitable than people from Uzbekistan. Certain people just seem hospitable from birth, as if it were in their genes or their blood. And others learn this from their parents. After they leave the impressionable age of childhood and are set in their ways, how can someone be taught to be kind to strangers?

This is the seemingly impossible task faced by any manager in the hospitality industry and especially in spas, where hospitality extends into more intimate, prolonged periods of contact between guests and employees than in any other situation. As someone who will potentially be seeking employment in the spa industry, you need to understand this problem that spa managers have and be prepared to offer a solution. You need to know that hospitableness is the number-one character trait for which the spa manager is looking, and at the same time, it is the most difficult trait to teach. If you can cultivate this trait on your own and then be willing to demonstrate your mastery of it in job interview situations and eventually while working in the spa industry, your chances at success will be greatly improved.

Take a look at the following points that may help you begin to develop a spa-hospitality mindset of your own:

- Just because spas are places of elegance, beauty, and at times wealth does not mean that you should assume an aloof or distant attitude, believing that wealthy or discriminating guests crave to be waited on by snobbish personnel. As Horst Schulze, past president of the Ritz-Carlton hotel chain, has said, "Elegance without warmth is arrogance."
- There is a fine line between personable and overly friendly, and there is an equally fine line between professional and aloof. It is up to you to strike the precise balance on both scales, always remembering that you are *both* an individual hospitably greeting another individual *and* a professional dealing with a paying client.
- Know that there is no cause for embarrassment or shame in the simple act of serving another human being. In fact, it is probably good for your soul. Many people find it difficult to assume a servile position, as they think it somehow reflects poorly on their own position in life. It is best, however, to leave this egotistical point of view at the door when you enter the spa to work. The more fully you can give yourself over to serving somebody else, the more quickly you will learn one of the more basic lessons in life—namely, we are all the same.
- You can borrow the hospitality customs from other cultures and establishments to help you develop your own skills. Asians, Polynesians, Southerners, and favorite aunts and grandmas are all famous for their ability to welcome guests and strangers into their homes or workplaces. Imitate them.

ACTIVITY

Hospitality Skills Role-Playing Game

With a partner, write out a script for guest hospitality (larger spas will often have a script that they expect therapists to follow). Then take turns being the customer and the spa therapist. Greet the "customer" at the moment he or she enters the spa and lead him or her through to the point at the beginning of the treatment, following the script as closely as possible.

SPA STRESS

It is ironic that modern spas, which owe their very existence to the concept of peace and tranquility, can engender so much stress and craziness among employees. Spas can be as bad as the most hectic of businesses, such as restaurants or even a stock exchange, with people shouting, voices being raised, and confusion reigning. Of course, all of this is exacerbated by the fact that it must remain strictly concealed from the guests, who expect nothing but calmness and serenity as they float from treatment to treatment on a cloud of bliss. This modern trend toward ultra-tranquility in spas may be a reaction against the noise and fast pace of our lives, but it was not always the case. In earlier times, spas were often the seat of much bustling activity, commerce, entertainment, and general hullabaloo. See the description of an ancient Roman spa in Chapter 1. The dichotomy between the front of the house and the back creates a tension in spas that makes them peculiarly prone to internal ruptures and strains. Strangely, it's the calm, cool collected image that spas create that makes them more stressful at times for the people who work there. From the "back of the house" point of view of the staff, spas can often feel like a battleground.

spa stress

the added on-the-job tension experienced by spa employees who are attempting to create a stress-free environment for guests

In order for you to work effectively in a spa, you will have to know how to deal with this particular type of **spa stress**. Because it usually cannot be seen by the guests, spa stress is a quiet kind of stress, and just like high blood pressure, which is known as "the silent killer," it can be deadly. Undue amounts of stress among employees can kill off the *esprit de corps* that is vital for a spa's success. This stress can lead to the gradual disintegration of a spa's reputation, no matter how well-established the business is. The first step in this downhill slide usually takes place when clients notice the negative attitudes of the staff and it begins to affect their experience.

For several reasons, spa guests are particularly sensitive to any disgruntlement on the part of the staff:

- They are hyper-aware of their surroundings because they are often disrobed, potentially embarrassed, and slightly on edge.
- They spend a large amount of time in one-on-one situations with therapists, which often leads to conversation and sharing of feelings.
- They tend to "bond" with their therapist in the intimate setting of the treatment room, potentially taking sides against others, be they other staff members, management, or owners.
- Spa guests frequently talk among themselves, weighing strengths and weaknesses among staff members and services. They do not hesitate to share information they've gleaned from therapists, thus spreading any rumors they may have heard.

It is vital, then, that you learn how to deal with this spa stress effectively and silence any negative rumblings before they reach guests' ears. If you want to prepare yourself for what the stress of spa work can truly be like for a therapist, take a look at the battleground scenarios below, try some of the related activities suggested at the end of this section, answer the review questions for this chapter, and practice until you understand viscerally how to deal with these conditions when they arise.

Battleground Scenarios

1. When you arrive at work one day, you discover that the schedule has been rearranged by the front desk, and you now have four back-to-back deep tissue massage treatments with only a few minutes to rest in between.
2. A new policy mandated by the spa owner now makes it a requirement to sell a certain amount of retail products each month. The staff threatens to revolt, and several co-workers want you to pick

sides. You're either for the therapists or for management.

3. You're in the middle of giving the spa's signature Balinese Ritual, complete with a soak in a hydro bath strewn with rose petals, when you see a cockroach climbing up the wall behind the guest as she reclines in the tub.
4. A co-worker bursts from her treatment room in tears and blurts that she cannot bear to work on a particular guest, who is overweight, has an unattractive skin condition, and is "just too gross." Your spa director wants you to take over while he deals with the co-worker.
5. Somebody puts upbeat music on the spa's central audio system and the client on your table complains that she wants it changed immediately.
6. A guest, already on your table, states that he wants "as much pressure as you've got, but only using Swedish massage techniques." He has declined to pay for the deep-tissue massage, which is on the menu for $15 more and for which the spa would pay you a higher fee.
7. The spa runs out of massage oil one day, and all the therapists are booked solid. The spa director is out to lunch, and you and your co-workers find yourself in charge of remedying the situation (Figure 15–4).

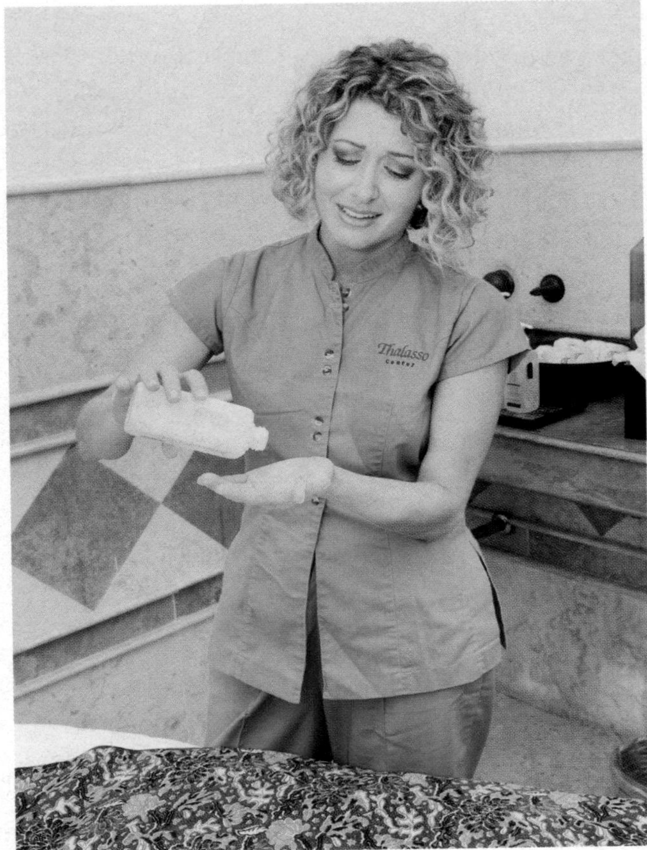

FIGURE 15–4 Spas can run short of supplies, leaving you stuck.

8. The spa software malfunctions and three guests are booked for exfoliation treatments at the same time in the spa's only wet room.
9. A guest begins dyeing her hair bright blue in one of the ladies' locker-room sinks and the chemical smell fills the entire area. She does not listen to the entreaties of the spa attendants or spa director. You are scheduled to give her a massage in 20 minutes and have already developed a rapport with her.
10. You are working in a day spa/salon, and the noise of chatter, gossip, and hair dryers is driving you and your clients crazy. Even though he has promised to soundproof your treatment room, the spa's owner has not come through yet, and it is increasingly difficult to create a serene environment for your clients.

You may have noticed that the scenarios listed above had a few common threads running through them. Essentially, each problem that a therapist has to deal with in the spa can be traced back to a thought process that goes something like this:

1. My manager/director/boss is causing a problem.
   or
2. This guest is causing a problem.
   or
3. This co-worker is causing a problem.
   or (least likely)
4. I am having a bad day.

ACTIVITY

Role Playing "Battleground Scenarios"

Role-Playing:
Choose one of the "battleground" scenarios above and act it out with a classmate. One person plays the therapist and the other plays either guest, spa director, fellow therapist, or front-desk attendant. Note: if performed in front of the class, these scenarios can be quite entertaining.

Notice the other-directedness of the first three and the unnecessary self-recrimination of the last. Spa therapists sometimes look for a way to blame others or needlessly blame themselves when things go poorly, rather than proactively seek ways to correct the situation without laying blame. If you can find a way to build your self-confidence enough to avoid this type of blaming, you will go far in the spa industry. Techniques can be taught. Skills can be learned. It is extremely difficult, however, to instill the proper attitude in an employee.

ATTITUDE IS EVERYTHING

The attitude you assume while on the job in your spa will determine the course of your career. Once again, it is important to remember the golden rule for spa employees: "Treat the spa and each of its guests exactly as if you were the owner. This is the most accelerated way to move forward in your spa career. No exceptions. No excuses."

This golden rule may be simple, but following it is difficult. It is extremely challenging to treat each guest as if you were the spa's owner. After all, you are *not* the owner, and if through your efforts the profits of the spa increase, how will that benefit you? Won't you be slaving away for someone else's profit?

Although it may seem counterintuitive at first, the truth is that you are always working for yourself. Though you may have somebody else telling you what to do, and a set of rules that you are supposed to follow, and a person signing a paycheck for you, you are, ultimately, doing what you are doing for your own benefit. You may not like it, but you are, in a way, choosing it.

There may come a time in your career when you decide that the circumstances in which you find yourself are of your own choosing, when you step into the role that you are already playing, accept it, make it your own, and then move onto the next level. Many, many massage therapists have been able to do this within the spa industry. There is unlimited upward potential into supervisory positions, management, training, and consulting for people who choose responsibility and cultivate the proper attitude.

This discussion does not imply that you need to move up the ladder in order to thrive and be happy. Doing the hands-on work of a therapist one-on-one with your clients is equally valuable. What is important to note is that you may never reach professional satisfaction or fulfillment, in a spa or at any job, no matter what your position, if you mentally place yourself outside the structure within which you are operating. The culture in which you find yourself when you work for a spa is one of discipline and service, and it is sometimes natural to fight against it. You may need to exert a conscious effort to overcome your own tendency to "rebel and repel." When you rebel against authority, you repel the very chance at success that caused you to seek work in this field in the first place.

Actions versus Attitude

Even if you agree that a mature, responsible, positive attitude is important, that might not make it any easier for you to cultivate one. How do you actually go about becoming the successful spa therapist you envision yourself being? Do you simply tell yourself, "Okay, now I'm successfully and happily going forward

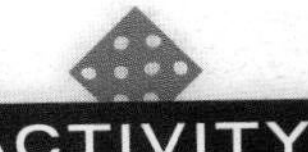

ACTIVITY

Following the Golden Rule for Spa Work

The following behaviors may feel unnatural at first, but if you try them, you will feel what it is like to care about the spa where you work as if it were your own. Doing so will hone your ability to follow the "golden rule" for spa work and increase your chances at becoming a valued employee.

Practice behaviors:

- Pretend for a day that you are actually the boss of your own corporation and that everything you do matters. People are watching you, judging you, emulating you, wanting a piece of you. How do you relate to others in this capacity? How do your behaviors change when you feel that you are responsible for others' well-being and livelihood?
- The next time someone "pushes one of your buttons" and gets you angry or upset, stop for a moment. Do not react in the way you feel compelled to react. Instead, examine your own feelings in that moment. In what ways does your wanting to feel "right" about the situation cause your anger? How would letting go of this desire help dissolve or diffuse the situation? How would this come in handy while working in a spa?
- Sit and have lunch with someone in school with whom you do not normally interact. Ask yourself why you do not normally interact with this person. What judgments have you been making? What do you learn through the experience?
- The next time you are bored, ask yourself what it is that you are avoiding doing. Get up and do it.
- To learn viscerally about service, volunteer for a day at a community soup kitchen, Habitat for Humanity, or a similar organization. Write a page or two about your experience afterward.
- Go to the most expensive spa in town and receive their signature treatment. Dress and act the part of a well-heeled client. Do not mention to anyone that you are "just a massage student." How does the staff treat you? How do you like it? What does this teach you about how you can treat others in the spa?

as a well-adjusted member of this marvelous spa team. Am I not truly blessed?" While it might help to talk to yourself in these positive terms, a truly positive attitude is cultivated through actions rather than just words. Sometimes, what you do speaks louder to yourself than what you say.

Comportment

Your on-the-job **comportment** can be defined as the dignified way in which you handle yourself in all situations, day to day, minute by minute, at the spa. While you are at work, you will definitely be "on," in the same way that an actor is on when she is acting before the camera or an audience. You will, in a sense, be playing a role. Truly talented individuals do this in a way that seems absolutely authentic and natural to the client. You may have noticed this in a fine dining establishment. The waiters often appear more relaxed and personable than at lesser restaurants, but their seemingly effortless friendliness is in fact a cultivated skill. It is not easy to be personable, warm, friendly, and attentive on demand, with perfect strangers, but the people who do it well make it feel easy. And this very high bar is your mandate in the spa setting, where guests harbor such high expectations—perhaps the highest in any industry.

comportment

the dignified way in which you handle yourself in all situations

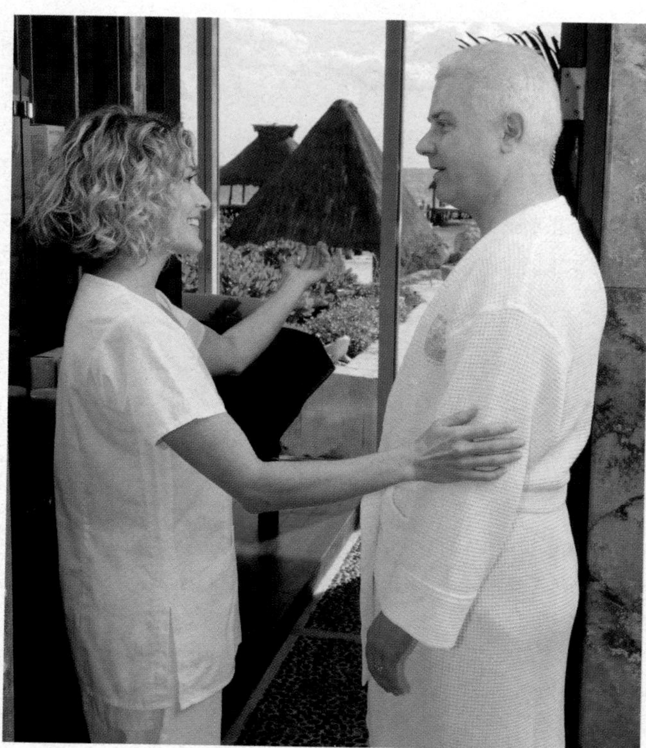

FIGURE 15–5 Effortless professionalism is something that must be cultivated over time.

How can you go about attaining this state of friendly, effortless professionalism? It is something that must be cultivated over time, and one of the best ways to achieve it is to model someone who does it well (Figure 15–5). Splurge on dinner at the best restaurant in town for the express purpose of learning about comportment from the waitstaff. Observe closely. Take notes. Copy them.

Professional comportment is especially important in times of stress. When the spa's laundry machines boil over and suds are streaming down the treatment room hallway, it is not time to run screaming for your life. It is time, rather, to look out even more assiduously for the welfare and comfort of the guests. In times of stress, proper comportment in the spa means you will:

- Remain calm.
- Help others first when you are not in danger.
- Refrain from causing undue alarm.
- Discreetly apprise the manager of any problems.
- Quietly contact the proper authorities if necessary.

Dress

When you work at a spa, you will most likely be expected to wear some kind of uniform. For some massage therapists, this will not be a problem. For others, however, wearing a uniform, which by definition makes them look quite similar

ACTIVITY

Improving Comportment Skills in the Spa

You can try these exercises to stretch your "comportment muscles" in the spa setting:

- Ask someone, out of the blue, if there is anything you can do for them. Then immediately do it for them.
- The next time somebody asks you for something, go out of your way and surprise them with your generosity, swiftness, and sensitivity.
- Guess what someone is going to want before they even decide consciously to want it, and then provide it for them.
- Act in a dignified manner in a situation that does not particularly call for it. The next time you are shopping at a drugstore, for instance, say to the clerk, "Would you be so kind as to help me find the Vaseline Intensive Care Lotion? Thank you ever so much."
- In whatever employee or student capacity you now serve, spend a day acting in the most dignified and respectful manner you know how. Behave as if everyone around you is a guest and you are a concierge at the Ritz. How do people respond differently to you when you act this way?

to everyone else, is akin to wearing a steel cage over their entire body. Creativity dies. Individuality dies. The soul shrivels up in a short-sleeved polo.

Even if you are not opposed to polo shirts and Bermuda shorts (or whatever outfit in which the spa deems it fit to deck out their crew), you would probably rather wear your own comfortable clothes. There is no doubt that you will look less individualistic in the spa's choice of clothes. And it would be wonderful if you were at a different stage in your life, a stage in which you were the one making the fashion statements and the fashion rules, a stage in which nobody else could enforce some kind of arbitrary code on your personal style. But that is not the stage you are going through if you are moving into the spa therapist workforce. You are instead moving into the stage of communal effort, and the more you fight against the outward signs of this communality, of which the uniform is perhaps the most visible sign, the more you will actually be struggling against your own success.

Go ahead. Give in. Just be one of the crowd for a change. What have you got to lose by exploring this aspect of your humanity? While your individuality may be one of your most prized "possessions," it is also something that you need to let go of at some point. Pitching in as part of a team of like-minded, like-intentioned—and yes, even like-uniformed—people to attain a specific goal (customer satisfaction and superlative spa service) is one way for you to get to know an aspect of your personality that has perhaps gone unexplored up to this point (Figure 15–6).

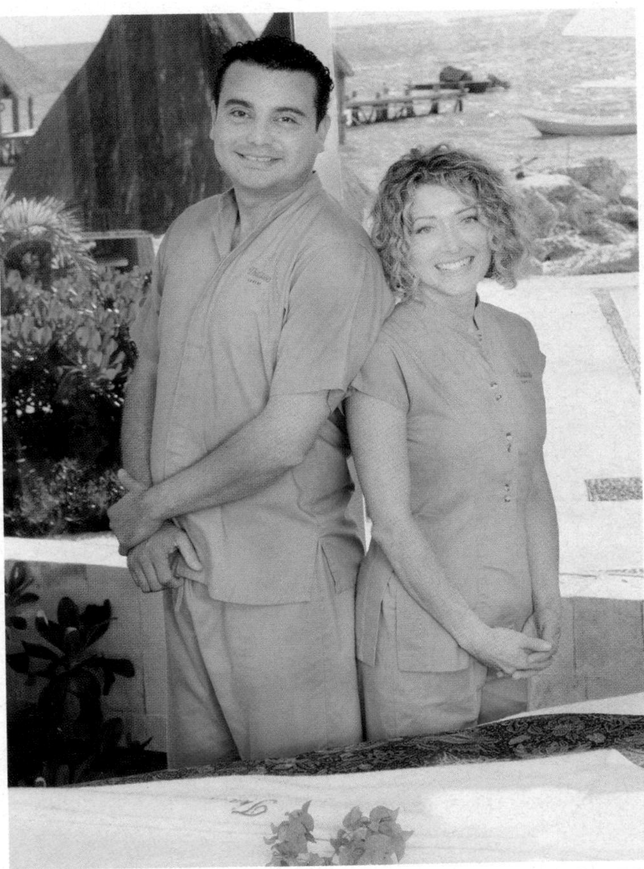

FIGURE 15–6 Wearing a spa uniform does not lessen individuality but rather reinforces a commitment to consistent customer service.

One other thing you should know about spa uniforms is that there has never been one made that can satisfy an entire staff of therapists. Certain employees are bound to be unhappy with the choice of color, or fabric, or dye in the fabric, or weave, or thread count, or country of manufacture, or philosophy of the company that manufactures it, and so on. It is absolutely impossible to get everyone to agree on one outfit. Therefore, though it might seem autocratic to you, it is in everyone's best interest for the spa director, owner, or manager to choose the uniform. Receiving input from the staff can sometimes be helpful but is often counterproductive as it sets up tensions between competing camps. Short sleeve or long? Cotton or breathable synthetics? Celestial blue or neutral beige? In this one aspect of your life, it is advisable to let others dictate your dress code for several hours each day.

Grooming

In addition to the dress code at spas, you will also have to adhere to the grooming rules (Figure 15–7). These are equally important, as there is often someone among the ranks who will agree to wearing a uniform but then atone for this self-perceived "sellout" through aggressive grooming strategies. To counteract this,

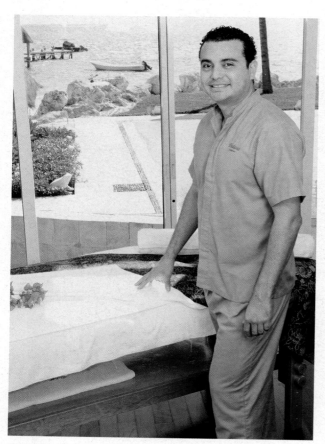

FIGURE 15–7 Spa therapists should give management no reason to question their grooming habits.

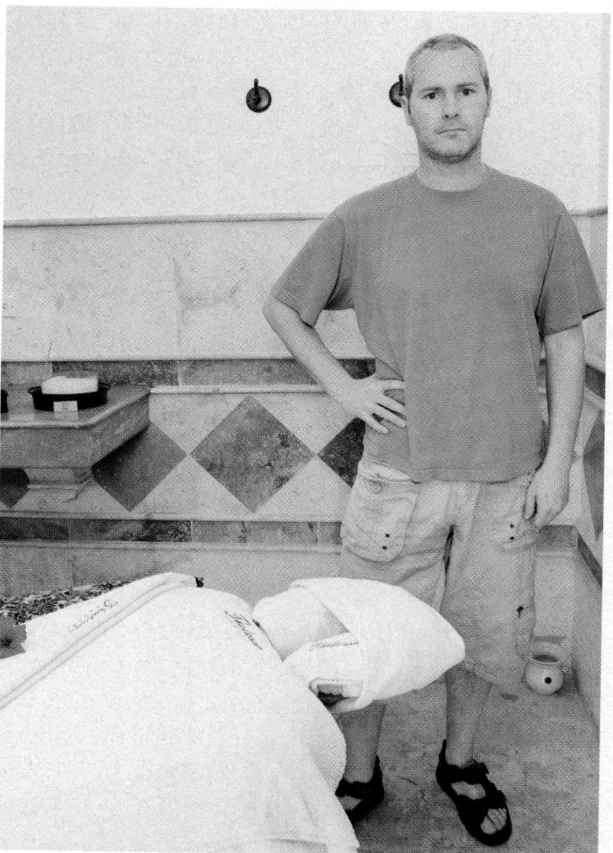

FIGURE 15–8 Poorly groomed therapists can make spa clients uncomfortable.

most spas have instituted a list of grooming rules. Some of the more common ones you are likely to run into as a spa employee include:

- No visible piercings except for one on each earlobe for women
- No facial hair on men
- Hair must be neat and tidy
- Hair off the shoulders for men
- Hair tied back or in a bun for women
- No visible tattoos (or only small, inconspicuous ones)
- Shorts must be mid-thigh or longer
- Shirts must have sleeves
- Shirts must be tucked in
- Uniforms must be kept clean and wrinkle-free
- Shoes must be clean and new-looking
- No sandals
- No gum chewing

Keep in mind that spas usually institute these rules out of fear—fear that letting one therapist express individuality through grooming would lead to an entire staff's being mismatched and untidy. This fear is very real for spa owners, and for good reason. Spas are in the tricky situation of having to cater to a discriminating, mostly clean-cut clientele, while at the same time having to hire from a pool of individuals who are often eclectic with their grooming habits (Figure 15–8).

Did You Know?

Top Behavioral Characteristics of a Successful Spa Therapist As Listed by Top Spa Directors

A group of twelve spa directors from top U.S. spas were gathered at a symposium and asked what the top characteristics were on which they judged massage therapy job candidates. Each director had his or her own view on the importance of various qualities, so none could be ranked as more important than another. These, in random order, were their responses:

- Team player
- Responsible
- Caring and open-hearted
- Open-minded
- Mature
- Good communicator
- Positive
- Calm under pressure
- Honest/trustworthy
- Able to follow instructions
- Passionate about doing spa work and massage
- Healthy/leading a healthy lifestyle
- Customer-service–oriented
- Sales-oriented
- Common sense
- Ability to accept change
- Humility
- Desire for continuous improvement—how many classes have they taken?
- History of success/longevity in positions
- Neatness/tidiness

One of your objectives, as far as attaining and retaining the spa work you desire, should be to give spa management absolutely no reason to question your grooming habits. Notice that this does not mean you cannot pierce, tattoo, and adorn yourself in any number of ways. It just means that nobody can see it in public while on the job.

SPA ETHICS

Much has been written about ethics for the massage therapist, and it is no wonder. Few professions allow so much private time to be shared between client and provider. The lines between familiarity and professionalism must be drawn and redrawn again and again by therapists in their treatment rooms with their clients. While ethics are a vital part of the massage profession as a whole, they play an especially crucial role in the spa, because spas become by default liable for any questionable ethical behavior on the part of the therapists who work in them. So, when you work in a spa, not only will you have your own reputation and that of your profession to uphold, but the reputation and financial well-being of your employer as well. This can be serious business. Spas have closed and careers have been ruined because of ethical issues. When it comes down to it, we can use plain language to describe the two basic ethical categories that are of primary concern in the spa environment: sex and money.

Sexual Issues

Spas sometimes create a carefree atmosphere in which certain guests, away from their normal lives for a time, feel at liberty to behave in ways that do not conform to their customary moral standards. In other words, they're looking to "have some fun." The most accessible employee at the spa with whom to have this fun will most likely be the massage therapist. How should you react?

One of the most powerful forces at work in humanity, and all life on the planet, for that matter, is sexuality. It is the drive to continue life, and it cannot be denied. There is no use trying to suppress it. Look what happened to the Victorians, with their tight bodices and copious Freudian syndromes. Some clients may find it difficult to ignore this drive when it surfaces during a massage or spa therapy session, and this is when your professionalism will be most needed. There are several ways to handle such situations, depending on the seriousness of the circumstances:

1. Ignore it. If the client simply exhibits signs of arousal but is not attempting to initiate any improper contact, perhaps it is unintentional. To save both of you embarrassment, proceed with the treatment.
2. Issue a verbal warning. If the client makes you feel uncomfortable in any way, communicate this verbally. Then proceed with the treatment if the client ceases the behavior.
3. Terminate the session. If the client makes you uncomfortable in any way and does not respond to a verbal warning, cease the session and leave the room.
4. Contact a supervisor or director. If you were forced to stop the session, report the incident to the spa supervisor, director or manager so that appropriate actions can be taken to avoid future incidents. Some spas have a policy of reporting any incident in the treatment room that made you feel uncomfortable. Always follow the guidelines of your particular spa.

There have been occasions when a therapist has been the guilty party and exhibited unethical behavior in the spa setting. You do not need to be reminded about what these behaviors are, because training in ethics is part of your core massage education. There are several considerations to take into account before you head down this path. If you were found to be engaging in unethical behavior in the spa, you could:

- lose your job
- get arrested and be put in jail

- be shamed publicly (one therapist was pulled out of the treatment room in the middle of a session and led away in handcuffs in front of the entire staff)
- be sued for all your money, plus the money that an insurer may have to pay on your behalf, making you uninsurable in the future
- find yourself unable to practice in your profession ever again, thus wasting the large investment of time and money you made in your education
- perhaps worst of all, lose faith in yourself

Speaking honestly, it has to be admitted that attractions do sometimes occur between client and therapist in the spa setting. Couples have met in this setting. Bonds have formed, marriages have taken place, children have been born and lives changed. If the first time you lay eyes upon your future spouse, he or she is lying on your treatment table prior to receiving a European Rose Clay wrap with ingredients from the south of France, well, there is no denying your destiny. There are certain steps you should take, however, to save yourself, your boss, the spa, and your guest/future spouse a great deal of grief.

- First, refrain from any unprofessional or overly familiar conduct or conversation while actually in the treatment room. Polite conversation, as you would engage in with any guest, is of course appropriate.
- Then, only at the guest's instigation, agree to continue this polite conversation after the treatment session is over.
- If both of you agree that you want to continue the conversation in a public space outside of the spa at some future time, then you can interact as two individuals instead of under the constraints of the client/therapist relationship.
- If you do meet socially, then do not meet professionally at the spa any longer, as this may lead to over-familiarity in a setting that is not appropriate.

Many people recommend that there be no social contact between staff and guests. In fact, many spas have that rule written down in their employee guidelines. In this case, it is best to try and follow these rules. But reality is reality. It has happened in the past and it will happen again in the future: hearts meet under diverse circumstances and there is no rule or regulation that can keep them apart. If you feel this happening, observe the precautions above and you may survive with job (and heart) intact.

Money Issues

As you read these words, a furious ethical debate is being waged within the spa industry regarding money. It has been waged for years, and it will continue to be waged for years to come. The battle is being fought on four main fronts:

- The ethics of retail sales
- The ethics of taking spa clients as private clients
- The ethics of accepting/asking for tips
- The ethics of appropriate compensation

The Ethics of Sales

A much more thorough discussion of this topic is found in Chapter 16, but here we will focus for a moment on the ethical side of this question. Is it ethically acceptable for therapists to sell retail products in the spa? To many people, this might seem like a silly question. Spa directors will say, "Are you crazy? Of course it's acceptable, and in fact retail sales is one of the primary components of a spa therapist's job description." On the other hand, many therapists will assert with equal fervor that "It is wrong and ethically reprehensible for a therapist to sell retail products. Would a doctor sell drugs directly to his patients? Why should I?"

You can imagine the tension that these two opposing views often cause in the management/staff relationship at many spas. Part of this strain is unnecessary. It can be stated right here and right now that there is in fact no rule in any major massage association's code of ethics stating that it is not permissible for therapists to sell products to their clients. So, in that sense, retail is not wrong. In another sense, however, it is sometimes suggested to therapists during their education that retail should remain outside their realm of expertise.

If you are firmly set against selling any retail products on ethical grounds, you may find it difficult to get or keep good work in the spa industry. Though there are certainly many spa therapist positions that do not require retailing, it is increasingly common for management to expect at least a modicum of effort from you on that front. As far as the development of your own career goes, it is crucial for you to understand the importance of retail sales, especially if you want to open your own spa-oriented practice some day.

Perhaps it is more useful to look upon this not as an ethical issue but as a practical one. Do you want to do what most spa directors and supervisors want you to do? Or not? If not, steer yourself away from that path, and make sure that you are scrupulously honest with yourself and with any spas where you apply for a job. Do not try and "fake it," pretending that you are willing to do retail sales just in order to get the job. Soon enough, your true feelings will become apparent, causing an uncomfortable situation for all involved.

The Ethics of Taking Spa Clients as Private Clients

This has been another area of strain between staff and management over the years. Is it ethically okay to treat the spa's clients outside of the spa? One thing is clear: It is absolutely wrong to solicit a client you meet in the spa, asking him if he would like you to give him a private treatment in his home. But what about those occasions when a spa guest solicits you? What should you say when she is asking you to please come to her home to give massages to her and her husband? On the one hand, you will be counting the money in your mind, quickly calculating that you will make a good deal more money in this manner than you would in the same amount of time working at the spa. On the other hand, is it right for you to take away the spa's business in this manner? And finally, what about the client? After all, wasn't it the spa director who said that the customer is always right? This guest is going to be getting private massages from somebody and paying good money for it. Why shouldn't that somebody be you?

What a dilemma! What should you do? Although you will have to look into your own heart and make your own decision there in the privacy of the treatment room, the best course for you to take is probably to follow these three easy steps:

1. Consider the spa's written rules on this subject. Is it strictly forbidden to accept outside clients whom you first met at the spa? If the answer is yes, then skip to step 2. If the answer is no, then go ahead and happily accept the request, giving the client your personal card so she can contact you at her leisure. If you do not know the answer, then you should find out from somebody what the prevailing attitude of management is toward this subject. Some spas have an unspoken rule that taking outside clients is forbidden, and management will tell you so if asked, but there is also an unspoken policy of in effect looking the other way if the clients remain happy and also continue coming to the spa. This "gray area" can be tricky to deal with, and you would be well-advised to consult a senior therapist on staff regarding the situation.
2. Tell the client that you would love to give her a massage in the comfort of her own home but then inform her about the rule against taking clients outside the spa. She may perhaps choose to ask your spa director personally if it is all right for you to give her a private treatment, or she may just take your answer at face value and the conversation will stop there. If you choose to avoid the spa's rule and "sneak" this person onto your private client list, you should be prepared to face the consequences if you are caught, which may include termination of employment. Also be aware that you will have to deal with the internal tension of knowing you are breaking the rules your employer has set.
3. Whatever the outcome of the situation, keep the spa's interests uppermost in your mind. If you do end up treating the client privately, remind her how happy you would be to see her at the spa again to give her one of the services it is impossible to administer at home. Without the spa, you would not have met this client in the first place. A grateful attitude and a mutually beneficial relationship are essential if you want to continue your employment. If you do not have the opportunity to treat this client privately, do not harbor a grudge against management. The rules are the rules. If you cannot abide by them, you are free to seek employment elsewhere. In the meantime, being the best spa employee you can be means overcoming the tendency to judge and blame.

The Ethics of Accepting/Asking for Tips

In spas, it is almost always appropriate to accept tips, but it is never appropriate to ask for them. Usually, the spa will have a written policy on this topic that clients can read in a brochure or on the list of services. It is not your job to solicit or collect tips for yourself. However, if a client hands you a tip directly, it is appropriate to accept it graciously. Often, clients will leave a tip for you at the spa desk or with the locker-room attendant.

Do not concern yourself with collecting these gratuities. Always perform your duties briskly and efficiently, especially when escorting the guest back to the front desk or changing area. Do not linger expecting a cash handout. If a client feels you waiting around, he may become uncomfortable.

Some therapists feel that it is not appropriate to accept tips. They argue that doctors and physical therapists do not accept tips, so why should massage therapists? If you are one of these therapists, then you have two options:

- Seek work in the medical or clinical fields, not the spa industry.
- When working in the spa, graciously accept tips anyway.

If you were to work in a spa and not accept tips, you would be upsetting normal operating procedures. By making an issue about your personal feelings on the topic, you can confuse guests and alienate other therapists. If you feel very strongly about it, you can decide to donate all of your tips earned at the spa to a certain charity, or you can distribute them to the locker-room staff. Of course, the option of leaving and seeking a job in a clinic or medical office is always open.

Because massage therapists work in so many fields, it is difficult to come up with one blanket rule that is appropriate for them all. Perhaps what is needed are separate designations for spa therapists, medical therapists, and others, each with an appropriate ethic regarding the issue of tipping. We do not have these designations available yet (at least not in the U.S., though they are in force in certain Canadian provinces), so for now, if you choose by default to define yourself as a "spa therapist" by accepting employment in a spa, you will do best to accept the practices in effect there. Go ahead, take the tip.

The Ethics of Appropriate Compensation

You might think it unusual to find a mention of compensation under the heading of ethics, but ask yourself this one question: Is it ethical for you to be compensated so well that you help to slowly, painfully put the spa right out of business? This is exactly what many therapists, either knowingly or unknowingly, do when they accept wages of 40 percent, 50 percent, or even more of the spa's total service revenue. Is it really fair for you to expect such high wages? Do you fully appreciate the huge overhead costs involved with running a spa? Have you educated yourself about the realities of doing business in the spa industry? Do you understand the spa owner's point of view as well as your own, and want to grow within the spa industry in a sustainable way, or are you there simply for your own profit, ready to move on once the business tanks?

Ask yourself these questions and consider your own personal ethics for a moment.

SPA ETIQUETTE

Etiquette can be defined as the rules governing socially acceptable behavior in a particular situation, and when it comes to etiquette in spas, much depends upon the type of spa, geographic location, guest demographics, and overall management strategy. Some spas are more laid-back and informal, such as many properties in the islands or in outback wilderness locations. Other urban spas are the epitome of chic and require a hushed, delicate demeanor on the part of their therapists. Wherever you find yourself, it is important for guest satisfaction, not to mention your own job security, that you always operate within the parameters of your spa's etiquette guidelines. Often, these guidelines are unwritten. At times, they are not even spoken of, and you will be left to your own devices to decipher and implement the underlying principles that guide many of the activities and interactions in your workplace. This is true not just for spas but for life in general. Note that columnist Emily Post became famous by explaining at length the usually unspoken rules governing our behavior in a wide spectrum of situations. When you are not sure about the proper etiquette in a given situation, aim for "polite yet personable." It is better to be circumspect and perhaps overly cautious, erring on the side of propriety, rather than to be too informal. In the following sections you will find seven points of etiquette for you to consider in each of three main settings in the spa: in the treatment room, outside the treatment room, and outside the spa.

Etiquette Inside the Treatment Room

An entirely unique set of etiquette guidelines exist for interactions between spa guests and therapists inside the treatment room. This is one of the rare circumstances when individuals come into such close contact after so brief an introduction. In a private massage practice, client and therapist usually have more interaction prior to the first service, and there is often an introduction or referral by another client. In the spa, client and therapist often meet just moments before their first session and have very little time, if any, to review an intake form or get to know each other. Therefore, your skills at handling the etiquette for this particular situation are of the utmost importance.

- Make sure that guests feel comfortable about the process of getting undressed and being undressed in your treatment room. Do not assume that they have disrobed in a small room with a stranger waiting outside before, and be aware that they may experience considerable anxiety regarding this process, which may be second nature to you. Verbal communication and a gentle demeanor are essential at this point. Explain the disrobing process thoroughly, saying, "You can disrobe to the level of your comfort, leaving on shorts or undergarments if you are more comfortable that way. I will leave the room while you disrobe and will knock before reentering."
- After your initial interchange regarding the massage or spa therapy you will be administering, leave it to the guest to initiate further conversation. If he wishes, the session should be performed in silence.
- Leave it to the guest to decide about music. Just because you're a fan of Native American flutes doesn't mean that silence or some other musical option are not appropriate for the guest. Even upbeat reggae, jazz, or soft rock are preferred by some clients. If you can change the music in the treatment room to suit the guest's preference, do so.

- The guest is always right about temperature. Even if you feel that 80°F is plenty warm enough, raise the thermostat further if the guest requests it and you are able to adjust the treatment room temperature. If not, add blankets or a table warmer.
- If the guest attempts to gossip with you about other spa guests or employees, refrain from engaging in the conversation, stating that it is against spa policies.
- Ask the guest on more than one occasion during the treatment whether he is comfortable. Often, guests will avoid complaint if not asked repeatedly to state their comfort level or ongoing satisfaction with the treatment while it proceeds.
- Steer guests gently away from over-confiding their private information to you. Though the circumstances of a massage or spa treatment lead to confidential sharing, you should not encourage a disclosure of private matters that could make the guest uncomfortable in retrospect.

Etiquette Outside the Treatment Room

When you are outside the treatment room, your interaction with guests should be as proper and hospitality-oriented as any other employee's. Just because you are a trained therapist does not mean that you can get by with less of a focus on proper etiquette when you are not actually administering therapy. Some therapists, when they first find employment at a spa, assume that they are somehow above the rules of conduct that apply to other non-therapist employees. Do not make this mistake. Follow the normal forms of etiquette outside the treatment room as well.

- Greet the guest with a firm, professional handshake when you first meet. Though you might think it is more gentle and "spa-like," a weak handshake does not inspire confidence.
- Lead the way to the treatment room. Even though it is customary for men to let women pass through doorways and other passages first and for hosts to allow their guests to go first, in this instance, you are the one who knows where to go and what awaits on the other side. Spa guests are more comfortable and reassured if you enter first.
- When you are done with the treatment and have left the room, stay close by so you can reorient the guest and guide her back to "reality." Do not allow the guest to flounder after leaving the treatment room.
- Unless it is against spa policy, offer a glass of water, ice tea, or fruit beverage after the session is over. This small gesture goes a long way in making the guest feel cared for.
- If you see a guest who needs assistance of any kind in any area of the spa, offer it immediately. If you are late for an appointment, tell the guest that you will send someone else to help with the problem, then proceed to the appointment.
- Never discuss a guest's problems or personal situation with other guests or fellow employees in the spa.

- Even when you think there are no guests present, behave in a decorous manner; spas are in some ways "glass houses," and your actions can be witnessed and commented upon by guests at any time.

Etiquette Outside the Spa

Though you may seldom come in contact with your spa's guests outside of the actual spa, it is still important to know how to act on such occasions. For that reason, keep these few etiquette guidelines in mind.

- Treat guests you see outside of the spa in the same manner you do inside, being both professional and personable.
- When meeting a spa guest in public, do not discuss other guests or the internal workings of the spa.
- If it is part of spa policy, call the guest several days after the appointment to see how effective the treatment was and how he is feeling. If it is against spa policy, do not make this call, but you may want to suggest this option to spa management if they have not considered it before, as it increases customer loyalty.
- Treat all the surrounding property, parking lots, and public areas the same as the spa itself, and behave in a manner consistent with spa policies while in these areas.
- Whenever you are wearing your spa uniform, even off property, you are representing the spa. Assume a professional, friendly demeanor and do not engage in any activities that would discredit the spa.
- When you run into spa clients outside the spa (in the grocery store, for example), refer to them by their last names ("Mrs. Smith" rather than "Betty"), as you are still on a professional standing with them even though you are outside of the spa.
- While representing the spa at off-site events such as health fairs, observe all dress, grooming, and comportment guidelines as addressed earlier in this chapter.

YOUR JOB DESCRIPTION AND BEYOND

When you work as a therapist in a spa, chances are good that you'll be asked to follow the guidelines written in a document called a **job description**. "What's that for?" you may wonder. "Why do I need someone to describe what I already know how to do—massage people?"

job description

document containing written guidelines and requirements for employees who are performing a particular job

As you are no doubt beginning to understand, becoming a successful spa therapist is about much more than just giving massages and spa treatments. In fact, that is just the tip of the iceberg, the visible commonality that makes the job seem so simple to the casual observer. Think of a champion race car driver or a top professional golfer. On the outside, they are doing precisely the same things that everybody else around them is doing. On the inside, however, they must be doing something different to consistently come out on top. What is that special invisible something? It has been called many things, such as talent, concentration, focus, flow and even the "X factor." What all these states have in common is that they describe a mental reality, as compared to a physical one. So, in the same way, what will make you a great spa therapist is not so much what you will be physically doing while performing your duties—although that is important and you'll need to have skill in this area. What really matters is what is going on inside your mind—how you are describing your actions to yourself, the inner narrative. What matters is your concentration, your focus, your flow, the elusive "**spa X factor**" of an excellent tuned-in therapist.

spa X factor
the invisible mental reality created by excellent tuned-in therapists who, through concentration and focus on their own inner narrative, attempt to continually improve performance

A good job description will help you achieve these states of mind in several ways:

- Just as a yoga teacher guides you into new awareness of your body during practice, a good job description will guide you into a new awareness of precisely what it is you are doing while working as a spa therapist.
- It will serve as a guidepost for all of those moments when you are not giving treatments and need to stock, refill, replenish, clean, and prepare the treatment space.
- It will instruct you in "relationship management," which is a crucial part of working in any spa, showing the proper patterns of interaction between you and other employees, clearly laying out who has authority over you and in what ways you are autonomous.
- It will give concrete guidelines regarding your responsibilities in other areas of the spa outside the treatment room, locker room, and front desk, outlining behavioral requirements and other duties while on the property at large.
- It will offer guidance regarding dress, deportment, and grooming.
- It will describe the proper role you will play for guests and what to do if improper conduct is encountered at any time by a guest or another employee.

When many therapists first see a spa therapist job description, they are surprised or even outraged. They think something like this: "According to what I see here, it looks like I will be expected to do many other things in the spa in addition to my massage and spa therapy work. This is not right. I went to school in order to learn specific skills, and I am here to heal and transform people, de-stressing them and improving their lives. I should not have to engage in menial tasks that will cause me to lose focus on my main intention. Won't these extraneous duties take away from my ability to perform the best therapy?"

The answer to this last question is an emphatic "no." Performing well as part of the spa team (see the section on teamwork at the end of this chapter) does not take away from your ability to perform well as a therapist. The two go hand in hand. When you are in the treatment room, your focus should be on your treatment and the customer-service interaction you are having with the guest. When you are not in session, however, it is important for you to keep your mind focused and to keep yourself engaged in the overall operation of the spa. The only time that you are not "on" is when you are backstage, behind the scenes, in the employee break room or cafeteria.

In order to be effective, a good job description must include enough information so that you are not left wondering about your responsibilities or your

Job Flow

Did You Know?

The following few paragraphs offer an example of a spa therapist's "job flow" as she moves from one part of her job description to another during a busy day. It is by necessity condensed and told in stream-of-consciousness from the therapist's point of view in order for you to better understand the sequence.

"Well, this session of craniosacral therapy is going really well and I feel some real progress with my guest today. She's already come in for three sessions this week, so she must feel the progress as well. Now, I just need to focus for the last five minutes of the session as we enter still point, that elusive quiet space where the body's rhythms slow down . . . focus, focus, focus. Ahhh. That's it.

"Time for the session to end. I'll let her have her space for a few minutes while I retrieve some water for her and see if my next guest is already in the waiting area. No, he's not there yet, so that gives me a little extra time with my last guest. Hmm, what's this? Somebody's left some used towels on the women's locker-room floor and none of the attendants has had a chance to pick them up yet. I'll just deposit them in the linen basket before any other guests wander through. That's it. Now, here's the water. Time to head back to my guest.

"Yes, I'll just give Mrs. Smith her water and assist her out to the lounge area. Everything okay with her? Yes. I've told her to make sure to take real good care of herself this evening since she's gone pretty deep into her own body and mind during our session today.

"Now onto the next client. Is he in the waiting room yet? No. Let's see, I'll visit the front to see if they have any news about him. Got to remember to stay out from behind the counter and let the receptionists do their job. No sign from the guest yet. A no-show? Hmmm, that gives me time to take care of some other business. I'll let the front desk know where I'll be, then head back to the supply room for some straightening up.

"It's good to have these few spare minutes to get our materials in order. During the day, we don't have a chance to pour mostly empty bottles of massage oil into newer ones, change the water in the hydrocollator unit, and retrieve extra sheets and towels from laundry downstairs. The spa used to have a staff of attendants who took care of this for us, but then the spa director explained how that was not necessary if we therapists pitched in together to do the side work. Now we each make $1 per hour more, which is not much, but it adds up.

"Hmm. What's that? Jamie from the front desk letting me know my guest has arrived, 15 minutes late. Not to worry. I'll be there. Have him escorted directly to my treatment room. It's a deep tissue massage, and it says on his intake form that he needs extra attention on his legs because he's an avid jogger. I'll explain that we might make the best use of his remaining time by focusing entirely on his legs to make it a sport-specific treatment. First I'd better pop into the herbal wrap room and make sure the sheets are soaking in the herbal solution because I have two back-to-back wraps coming up after this gentleman. Here we go."

relationships to the other individuals with whom you come into contact at the spa. Thus, the job description must by definition include several components:

- what you do
- what you do *not* do
- who your supervisor is
- whom you supervise
- the special ways in which you focus on guests

- the elements of customer service emphasized in your position
- those duties beyond your core responsibilities you should learn to master
- your proper interactions with all levels of co-workers
- an understanding of how your efforts contribute to the overall mission of the spa
- an understanding of how your efforts on the spa's behalf influence your progress along your own personal life and career paths

Take a look at the massage therapists' job description on the following page. The Mii amo Spa at the Enchantment resort in Sedona, Arizona, is not only one of the most stunningly beautiful spa settings in the world, it is also renowned for the quality of its treatment staff. Set in a dramatic red rock canyon which is still held sacred by Native Americans, the resort conjures up feelings of spirituality in many guests, and the spa offers several avenues through which to explore this. Mii amo has a Native American Program Director on staff and several treatments with a focus on consciousness exploration. Some of the staff therapists have advanced certifications in modalities that open guests' minds, hearts, and emotions to new experiences. Yet, in spite of the spa's serious emphasis on advanced modalities and Native American–influenced spirituality, the very first line in the job description for therapists on staff includes these words: "The Massage Therapist . . . is involved in the operation of the spa and guest service."

Notice the key words in that sentence: "operation" and "guest service." You can see by this how important those two areas are to the spa's management. Even though the therapists' first priority is to provide high-quality therapy, of equal value to the spa is their ability to provide operational support and first-class guest service. What does this tell you about where your own priorities should be when you go in for a job interview at a spa? What will the spa director be looking for in addition to good hands-on technique? How can you prepare yourself for a position that has such a major focus on service and operations?

TEAMWORK, TEAMWORK, RAH! RAH! RAH!

How many professionals can say they are as independent as massage therapists? Almost everyone needs some kind of support structure: The chiropractor needs a receptionist and billing specialist; the librarian needs an assistant; even the lone telephone repairman needs a telephone company to work for. But as a massage therapist, you have the ability to work completely free of all other professional support. Once you have your table and your phone, you are in business. This fierce independent streak is one of the main reasons, consciously or unconsciously, that many people pursue the career of massage in the first place. The moment you walk through the door of a spa your first day on the job, however, that independence will vanish. For as long as your work in the spa industry, you will be irrevocably part of a team.

It is important to remember this.

When you are behind closed doors, alone with one client at a time all day long, it is easy to forget that you are part of a team. There, with the music playing, the lights down low, and your hands on one person who appreciates you (only you!), a

Did You Know?

Job Description for Mii amo Spa at the Enchantment Resort, Sedona, Arizona

Job Title: Massage Therapist
Department: Mii amo Spa

Level: V

Basic Function

The Massage Therapist provides professional massage at the Spa, and is involved in the operation of the spa and guest service. The Massage Therapist will provide the type of treatment requested by the guest. This will not be changed at the Massage Therapist's discretion without consent of the guest. All massage therapist job descriptions & SOPs [Standard Operating Procedures] apply to this position.

Work Performed

- Read and adhere to schedule postings in regards to shifts, room assignments, and the computerscheduling system.
- Provide professional massage (accordance with accepted industry practices) and consistent manner at the spa. Provide all guests with consistent services even when booked by the hour for a six-and-a-half-hour period. Massage & treatment durations include 60, 75, and 90 minute. Be qualified for 80% of the massage & treatment services offered (100% of "Mii amo" treatments) at Mii amo.
- Assist and perform daily prep work duties such as restocking rooms, refilling bottles, helping team keep prep rooms clean and organized, and keeping rooms clean. During down time, assist with duties as directed by Director of Spa Operations or Treatment Supervisor.
- Lead by example and be an effective role model for guests and staff. Maintain a co-operative team attitude with co-workers.
- Be prompt with appointments, quality of work, and attitudes with guests. Begin services on time and perform all services within the time frame established for each treatment.
- Properly educate guests in regards to all massage and treatments. Promote spa and all services, products and programs.

Supervision Exercised: None
Supervision Received: Treatment Supervisor and Director of Spa Operations

Responsibility & Authority

- Exhibit proper use of product and abide by all product control guidelines. Maintain and ensure adherence to service standards.
- Maintain & reinforce a safe work environment by filling out maintenance request forms and suggesting improvements of procedures, etc.
- Read and adhere to scheduled postings and memos in regards to shifts, room assignments, and the computer scheduling system.
- Be informed about policy, procedures, and communication. Read all memos and staff communications. Attend training and meetings as requested.
- Wear proper uniform and maintain a high standard in regard to personal appearance as outlined in the employee handbook.
- Keep an open communication to other staff and management.
- Keep communication with guest to a minimum, as well as on a professional level, only to be initiated by the guest. At no time will the solicitation of gratuities be tolerated.
- Therapist is empowered to determine when to terminate a massage in the event it becomes unprofessional and/or uncomfortable for either party.

(Continued)

Job Description for Mii amo Spa at the Enchantment Resort, Sedona, Arizona *continued*

Did You Know?

Minimum Requirements

Essential: Current (National) Certification with a minimum of 500 hours of training in Massage Therapy required. National Certification is preferred.

Must possess basic computer knowledge. Must possess good communication with guests and staff. Ensure that the guests feel comfortable during treatment. Must be able to adhere to hotel policy and procedure.

Physical Requirements

Lifting up to 50 pounds

Be able to maintain a schedule of:

- 10 % Sitting
- 20 % Bending
- 50 % Standing
- 20 % Walking

Manual and Hearing Dexterity

Approved by

I have reviewed and understand this job description.

____

Employee Signature/Date

Job description courtesy of Mii amo Spa at Enchantment resort, Sedona, Arizona. Used with permission.

certain rebel voice begins to speak softly into your ear: "Hey, it's you this client is paying to be with. And it's you who should be receiving more of the money. The rest of this place is basically a fancy hotel. Without you, there is no spa! Shouldn't they be paying you more? Shouldn't you be allowed to make your own schedule? And what's up with all these rules and regulations and the constant cheerleading? Teamwork, teamwork, rah rah rah. You don't need any of it. You're independent, strong, a lone wolf."

Sound familiar? It is an all-too-common refrain within the minds of spa therapists or would-be spa therapists. However, the reality is exactly the opposite of this fantasy. Without the spa, there would be no clients. There would be no job. There would be no therapists needed.

You can rest assured that behind the closed door of her office, the spa director of such a crew is having similar fantasies about running an enterprise that does not have to deal with the whims, stubbornness, and fierce independence of a bunch of ungrateful, lone-wolf rebels. The spa–therapist relationship is a symbiotic one. It runs in both directions.

Which brings us once again to the golden rule of spa work: Treat the spa exactly as if you owned it. This is the most accelerated way to move forward in your spa career. No exceptions. No excuses.

If you were indeed the owner of the spa, you would want all the people working there to combine their efforts, present a united front, and become through

ACTIVITY

Write Your Own Job Description

One significant process that may help you understand the true requirements of your future job as a spa therapist is to write your own job description. Imagine yourself working in the most ideal spa environment in the world. This is your dream spa job come true, with all the pieces falling into place. The facility, your supervisor, the ownership, your co-workers, the equipment you use, the products you apply and recommend, and the guests themselves are the best you can imagine. You've just been told that you are in charge of creating the new job description for the therapists on staff. Using every ounce of your creativity, write a job description that fulfills your personal vision of what it should be like to work in the ideal spa. Feel free to improvise and be idealistic regarding your personal goals and the mission of the fictional spa you create. You can name the spa if you wish, and give it a geographic location if that helps make it easier for you to envision. Some questions you might ask yourself:

- How many other therapists does the spa have on staff?
- Which therapies do you perform?
- How extensive is the training?
- Are you paid for training?
- Who is your supervisor? What kind of controls does this person have over you?
- How often do you take breaks? What is the time between services?
- What policies are in place to avoid on-the-job injuries and repetitive stress?
- What channels are available to address problems you or other therapists have with management? With guests?
- How is your performance monitored? What feedback do you get? How are pay raises given?
- What are your retail responsibilities?

synergy something greater than the sum of their individual talents. This is the mission and this is the goal. How do you achieve that?

You might at first think it would be difficult to blend into a team if you spend 95 percent of your time at work behind closed doors away from the rest of your co-workers. This is not true. Ask anyone who works on the hospitality staff at a spa, at the front desk, or in management, and they will tell you that a team-oriented attitude on the part of the massage- and spa-treatment staff is absolutely essential for the overall functioning of the spa. Everything you do and say behind closed doors during that vast amount of quality time spent with the guests reflects mightily on the perceptions people have of the spa. It also impacts the way in which other employees view you and view each other. As a spa therapist, you are in a real sense setting the underlying tone of the entire operation. Although, as we've said before, it is counterproductive to think of yourself as a "rock star" and somehow above other people on the staff, it is wise to remember that your words and actions have a magnified impact simply because you spend more time with the guests than anybody else on staff, by a large margin.

A Team with a Mission

True teamwork can only be achieved if each separate player is dedicated to the stated mission of the overall enterprise. Thus, it is important to know what that mission is. This is what mission statements are all about. When you first walk into a spa and see a **mission statement** posted on the wall in the employee lounge,

mission statement
a summary describing the aims, values, and overall plan of an organization or individual

you might think it is irrelevant, or a ploy by management to keep people in line. Actually, when crafted skillfully and used effectively, mission statements can be important tools to improve the spa's overall functioning and, ultimately, its success.

The core components of a spa's mission statement can include references to some or all of the following categories:

- **Philosophy:** What are the strengths, beliefs, core values, aspirations, and philosophical priorities of the spa?
- **Customers and market:** Who are the spa's customers, and from what demographic market do they primarily come? How is this market reached?
- **Products and services:** What are the spa's most important products and services?
- **Commitment to success:** What plans does the spa have to achieve profitability tempered with sustainability?
- **Larger community:** What image and impact does the spa wish to project into the community at large?
- **Employees:** What is the spa's attitude toward employees?

Team Members

To truly understand the mission of any team, you need to know the roles and responsibilities of all the players. In a spa, this can be confusing. When you get your first spa job, you might be amazed at the wide range of specialists employed there. To play your part in the spa's mission, you'll need to interact effectively with each of these other people. Here, then, are some brief job descriptions for spa positions, with some suggestions as to how you as a massage therapist can best work with them as part of a successful team.

Locker-Room Attendants

Locker-room attendants are responsible for guest comfort from the moment the guest is "handed off" from the front desk. They are the intermediate stop between a guest's entrance to the spa and entrance into your treatment room. So, in that sense, they are important to how the guest is going to perceive what happens next. If the locker-room attendant is lackadaisical or inattentive, a guest's entire experience can be colored in the negative, thus making it harder for you to set things right and form a good impression through your hands-on work.

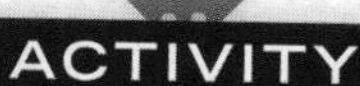

ACTIVITY

Create a Spa Mission Statement

Create a mission statement for a fictitious spa, incorporating the qualities listed above that you feel are most important. Make it appropriate for the ideal spa in which you would one day like to work. It should be 3 to 4 sentences long and should be something you actually believe yourself, or else others will not believe it. Get to the core values and avoid simply bragging about what a great spa this is. Some people believe the best mission statements are collaborative efforts between several or all members of the team. If you would like, work with a group of classmates to create a mission statement for your ideal spa.

Typically, a locker-room attendant's job is not excessively difficult. They hand guests towels and assign them a locker, leading them to the appropriate area and perhaps giving a short tour of the facilities. They also keep the locker, shower, bathrooms, and treatment areas clean. These simple tasks, however, can be performed either with enthusiasm or with disdain.

Relationship with Massage Therapists: Your job is made easier if the locker-room attendant is performing his well. Therefore, it is a good idea for you to assist in making the locker-room attendant look good and feel good about his job. When you are talking to a guest who has just been "handed off" to you via the locker-room staff, for example, you can say, "Has [locker-room attendant's name] been taking good care of you? He's the best." On other occasions, you can reaffirm your willingness to work with this person by freely doing a few chores for him. Picking up a used towel when it is not your job to pick it up goes a long way toward creating good therapist–attendant relations.

Spa Technicians

Typically, "spa techs" are in charge of performing jobs auxiliary to the core therapies, such as setting up treatment rooms and supplies, keeping staging areas well-stocked, and assisting therapists and supervisors in anything they may need. In some spas, they actually perform such non-massage services as herbal wraps. This depends upon the licensing laws of your state or province.

Relationship with Massage Therapists: Some spa attendants have the attitude that they are performing similar tasks as the therapists on staff, so why shouldn't they be paid the same? This can lead to jealousy problems, so it is a good idea to have an open line of communication between yourself and the "spa techs." Often, these individuals, with the right encouragement, will find that they would like to pursue a course of massage studies themselves and earn the right to the higher-paying positions.

Front Desk

These employees greet guests and set them up for their experience at the spa. Often, they are the first individuals that guests meet when they come in the door. In small spas, this position could be filled by the receptionist. They answer the phone, deal with guest questions, check guests in for their appointments, and often collect payments for services rendered. They often also make reservations for guests who call in or walk up to the desk, though this can be handled by reservation specialists in larger spas.

Relationship with Massage Therapists: One thing you want to remember is not to crowd the front-desk staff. Their desk is their domain, and frequently this domain is breached by therapists curious to know their schedules for the day. Resist the temptation to lean over or actually head behind the desk yourself to get information from the computer screen. This will create tension. It is best to form a relationship of mutual respect with these employees. Respect what they do in their space, and they will be more likely to respect you. How would you feel if a front-desk attendant walked into your treatment room during the middle of a session? Not good.

Keep in mind that these individuals may also be instrumental in closing any retail product sales in the spa. It is important for you to be on good terms with them so that they promote your interests in this regard, giving you credit when you have initiated a customer purchase but did not have time to close the sale yourself. Larger spas may have a dedicated retail specialist in the spa shop, and you should make similar efforts to gain the trust and support of this person.

Reservation Specialists

These employees work behind the scenes in larger spas, often in a room behind the front desk, booking massage and spa service reservations full-time for guests on the phone.

Relationship with Massage Therapists: Although it is sometimes not even necessary to get to know these folks because they are hidden away, you would be wise to make an effort to do so. Who do you think is lining up your appointments? Who do you think is talking to guests about which therapists are best? Who is trying to juggle multiple schedules and multiple requests at the same time? Who has control over part of your life? That's right, the reservationist. Smiles, praise, and personal touches like an unsolicited chair massage during a break go a long way toward making reservationists more sensitive to your happiness.

Supervisor

Most often, a "spa therapist supervisor" or "massage supervisor" or "services supervisor" is a therapist who has moved into this position after a certain period of employment at the spa. She can be in charge of setting up trainings, creating weekly schedules for the staff of therapists, and even payroll. The amount of managerial work the supervisor takes on depends greatly on the size of the spa and the role played by the spa manager or director. Some supervisors take on a great deal of responsibility.

Relationship with Massage Therapists: Because this person usually has risen from the ranks of the therapists, the supervisor quite often lends a sympathetic ear to the staff's concerns and complaints, acting as a liaison between the therapists and management when it comes time for negotiations of any kind. This position can also be coveted by many on the therapist staff, so she may be defensive at times with certain individuals. On the one hand, you will find it easy to relate to this individual because of your shared background in massage therapy. On the other hand, the supervisor may be trying to distance herself from the therapists while moving up the corporate ladder. It will be your task, then, to befriend that side that is sympathetic to your own position. Praise the climber. Befriend the therapist.

Spa Manager

The definition of a spa manager is quite broad and can range from a supervisory role with limited authority all the way to *de facto* spa director. The manager is usually responsible for the daily operations of the facility and staff. At larger properties, there is often a **manager on duty (MOD)** during off-hours, weekends, and nights, who sleeps on-site and is available in emergencies. This person can be from any department and does not need to be particularly well versed in spa services. The most important function of the manager is to keep things running smoothly. Some spas have both a manager and a director. Some spas have just one or the other.

manager on duty (MOD)

manager on-site after hours, sleeping over at (spa) facility to handle all concerns or emergencies should they arise when no other managers are present

Relationship with Massage Therapists: When the manager has risen from the ranks of hands-on staff, he is often customer-oriented and a good "people person." Spa managers who have come to the position from other management channels, perhaps even outside the spa industry, tend to be highly organized and detail-oriented, yet sometimes less well-versed in the essence of the therapist–guest interaction, which can lead to some communication problems. You have to determine with whom you are working and then act accordingly. For the therapist/manager, make it a point to discuss your dedication to the healing arts and your clients. For the manager/manager, make it a point to let him know how organized and detail-oriented you are. Show the manager some S.O.A.P notes, share your detailed client intake forms, meticulously take care of your treatment room, and stay strictly on schedule. In this way, you will forge strong bonds with the person in charge of making things run smoothly at the spa. If the manager knows that he can count on you, it can make your life easier and perhaps even improve your chances at success within the organization.

Spa Director

This position is often filled by the owner in smaller spas. In all spas, it is the position of highest authority within the spa itself, though an even higher authority may exist elsewhere, such as a general manager at a resort property or an owner at a large day spa. The spa director sets up guest expectation through maintenance of a certain ambience and underlying philosophy. She is often in charge of employee training, heads up guest relations, reports to the owner/board, is in charge of financial record keeping and is responsible for overall success, has the final word on who gets hired and who gets fired, and is the ultimate arbiter of any disputes. In smaller facilities, she may also be the PR and marketing/communications director, fundraiser, and even a hands-on operator, most often an esthetician or massage therapist.

Relationship with Massage Therapists: Like it or not, you as an underling of this person may very well have the tendency to think of the director in parental terms: the boss. The matriarch. She rules the roost. Therefore, she operates in another world than the one with which you are familiar, and can thus be judged as an "other."

This is a mistake.

Casting the spa director into a parental authoritarian role is an unconscious tendency. Most of us do the same thing with our bosses in any job. Yet even though the situation is so common, it is counterproductive to your ultimate goals in the spa industry. You want to grow and be successful. Perhaps you want to open your own spa one day. At the very least, you want an opportunity to improve your earnings and increase your job security over time. By creating an ongoing antagonism between yourself and the "authority figure," you undermine these goals.

How do you avoid this problem? Basically, you have to put yourself in the spa director's shoes. Think of her situation, how difficult it is to manage a staff of people and keep the guests happy at the same time. Know that much of what you might experience as "standoffishness" is actually a defensive reaction to protect herself from the constant squabbling of all those surrogate children on the staff. Instead of subtly working against the director, support her, in the same way in which you support any other person on the team. Align your mission with the director's mission within your own mind, and you will more swiftly move to her level: a level of authority. This does not mean that you will necessarily move into a management position in the spa industry if you do not want to, but it does mean that you will learn to manage your own career more capably, wherever it may take you.

Hospitality Specialists

Be they called *spa concierges, hostesses, guest specialists,* or *spa program coordinators,* these employees arrange guests' experience at the spa, often acting in an assessment capacity during the intake process when guests first arrive. They query guests regarding their situations and build programs to suit their needs, including the most appropriate therapies, esthetic services, and—in some spas—medical, fitness, and nutrition services as well. In smaller day spas, this capacity is often filled by receptionists or front-desk personnel who are responsible for guiding guests into the spa experience.

Relationship with Massage Therapists: Hospitality specialists play an important role in the spa. They can make the difference between a guest signing up for just a massage or an entire "personal path spa package," as is offered at one successful day spa in California. It is their job to know as much as possible about each therapy and each therapist, to better match guests with the right provider and service. So, it just makes sense for you to let these employees know as much about you as possible. Give them multiple free treatments. Talk to them about the ways in which your services are high-quality. Give them information about your background and training and relevant personal history. In this way, they will be better able to sell your services to guests.

Food and Beverage

These employees are responsible for procuring, cooking, and serving food and drinks to the guests. They include chefs, purchasing managers, waitstaff, and kitchen help.

Relationship with Massage Therapists: Though you will not normally work directly with food-service personnel, you never know when a guest is going to need something from the kitchen or when you yourself will need something. If you form alliances with the kitchen and dining room folk, you can smooth out any special requests that might come up. Also, these employees have a great deal of contact with the guests, and it will help your cause in the spa if they speak highly of you. Let key waitstaff and chefs (especially chef instructors at larger spas) get to know you and what you do. Guests will learn about you more quickly that way, which is especially important in destination and resort spas where you have a limited window of opportunity to work with guests.

Maintenance

The maintenance department is in charge of keeping the spa's entire physical facility in proper working order. In larger facilities, they are on staff. In smaller spas, they are often hired contractors.

Relationship with Massage Therapists: In some larger spas, to get things fixed when they are broken (such as the air-conditioning in your treatment room)

Did You Know?

The Ten Core Retail Concepts for Massage Therapists

The 10 core retail concepts for massage therapists are:

1. People need to purchase products
2. People purchase products from other people
3. Buying from knowledgeable professionals is preferable
4. Selling products is not unprofessional
5. Other health professionals sell products
6. Massage therapists are permitted to sell products
7. The products offered in spas are beneficial for clients
8. Home care completes spa services
9. Not selling spa products is a disservice to clients
10. You do not need to be a salesperson to sell

example, you need to purchase some kind of clothing to wear in order to go out in public. You need transportation. You need food. You need shelter. In addition to the basic necessities, you also choose certain items to buy because you feel they would be beneficial or pleasurable. Shopping malls are filled with people who consider it fulfilling in one way or another to spend time shopping and purchasing. Without the ability to purchase needed or desired items, people are hampered from functioning fully in society.

Retail Concept #2: People Purchase Products from Other People

Where do people purchase products? You may have an image of large, impersonal stores owned by corporations. However, these corporations are owned by individuals, either shareholders or families. Many people work in these stores, and their jobs depend upon a steady flow of people coming in and making purchases. In smaller stores and markets, you can personally meet the people who are selling the products. The fabric of our society depends upon this interchange of buying and selling. You may feel that you are excluding yourself from this interchange (at least the selling end) by choosing not to sell anything. Instead, like most people, you work to earn your money in the form of a paycheck. If you look closely, you will find that you are still selling something—your time. If you work for a paycheck, you are selling time for money, and other people are buying your time.

Retail Concept #3: Buying from Knowledgeable Professionals is Preferable

The items available for sale in spas are often available elsewhere. Skin creams, oils, body scrubs, moisturizers, aromatherapy products, and more can all be purchased in retail stores. You, as a trained massage therapist who is familiar with the skin and the human body, are probably much more knowledgeable than the person at the retail store where these products are sold. Your opinion counts when it comes to telling people which items are best for them. Letting people know the benefits of certain products is a way to take responsibility for their well-being after they leave the spa. Sometimes, the products for sale in spas are only available in a professional environment (certain supplements and high-powered facial exfoliators, for example); if you fail to let clients know about these products, they may buy inferior ones at other outlets.

Retail Concept #4: Selling Products Is Not Unprofessional

Perhaps you feel that selling products would make you appear unprofessional. This is simply not the case. When done with the correct attitude, selling can actually enhance your professionalism. When clients see products all around them in the spa that they know are for sale, they expect to be approached with some information about those products. If nobody on the spa's staff takes the time to inform them about the use and benefits of the products, clients sometimes feel that the service level of the spa is unprofessional.

Retail Concept #5: Other Health Professionals Sell Products

Many health professionals, including doctors, chiropractors, and physical therapists sell products to their clients. Health professionals are in a unique position to help people by recommending products and equipment that really work. As long as the sale of these items is up-front and transparent, rather than kept as a hidden cost within treatments, patients often perceive them as an added benefit. Education is an important component of any sales within a health care environment, and many clients expect some of that same education in a spa setting.

Retail Concept #6: Massage Therapists Are Permitted to Sell Products

Nothing is written in the bylaws or code of ethics of any professional massage association that restricts or prohibits massage therapists from selling products to their clients. You can search through all the rules and regulations, and you will never find one against selling. As a massage therapist, you will not get in trouble if you sell products to your clients, as long as those products are legal. Of course, you are not permitted to sell pharmaceuticals or medical devices to clients, but spas do not offer these items. Certain items for sale in spas are meant to be recommended by estheticians, who have a more specified understanding of the skin and complexion. Leave these items to the estheticians. You can recommend everything else without any fear of overstepping your scope of practice or committing some breach of ethics in your profession.

Retail Concept #7: The Products Offered in Spas Are Beneficial for Clients

Everything offered for sale in a spa has a benefit for the clients who will use them (Figure 16–1). With normal use, the products will not harm the clients, as long as they follow the directions provided. Clients' skin is cleansed, moisture levels increased, appearance enhanced, and some products even promote improved circulation, remineralization, or detoxification. You are doing nothing to hurt people if you suggest that they buy spa products. People love to buy spa products, and they will purchase similar (and perhaps less effective) items somewhere else if they do not purchase them at the spa.

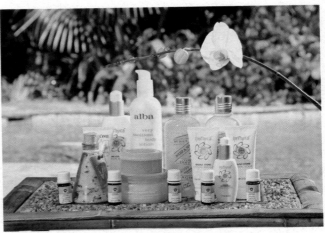

FIGURE 16–1 Repeat after me: "Spa Products are Beneficial. They do not hurt people. People love to buy them."

Retail Concept #8: Home Care Completes Spa Services

Many spa services are not completely effective unless they include a home-care component that clients can use to extend and enhance the benefits of the service you offer in the spa. The effectiveness of spa cellulite treatments, for example, is greatly augmented if the client takes home supplements and creams containing active topical ingredients. Even a simple body scrub is enhanced if the client can continue to cleanse and exfoliate the skin at home with the proper product. Of course, in order for clients to experience the benefits of home care products, they must be convinced to buy them. Leaving them on the shelf near the front door of the spa is not sufficient incentive. You as a spa therapist will have a responsibility to educate clients about the benefits of home care and to recommend appropriate products.

Retail Concept #9: Not Selling Spa Products Is a Disservice to Clients

If your own fears cause you to avoid your responsibility to educate clients about the benefits of spa products, you are actually doing those clients a disservice. Your reluctance to sell will perhaps keep people from discovering a new and more effective way to maintain their health and well-being. The products offered in spas are often of higher quality than those found in drug stores or at beauty counters. And, of course, some spa services are incomplete without a home-care component, as was already mentioned.

SPA CAUTION

Do not let your own fears stand in the way of a client's need for therapeutic products that can actually help improve health and well-being. Make a commitment to help the spa's clients by overcoming your own fears.

Retail Concept #10: You Do Not Need to Be a Salesperson to Sell

You may be afraid of becoming a "used car salesman" if you ask a client to buy something in a spa. You wish at all costs to avoid defining yourself as a salesperson. This, in fact, may be one of the reasons you chose massage therapy as a career. You want to comfort people and care for them, not make them uncomfortable by trying to sell them something. Therefore, the only way you can feel

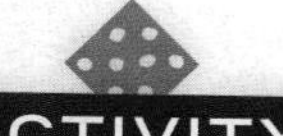

ACTIVITY

Perceptions of Sales People

What do you think of when you hear the word "salesman?" At a recent spa conference, participants were asked exactly that question. Here are a couple of their responses:

- used car salesman
- slimy

What do you think of when you hear the word "salesman"? Fill in a few descriptions of your own.

- ____________________
- ____________________
- ____________________

Now, take a moment and think back to the last time you actually interacted with a salesperson. Was it at a local store? A customer representative on the phone? How was that interaction? Was it really as negative as the images that first come to mind when you hear the word "salesman"? Most people who try this exercise report that the reality is not as negative as the preconceived notion. Now, write down what it was actually like to speak with a salesperson:

- ____________________
- ____________________
- ____________________

When you sell products in the spa, you can make your interactions with clients positive by focusing on customer service and fulfilling their needs, not just making a sale.

good about selling people things is if you believe it will give them great benefit. When you approach sales in the spa, then, it is important that you focus on the needs of the client more than on selling the product. You do not need to be a salesperson to sell. You only need to educate clients and offer them the opportunity to purchase. Do this by transforming negative impressions of spa sales into positive ones (see Table 16–1).

WHY SELLING IN THE SPA SETTING IS PERCEIVED AS NEGATIVE BY MASSAGE THERAPISTS	WHY SELLING IN THE SPA SETTING SHOULD BE PERCEIVED AS POSITIVE BY MASSAGE THERAPISTS
forces clients to buy	helps clients with home care to continue benefits of spa treatments
you have to be a "salesman" to sell	you can help clients by educating them about spa products
other health professionals do not sell	actually, many doctors and other health professional offer superior products to patients
massage therapists are not allowed to sell products	no laws, rules, regulations, or codes of conduct exist that prohibit massage therapists from selling products
shyness	sales offers the opportunity to grow personal communication skills that benefit therapists

TABLE 16–1 Bad vs. Good Perceptions of Spa Retail Sales by Massage Therapists.

Did You Know?

The MLM Conundrum

Interestingly, massage therapists seem to have no problem selling products to their clients if the products are part of a direct-distribution network, also known as "Multi-Level Marketing," or "MLM." Many therapists have been caught selling MLM products directly to clients in a spa and taking all the profits for themselves, sometimes getting fired in the process. They refuse to sell the recommended products on the shelves, but they have no problem selling the products they secretly bring to the spa in their own purses or backpacks. Why is this so? They do it because they truly believe in these products. Most people who become massage therapists have a sincere desire to help other people lead healthier lives. When they find a product in which they truly believe, they want to spread the news. The root problem behind therapists' reluctance to sell most spa products is that they do not believe in them.

MLM companies do an excellent job of convincing people about the effectiveness and health benefits of their products. In fact, they often turn people into "converts" who spread praise for their products far and wide. These companies capitalize on massage therapists' deep regard for their clients' health.

Often, massage therapists develop an emotional bond with the MLM products. On the other hand, therapists usually do not form such a bond with the products sold in the spa, and often they do not believe in the products' effectiveness. Unfortunately, therapists are not convinced by managers, trainers, or vendors that the spa's products are superior and offer deep health benefits.

The most effective way for most massage therapists in the spa setting to become better salespeople is to find a way to create an emotional bond between themselves and the products they are required to sell. It is the responsibility of spa owners, spa directors, and product vendors to convince therapists that the products offered for sale in the spa are deeply beneficial to their clients' health. It is the responsibility of spa therapists to follow up on that belief with positive sales for the spa.

THE IMPORTANCE OF SALES IN THE SPA

Retail sales are vital to the success of almost every spa operation. Many therapists do not realize that spas need the profits from retail sales just to remain in business. As most spa owners, directors, and managers have learned, the amount of profit earned by offering spa treatments can be quite small. In fact, many spas would have no profit at all if they had to rely on treatments alone. So, how do they survive? The answer to that, of course, is retail. Many spas that otherwise would have to go out of business rely on the profits they make from their retail sales. These retail sales are crucial, and that is why spas place so much emphasis on this part of the business, with many spas businesses aiming for a **sales to service ratio** of 20 percent or even higher. Massage therapists, estheticians, and cosmetologists are the spa's front-line sales force, the ones with whom clients spend a large majority of their time. While estheticians and cosmetologists have little problem recommending and selling products, massage therapists are sometimes unwilling to do so. It is no wonder, then, that spa directors and owners are so often frustrated with their therapists. If you follow the suggestions in this chapter and take them to heart, you'll improve your chances for finding success in the spa industry through helping owners and managers reach their goals.

sales to service ratio

the percentage of money that comes into the spa in relation to the amount coming in from actual treatments. It can be measured per-therapist or over the entire spa per unit of time. For example, if a therapist sells $10 worth of products for each spa treatment given, and the treatments cost $100, then the sales-to-service ratio is 10%.

ACTIVITY

Expense Reduction

Take a look at Table 16–2 for a list of expenses that spa owners face when they provide services to their clients. Fill in your best estimates for the costs involved in terms of percentage. For example, if the spa charges $100 for a body wrap and massage combination treatment, and you believe the therapist should be paid $50 of that, then the cost for "therapist commission" would be 50 percent. Go on down the list filling in the items to the best of your ability. These do not have to be completely accurate figures for you to understand the lesson here. Once you've given your best estimate, add up the numbers, then subtract the total from 100 percent. That is the percentage of profit left over for the spa. Because there are so many expenses involved with running a spa, the percentage of profits you come up with might even be a negative number. This is no coincidence. Spas are extremely expensive to run.

Another way to look at the expenses incurred by spas is on a monthly basis, as in Table 16–3. Some people find this easier to estimate. Take the same costs, but guess how much they would amount to over an entire month. For example, if the spa is leasing a building on a major road, chances are the lease payments are several thousand dollars per month. We'll leave out the furniture and equipment, because depreciation over time makes it too hard to estimate. Try doing this for a 3,000-square-foot day spa in a medium-sized city, with 6 treatment rooms and a staff of 10 therapists, 6 support staff, and 1 owner/manager, doing 30 total hours

EXPENSE	ESTIMATED % OF COST OF TREATMENT
therapist's commission	%
support staff pay (front desk, etc.)	%
salary to owner/managers/director	%
product/supplies (oils, seaweed, etc.)	%
laundry	%
cleaning service	%
insurance (workers' comp. etc.)	%
taxes (payroll, property, business)	%
utilities (phone, electric, water)	%
overhead (rent/lease/mortgage)	%
overhead (furniture, fixtures, and equipment)	%
marketing, advertising, promotion	%
misc. (computer software, legal advice, etc.)	%
TOTAL	%
100 − TOTAL =	% PROFIT

TABLE 16–2 Fill in Your Best Estimates for Each Cost Incurred by a Spa.

(Continued)

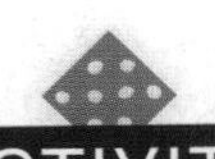

ACTIVITY

EXPENSE	ESTIMATED MONTHLY $ TO RUN SPA
therapist's commissions	$
support staff pay (front desk, etc.)	$
salary to owner/managers/director	$
products/supplies (oils, seaweed, etc.)	$
laundry	$
cleaning service	$
insurance (workers' comp. etc.)	$
taxes (payroll, property, business)	$
utilities (phone, electric, water)	$
overhead (rent/lease/mortgage)	$
marketing, advertising, promotion	$
misc. (computer software, legal advice, etc.)	$
TOTAL	$
TOTAL ÷ 900 =	$

TABLE 16–3 Fill in Your Best Estimates for the Monthly Costs Incurred by a Spa.

of treatments per day. This makes a total of 900 treatment hours in the month. Once you've determined the total amount of all the expenses added together, divide that by the number of treatments, 900. This is the amount the spa would have to charge for each hour of treatment given, just to break even.

BECOMING POSITIVE ABOUT SALES

Once you feel comfortable with the ethics of selling beneficial products to clients in the spa setting, you can begin to focus on the details of making those sales happen. The first detail you should focus on is your own attitude. Perhaps the biggest block that most massage therapists experience related to selling can be summed up in these few words: "I just don't feel like it." Even if you are convinced that sales are good for the spa and you are open to trying to sell, you may still feel like your heart is simply not in it. It feels difficult, if not impossible, to build up the necessary enthusiasm to approach clients on the topic. This, unfortunately, usually appears to spa directors like reluctance or rebellion. In reality, it is fear.

You may quite likely be scared to death at the idea of approaching another person and asking her to buy something. The main types of fear that sales bring up are:

- the fear of rejection
- the fear of change
- the fear of success

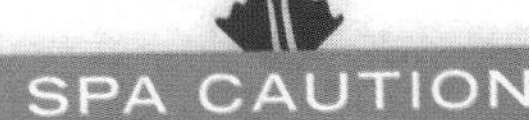

SPA CAUTION

Avoid the tendency to label spa owners and spa directors as greedy. This is typical among therapists. Instead, do your homework to discover the expense and hard work that is actually involved in operating a spa business. The experience may humble you.

The Fear of Rejection

Every time you approach someone about buying a spa product, there is a chance the client will refuse. Chances are that you became a massage therapist precisely because you prefer not to experience this kind of rejection. You'd rather have a positive interchange with each client and not risk tainting it with a sour note at the end if the person is simply not interested in purchasing the products. This fear is natural, and it creates reluctance on your part. In order to counter this fear, it is important for you to understand these two basic facts:

- Clients do not mind being approached to buy things in the spa. They come into the spa expecting there to be products for sale. Some clients might even be disappointed if you do not give them the opportunity to buy.
- The only time a sales pitch annoys spa clients is when the pitch is presented by a reluctant therapist full of fear and uncertainty. If you are calm and confident and not afraid of being rejected, you can present the product simply to the client and let her make up her own mind to purchase it or not. This is *not* an imposition. The way you achieve this effortless sale is to "release the charge" with which you have invested the act of sales, and the way you do that is to practice the three-step spa sales rules (see "The Three-Step Spa Sales Rule" sidebar section later in this chapter).

The Fear of Change

Another, perhaps more subtle, fear that you may experience concerning spa sales is the fear of change. You may fear that if you begin trying to sell things, you will become a salesperson, and salespeople do not care about people as much as they do about profits, right? Not necessarily. You can be a conscious and caring therapist and still offer products for sale to your clients in the spa. If you fear that selling things will change you into someone less conscientious and caring, that will lead you to fear success itself.

The Fear of Success

It may be difficult to imagine that you are secretly afraid of increasing your income and gaining more prosperity, but this is all-too-common among massage therapists, and it often translates into a reluctance to engage in spa sales. Your reasoning may go something like this: "If I become an expert in sales, I will focus my energy on that aspect of the business. I'll forget why I became a massage therapist in the first place. I'll be a sellout. All the money I'll be earning will only serve to make me unhappy, like all those rich miserable people I see on television."

Many therapists unconsciously harbor fear-of-success thoughts. There are two steps you can follow to overcome them. First, you need to realize that selling spa products to spa customers is part of the job description. Fearing that you will become too successful at it is like a chef in a restaurant fearing he will become too good at selling food to his customers. The two go hand in hand: the cooking and the selling of the food can be compared to the administering of spa therapy and the selling of products to extend the service into clients' homes. Second, you can work within your own comfort zone at first and gradually build up to higher sales levels. Start out selling just one product to one client. See what it feels like. You may actually be more afraid of the unknown than of success itself. Once you feel what it is like to sell successfully, you may find that you enjoy the sensations that come with helping the client receive more benefits, helping the spa increase profits, and helping yourself increase your prosperity. Give it a shot.

sales commissions

a percentage of the total dollar amount sold given in compensation for making the sale

straight commission

compensation equaling a set percentage of the sales price of all items regardless of how many items are sold in a given sales period

sliding commission

increasing percentage of sales commissions offered as specific total sales levels are reached in a given sales period (e.g., 10 percent commission to start, 15 percent on sales over $500 per month, etc.)

markup

the amount above the wholesale cost of a product charged to retail customers

private label

items manufactured by one company for sale by another, with the label of the retailer on the item and no sign of the manufacturer visible to the purchaser

GETTING PAID FOR SALES

One spa owner did a study of sales in her spa and found that 93 percent of the customer's decision to buy was based upon recommendations by spa therapists. To compensate them for this astounding influence they have on the guests, spas typically pay therapists for their sales through a commission structure. **Sales commissions** can be defined as a percentage of the total dollar amount sold given in compensation for making the sale. This percentage varies from spa to spa. Even within the same spa, different therapists, estheticians, manicurists, and other technicians can receive different commission rates for their sales. These differences can be affected by seniority, by the type of product sold, and even by the amount of product sold by a particular employee. The two main commission structures used in most spas are "straight" and "sliding."

In a **straight commission** structure, therapists are given a specific percentage of the sales price of each item they help sell. For example, if you sell a jar of chamomile body scrub for $16 and receive a 10 percent commission on the sale, you would receive $1.60, regardless of how many jars you sold in a particular sales period. If, on the other hand, the spa had a **sliding commission** structure, you might receive 10 percent for the first $500 of products you sell in a sales period, but then once you'd reached that level you would receive a higher percentage, such as 15 percent. In this example, if you sold another jar of body scrub after reaching the $500 mark, you would receive $2.40 for the sale. Some spas offer another tier in their commission structure. In this example, sales above $1,000 would earn you a 25 percent commission ($4). Fifteen to 20 percent is commonly the highest spas can go with their commission structure and still remain profitable, while 5 to 15 percent is typical. However, certain spa products have a higher **markup**, and in this case therapists can receive a higher commission rate.

Often, the spa's **private label** items (Figure 16–2), which are cheaper for the spa to buy, carry a higher commission rate. Private label items are manufactured

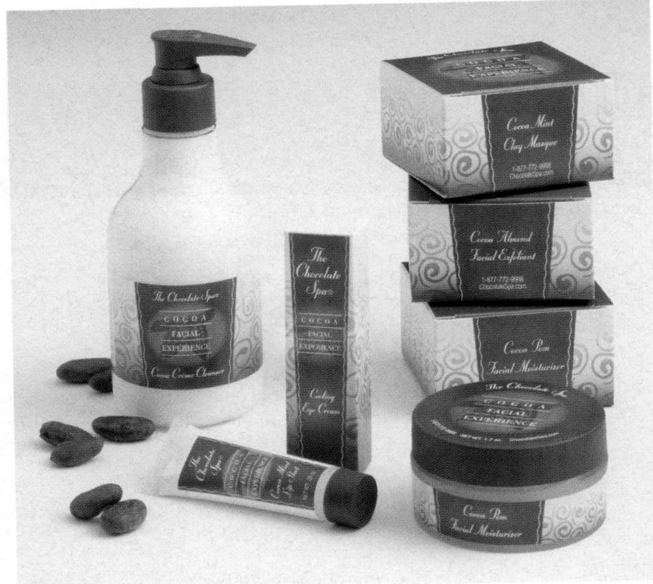

FIGURE 16–2 Spas make higher profits by selling high quality private label products.

by companies that specialize in creating products to sell under the brand name of other businesses. Many spas offer private label items for sale on their shelves. In fact, a large majority of spa-branded products are manufactured by private label manufacturers. These products are usually just as high-quality and therapeutic as the name-brand products on spa shelves. Because they usually have higher profits built into the pricing and because they increase the spa's visibility by having the spa's name on the label, these products are what spa directors and owners hope to sell first. If you as a therapist try these products for yourself, find them effective, and believe in them, it will be easy for you to sell them to the spa's clients, and you may earn a higher commission for doing so, as compared to selling products from name-brand companies.

SPA SALES PROTOCOLS

When it is time to sell a spa product to a client, some therapists become tongue-tied. What do you actually say? How do you approach the issue? Obviously, it is not appropriate to just blurt out, "Please buy this. The spa director wants me to sell it to you." What, then, are you supposed to do? Most massage therapists are against the idea of "hard selling" spa products to their clients. This attitude, however, often inhibits them from doing any kind of selling at all. "**Soft selling**" is an alternative to the hard sell, and many therapists would be quite talented at it if they could overcome their general reluctance. The technique of soft selling has worked in many spas. Soft selling, which means non-aggressive selling, can be broken down into three basic components: relation, education, and cooperation. Each one has its own approach, described below. Regardless of which sales approach or script you use, the proper use of certain key communication techniques are crucial, as demonstrated in Tables 16–4 and 16–5.

soft selling

the understated use of relation, education, and cooperation to sell items, as compared to aggressive, pushy sales tactics

VERBAL COMMUNICATION TECHNIQUES	DESCRIPTION	PROPER TECHNIQUE	IMPROPER TECHNIQUE
Diction	the clear, articulate pronunciation of words to get across a message	speak slowly and clearly	speak rapidly, mumble
Clarity	easy-to-understand words and sentences	speak about the treatment or product in clear, simple terms	confuse or irritate clients by speaking about treatments or products in overly technical or "mystical" terms
Brevity	use of the fewest words possible to get the message across	tell clients what the product can do in a few short sentences and let them decide	ramble on about product, treatment, or even unrelated items
Uniqueness	use of your own words to describe benefits of product or, if using a script, personalizing it	be yourself and let personality shine through	act like a robot giving the same tired sales pitch to every client

TABLE 16–4 Verbal Communication Techniques.

NON-VERBAL COMMUNICATION TECHNIQUES	DESCRIPTION	PROPER TECHNIQUE	IMPROPER TECHNIQUE
Posture	stand straight without slouching, hands out of pockets, facing client	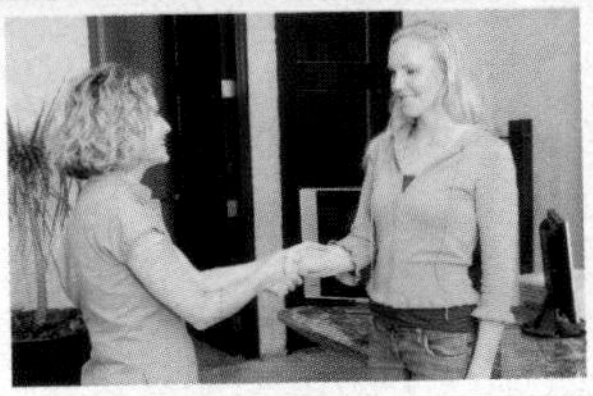	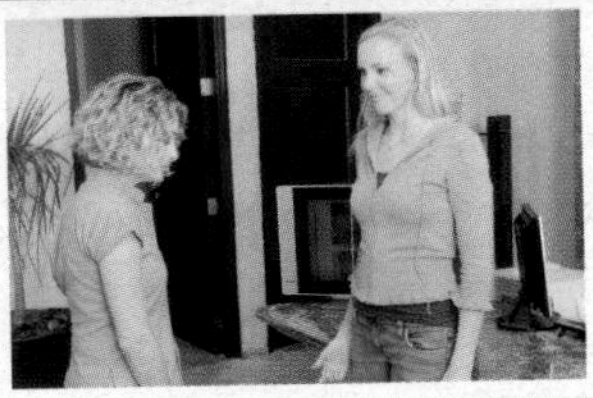
Eye Contact	look often and directly into the client's eyes when selling	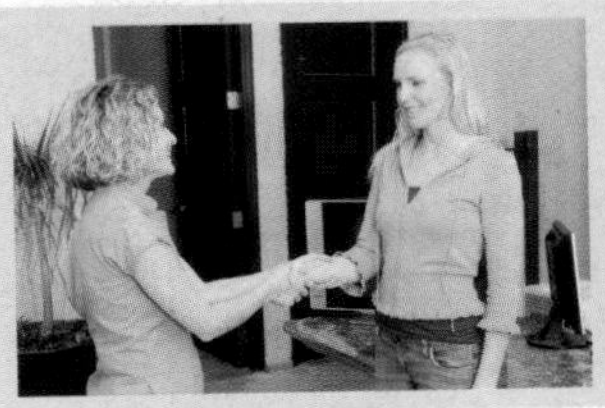	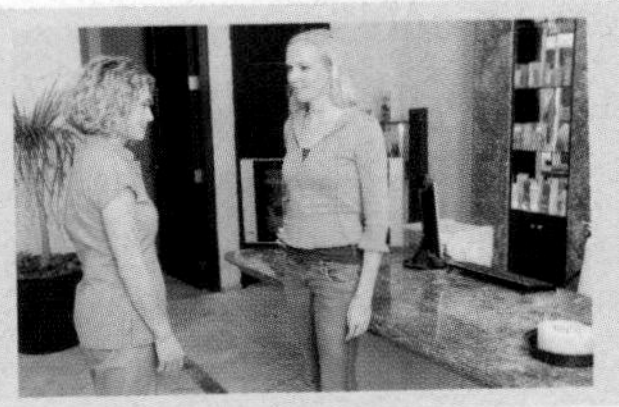
Handshake	both males and females should offer a firm handshake that shows self-confidence	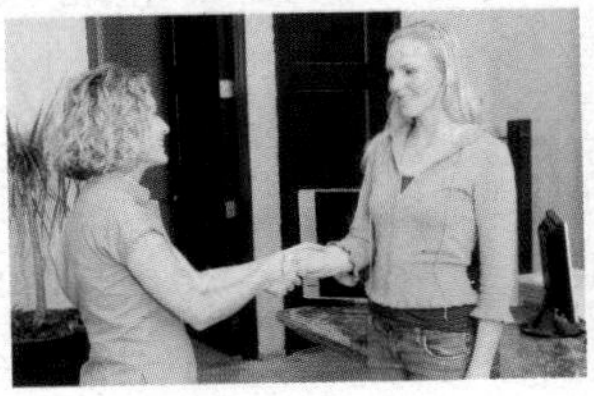	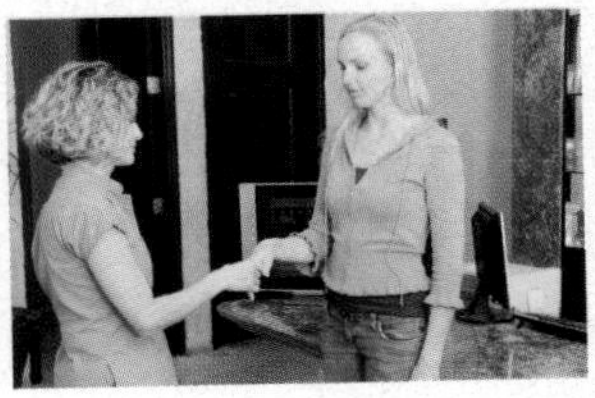

TABLE 16-5 Non-Verbal Communication Techniques.

Soft Selling Component 1—Creating a Relationship with the Guest

What many massage therapists are most afraid of is alienating another human being, especially one with whom they are supposed to be forming a healing, therapeutic relationship. While hard selling somebody a product they do not want and forcing something upon them against their will may indeed alienate people, soft selling does just the opposite. Therapists who practice soft selling seek first to understand. Selling is secondary to the relationship they form with the client. For this type of selling to be successful, communication is key.

Soft selling, then, is not about telling clients what they should buy. It is about asking clients what they want. It is about finding out what they need to feel better about themselves, to feel healthier, more youthful, more attractive, and more proactive with their own well-being.

What does soft selling look like in the spa? If you were to peer inside the treatment room while a talented therapist successfully applies soft selling techniques, you would see what looked like a discussion between friends or acquaintances. The therapist would be concerned about the guest's health, about the quality of her skin, about how the client feels in general. Most noticeably, the therapist would be asking lots of questions.

Take a look again at Retail Concept #2: People purchase products from other people. This concept can be broadened to read, "People are more likely to purchase products from other people with whom they have a relationship." The very

SPA ETIQUETTE

Clients are likely to purchase spa products from those therapists who make the extra effort to forge a professional relationship based on courtesy and respect. While it is not appropriate for therapists to ask personal or intrusive questions, it is appropriate to show curiosity and caring when it comes to finding out about clients' goals and how the spa's products and services can help achieve them.

best therapists and estheticians in spas truly focus on their clients' needs and concerns. They make the clients feel cared for. Selling them beneficial products is just one way of doing that. For these top-notch therapists, sales is not just about making money. It's about serving the client, understanding the client, and creating a professional yet friendly relationship with the client. Not surprisingly, the therapists who do this end up reaping much greater rewards for themselves as well.

Soft Selling Component 2—Educating the Guest

If you're like most massage therapists, you enjoy educating your clients about their bodies and their health. Selling spa products is a perfect opportunity to do just that. Built into the natural interchange that occurs with every sale in the spa is a chance to educate, inform, and enlighten clients about their own bodies. Even the simplest product, like a body scrub, can be sold with this in mind.

When you are educating clients about their bodies and their health, it is natural to emphasize the benefits of the products for sale in the spa. Therefore, it is especially important to have a thorough understanding of the benefits of the retail items available. This understanding comes from several sources: trainings offered by the vendors of the products, trainings given by the spa, and advice from co-workers. There is no substitute, however, for firsthand experience. Spa guests will respond much more readily to a personal recommendation from a therapist who actually uses and enjoys the product. Spas often offer a discount to therapists so that they can test each product personally. The cost involved is quickly recouped with the sales made by enthusiastic therapists.

Putting the emphasis on the benefits of spa products naturally shifts the emphasis away from the price. In fact, there is initially no need to focus on the price at all. Many therapists sabotage themselves by worrying that spa clients cannot afford the items. Spas, however, are not famous for being cheap. People expect to pay well for high-quality products. Focus on education first, explaining why the product is high-quality. Price is secondary. Let price come up naturally at the end of the conversation, if at all. Many clients are perfectly willing to take therapists' recommendations regardless of price.

Soft Selling Component 3—Cooperating with Your Team

Therapists who sell in the spa never sell alone. They are part of a larger team that facilitates sales together. The more sales that are made, the more likely the spa is to survive and thrive, thus ensuring a livelihood for all employees. Spa staffs that achieve sales goals and provide excellent service to clients while doing so have high self-esteem and *esprit de corps*. When therapists think of themselves as lone guns or independent salespeople, they put pressure on themselves and feel a heavy burden of responsibility for making sales. They feel that if they fail or are rejected, they alone are to blame. If, on the other hand, they were to focus instead on making the sales so that the spa's overall success is enhanced, their approach would be more selfless, more lighthearted, and definitely more likely to succeed.

You can take much of the sales pressure off yourself as a spa therapist if you connect with your co-workers and try to do the best job you can for them, rather than just for yourself. This sometimes translates into actual income for other staff members. Some spas pay a **pooled commission** to front-desk and reception staff for non-spa-product items. So, if you were to recommend a certain book or tape to one of your clients and she was to buy it later in the spa shop, that sale would put money in the pockets of your co-workers. The front-desk staff, on the other hand, can look out for the therapists' best interests by making sure that guests give credit to the proper person for spa product orders.

pooled commission

a percentage of income from the sale of certain items that is pooled together, then split evenly among front-desk and reception staff members; usually consisting of non-therapy items such as candles, books, etc.

The Three-Step Spa Sales Rule: Show, Describe, Offer

Regardless of which soft selling techniques you use or which scripts you follow, it will help sales and make your efforts more natural and honest if you follow the "Three-Step Spa Sales Rule." Following these steps will help you retain your integrity as a therapist while at the same time making clients comfortable in a sales environment. The steps are (1) show the product, (2) describe the product, and (3) offer the product.

Step One: Show the Product

Clients should be able to see products prominently displayed when they enter the spa space or the treatment room. Some spas conceal retail products behind counters or inside cupboards, and when the treatment is finished, the products "magically" appear atop the counter at checkout, and the front-desk person engages in a hard sell. This is an attempt to trick the client into buying when she is most vulnerable, and spas that engage in this practice quickly develop a poor reputation. Before you accept employment at a spa, be sure to inquire about their sales techniques, and make sure they show the products to clients prior to trying to sell them.

Step Two: Briefly Describe the Products during Treatment

After clients have seen the retail products that are plainly on display at the spa, you can reinforce the fact that they are for sale by mentioning it during the treatment. Try saying something like this: "I'm glad you're enjoying this body butter. It's excellent for dry skin. We have it for sale here at the spa on the front shelf when you come in."

Step Three: Offer to Sell the Product

After the treatment, make a clear but non-aggressive offer to sell the product to the client. Say, "If you'd like this product for home care, I can have one ready for you at the front desk." You do not need to be pushy, but if you do not follow up with a straightforward offer, the client may be confused and not understand if you are actually selling the product or not. This step is called "closing the sale," and it is the scariest for many people because it is the time when fear of rejection can arise. With more practice, this fear will subside and you will be able to simply and clearly ask the client if he is interested in buying the product or not.

Remember these three simple steps—show, describe, offer—and you will find it much easier to sell with integrity.

ACTIVITY

The Sales Game

You can combine all of the skills and suggestions from this chapter into a "sales game" that will help you overcome some of the blocks you may encounter when trying to make selling more natural. The first version of this game can be played with just two other classmates, while the second version requires participation by the whole class.

Pair up with a partner and ask the third person to wait in another room, out of earshot. Then you and your partner play buyer and seller. This game is real, selling something real and using real money, though the amount should be kept minimal—a few dollars at most. The object itself and the amount of money are not that important. It will help, however, if you choose something that might possibly be found in a spa.

The object is simple: the seller tries to get the highest price from the buyer, and the buyer tries to get the lowest price from the seller. You will meet somewhere in the middle, and the sale will take place.

Before playing this game, review the soft selling components: relation, education, and cooperation. Also, review Tables 16–4 and 16–5 to remind yourself of the proper verbal and non-verbal communication skills that will make the sale more successful. Then, have some fun. Hold the item up for sale and tout its marvelous benefits. Ask a price that may seem too high at first. Then, be willing to negotiate if your partner does not seem too interested.

After you've settled on a price and money has actually changed hands, call the third person into the room. Then, the person who just played the buyer becomes the seller of the same object, and the new person becomes the buyer. Do not tell the third person how much was paid for the object in the previous transaction.

When you have finished, all three participants should take a moment to contemplate the insight gained from this experience. If you purchased the item yourself for use in this game, was the price you paid more or less than the price you received? How did that make you feel? Did the second person to buy the object pay more or less than the first person? How did that make you feel? Perhaps through this exercise you'll come to understand that although the object has a value of its own, the price you agree upon has more to do with the emotion of the moment and the interaction of the two people involved in the transaction. This is important. Part of sales is providing a rewarding emotional experience for the buyer, regardless of the price.

Sales Game Version 2 for the Whole Class

For the group version of the sales game, you will take part in a type of auction. Each student brings an object to sell and gets up in front of class to do so. Once again, pay attention to verbal and non-verbal communication skills. Review the material in this chapter before making the presentation. Ask for a fair price that you believe to be on the low end of the object's value, and see if you can get anyone to bid on your object. If someone does, ask if there is a higher price somebody would be willing to pay. When no higher offer is forthcoming, exchange the object for the money. After everyone has taken a turn, the group critiques each other's technique. This can be fun. The objects can be anything at all, not necessarily spa related. The point of the game is to hone your sales skills and get you more comfortable making a sales presentation. Keep in mind that the more expensive the item, the more difficult it may be to sell, unless you are offering a very good price. Do not choose an item that costs just a few pennies, as that is too easy to sell and will not give you the emotional impact of making an actual sale.

(Continued)

ACTIVITY

Typical Problems to Avoid

Here are a few typical problems to watch out for when making your sales pitch in these games:

Therapist's Sales Pitch: I've got a fantastic bar of all-natural herbal soap here. It's made from organic ingredients and has ground herbs inside it to exfoliate your skin while it cleans. It's only $5.95.

Problem: The therapist forgot to actually ask the person to buy and close the sale. Verbally say the words, "would you like to purchase this today?" You've got to *ask* people to buy.

Therapist's Sales Pitch: This body wash is a little pricey but it's better than the stuff you can get at the department stores. Would you like to buy some?

Problem: Therapist made price an issue instead of focusing on quality and letting the client decide what is expensive and what is not.

Therapist's Sales Pitch: People say that this moisturizer I'm using on your skin is the best one on the market, and you can only get it here. It's on sale this month. Would you like to purchase one today?

Problem: Therapist gave secondhand information from "other people" instead of a personal recommendation that she has used and enjoyed the product.

Therapist's Sales Pitch: Yes, the music playing in the spa is for sale on CDs. They're available in the spa gift shop.

Problem: Because the therapist knows he will not receive a commission on this particular item, he does not make the effort to escort the client to the gift shop and display the product. This is not proper teamwork and does not foster a positive environment in the spa.

TYPES OF PRODUCTS FOR SALE

As a massage therapist working in a spa, you may think that the most natural items to sell are the ones you apply directly to clients' skin. However, while selling the massage lotion that you use in the treatment room may seem natural and obvious, it is not always easy. Most people do not have the same need for massage lubricant that you as a professional do. Others may think that oils and creams for actual treatments at home are too messy or complex to apply. It will be up to you to educate clients about the important benefits of each product. In addition, the spa environment offers several alternative products for massage therapists to sell (Figure 16-3). The main retail product categories are listed below, with some ideas about how to sell each. Also, Table 16–6 lists these products and techniques in condensed form for reference.

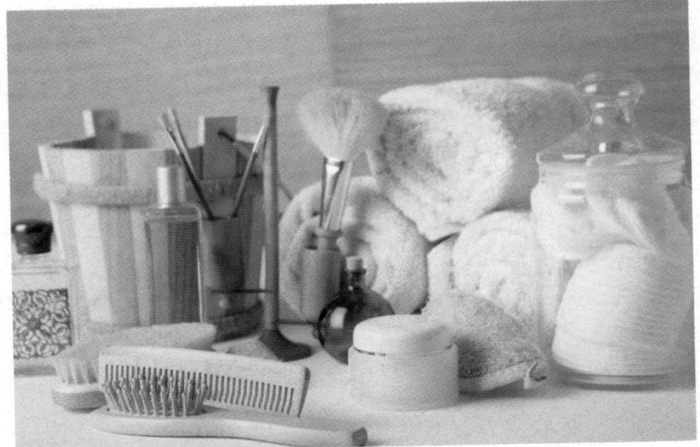

FIGURE 16–3 Therapists can sell the items they use in the spa . . . AND they can sell non-treatment items as well, like candles, lipstick, bathrobes, and more.

Moisturizers

As a massage therapist, you see firsthand how thirsty the skin can be. Moisturizers are especially important

TYPE OF RETAIL SPA PRODUCT	BENEFITS	SALES TECHNIQUE
Moisturizers	helps preserve healthy and attractive skin, especially in dry conditions	Talk about the benefits of specific ingredients with which clients may not otherwise be familiar. Customize suggestions to clients' skin type.
Exfoliants	removes layer of dead skin cells to leave skin attractive and better able to absorb therapeutic products	Educate clients about grain size, effects of specific exfoliant types, and origin of materials.
Body Wash	cleanses skin	Inform clients how the spa's body wash works synergistically with exfoliants and moisturizing products.
Herbs, Clays, Seaweeds, Muds	moisturizes, nourishes, remineralizes, detoxifies, cleanses skin and entire body	Emphasize the benefits of natural products, educate on proper home use techniques to bring these benefits into everyday life.
Weight Loss and Cellulite Reduction	extends the effects of in-spa treatments through assisting in elimination and metabolism	Stress the need for home-care follow-up in order to make these treatments effective.
Supplements	strengthens clients' overall health and well-being from the inside out	Educate clients about the importance of supplements generally, the quality of the spa's brand, and their enhanced effects when combined with spa treatments.
Massage Tools	brings the pleasures of massage home for the client	Therapists can recommend those tools they personally believe in and use.
Sunscreens	protects against harmful rays from the sun	Clients need to be reminded about the importance of proper protection, and therapists are in a good position to do so. A perfect opportunity for education, especially regarding proper application.
Non-Treatment Items	adds convenience for spa guests who would need to go elsewhere to purchase these spa-related, health-promoting, or uplifting items	Remind clients that they can "take the spa home" through any number of inspirational items or memorabilia.

TABLE 16-6 Typical Retail Spa Products for Sale.

in dry, desert areas. You can experiment during the massage or other body treatment to find out which moisturizing agent is most appropriate for the skin of each particular client. The spa treatment room and the massage room are perhaps the only places where people have the opportunity to discover which products work best over a large area of skin.

Exfoliants

Many people are comfortable using exfoliants at home, usually in the shower. When applying a body scrub, sea salt glow, or similar treatment, you can inform clients about the special benefits of the products you are using. Are these salts from the Dead Sea? Which particular minerals make them most effective? What size grain is most appropriate for each skin type? The added information will make it more comfortable for clients to buy. You can also add essential oils to the exfoliant and educate clients about their effects.

SPA VISION ASSESSMENT

Answer yes or no to the following questions.

1. Do you know who your customers will be? Have you narrowed down your target audience?	Yes	No
2. Do you know what your spa will look like and the environment you will present to your clients?	Yes	No
3. Have you determined whether to set pricing low to attract customers or high to create exclusivity?	Yes	No
4. Have you imagined a particular theme for the spa and determined how to create it?	Yes	No
5. Have you determined what product lines you will carry, either a known brand or your own label?	Yes	No
6. Have you thought of a name for your spa that will uniquely express your offerings?	Yes	No
7. Have you brainstormed with anybody in the spa industry who may be able to guide you?	Yes	No
8. Have you visited other spas to determine what will work in your own spa?	Yes	No
9. Do you have at least one marketing strategy in mind that will set your spa apart from the rest?	Yes	No
10. Is your desire to open a spa so strong that you can think of nothing else much of the time?	Yes	No

Add the total number of "yes" answers = ______

EMOTIONAL ASSESSMENT

Answer yes or no to the following questions.

1. Are you emotionally prepared to be in charge of other people's schedules, training, and discipline?	Yes	No
2. Do you feel secure and confident enough to ask for other people's money or risk your own?	Yes	No
3. Are you willing to shoulder the responsibility of having no one to answer to and no one to blame?	Yes	No
4. Are you ready to have others critique and rate your spa business publicly, in the media, etc.?	Yes	No
5. Are you comfortable selling items to clients? Are you willing to focus on retail endeavors?	Yes	No
6. Have you developed your communication skills and feel comfortable marketing your business?	Yes	No
7. Are you emotionally prepared to potentially fail at your spa venture? Do you have a backup plan?	Yes	No
8. Do you have friends, family, or colleagues who will support you in your vision?	Yes	No
9. Are you emotionally prepared to let go of doing hands-on therapy in order to take care of business?	Yes	No
10. Are you emotionally prepared to let go of some responsibility and delegate?	Yes	No

Add the total number of "yes" answers = ______

Now, add the final numbers from the three categories above to determine your "preparedness stage" = ☐

26–30 **(stage 5)** = You are ready to begin the first concrete steps to put your spa together.

21–25 **(stage 4)** = You are committed to your spa project idea. Continue looking into the possibility of opening your spa.

16–20 **(stage 3)** = You are almost ready to begin but will benefit from more time to develop your ideas.

11–15 **(stage 2)** = You are on the fence and may not have sufficiently considered all the details of opening a spa at this time.

0 –10 **(stage 1)** = You are simply toying with the idea of opening a spa at this time.

Note: Do not be discouraged if you find yourself with a low preparedness level. As you grow toward your goal of opening a spa, complete this profile again six months or a year from now. Your level of preparedness will of course shift over time. Use this self-assessment as a guide to move you in the right direction.

FIGURE 17–2 Spa ownership preparedness profile.

Information Gathering

Depending upon your stage of spa ownership preparedness, you will find certain resources to be more helpful than others. As you sift through the large amount of available information, you'll be able to refine your search by focusing first on those items most suited to your stage. Resources include consultants, trainers, videos, DVDs, books, workshops, magazines, expos, conferences, and more. The challenge is to find the right resources for your particular situation. With so many options available, therapists are often faced with an unexpected problem—information overload.

Once you have determined your current preparedness stage, you can begin to assess what steps you need to take to move to the next stage. Take a look at Figure 17–3 to discover the resources appropriate to each stage through which you may likely pass as you progress toward putting together your own spa.

Books and Magazines

Perhaps you have only toyed with the idea of opening a spa, or the idea is on the back burner in your mind. But you still feel somehow drawn toward the spa industry. The first place to look when you begin exploring the spa world is the many books and magazines available. Many magazines offer free or inexpensive subscriptions, and you'll find surprisingly detailed information in their pages (see Table 17–1). You can spend many hours researching the industry through magazines, getting to know the equipment most spa owners use, the products they offer their guests, the layouts and designs they choose for their spaces, and more. As you read and research, put together a file of the items that interest you. Cut out photos of spas that seem most attractive to you.

If the research you do in spa magazines stimulates your interest further, the next step is to explore the pages of a book or two that will give you some more concrete ideas regarding what it's really like to operate a spa on a daily basis. *Spa Business Strategies: A Plan for Success* by Janet M. D'Angelo is helpful in this regard.

Videos and DVDs

If the initial research you do through books and magazines leads you to explore further, you may find yourself, like many therapists, excited about opening

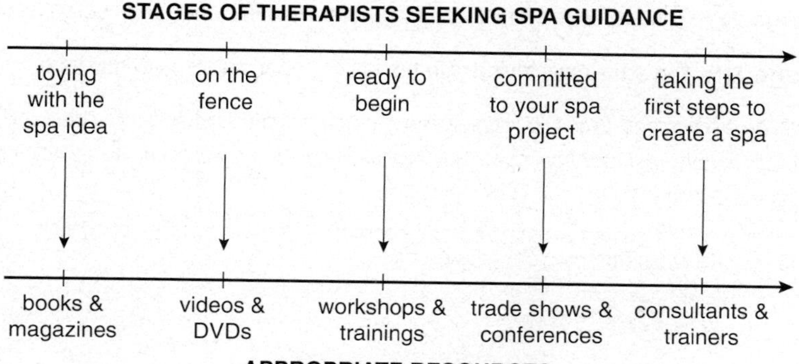

FIGURE 17–3 Appropriate resources for therapists seeking spa guidance.

MAGAZINE	DESCRIPTION	INFORMATION
American Spa	Features the newest spa products and equipment, latest techniques in skin, nail, and hair care, business growth, marketing, décor, equipment, and industry news.	http://www.americanspamag.com (866) 344-1315
Spa Finders	Focuses on luxury spas, but the best spa bargains are also explored, plus the latest on health and medical issues, furnishings and fixtures, and day spa news.	http://www.spafinder.com (866) 436-2456
Professional Spa	Focuses on the international spa market and trends from around the world.	http://www.professionalbeauty.co.uk 01371 810 433
Healing Lifestyles & Spas	Profiles spas and lifestyle choices among spa guests and those interested in wellness.	http://www.healinglifestyles.com (724) 465-0643
Day Spa Magazine	Features the latest trends, products, equipment, management tools and operations techniques, and positioning and marketing, plus legal, regulatory, and financial issues.	http://www.dayspamagazine.com (800) 624-4196
Dermascope Magazine	Industry leaders in spas and salons share knowledge and experience on latest trends, equipment, techniques, operating procedures, marketing strategies, and legal and financial issues.	http://www.dermascope.com (800) 961-3777
Skin, Inc. Magazine	A business guide for face and body care specialists, as well as owners/managers; includes information on finance, retailing, marketing, treatments, and more.	http://www.skininc.com (800) 469-7445
Spa Management Journal (& Medical Spa Journal)	Features the latest information on spa management; it's the only magazine specifically for owners/managers.	http://spamanagement.com/ (514) 274-0004

TABLE 17–1 Spa Magazines.

a spa of your own, but still uncertain. At certain moments, the idea seems brilliant, while at other times it seems like a foolhardy mission doomed for certain failure. You are on the fence, going back and forth, waffling. Therapists at this stage are in a "manic-depressive" state of mind regarding their spa dreams, sometimes exuberant, sometimes discouraged. This is not the time to invest in an architect or a high-priced consultant. Though you may, in the midst of an exuberant moment, be tempted to hurtle forward and overextend yourself, it is best to pull in the reins a little. The best resource to focus on at this time is videos and DVDs. You can find these resources online at any of the massage and spa distribution companies' Web sites. For instance, search Massage Warehouse's site (http://www.massagewarehouse.com/) for choices in spa training media.

Workshops and Training

Eventually, if your interest level remains high and you finally jump off the fence, you'll enter the "ready to move forward" stage. At this point, you'll want to make personal contact with some other professionals who have gone before you and know the ropes when it comes to getting started in the spa business. Hiring these professionals on an individual basis can be quite expensive, however. Therefore,

TYPE OF EDUCATION	ORGANIZATION	DETAILS	CONTACT
in-depth training	The American Spa Therapy Education & Certification Council (ASTECC)	many levels of training offered, from hands-on modalities to theory to management	http://www.asteccse.com (888) 241-2095
management training	Preston Wynne Success Systems	successful day spa operators show you pitfalls and processes to open and manage a spa, including budgets, compensation, etc.	http://www.pwsuccesssystems.com (877) 256-3513
classes in massage schools	Touch Training Directory (ABMP)	hundreds of schools listed; check for those offering spa courses	http://www.massagetherapy.com click "careers in massage and bodywork"

TABLE 17–2 Choices in Spa Education.

SPA TIP

You can move forward through Stages 1 and 2 of spa ownership preparedness, investing in books, magazines, and video trainings with no fear of overextending yourself financially. However, moving on to the more costly aspects of preparing to open your spa in Stages 3, 4, and 5 requires a substantial commitment of time and money and should be undertaken with caution.

most therapists at this point elect to enroll in some kind of workshop or training where they will join others in a learning environment (Table 17–2). These workshops and training programs can be quite enjoyable because they include an immersion in spa treatments and philosophy. You will not only learn and perform spa modalities, you will also receive them, so in that sense, attending the training is like visiting a spa. Depending upon your goals, the training you choose will emphasize either hands-on techniques, business development, spa management, or a combination of these.

Before making the investment in one of these programs, make sure that you feel strongly about building a spa. Too many therapists get overexcited at this early stage and end up spending more money than they should. They sign up for classes or workshops because it's the easiest thing to do. Making concrete plans and assessing your current situation is more difficult, but more important.

Tradeshows and Conferences

At a certain point, you'll leave behind all doubts and become fully committed to your spa plans. You've passed the Spa Ownership Preparedness Profile with flying colors, and you are making concrete progress in the real world toward creating a spa business. Now is the time to immerse yourself in the spa industry as fully as possible. Too many therapists enter the business as outsiders, afraid or unwilling to join the professional community that is waiting there to guide and assist them. Amazingly, some therapists decide to open a spa without ever having visited a spa themselves. This can lead to some unrealistic thinking.

The best place to begin your exploration of the spa industry is at those events a majority of spa professionals attend. This may sound simple, but with so many trade shows, conferences, and expos out there, you may find it difficult to narrow your choices down to one or two that merit your attendance. Conferences can be expensive, and few therapists have the resources to attend them all. Table 17–3 features a list that will help you determine which events are most appropriate and important for your circumstances.

TRADE SHOW	DESCRIPTION	CONTACT
Day Spa Expo	a trade show and education forum focused exclusively on the day spa sector	(800) 859-9247 http://www.dayspaexpo.com
International Salon & Spa Expo	primarily focused on those spas that incorporate salon and beauty services	(800) 468-2274 http://www.probeauty.org/isse/
Cosmoprof North America	same group that holds huge conferences worldwide for spa and beauty professionals	(800) 557-3356 http://www.cosmoprofnorthamerica.com
Spa & Resort/Medical Aesthetics Conference & Exposition	held in two locations each year—New York City, Miami Beach, and Los Angeles—with exhibitors, teachers, and vendors specific to the spa industry	(877) 271-6789, (888) 267-3793 http://www.sparesortexpo.com
International Esthetics, Cosmetics & Spa Conference	large show, inexpensive, with a 50/50 salon/spa focus, held twice per year (in Las Vegas and Florida)	(800) 624-3248 http://www.iecsc.com
International Spa Association (ISPA) Convention	largest gathering of spa professionals worldwide, featuring more than 2,500 attendees representing 73 countries; this is where all the spa owners and directors go (expensive but worth it if you are investing a great deal in your spa)	(888) 651-ISPA http://www.experienceispa.com
Spa Evolution	produced by a Canadian spa association; this show is great for anyone thinking of operating a spa in Canada	(800) 704-6393 http://www.leadingspasofcanada.com

TABLE 17–3 Spa Trade Shows and Conferences.

Consultants and Trainers

Depending upon how extensive your spa project is, you may find that you need some one-on-one coaching to help you attain your goals. If you are simply converting a massage practice into a sole-practitioner spa, the expense of hiring a consultant or private trainer is probably not warranted. If, however, you are hiring employees, constructing a new facility, or purchasing a significant amount of equipment, you may be in need of your own private expert to help you out. Often, therapists only realize this when they are in the middle of the spa project, and the consultant is called at the last minute to help save a failing venture. Consultants can be of service at every stage of spa development, however, and it is best if you explore your consulting options as early as possible if you think your project might benefit from this kind of expertise.

Consultants are not cheap. Some work on a monthly retainer basis, and others charge by the day or by the project; in any case, you should be prepared to spend thousands of dollars. See the section on consultants later in this chapter.

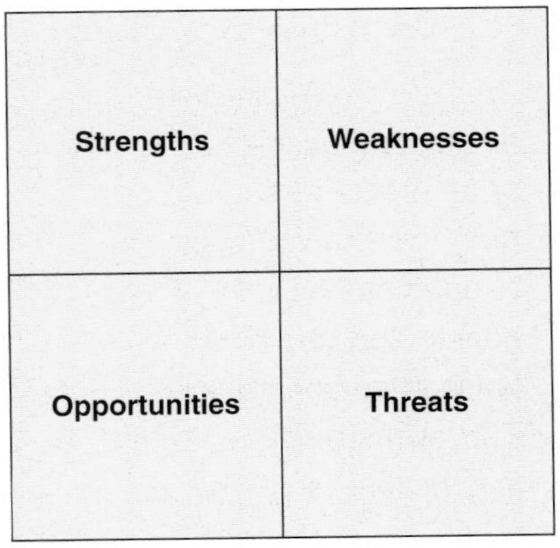

Strengths	Weaknesses
Opportunities	Threats

FIGURE 17–4 The SWOT analysis, which stands for: Strengths, Weaknesses, Opportunities, and Threats, can help determine your potential for building a spa business.

Self-Assessment

Using a self-assessment tool such as SWOT that provides insight into your current real-world potential for building or growing a (spa) business will help you identify key issues that you should consider. SWOT stands for *strengths, weaknesses, opportunities, and threats.* Creating your own **SWOT analysis** is simple. Start with a blank sheet of paper, which you divide into four quadrants (Figure 17–4).

SWOT analysis
a self-assessment tool that provides insight into your current real-world potential for building or growing a (spa) business

The items in the upper two quadrants correspond to the internal side of your business's potential (the part inside of you that depends upon your attitude, resources, and skills), while the bottom two quadrants relate to the external side (the part outside of you determined by factors already in motion, such as where you live and where you plan to grow your business). This completely honest internal/external snapshot of yourself and your plans will give you a firm basis upon which to grow your spa vision.

You do not need to include a great deal of detail in a SWOT analysis. Simple words and short phrases that honestly sum up your current situation are best. This is just a snapshot that will, you hope, reveal the big picture. If the SWOT assessment opens your eyes to certain challenges or opportunities on which you hadn't focused before, you can take time afterward to study them more deeply. Then, in the real world, you can take the necessary actions that will reduce the threats to your spa business and help you take advantage of the opportunities.

Strengths

In the upper left box, list all of your strengths that will help you build your spa business. Write down anything a customer wants that you will be able to provide. Brainstorm what you can provide that your competitors do not provide. Will you have a better location? More appealing products? More highly trained staff? Include anything (including personality traits, experience, attitude, etc.) that will help you reach your goals. You can edit later.

ACTIVITY

Create Your Own SWOT Analysis

Create a SWOT analysis for the spa business or one-room spa practice that you hope to open one day. Be honest and to-the-point when analyzing your own strengths and weaknesses. The SWOT is not meant to make you look good, but rather to help you discover areas that need improvement and areas of strength on which to capitalize.

Weaknesses

In the upper right box, list weaknesses—qualities you don't have, things you can't do or don't like to do, or skills or resources you do not possess. Be honest. This document is only for your own information. You are not being graded.

Opportunities

In the lower left box, list opportunities you perceive in your particular market. What are your potential future competitors not doing? What kind of spa atmosphere or offerings are not being provided that you could perhaps develop? What could make things better for existing spa customers, more affordable, convenient, or attractive? Also, what legal, political, technological, and cultural factors might fall in your favor as you develop the business?

Threats

In the lower right quadrant, list any threats you perceive that could derail your spa business plans. What developments could make you obsolete or shut you down? What are your competitors doing that will change the marketplace? What economic or demographic forces might shift? How could things go wrong?

Demographics

demographics
the characteristics of human populations and population segments, especially when used to identify consumer markets

Demographics can be defined as the characteristics of human populations and population segments, especially when used to identify consumer markets.

Have you given any thought as to who, exactly, your clientele will be once you open that dreamed-of spa? How can you hope to choose the right location if you do not know where your future clients live? A common mistake therapists make when they open spa businesses is to assume that everyone in the world

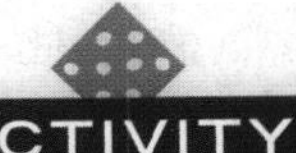

ACTIVITY

Narrowing Down Your Target Clientele

To help you narrow down the list of potential clients for your new spa, try this exercise. Use the 10 specific characteristics listed below and narrow each one down to describe the type of person you hope will most frequently visit your spa.

CHARACTERISTIC	DETAILS OF YOUR TARGETED SPA CLIENTELE
1. income level	
2. age range	
3. hobbies/pastimes/interests	
4. fitness level	
5. gender (% men vs. % women)	
6. ethnicity	
7. location (by town, region, etc.)	
8. publications/books read	
9. main goals for spa visits	
10. spa products used at home	

Now that you have a clearer picture of who your clients will be, how can you communicate with them? The topic of marketing your new spa services will be covered in the next chapter.

will want to be their customer. This shotgun approach to finding clients is not the most effective.

Paradoxically, you need to narrow down the list of potential clients for your new spa in order to increase their number. The tighter the focus you have on a particular niche, the more likely it is that you will be able to reach members of that niche and fill up your treatment rooms with them.

FINANCIAL ANALYSIS

When you start heading down the road toward spa ownership, you may be tempted at first to handle the entire project on your own, from financing to construction to hiring a staff and planning the grand opening party. However, you should be aware that the personality traits (perfectionism, attention to detail, self-direction, a deep sense of responsibility for others' well-being) that help you become a highly skilled and sought-after massage therapist may in fact be impediments when it is time to switch roles and become a business owner. In order to successfully run a spa that has more than just one employee (you), it will be necessary to learn how to delegate responsibility, and the very first item you can delegate is also one of the most crucial ones—coming up with the capital

SOURCE OF FINANCING	DESCRIPTION	POSITIVE FEATURES	NEGATIVE FEATURES
Cash	from friends	easily accessible, faith in your abilities even if you are untested in business	potential strain on friendship if unable to repay loan in a timely manner
	from family	family members believe in and support your dream, willing to give the business longer to succeed	may put strain on family members if not repaid, may cause borrower to be lax in repaying
	from savings	no interest payments, immediate full ownership, pride of being able to pay up front	depletes emergency funds, lowers creditworthiness due to lack of capital, unable to use cash elsewhere or invest it
	from other business	keeps the spa going during early lean times	can make the spa business dependent upon your other business and never become self-sufficient
Bank Loan	money loaned by financial institution, usually after proof of collateral	decent interest rates	difficult to obtain without collateral or a personal contact at bank
Home Equity Line of Credit	a loan or line of credit that uses the equity in your home as collateral	easy to acquire if you have sufficient home equity, low interest, perhaps tax-deductible	puts your home at risk
SBA Loan	Small Business Administration makes loans available to qualified individuals	competitive rates, extended payback period, covers depreciation of assets	can be a long, complex process to secure such a loan
Credit Cards	an individual's revolving credit line used to finance spa startup equipment and supplies	easy access to money, low payments	high interest rates, missed payments can lower credit rating, temptation to overspend because of ready availability
Lease	a contract granting use or occupation of property during a specified time for a specified payment	frees up cash for other uses, possible payoff feature at end of lease term	non-cancelable

TABLE 17–4 Financing Sources for Spa Businesses.

to start the business. There are six main ways that therapists go about getting money to open up their spa operations. There are advantages and disadvantages to each choice. Table 17–4 describes these financing options.

All of these financing options (except for your own savings) require you to engage the confidence and support of other people. Many therapists prefer to ask friends or family first, and that is often a good choice, but it can also lead to a less-than-professional beginning to a spa project. If you do not have a banker, loan officer, or credit company watching your progress and expecting timely payment, you may not try as hard to make the spa a monetary success as soon as possible. Many therapists do obtain financing, in spite of the obstacles, and leasing is becoming especially popular. According to one spa industry expert, 80 percent of all spas use some form of lease to finance all or part of their setup costs. Some leasing companies actively seek entrepreneurs looking to start a spa business. You can find them at spa trade shows and conferences.

Working with a Partner

One other popular option for financing a spa is to go into partnership. Often, people with funds to invest formulate a dream to one day open a spa, and they seek out someone with the skills to help make that dream a reality. Conversely, therapists with the skills and ambition often lack the funds. The financier and the hands-on expert then go into partnership. This is called the *business partnership*. Or, sometimes, spouses decide that a spa business is a good idea. The wife may be a therapist or esthetician, the husband a businessman, and they pool their efforts into a common business. This is an example of the *spousal partnership*, which is quite common in the spa industry. Alternately, two friends who have known each other for years embark upon a spa business, one with the money and the other with the skills. Or two friends with an abundance of skill and ambition, but no funds, go into business together. These are examples of the *friendship partnership*. All of these types of partnerships, while they sometimes work well, are also prone to be problematic for several reasons. Be careful if you plan to embark on a spa partnership. Realistically assess your chances at success and consider some of the potential pitfalls of each scenario before you begin.

Challenges with the Business Partnership

Sometimes, what seems at first like a dream partnership is not really a partnership all, but rather a way for an astute businessperson to get more work out of you than he is paying for. If you are approached by a financier with the idea of opening a spa business, be cautious regarding what you agree to do to uphold your end of the bargain. You may end up running the entire operation without receiving sufficient equity in return. **Equity** can be defined as ownership interest or financial stake in a (spa) business and/or property. What you want from this kind of partnership is to build up your own equity in the business through your hard work. This is known as **sweat equity**, a financial stake in a (spa) business that has been earned through time and labor rather than investment of capital. In a partnership, you need to think in terms of building up some kind of ownership stake in the business rather than just working for money. If you are not building up such a stake, you are in a boss–employee relationship, not in a true partnership. Beware.

equity

ownership interest or financial stake in a (spa) business and/or property

sweat equity

a financial stake in a (spa) business that has been earned through time and labor rather than investment of capital

Challenges with the Friendship Partnership

When two friends get together and decide to open a spa, in spite of a lack of funds and/or experience, they either fail or they become so enthusiastic that they make the venture work in spite of themselves. Either outcome has its challenges. If they fail, the friendship may sour. And if they succeed in spite of themselves, they may be left with a thriving business that they have no real skills to manage. In this case, they will have to be wise enough to seek consultants and trainers who can help them. See the “Consultants” section on the next page. A signed legal contract will help define the parameters during a working relationship and afterward in both the business partnership and the friendship partnership. You will be wise to create one in either case, in spite of the natural tendency for most therapists to be "nice" and avoid the technical or even adversarial language found in many business contracts.

Challenges with the Spousal Partnership

Spouses going into the spa business together are sometimes the strongest teams of all. Their partnership is based on a history of financial trust and an intimate knowledge of each other's strengths and weaknesses. However, if one partner is stronger in business and the other in hands-on service for the clientele, an imbalance of power can develop that is difficult to resolve. One partner tends to look exclusively at the bottom line, while the other focuses on the level of service and luxury for the clients. The relationship can become like a microcosm of what happens at larger spas on a daily basis, with ownership/management operating from one perspective while the hands-on staff operates from a completely different perspective. Couples need to be expert communicators to avoid this trap.

CONSULTANTS

spa consultant

a hired contractor with expertise in helping entrepreneurs set up or improve a spa business; some are generalists, while others specialize in equipment, products, layout, employee relations, etc.

A **spa consultant** will help you in innumerable ways to improve your chances at success, and it is always best to consult with someone who knows how to maximize space in each area of the spa. Your consultant can be a paid professional or an experienced friend who has already set up a spa and is familiar with the pitfalls. One thing is for certain about spa consultants: They are not in short supply. The spa business, it seems, has launched a thousand consultancy ships over the past several years. One good thing about many spa consultants is that you can retain as much or as little of their services as you need for your particular project, contracting for those parts of the project in which you feel weak. For example, you could hire a consultant to help with menu planning, retail issues, and staffing only, and do all the layout and design yourself.

A good place to start in your search for a good consultant is the International Spa Association Web site at http://www.experienceispa.com. They have a section devoted to consultants, and you may be able to find the person you're looking for there. Another resource is http://www.spatrade.com. Give them both a try and see if you can find someone to match your needs.

The questions you will want to ask potential consultants include the following:

What is your background? Certain consultants were nowhere near the spa industry until they suddenly saw a lucrative opportunity and jumped in. Some of these individuals may have strong business backgrounds, but their depth of experience and network of valuable contacts is probably lacking. Many of the best consultants worked their way up gradually through the ranks from spa employee to manager to director, and sometimes to owner, before feeling capable of offering well-rounded advice to clients.

Whom have you helped? You'll want to get a list, complete with references you can contact, of spa projects the consultant has helped bring to fruition. Make sure to call those references.

What is your fee structure? Of course, you'll want someone who is flexible. Ideally, the candidate will live in a geographically desirable area, close enough to you that a site visit won't costs thousands in travel expense. Some consultants use a monthly retainer, while others bill by the hour. These rates vary widely. For most therapist-owned spas, finding someone in the $100-per-hour range would be reasonable.

Last, do you like the consultant's style? She may very well have a profound effect on your finished spa. You'll want your consultant's sensibilities to be as closely attuned to yours as possible, while still leaving room for some creative divergences.

There are three main categories of spa consultants: trainers, full-service consultants, and vendors/suppliers.

Trainers

Often, the very same people who teach workshops and offer trainings are also consultants. These individuals are often the most reasonably priced and most willing to work with individual therapists and small business owners. Their primary expertise is often hands-on training, but they can also offer advice on layout, design, purchasing, hiring, and more.

Full-Service Consultants

These consultants work primarily with large developers who are building multi-million-dollar spas. They offer management training, architectural services, hiring and training services, purchasing, and more. Often, these consultants have worked for years at major spa properties and now help others launch their own larger projects.

Vendors/Suppliers

You can also take advantage of the consulting services provided by vendors and suppliers of spa equipment and products. These services are often billed as "free," but what that really means is "free for people who are purchasing products and equipment." Still, this can be an economical option. If you are going to be spending the money on products and equipment anyway, why not get some consulting with the deal? One word of advice: The consulting you receive from vendors and suppliers will always be prejudiced in favor of the particular products and equipment being offered. Try to make your decisions about your products and equipment before you engage this type of service so you will not be unduly swayed by your consultant's opinion. Vendor/supplier consultants can also be found on the ISPA Web site.

Often, consultants are a mixture of the three types listed above. You may find someone who offers consulting in conjunction with a particular brand of products, but also works independently and will be glad to help you get your spa off the ground, even if you do not purchase those products. You have to find the right fit for your particular circumstances, and to do that, it pays to shop around. Talk to several consultants. Ask for references from past clients. Make your own decisions.

CREATING A SPA BUSINESS PLAN

Remember, if you are not sure about taking that next big step of opening your own spa, it probably will not hurt to wait, at least for a little while. Or, start out on a smaller scale than you had envisioned at first. Many therapists start out in one room and gradually build up a successful business, and this organic-growth model of the therapist-owned spa may be the best one available (see profile of Becky Zwickl). However, when you move beyond this model and envision a larger operation, a business plan becomes crucial. Creating a professional business plan for your proposed spa business is important for three main reasons:

- It is a tool to focus your own ideas about the details of the business.
- It is a conceptual summary to share with potential investors, advisers, and employees.
- It is a sales pitch for your future business, letting others know how and why your spa will be better than others.

If you plan to secure financing from a traditional source such as a bank, you will need to be able to show that you are serious about the financial side of your spa dream. This is where a business plan is indispensable. Stated simply, a **business plan** can be defined as a written document outlining the details of a proposed business venture, including information such as financial strategies, products and services to be provided, estimated market, profits, key team members, and return for investors. Once you have written your business plan, you can show it to potential lenders and backers. The plan will almost certainly change over time as you build toward the opening of your business, so do not be overly concerned if the first draft of your business plan does not include every single detail of your completed vision. You can add to the plan as you go along. The following components are usually included in business plans:

- Introduction
- General Information about Your New Business
  - Description of business
  - Personnel
  - Competition
  - Marketing plan
  - Operating procedures
  - Insurance, licensing, and related issues
- Financial Information about Your New Business
  - Equipment and supply list
  - Loans and loan applications
  - **Balance sheet** (assets and liabilities)
  - **Breakeven analysis**
  - **Pro forma** income projections including **profit and loss (P&L)** statements
  - Projected **return on investment (ROI)** for investors
- Supporting Documents
  - Résumés of all principals
  - Recent tax returns of principals
  - Lease or purchase agreement for spa location
  - Licenses
  - Letters of intent from suppliers, vendors, service providers

business plan
a written document outlining the details of a proposed business venture, including information such as financial strategies, products and services to be provided, estimated market, profits, key team members, and return for investors

balance sheet
a summary of a company's financial condition at a specific point in time, including assets, liabilities, and net worth

breakeven analysis
a calculation of the approximate retail and service sales needed to cover costs, below which the spa business would be unprofitable and above which it would be profitable

pro forma
used to describe elements of a financial plan that are estimated or projected and not expected to be completely accurate, such as budget projections and P&L statements in advance of the opening of the business

profit and loss (P&L)
a financial document published by a company showing earnings, expenses, and net profit

return on investment (ROI)
the income that an investment provides

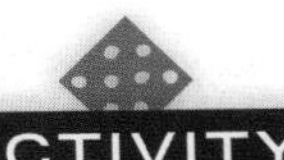

ACTIVITY

Writing Spa Business Plans

Write the introduction to the business plan for a spa that you might one day like to build. Alternatively, the entire class can participate in this activity by breaking into groups of two or three students. The instructor will provide the name, location, type, and approximate size of a spa, and each group of students writes one portion of the business plan for this spa.

CREATING A DEDICATED SPA SPACE

Many therapists, when they first begin offering body scrubs and wraps in their massage rooms, are tempted to use the term "spa" to describe their newly revamped offerings. While it is important and appropriate to capitalize on the continuing popularity of spas by using the word "spa" to describe your business, it is nevertheless unethical to do so if you are not, in reality, operating a spa. So, how do you know when you can ethically and legally use the term "spa" as part of your business name? Once again, it has nothing to do with the size of your operation. Many therapists have started with one room and called their business a "spa." Becky Zwickl, for example, began her business in *half* a room, taking the back portion of a garage and turning it into a multi-modality treatment center which she dubbed "Becky's Day Spa." (See her profile later in this chapter.) Today, Becky's Day Spa takes up over 2,000

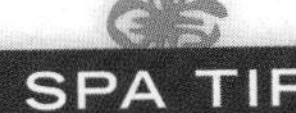

SPA TIP

If you embark on the creation of your own spa business plan, it may be helpful for you to take a look at examples of real plans that have been used to launch other businesses. You can find many at http://www.bplans.com.

SPA TIP

A spa business plan is not a place for dreaming, cheerleading, or lavish self-praise. It should be a sober document containing facts, figures, estimates, plans, profiles, backgrounds, and realistic assessments of profit potentials. Do not say, "This is going to be the greatest spa ever built and attract a huge number of clients to the original location, after which we will franchise and make millions of dollars." Savvy investors will know immediately that you do not have a realistic grasp of the marketplace. Instead, do your homework and propose a reasonable business model with a reasonable chance at success.

Other mistakes to avoid when crafting your business plan include:

- Requesting people to sign a non-disclosure agreement.
  Most people will not sign one at this stage, and asking them to do so will appear paranoid and/or amateurish.
- Overstating your qualifications.
  If you try to make yourself and your team members look more experienced or qualified, people will eventually find out, and by then you may owe them money. Not a good idea.
- Focusing too much descriptive detail on the spa market.
  Potential investors already have an idea of the marketplace (perhaps a much more realistic one than you yourself have). Spend more time in the business plan describing your plans, concrete goals, benchmarks for success, and what makes your team special enough to implement them.

square feet of prime real estate in Scottsbluff, Nebraska. She has also opened a second location, and now she is bursting at the seams, in need of even more space. Becky used the word "spa" to describe her original one-room operation so that people would know immediately what types of items she had on her menu and what kind of service they could expect. She didn't need a Vichy shower, an expensive hydrotherapy tub, a full-time receptionist, or even a waiting room. What she did offer, however, was a full menu of spa services in a dedicated treatment space.

Many therapists have compromised on the name of their business, opting for titles such as "Therapeutic Massage and Day Spa," which highlights the focus on massage while still alerting potential customers to the spa services offered. This option works well in many instances, but you should remember that in order to call a business a "spa," you need three basic ingredients, all of which Becky Zwickl, along with thousands of other therapists, had before they opened their own spa businesses to the public. Those three ingredients are:

- the therapeutic use of water
- a dedicated space
- a well-developed spa services menu

Note that these three ingredients are in addition to the basic supplies and equipment needed to create a spa experience for clients.

Because spas have their origins in the therapeutic use of water, therapists need to remember to make the healing properties of water available to their clients in any spa, no matter how small, even in a single room. The source of water can be a sink down the hall outside of this single room. Add a heating unit and insulated container to keep products and towels hot, and that is all you need.

In order to realistically call your place of business a "spa," you must have, at the very minimum, a treatment space that is dedicated to the offering of spa services. This does not necessarily mean that you are operating your spa business out of an expensive building or that you need any infrastructure at all. Some therapists successfully offer spa services to clients in their own homes or at "spa parties." What you need, essentially, is a dedicated "mental" space that will allow your clients to feel that they are receiving a true spa experience while in your care. Your mindset must be a spa mindset. You must live and breathe the "golden rule for spa employees" as stated in Chapter 15: "Treat the spa and each of its guests exactly as if you were the owner." In this case, you *are* the owner! The spa is your business, regardless of where it is set up, and you owe it to your clients to be a dedicated spa owner. Even if you own no real estate, you do own the spa concept that you are creating for your clients, and you must take responsibility for that.

Enterprising massage therapists have been able to create serviceable spa spaces out of half a garage, large bathrooms, converted ambulances (mobile spa on wheels), walk-in closets, and many other unlikely locations. This "economy spa" route may be the wisest course for you to take if you are on a tight budget. However, some therapists have money to spend on their spa spaces, either from investors, loans, or savings, and they are ready to go out in search of more elaborate venues for their new businesses. Therapists in this position should keep three main points in mind: location, price, and condition of the property.

Choosing a Spa Location

Choosing a location for your spa is a weighty decision. You've been told countless times that only three things matter when it comes to a service or retail business: location, location, and location. It is only natural, then, that you will feel pressure to find the choicest location for your business.

When it comes to spas, most owners want to locate their businesses in such a manner as to be convenient for their most likely customers. This does not mean that all spas need to be located in the swankiest part of town. But it does mean that your spa should be located where your targeted customers live, shop, commute, or otherwise congregate on a consistent basis. See the Demographics section and the Did You Know sidebar, "Narrowing Down Your Target Clientele," earlier in this chapter for more information on this topic.

Some of the questions to ask yourself as you are scouting possible locations include the following:

- Do you want walk-in customers, or would you like to focus exclusively on pre-booked appointments? Spas that cater to a walk-in clientele need to be located in well-traveled areas, often those spots that attract tourists and pedestrian shoppers.
- Do you want to create a more therapeutic and medically oriented image, or a luxury- and beauty-oriented image? This will help determine the type of location you choose if your spa will be part of a larger existing building.
- Do you want the physical location to somehow reflect your esthetic values or the core philosophy of the spa? Some spas have themes that reflect nature, a culture, or other specific idea, and their owners want the spa's location to be a part of that image.
- Do you want to deal with other parties when it comes to sharing the physical space? Certain spa location options necessitate more interactions than others. Spas that share space in a converted house, for example, will need to deal with landlords and other tenants.

Table 17–5 describes some of the most typical locations for new spa businesses, with the advantages and disadvantages of each.

Finally, do not underestimate the power of "energy" when it comes to choosing a location for your spa. Many therapists are attuned to the invisible energy fields at play in human interactions, using them as part of their repertoire of treatment options in modalities such as Reiki and polarity. People intuitively understand that some unseen force seems to keep the public away from certain buildings while attracting it to others. The mechanics behind this phenomenon cannot be explained satisfactorily by anybody. Still, most people would agree: Some places are better for business than others. So, when you head out looking for a space to open your spa, pay attention to your intuition. All other factors being equal, choose the location that feels right.

SPA LOCATION	ADVANTAGES	DISADVANTAGES
in a store front	usually has high visibility for walk-in traffic, spa owner not responsible for building, relatively simple build-out	lack of equity in building, limited creative control over how the business looks to clients from the outside
as a stand-alone building	potential equity in site, prestige image, complete control	spa owner responsible for building, including insurance, damages, upkeep, parking, etc.; often expensive
in rooms of a converted house	homey atmosphere without the cost of buying/leasing an entire house, camaraderie with other tenants, potential synergy with other tenants in like-minded businesses	have to deal with other tenants in close quarters, no guarantee of synergy with other tenants and their businesses, potentially second-tier image if house is not kept up by owner, lack of control over total environment, lack of equity
within a fitness environment	built-in clientele, motivated clientele who want to look their best (often conducive to multiple treatment packages, especially for slimming, etc.), educated clientele who know benefits of stretching and massage and want to improve results of their exercise programs	noise, atmosphere not conducive to relaxation, often second-rate ownership opportunity or none at all (fitness club owner retains equity), clients unresponsive to spa modalities in this atmosphere
within a medical arts building	high prestige among therapeutically inclined clients, potential networking with health care providers, potential insurance work for referrals, ability to offer medical spa services if physician present	some clients are intimidated by a medical environment, lack of equity in building, potentially subject to ostracizing by medical providers who look down on spas
within a salon environment	built-in clientele motivated to look their best, cross-selling of services with esthetic/cosmetic staff	potentially noisy and busy atmosphere not conducive to spa work, some clients not educated about therapeutic benefits of spa modalities and expect only superficial pampering
within an office park	often affordable rent, proximity to workers	can be hard to find, environment not normally associated with spa work, lack of equity in facility

TABLE 17–5 Spa Location Options.

Understanding a Spa's Price

Of course, when purchasing, renting, or leasing a location for your spa, you will want to make the best deal possible. But how, exactly, will you know what is a good deal and what is not? How can you compare the price of a 2,080-square-foot converted Victorian house on a side street with 1,100 square feet of raw space in a medical arts building? Many factors come into play.

First, determine the *cost per square foot per month* of the facility you propose to occupy. This can be determined by dividing the monthly cost of owning or leasing the facility by the total square footage. Keep in mind that some facilities have hidden costs, like insurance and taxes. Get all the information before you make your decision. Purchasing a site gives you the benefit of equity in the property itself, but it also saddles you with more of these hidden costs. Leasing or renting will let you off the hook for some of these expenses, but you will be left with no equity in the property.

Next, estimate how much potential income you could make from each property each month, including retail sales, which will depend upon the number of

	PROPERTY A	PROPERTY B
TYPE OF PROPERTY	EMPTY OFFICES IN MEDICAL ARTS COMPLEX	CONVERTED HOUSE IN MIXED-USE RESIDENTIAL/COMMERCIAL AREA
monthly rent/lease/mortgage/insurance/taxes	$1,400	$2,400
square footage	1,100	2,080
cost per square foot per month	$1.27	$1.15
projected income per month	$9,000	$17,000
projected income per square foot per month	$8.18	$8.17
potential profit per square foot per month	$6.91	$7.02

TABLE 17–6 Property Comparison for Choosing Spa Locations.

treatment rooms and the location (spas in more upscale areas can usually charge more for services). Then, divide that figure (your potential monthly income) by the total square footage to come up with your *potential income per square foot per month*.

Then, take the *cost per square foot per month* and subtract it from your estimate of *potential income per square foot per month* for each property. The resulting number is your hoped-for monthly profit from each square foot of the spa. Now, you can compare the monthly profit numbers for each facility and reach a more informed decision.

Table 17–6 shows an example of relative cost comparisons for two very different properties that have surprisingly similar profit potentials.

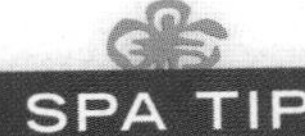

SPA TIP

When you are deciding upon potential locations for your spa, look at each property from your targeted clientele's point of view rather than just your own. When you are especially excited by a site's beauty, quirkiness, or unique charm, it may mean that you would be happy as an owner of that location, but it does not necessarily mean your clients will be happy as customers. Ask yourself these questions: Is it safe? Well-lit? How's the parking? It is easy to find? Does it have a clean, hygienic feel? Will the neighbors be friendly toward your clients?

Judging the Condition of a Property

Regardless of where it is located or how much it is going to cost, you have to consider what condition a potential spa facility is in and the cost of getting it up to par. It is not always the visible structures that will take more money to fix, but rather the hidden infrastructure. **HVAC**, plumbing, electrical wiring, foundation, and other behind-the-walls components of a structure can be expensive to repair, though they are mostly invisible when you first visit a property. On the other hand, what may seem like an expensive change might really be quite cheap. It is often a simple matter to move, demolish, or build a wall, creating an entirely new floor plan for just a few hundred dollars.

HVAC

heating, ventilation, and air-conditioning

Layout and Design

When it comes time to lay out the plan for your new spa space, you will need to be thinking like a businessperson rather than a therapist. The key element you will want to keep in mind when making every decision is **revenue-generating space (RGS)**. RGS is the holy grail of professional spa designers, and they keep it in mind when building anything from tiny day spas to mega-large resort spas. Basically, by focusing on RGS, you are focusing on the future success of your spa. So, how does RGS work? What it means is that you need to ask yourself an important question about each and every square foot of

revenue-generating space (RGS)

the square footage inside a (spa) business that generates revenue—examples include treatment rooms and retail displays—as compared to those spaces—such as hallways, relaxation areas, and waiting rooms—that do not normally produce revenue

SPA TIP

Raw Space vs. Finished Space

Some therapists are excited when they discover a location that seems already set up to be a spa, such as a former doctor's or chiropractor's office. This often seems like a good, economical choice. But consider the advantages of choosing **raw space** to build your spa:

- You won't be tempted to leave things the way they are just because they are already there.
- Walls are cheap to build.
- You can turn a raw space into a more precise replica of your vision for the ultimate spa.
- You will be able to think of your clients first and make the space better for them.
- You'll have many creative options (for example: one therapist chose to lease raw space that used to house a bank, with only one room still left intact, the vault, which she planned to change into a treatment room).
- You can focus more on the location of the space instead of searching for the perfect pre-setup spa, which may not be in the best area.

raw space

unfinished interior of a building, often with no walls or flooring, that will need a good amount of construction to render into a usable (spa) business environment

the space you are proposing to turn into a spa. That question is: Will this square foot generate revenue of any kind at any time, or is it "dead space" that I will have to pay for in rent and utilities but which will produce no income for me? The most obvious RGS in the spa is, of course, the treatment room. Every time a treatment room is filled with a client and a practitioner, revenue is being generated there. But the waiting room where clients sit prior to the treatment and the hallway clients walk down to get to the treatment room are usually not RGS. As you set about designing the layout of your spa space, even if it is only a couple rooms, it will pay to keep asking yourself the following questions:

- Will this space generate revenue or not?
- Is there a way to convert this potentially dead space into RGS?
- How can I make this common area or waiting area or resting area into RGS?
- How can I add to the RGS potential of these square feet through retail options?
- How can I make this space multi-purpose so that it can generate revenue more consistently?

If you take a look at Figures 17–5 and 17–6, you will see that the non-RGS area in this particular spa layout actually amounts to nearly half of the square footage. What otherwise looks like a perfectly acceptable layout and indeed does work for some therapists contains some hidden lost revenue because of its dead zones. So, what can you do when you are devising the layout of your own space? The following rules will help steer you clear of the most common mistakes, especially when it comes to missed revenues.

- Keep rooms multi-purpose so as not to schedule yourself into a box. If you can perform every treatment in every room, then you will never have to turn down an appointment because of lack of proper equipment or facilities.
- Get the square footage right before you begin build-out in order to eke out as much RGS as possible from each area. Plans may change during construction, but at least you will have an idea to guide you.

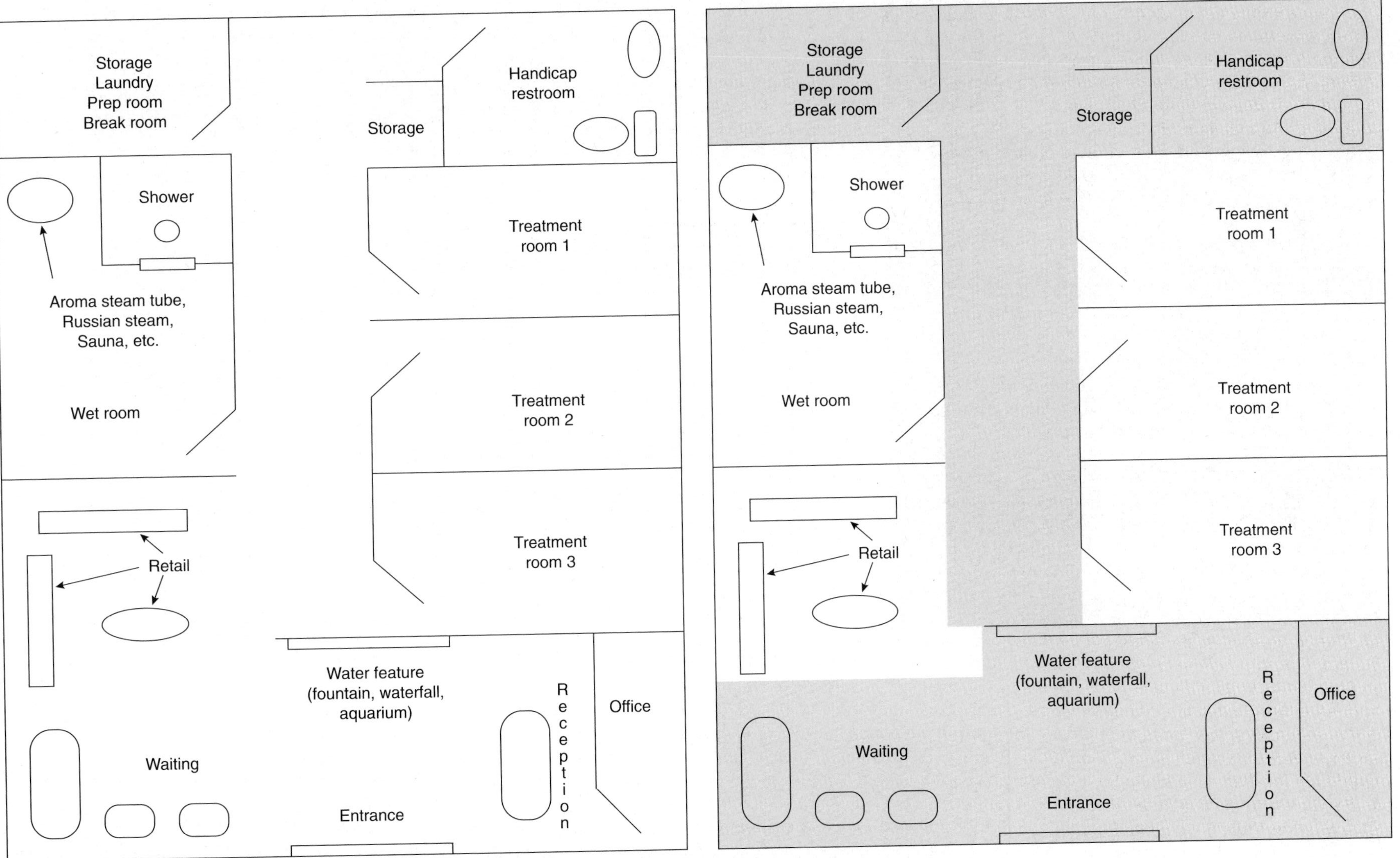

FIGURES 17–5 and 17–6 Looking at a small spa layout with non-RGS in green highlights the potential loss of revenue.

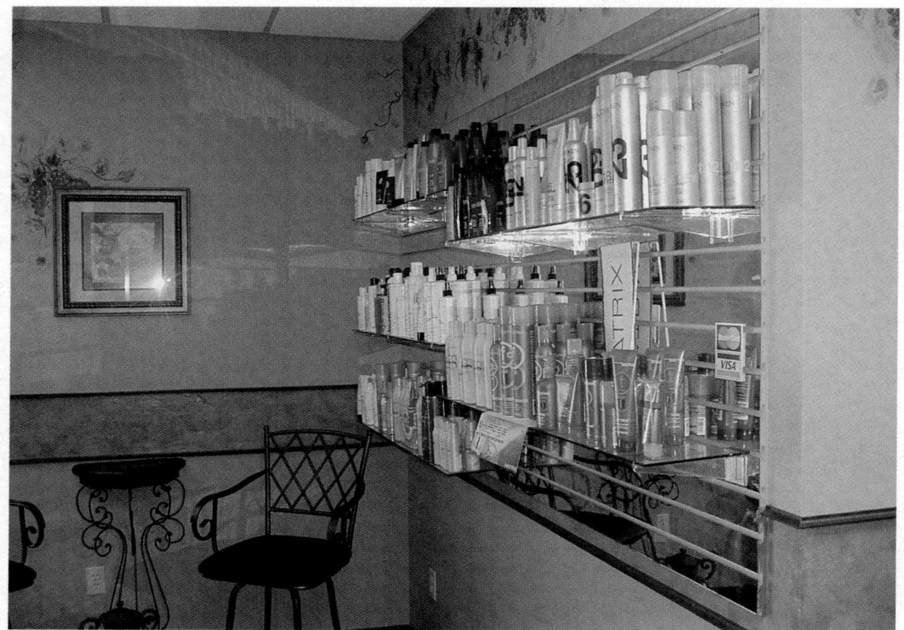

FIGURE 17–7 Placing products in otherwise empty spaces boosts RGS. The "Wall of Lotions & Potions" at Becky's Day Spa in Nebraska.

- Capitalize on RGS by turning typically non-revenue-generating spaces into hotbeds of profit, for example by placing products along the wall in an otherwise empty hallway (Figure 17–7) or using waiting areas to do spa foot treatments.
- Do not overspend on fancy exotic equipment that may not be profitable in the long run. Remember, most spas make 80 percent of their profit from the two standby treatments: massage and facials. By not including that high-end hydro tub, you will have room for an extra massage or facial room.
- Get good advice before installing expensive plumbing, heating, flooring, etc. You may know what you are doing, but is best to get other opinions also.

Now that you know some of the general rules for setting up a spa space, it is time to consider some of the particulars involved with each distinct area of the spa, including plumbing and electrical, HVAC, FF&E, treatment rooms, wet rooms, reception areas, changing rooms, lockers, and "back of the house."

Plumbing and Electrical

Even if you go to the expense of hiring a seasoned architect to lay out your spa space, you will possibly still be left with an improperly outfitted facility. The reason for this is that many architects are not familiar with the particular needs of spas. Two of the areas that are least understood are plumbing and electrical. So, before you push forward and make a big investment, make sure that you are receiving spa-specific advice when it comes time to install pipes and wires.

If you install equipment such as Vichy showers or Swiss showers, the drainage in the floor is going to have to be spacious enough to take the extra flow from these mega-showers. This usually means installing a three-inch drain instead of the normal two-inch PVC used in much of construction today. Not knowing this could end up costing you a great deal of money in reconstruction when you end up with big puddles on your floor. Another problem specific to wet rooms is improperly insulated flooring. Rubber matting needs to be installed beneath the tiles on the floor and a couple feet up the walls to prevent damage due to seepage.

When wiring is installed, electricians will need to know how many amps each piece of equipment draws and exactly where they will be placed. Electricians will also have to consider how to best light the treatment areas in order to create the most soothing effect. Sconces, recessed crown molding lights, and other forms of up-lighting are the preferred method.

Heating, Ventilation, and Air-Conditioning (HVAC)

One of the most common complaints from both spa clients and employees concerns heating, ventilation, and air-conditioning (HVAC). Therapists usually complain that spa rooms are too warm while guests, who are lying still on a table and often covered in water or products, complain the same rooms are too cold. If the HVAC is not well-thought-out in advance, your spa might end up with a single thermostat that controls both the reception area and the treatment area, a sure recipe for discomfort and complaints. Ideally, separate thermostats should be installed in each treatment room, if this is possible. That way, clients can request a temperature change without affecting the rest of the spa. Therapists need to know that good customer service calls for a thermostat set where the guest deems it most comfortable, not where the therapist deems it most comfortable. This will most often be a slightly warmer temperature than the therapist would desire. When it comes to wet rooms, the temperature has to be even warmer than in massage rooms. So, even if it is not practical to install individual thermostats in each room, it is highly recommended to at least have separate distinct zones for the wet rooms and the rest of the spa.

When it comes to air handlers, blowers, and furnaces, spa designers and construction personnel need to know where to place sometimes-noisy pieces of equipment, and if they cannot find a location sufficiently distanced from the treatment rooms, then they have to install adequate insulation.

Furniture, Fixtures, and Equipment

Many therapists have only a vague idea about the **furniture, fixtures, and equipment (FF&E)** they will need to open their new spa operation. While a high-end multi-purpose treatment table is top on most therapists' lists when it comes to outfitting the spa, you will also need more mundane items such as desks, chairs, lamps, waiting-room furniture, and telephones. Some spa spaces will also need to be outfitted with bathroom fixtures, cabinetry, flooring, and

furniture, fixtures, and equipment (FF&E)

term used to describe the items that need to be purchased and installed in a building in order to start up a (spa) business wall coverings. There is a great deal involved. Make sure to include this category in your budget because if you do not, the surprise costs may overwhelm you. FF&E is usually calculated as an addition to spa equipment itself such as hydrotherapy tubs, pedicure stations, and treatment tables.

Treatment Rooms

The treatment room is where you, as a massage therapist, spend most of your time, and so naturally you want the space to be as commodious and comfortable as possible. On the other hand, as a spa owner, you will want to maximize your RGS, and so if it is possible to build three smaller treatment rooms instead of two larger ones, you may be tempted to do so. The general rule is that a 12' × 10' room (120 square feet) is the bare minimum in which to comfortably practice spa therapy. If the particular room is going to be used exclusively for massage, which is not recommended, it can be slightly smaller. As already mentioned, it is always preferable that each treatment room be furnished and equipped in such a way that most if not all of the spa's treatments can be offered in it.

Treatment rooms need to be as sound-proofed as possible, especially if the spa is part of a salon or other potentially noisy environment. As discussed in the "Spa Sounds for the Massage Room" section later in this chapter, a white-noise generator and music can be used to help create the right environment, but if you are building the room from the ground up, installing insulation will be very helpful and is a good idea.

Reception

The reception area in your spa should be utilitarian and attractive. It does not need to take up much space. You will have your computer or appointment book there, a telephone, a credit card terminal, and a cash drawer (Figure 17–8). In addition to providing a space in which to book appointments, greet guests, and answer phones, the reception area should also be the hub for your retail sales. In fact, impulse purchase items can be arranged on the counter to increase those sales.

A one-person reception is sufficient for most therapist-owned day spas, but some of the larger ones will need space for two or three receptionists, especially

SPA CAUTION

The Meditation Garden Money Pit

You may have visited a wonderful destination spa and been impressed with their faux-Buddhist meditation garden or luxurious tranquility haven or other similar non-revenue-generating space that looks extremely cool but does not add to the potential profit of the business. Do not be seduced by these tranquil traps. The spas that build them often have large budgets. Many therapists think, "I'll create a little oasis with herbal teas and plush lounges people can recline onto and wear headsets playing New Age music and positive visualization tapes." Watch out! If you do not have extra money to throw away, make as many of your square feet as possible into RGS. Of course, it is nice to provide a comfortable waiting space in your spa, but your main meditation gardens will be your treatment rooms, and your clients can rest luxuriously while they are in them.

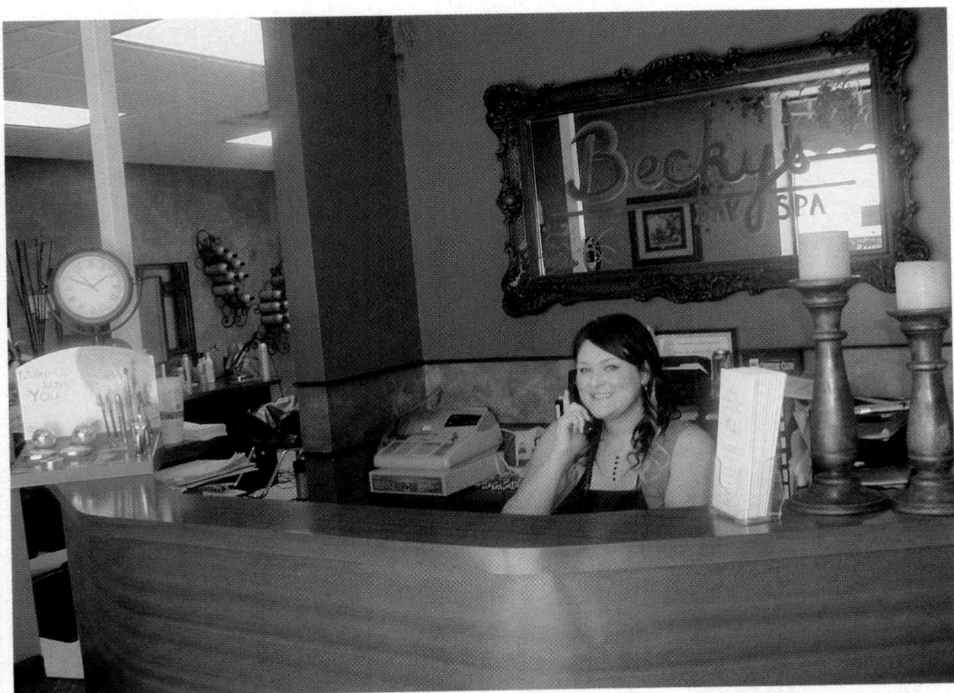

FIGURE 17–8 The reception area in a therapist-owned spa can be simple, efficient, and attractive.

if salon services are being offered. Typical setups for the reception area include a podium or high counter behind which receptionists sit or stand, located directly inside the front entrance of the spa. The counter does not have to be made from expensive marble imported from Italy, like the counters in some larger spas. Simple, attractive structures work well.

Changing Rooms and Lockers

Many therapists do not consider the options for changing areas or locker rooms when they are designing their spa spaces. Instead, they assume that clients will be happy changing in the treatment room itself, just as they are in a single-room massage practice. If you are creating a multi-room spa, however, many clients will expect someplace to change, to shower, to dry their hair, and even to shave. In short, they expect a locker room.

You have to be careful when you consider the inclusion of a locker room or changing area, because this is definitely not RGS. Therefore, you will need to strike a good balance between creating a requested amenity and avoiding a waste of money and precious square footage. Some small therapist-owned spas compromise on this issue and create a single-person changing and bath area. This is larger than a bathroom and has a few lockers included, but only one person at a time can use it. Some spas have two of these personal changing areas, one for men and one for women.

Some spas feature changing areas that accommodate more than one guest. These need to be quite a bit larger, usually at least as large as a treatment room. Many spa owners make the mistake of installing too many small lockers instead of just a few larger ones in these spaces, making them uncomfortable to use.

SPA TIP

Restricting Therapist Access to Reception

It is important to restrict the flow of employees in the reception area, especially curious therapists who are always concerned about their next appointments. If you can, provide another computer terminal or a written record of appointments somewhere away from the reception area so that therapists and others do not bother the guests and front-desk employees.

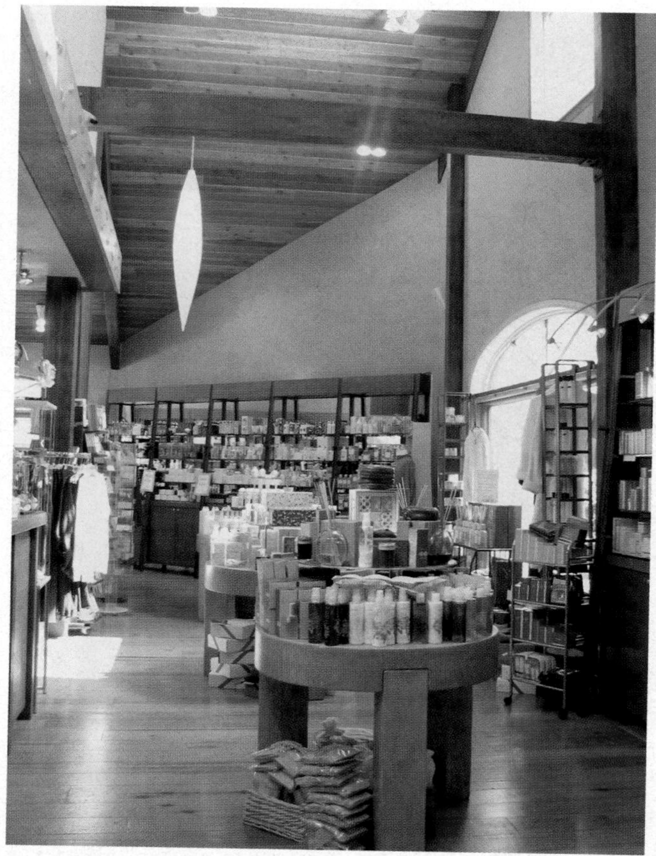

FIGURE 17–9 Retail items should be located in an attractive, easily accessible area.

If you do end up creating a locker room/changing area in your spa, cut the number of lockers you think you'll need in half and make them twice as large. You will probably not have to worry about this option if you are a therapist building a smaller spa, but should you become involved with a larger-scale operation, it will help to keep this in mind.

Retail

The most important thing for you to remember regarding retail when you are setting up your spa space is to make the retail areas as customer-friendly as possible. This usually means locating retail items in an attractive, easily accessible area (Figure 17–9). The most common location is adjacent to reception so that employees can monitor inventory and answer any questions clients may have regarding the products. The five key elements outlined in Table 17–7 will guide you as you develop ideas for your own retail area.

Back of the House

Many therapists, used to doing straight massage work, do not need to create a back-of-the-house area when treating their clients. A simple treatment room with an area for clients to hang their clothes and a shelf for the therapist to store oils and massage tools is enough. Therefore, when building a spa, they often overlook the need for a behind-the-scenes area, and so they neglect to design it into the space. In spas, though, what

SPA RETAIL AREA DESIGN ELEMENT	DESCRIPTION
accessibility	You'll want to make sure that your retail area is an organic part of your overall spa environment. Therefore, it should *not* be tucked away in a corner or cordoned off behind the reception desk. Guests should be able to flow into the retail area as a simple, natural part of their experience at your spa. Ideally, people with disabilities should be able to access every part of the retail area as well. Why not make retail as **ADA-compliant** as your bathrooms?
ubiquity	Retail products do not need to be restricted to one small area of the spa. Retail displays can be sprinkled throughout, even in the treatment rooms and hallways.
quality shelving	The actual surface upon which your retail products sit should be high-quality and attractive, as it reflects directly on the products you are displaying.
touchability	If people can touch, smell, and otherwise experience products, they are more likely to purchase them. Therefore, it is wise not to lock them up inside glass cases, except for extremely small, valuable products.
lighting	The way retail products look significantly affects the way people feel about buying them. It is a good idea to invest in track lighting or spotlights in order to maximize the appearance of your items.

TABLE 17–7 Spa Retail Area Design Elements.

clients do not see can be as important as what they do see, and you will have to create "back-of-the-house" or "off-stage" areas for your spa to be successful. These include preparation areas, laundry areas, employee break areas, and office space.

ADA-compliant

in conformance with regulations of the Americans with Disabilities Act; usually used in reference to physical facilities of a (spa) business being set up to accommodate people in wheelchairs and with other physical restrictions

Preparation Areas

Think about the herbal wrap treatment (Chapter 8) for a moment. In your spa, you will not want your client to watch while you prepare the herbal solution, soak the sheets, and wring them out wearing bulky rubber gloves. Instead, you will want this to happen out of sight, as if by magic. In order to accomplish this, you need to include a preparation area, sometimes referred to as a *staging area*, in your spa plans. The preparation area can be as simple as a small closet. It can even be inside the actual treatment room, if space is at a premium. You can create an off-stage area with the use of a screen or curtain.

The preparation area can also be used for storage where towels, products, and equipment are kept out of sight. It is also desirable, but not necessary, for the prep area to include a sink. In this area, you can, for example, mix seaweed to be used in a masque, heat the mask for application, blend aromatherapy oils to be applied after the masque, and store the dirty towels used to remove the seaweed masque. The spa preparation area will be used extensively in this manner for many treatments.

Laundry Areas

Your preparation area may also include a washing machine and dryer, or the laundry facilities can be kept in a separate room. Do not make the mistake of underestimating the amount of laundry you will do. A general rule of thumb for spa treatments is that they require triple the number of towels and sheets as do straight massage services. The laundry area may need extra insulation in the walls and perhaps the ceiling so the sound of the machines cannot be heard in the treatment rooms.

SPA ETIQUETTE

If any spa employee smokes while on break, he must be required to wash especially thoroughly before interacting with guests once again, because the aroma lingers on fingers, skin, and clothes, making for an unpleasant guest experience.

Employee Break Area

Even the most personable of spa staff members with great customer-service skills need a place to spend time on-site out of guests' view. A small break room, which can be just a table in the laundry area, will serve to let therapists, estheticians, receptionists, and others sit and relax without the need to be "on" for the guests. This area can also include employee lockers, an eating area, a microwave, and a refrigerator.

Office Space

Ideally, your work space or the work space provided for the spa manager will be out of guests' view. This space should be as small as practicable because it is non-RGS. Some therapists forget completely about planning an organizational space for their spa, though, and end up doing paperwork at the reception desk in full view of the staff and clientele. This is not appropriate. At the very least, you should plan on having your paperwork tucked someplace out of view, behind a screen or in a cabinet. A messy spa that mixes back-of-the-house details with the guest's experience will seem less than professional.

Spa Flow

Did You Know?

When you are first laying out the space for your spa, you may get lost in your own designs, losing sight of the forest for the trees, and you will not be able to see some of the most obvious problems that typically come up regarding the *flow* between one area of the spa and the next. To overcome this tendency, you will need to switch your perspective to that of your future guests and ask yourself the following questions. Pay special attention to the answers because they will impact important decisions about the construction of your space.

- Where will my guests go when they first walk in the door?
- Will they feel welcomed?
- What will they do next?
- Will they know what is expected of them?
- How does the waiting area of the spa flow into the changing rooms or treatment areas?
- Will the waiting room be in a public area out near the reception desk, or will it be inside, behind a wall?
- Will men and women share the same waiting room?
- If clients have back-to-back treatments scheduled (e.g., massage followed by body scrub), will they move from one room to another or stay in the same room?
- What will they do while the therapist is changing the sheets on the table?
- How do they get from the treatment room to the locker room if they want to shower afterward?
- Will they be wearing a robe at that time?
- Where will their clothes be?
- What if they need to use the restroom during a treatment?
- What if they need to move from a wet room to a massage room, or vice versa?
- Will the bathroom (and other spa areas) be easily accessible to those with disabilities and conform to the rules of the Americans with Disabilities Act (ADA)?
- Where will my employees be when they are eating, on break, etc. so the guests will not see them?

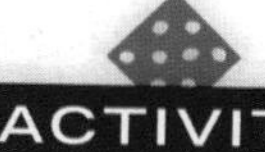

ACTIVITY

Designing Your Own Spa

Many therapists have entertained the idea of creating a functional one-room spa treatment space, but few elaborate upon this idea before creating it. Rather, they plunge right in and proceed by the process of trial and error. While this has worked well for some therapists, others are left with a hodgepodge of haphazardly selected elements in their spa treatment rooms. It is best to begin with an overall design plan. This plan need not be expensive. In fact, you can do it yourself for free. In this activity, you will design your own one-room spa treatment area on paper. This design may be based upon an area in your home, a stand-alone business space, or a room in someone else's place of business. This drawing can be artistically rendered in color or simply sketched out in pencil, but it must:

- include the therapeutic use of water
- engage the five senses
- feature space for retail display
- have plenty of storage space for towels, equipment, and products
- incorporate a versatile treatment table that will make the room multi-purpose
- optionally incorporate heating units such as a steam tent or heating capsule

CREATING A WELL-DEVELOPED SPA SERVICE MENU

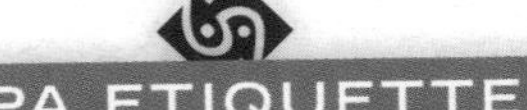

SPA ETIQUETTE

If you operate a one-room sole-practitioner spa with no receptionist, it is still preferable to create some kind of waiting area or antechamber in which to greet clients. Spa guests expect to feel invited in and taken care of. If you have no space for a separate greeting area, dedicate one area of your room to client comfort—with a chair where the client can sit down for a consultation, to sip a cup of tea, or to fill out an intake form.

To be officially classified a day spa, as defined by the Day Spa Association, a business must offer several distinct modalities in addition to massage therapy. Among these offerings are body packs and wraps, exfoliation, cellulite treatments, body toning/contouring, waxing, hand and foot care, cleansing face treatment, homecare program, aromatherapy, and some form of hydrotherapy, including steam and sauna. You should consider offering at least half of these modalities before including the word "spa" in your business name. Clients will understand if you do not have an elaborate menu of exotic treatments, but they often become irate when they find that what is advertised as a spa is actually a hair salon with a massage room attached or a massage room with a plug-in foot bath in one corner. Do your clients a favor by thoughtfully planning out a menu that contains the essence of spa, even if that menu contains just half a dozen items. Remember, these items can be combined creatively to make spa packages.

Therapists are usually eager to forge a unique menu of services to offer at their spas (Figure 17–10). In fact, creating the service menu is often the first step therapist/owners take as they approach their spa business ventures. Hands-on techniques are familiar to them, and they feel comfortable dealing with this aspect of the business. As we have seen, though, many other preliminary steps must be completed before the menu of services can be offered. So, while the service menu may be one of your initial motivations for creating your spa in the first place, you must put it in perspective and spend an equal or greater amount of time setting up your business plan, your employee manual, your marketing materials, and other crucial ingredients to your spa's success. Then,

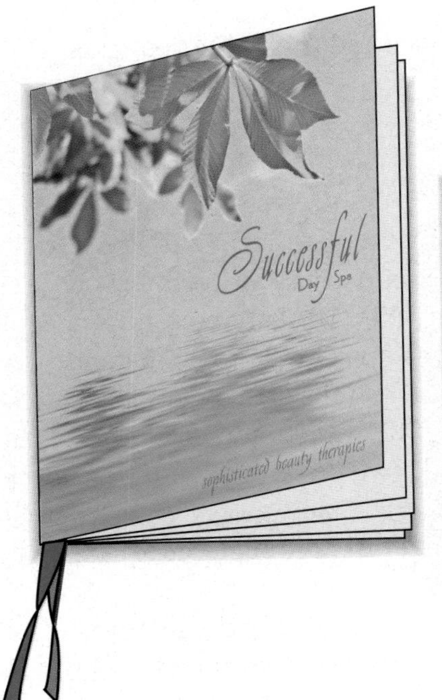

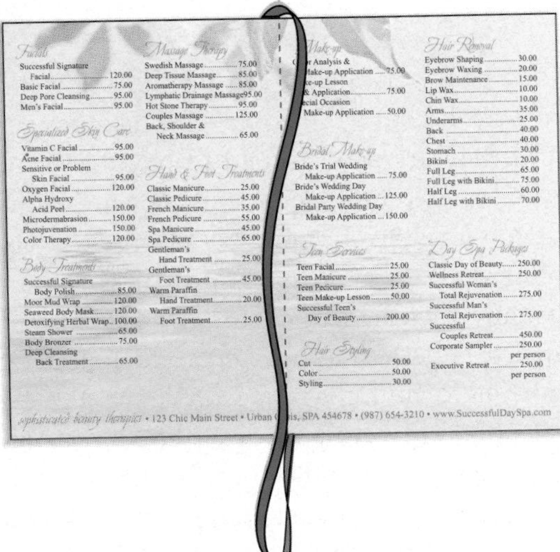

Facials
Successful Signature Facial 120.00
Basic Facial 75.00
Deep Pore Cleansing 95.00
Men's Facial 95.00

Specialized Skin Care
Vitamin C Facial 95.00
Acne Facial 95.00
Sensitive or Problem Skin Facial 95.00
Oxygen Facial 120.00
Alpha Hydroxy Acid Peel 120.00
Microdermabrasion 150.00
Photojuvenation 150.00
Color Therapy 120.00

Body Treatments
Successful Signature Body Polish 85.00
Moor Mud Wrap 120.00
Seaweed Body Mask 120.00
Detoxifying Herbal Wrap 100.00
Steam Shower 65.00
Body Bronzer 75.00
Deep Cleansing Back Treatment 65.00

Massage Therapy
Swedish Massage 75.00
Deep Tissue Massage 85.00
Aromatherapy Massage 85.00
Lymphatic Drainage Massage 95.00
Hot Stone Therapy 95.00
Couples Massage 125.00
Back, Shoulder & Neck Massage 65.00

Hand & Foot Treatments
Classic Manicure 25.00
Classic Pedicure 45.00
French Manicure 35.00
French Pedicure 55.00
Spa Manicure 45.00
Spa Pedicure 65.00
Gentleman's Hand Treatment 25.00
Gentleman's Foot Treatment 45.00
Warm Paraffin Hand Treatment 20.00
Warm Paraffin Foot Treatment 25.00

Make-up
C r Analysis & ake-up Application 75.00
ke-up Lesson & Application 75.00
ecial Occasion Make-up Application 50.00

Bridal Make-up
Bride's Trial Wedding Make-up Application 75.00
Bride's Wedding Day Make-up Application 125.00
Bridal Party Wedding Day Make-up Application 150.00

Teen Services
Teen Facial 25.00
Teen Manicure 25.00
Teen Pedicure 25.00
Teen Make-up Lesson 50.00
Successful Teen's Day of Beauty 200.00

Hair Styling
Cut 50.00
Color 50.00
Styling 30.00

Hair Removal
Eyebrow Shaping 30.00
Eyebrow Waxing 20.00
Brow Maintenance 15.00
Lip Wax 10.00
Chin Wax 10.00
Arms 35.00
Underarms 25.00
Back 40.00
Chest 40.00
Stomach 30.00
Bikini 20.00
Full Leg 65.00
Full Leg with Bikini 75.00
Half Leg 60.00
Half Leg with Bikini 70.00

Day Spa Packages
Classic Day of Beauty 250.00
Wellness Retreat 250.00
Successful Woman's Total Rejuvenation 275.00
Successful Man's Total Rejuvenation 275.00
Successful Couples Retreat 450.00
Corporate Sampler .... 250.00 per person
Executive Retreat .... 250.00 per person

sophisticated beauty therapies • 123 Chic Main Street • Urban O is, SPA 454678 • (987) 654-3210 • www.SuccessfulDaySpa.com

FIGURE 17–10 Therapists are usually eager to forge a unique menu of services for their spas.

when it comes time to begin work on your service menu, you can take it one step at a time in the following order:

1. Choose appropriate therapeutic products.
2. Set realistic, competitive prices.
3. Determine the correct treatment order for all guests using your services.
4. Create exciting multi-treatment packages to entice your customers.

Choosing Products

The most obvious choice to make when it comes time to pick the products you will use in your spa are the ones with which you become most familiar while going through massage school. While this may be the easiest route, and the products may be high quality, you should consider trying some other spa products as well. A wide range of manufactures offer hundreds of quality products in spas around the world, and if you do not experience some of these firsthand, you will probably not be able to make an informed decision. It is important, therefore, to visit spas yourself and to sample spa products from different companies. The opinions of other massage therapists and spa professionals is also important. A good place to experience many spa products is at the trade shows (see table 17–3), where you can touch and smell hundreds of creams, essential oils, massage lubricants, exfoliants, seaweeds, muds, herbs, clays, and more. Ask the manufacturers to give you the names of current customers so you can hear the opinions of your colleagues.

SPA TIP

If you sell branded products, you will be promoting that brand to your customers more than your own spa's brand, and that is why many therapist/owners are choosing to switch over to private label products, which we discussed in the previous chapter. With private label, you can make a much bigger profit margin on similar items while at the same time promoting your spa and your own brand instead of another company's brand.

Choosing the right products is crucial. Spa products that are less than therapeutic or less than completely pleasing to the client will lower your chances for success. Some questions to ask before you choose a spa product line include:

- Is it composed of natural ingredients, with a minimum, if any, number of chemical additives or enhancers?
- Is the brand one that will be recognized and trusted by your clients?
- Do your colleagues recommend it?

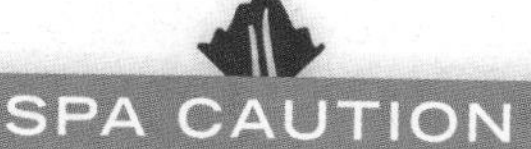

SPA CAUTION

Be aware that many spa product companies will be quite eager to give you free products, incentive pricing, and bonus discounts for volume sales if you agree to sign an exclusive contract with them. Do not be overly eager to tie yourself to certain vendors when you first start out, however. Keep your options open and work with a handful of product companies to see which ones offer the best fit and give you the most support.

Pricing

Rule number one regarding the pricing of your spa services is this: Do not undersell yourself. People expect to pay premium prices for premium services, and they are accustomed to paying well at spas. Spas are not cheap. People want spas to be special, and they are willing to pay for it. Some therapists feel uncomfortable charging people what other spas in the area charge and instead offer services at a discount, thinking they will attract more customers. This usually backfires, as customers tend to wonder what is wrong with the "cheap" spa. It is best to use great products, provide top-quality services in a nice atmosphere, and charge accordingly. Table 17–8 lists the suggested prices for a selection of treatments described in this book.

These prices reflect a relatively wide range because of the differentials in various markets. In general, you would not charge the same for a massage or spa service in a rural area as you would in a large city. Wherever you are located, try

EXFOLIATION SERVICES	CLEANSING FACE MASSAGE	SPA FOOT TREATMENT	HERBAL WRAP	AROMATHERAPY WRAP	BODY WRAPS	CELLULITE TREATMENT	SCALP TREATMENT
\$40–\$60 ½ hr	\$40–\$50 ½ hr \$65–\$80 hr	\$35–\$45 ½ hr \$50–\$70 hr	\$45–\$65 ½ hr	\$35–\$45 ½ hr \$50–\$70 hr	\$85–\$125 hr	\$90–\$120 1½ hrs	\$30–\$40 ½ hr

TABLE 17–8 Examples of Prices for Spa Services.

to push the envelope toward the upper end a little when it comes time to create your own pricing structure. If you would like to help people who cannot afford spa services, dedicate one day a month or one day a year to charity and give your services away for a worthy cause, but during normal business, charge well for super service.

Treatment Order

You will no doubt want to explore your own creativity when putting together a menu of spa services to offer your clientele. You know your clients best, and you know your own skills best. This is your chance to grow and explore new possibilities. However, as you're developing your menu, keep in mind that there are a few rules to follow regarding treatment order and combination.

- Rule #1: Exfoliation First
  It is a good idea to exfoliate before other treatments such as wraps and massage because exfoliation opens the pores to receive the full benefits of the product application to follow. If you were to exfoliate after a treatment, it might take some of the benefit away by sloughing product from the skin.

Tips For Pricing Spa Services

Did You Know?

The following are some other ideas for pricing that may help you.

- Create a Price Sheet
  Create a removable price sheet that you can change periodically without going through an expensive reprinting of your entire menu.
- Create Packages
  Offer package pricing for various combinations of treatments (see suggestions below).
- Offer Series
  Give clients the option of signing up for a series of treatments for a discount if they pay in advance. An example could be a series of 10 cellulite treatments, normally \$110 each, for \$900.
- Increase Prices
  A good time to raise prices is in October, when people are getting prepared to spend money during the holidays. You need to periodically raise prices in order to keep up with rising business expenses and the cost of living.

- Rule #2: Body Wrap Next
  Because oil, lotion, or cream on the skin would impede the penetration of herbs, seaweeds, clays, or other products, wraps should be performed before massage and other spa services, except for exfoliation. So a potential treatment order might look like this: (1) exfoliation, (2) seaweed wrap, and (3) massage.
- Rule #3: Massage Last
  Massage comes after exfoliation, body treatments, and wraps.
- Rule #4: Extend Services
  Create longer services out of shorter ones by combining them in ways that make sense. For example, for any exfoliation or wrap service, simply extend the application of hydrating lotion, massage cream, or body butter for an extra 30 minutes into a longer massage—and charge extra.
- Rule #5: Create Signature Services
  Your signature services will be spa treatment experiences that you develop for your own spa and for which you become well-known. The more distinctive these services, the better. Not just a new combination of existing treatments, signature services add something extra. Whether it features a special room with personalized ambience, a different twist on an old favorite, or a customized blending of products in a brand-new way, the experience should be unique. An example of this from an Ayurvedic spa menu might be a two-and-a-half-hour two-therapist synchronized exfoliation, massage, and third eye meditative Shirodhara treatment. Another example is the "Rain Forest Massage" using a Vichy shower to deluge the client with warm water while applying a massage using specialized essential oils.

Spa Packages

Most spas offer treatment combinations of one kind or another. These are often the spa's signature services, with exotic names and special package pricing, complex full-day affairs featuring half a dozen spa services plus a gourmet lunch, although they can be as simple as combining a half-hour exfoliation with a massage. As a general rule, the package price is lower than the sum of the separate services included in the package. For example, a $40 exfoliation combined with a $60 massage and an $80 wrap might be $150, instead of $180. See Table 17–9 for more examples of some treatment packages.

You will definitely want to include some treatment combinations at your own spa in order to set your business apart and give customers an incentive to order a greater number of services. These combinations can be changed periodically to reflect changes in your spa, the addition of a new product line to your offerings, or seasonal specials. For example, a "Warming Winter Wrap and Massage" combination offered December through March can feature herbal wrap therapy, warming essential oils, cups of hot tea, and a warmed herbal neck pillow the guest can take home. Use your imagination to create packages that entice customers to return and discover new offerings.

PACKAGE NAME	INCLUDED TREATMENTS	TREATMENT TIME	PRICE
The Rose Glow	body polish rose clay wrap 1 hour massage	2½ hours	$195
Marine Detox Treatment	salt glow seaweed body mask detoxifying massage	2½ hours	$195
Head-to-Foot Total Indulgence Package	cleansing face massage ½ hour spa foot treatment aromatherapy wrap	2 hours	$125
The Eastern Purifying Experience	Ayurvedic body scrub herbal wrap 1 hour warm oil massage ½ hour spa foot treatment	2½ hours	$145
The Royal Spa Day	body polish black Baltic mud wrap 1 hour massage 1 hour cleansing face massage 1 hour spa foot treatment	4½ hours	$295

TABLE 17–9 Spa Treatment Packages.

A CONSCIOUSLY CREATED SPA ENVIRONMENT

It is not necessary to compete with top spa properties that offer lavishly appointed treatment areas with picture windows opening onto fabulous views. Your own spa treatment room can feature four plain walls. Basically, to create a spa environment, all you need to add to those four walls are items that engage the five senses: lighting, sound, aroma, taste, and texture (Figure 17–11). Once you have created that space, you can offer the spa modalities you've learned in this book to your clients, along with your massage skills. Refer to "Setting Up the Spa Dry Room" equipment and setup explanation in Chapter 3 for more information on this topic.

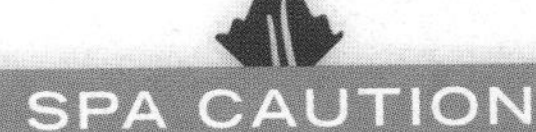

SPA CAUTION

Always keep the contraindications for each individual treatment in mind, even when several of these treatments are blended together as part of packages or spa days. Each package should be tagged with the total of all contraindications from all of the treatments contained within it, and all spa personnel should be aware of these contraindications as they pertain to packages.

Spa Lighting for the Massage Room

Many therapists, even if they do not offer spa services to their clients, create a spa-like atmosphere in their massage rooms through the use of artful lighting. As you can see in Figure 17–12, all it takes is a little creativity and some inexpensive material to completely change the ambience in almost any treatment room. In this example, the therapist used two layers of thin fabric attached to the drop ceiling to cover the fluorescent lights. An alternative to this is to use a similar piece of cloth and drape it over a floor lamp or a table lamp.

If you have the opportunity to run electrical wiring for your treatment room, install a rheostat (dimmer) switch so that you will be able to adjust the intensity of the light. Another option is to install a wall sconce to deflect light upward and away from the treatment table. You can even place lamps on bottom shelves and beneath tables.

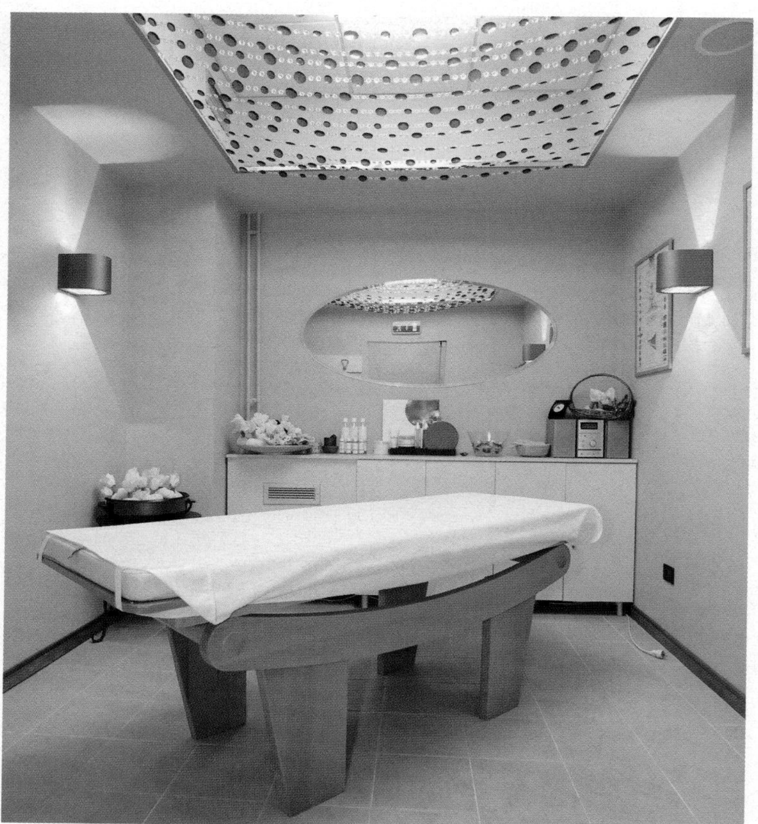

FIGURE 17–11 Spa treatment rooms should engage the five senses.

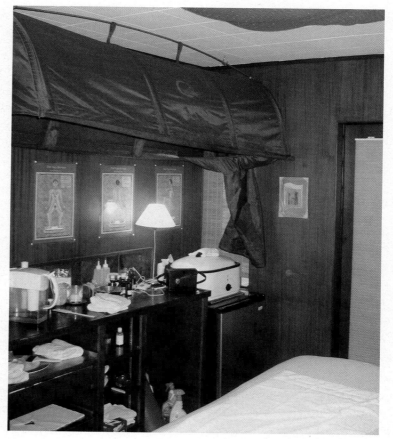

FIGURE 17–12 Therapists can do a lot with a single spa treatment room. Notice the "Steamy Wonder" (green) hanging over the work area and the colorful fabric covering the ceiling lights. Warming units, essential oils, colorful artwork and a small fridge add sensory touches.

Spa Sounds for the Massage Room

One of the main objectives in modern spas is to create an oasis of tranquility for guests. This can be accomplished in a massage room, but not if the environment is too loud or chaotic. Acoustic distractions are the worst for many clients because they cannot be easily shut off. Visual distractions are erased by simply closing one's eyes. Specific aromas can be altered or avoided altogether. Taste and touch are not usually an issue. When it comes to sound, however, your clients have little control. It is up to you to help them achieve the tranquility they seek by controlling the acoustic environment of your spa treatment room.

The most obvious way to control sound is to play music. Although most clients will agree that soothing music is ideal, some prefer other choices, including upbeat music, silence, and white noise. A **white-noise generator** is an inexpensive machine used in some spas to generate a mixture of sound waves extending over a wide frequency range (low-level background noise), making unwanted noises and voices less audible and the atmosphere in the treatment room more enjoyable.

Some therapists ask their clients if they would prefer to wear stereo headphones while receiving spa treatments. This technique blocks out much background noise, but it can be bothersome dealing with tangled wires. As an alternative, some treatment tables have stereo speakers built into them so that the vibrations from music travel physically into the client's body as well as the ears. This of course makes the treatment table more expensive, but it is a good option for those therapists creating a spa space in an area with significant unwanted noise.

Another appropriate sound for the spa treatment room is the sound of running water. Water, as you learned in Chapter 1, is the very essence of spa, which many people equate with *sanitas per aqua,* or health through water. Fountains, miniature waterfalls, burbling bowls atop tables, wall-mounted cascades, and free-standing floor units have all been used by therapists to lend their treatment rooms a spa feel (Figures 17–13 and 17–14).

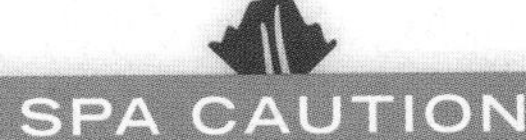

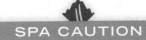

SPA CAUTION

When using fabric to cover and enhance lighting in your treatment room, make sure that the material does not come into direct contact with the bulbs. Maintain at least six inches of space between the material and the light itself to avoid potential fire hazards.

white-noise generator

an inexpensive machine used in some spas to generate a mixture of sound waves extending over a wide frequency range (low-level background noise), making unwanted noises and voices less audible, which renders the atmosphere in the treatment room more enjoyable

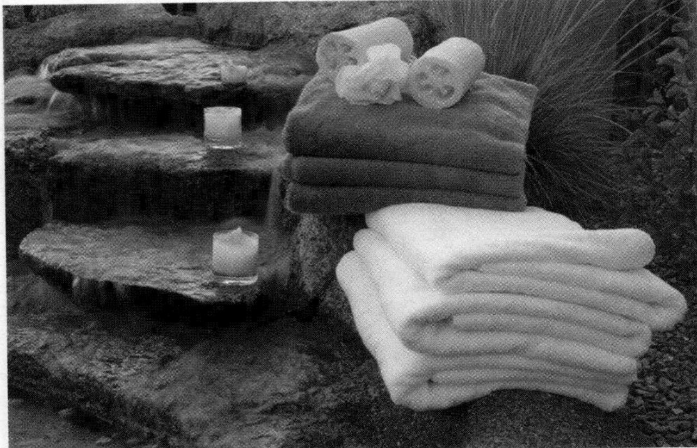

FIGURE 17–13 Water plays an important part in many therapists' one-room spa setups.

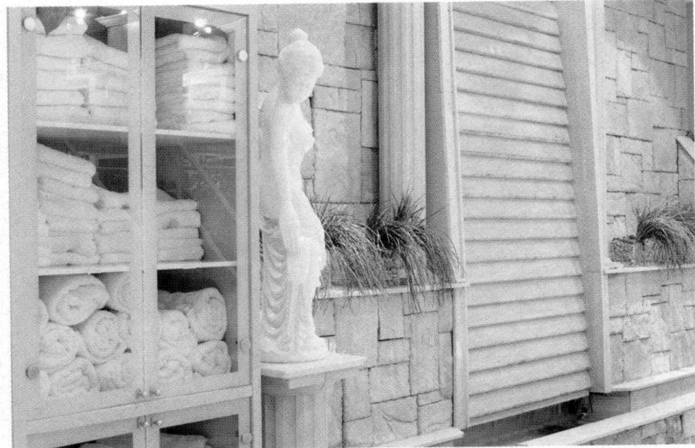

FIGURE 17–14 Water fountains and waterfalls can also be used effectively in spa waiting areas.

Spa Aromas for the Massage Room

Upon entering many high-end luxury spas (or simply walking by their entrances), the first and most powerful sensation you experience is the strong "spa smell." What exactly does that aroma consist of? Usually, its main constituents are sea-based products, boiling herbs, and essential oils, either in pure form or burned in candles. It is a distinctly organic scent, and quite pleasant. If you can recreate a version of this scent in your single treatment room, you will go a long way toward giving clients a total-sensory spa experience.

There are several ways to achieve this aroma in your treatment room. Many different types of aromatherapy diffusers are popular, even if you are not offering aromatherapy treatments on your menu. These include electric fan types, clay models used with candles, light bulb rings, and steam distillation units. The practice of using aromatherapy oils in treatments, even without a diffuser in the room, is enough to leave a lingering therapeutic scent in the air. Also, scented candles made with essential oils are used effectively for their scent and their light by many therapists, though caution must be exercised whenever an open flame is present.

Even though aromatherapy may seem like the obvious choice when it comes to creating aroma, probably the single strongest ingredient in that telltale "spa smell" remains seaweed, and this is one that many therapists overlook in their single treatment rooms. Even if you do not offer thalassotherapy treatments on your menu, you can still feature the scent of seaweed in your treatment area by adding small amounts of packaged seaweed treatment powder to a bath, a crock-pot, or a bowl of hot water.

Herbs in general—and specifically any blend of herbs that is used in the detoxifying herbal wrap (see Chapter 8)—create another distinctive scent in spas. Once again, even if you do not offer the detoxifying herbal wrap on your menu, you can still place an ounce of herbs in a small muslin bag and soak it in hot water to add an herbal scent to your treatment area.

Incense, though many people enjoy it, is not usually part of the aromatic environment in spas, except perhaps for those spas with Asian or Indian themes. The smoke emitted by incense is not enjoyed by all clients, and in the enclosed space of a treatment room, it can often be overpowering. Stick to the suggestions above in order to create a true spa atmosphere.

Spa Tastes for the Massage Room

While you may not usually think of taste as being central to a spa experience, this sense is actually quite important at larger spas that offer their guests nutritious food, healthy snacks, and many alternatives to the salt-, caffeine-, and sugar-laden items consumed by most people most of the time. You can also offer clients simple spa-inspired taste experiences in your treatment room. Something as simple as a glass of cool spring water with a twist of lemon or a freshly brewed cup of herbal tea can add a special extra level of sensory enjoyment for your clients. Other options include baked treats such as muffins, snacks like unsalted popcorn, vitamin waters, juices, iced herbal tea, and fresh fruit (Figure 17–15).

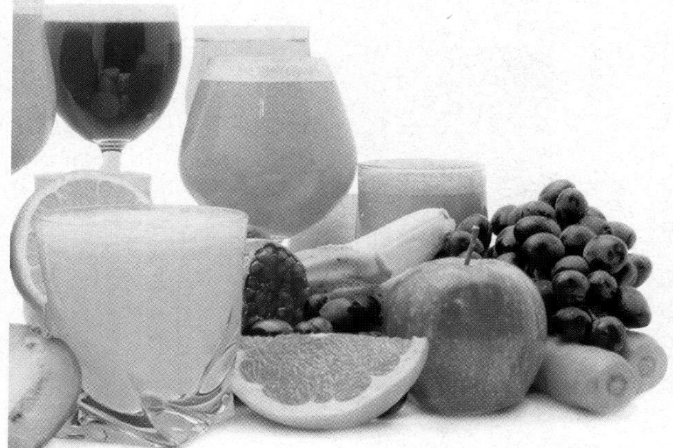

FIGURE 17–15 You can also offer clients simple spa-inspired taste experiences in your treatment room.

Spa Textures for the Massage Room

Finally, do not neglect the sense of touch when it comes to outfitting your spa treatment room. Of course, while in this room, you will spend a good deal of your time in direct physical contact with clients, but this does not mean that you should neglect the other tactile experiences your clients will have there. People expect a certain level of luxury when they enter a spa sanctuary, and you can provide this for them with something as ordinary as a towel. Objects like towels (and robes and slippers and sheets) that come into contact with your clients in the spa treatment room should be chosen for their quality. Plush, soft fabrics with high thread counts can help make your space more spa-like (Figure 17–16). Special textures can also be incorporated into other items in the treatment room, including the multi-purpose treatment table, which can be covered in **Ultraleather™** or another supple finishing fabric for a small percentage increase in overall cost of the equipment. Even the texture of such unlikely surfaces as the shower floor can make a big difference, as illustrated by one therapist's choice of natural river stones (Figure 17–17).

Ultraleather™

high-end fabric that can be used to upholster treatment tables, especially appropriate for use in spa rooms because of its plush, luxurious feel

Spa Retailing for the Massage Room

Although it was the focus of the previous chapter, spa retailing is important enough to mention again here. In the one-room spa environment, you will be solely responsible for your own retail success. Although it may seem difficult or not worth the trouble, you can definitely make retail work for you, even in the most cramped environment. A single shelf is enough from which to sell dozens of items. This shelf can fit along one wall in the treatment room or waiting area.

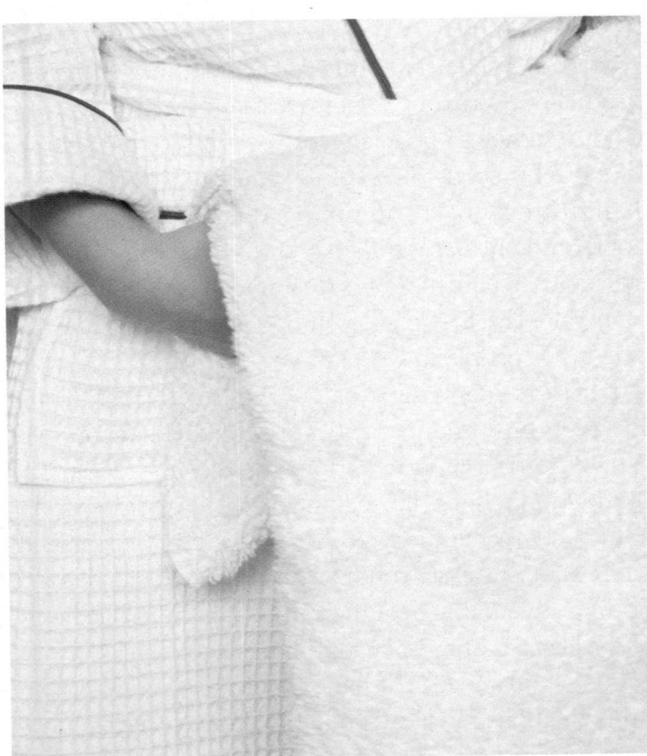

FIGURE 17–16 Plush, soft fabrics with high thread count can help make your space more spa-like.

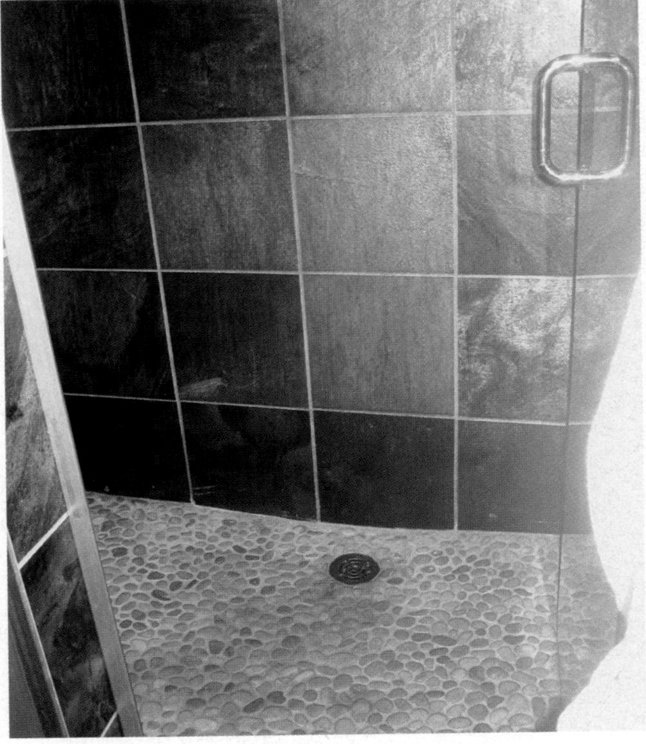

FIGURE 17–17 The texture of such unlikely surfaces as the shower floor can make a big difference in how your spa feels.

It should be well-lit, and price tags should be attached to the items so there is no mistake that they are for sale. Do not hide your retail selections away. If you stock your treatment room with items that you personally like to use and highly recommend, your clients will naturally want to find out more and purchase them. You can use the same sales protocols you learned in the previous chapter to sell retail items in your one-room spa treatment space.

CREATING A TEAM

Once you have created a physical location for your spa, designed a functional interior space, settled on the right theme, and filled it with the proper equipment, you will need to find some people to help you run it. This is sometimes the hardest part. While a multi-purpose massage table is a static entity that can be fixed in place and relied upon, humans can sometimes be less predictable. See the profile of Becky Zwickl in this section.

Regardless of the pitfalls involved, the therapist who becomes a spa owner must rely upon the skills and hard work of other people, or else she will fall prey to an exceedingly common predicament called the **owner/slave syndrome**. Many therapists, estheticians and other hands-on practitioners who open spas end up slaving away to support their own businesses, turning the spa into a glorified extension of their own private practices. This is not the point of opening a business. The point of opening a businesses is to create value in the business. In order to do that, you need to become skilled at hiring, training, and compensating other people.

owner/slave syndrome

tendency for therapists and other hands-on practitioners who open spas to rely upon their own work to support the business rather than build their spa's brand through the work of employees

Hiring

Massage therapists, by definition, are people who like to achieve specific results (relaxation, healing, stress-relief, etc.) through their own efforts and on their own terms. Often, they are not the type of people who feel comfortable delegating responsibility, because they feel that "if you want to get a job done right, you have to do it yourself." While this may be an admirable quality in any professional, it is not conducive to running a successful spa. One of the keys you will have to learn in order to make your spa business successful is to let go of some of the need to do everything yourself. The first place you begin doing this is when you start the process of hiring other people to work for you.

The therapists who grow their businesses gradually begin the hiring process organically and incrementally over time, finding people to work for them one at a time through personal referrals, word-of-mouth, and business connections. The therapists who have investors and more financial backing from the start, however, may find themselves suddenly in charge of hiring 10, 20, or even more people all at once to staff their new facilities. In this case, you may need to fall back on some more aggressive tactics, including advertising, seeking candidates at local schools, combing the Internet job listing sites, and hiring headhunters or recruiters.

Don't place all your attention on hiring just the hands-on staff. Though you are a therapist yourself and your inclinations may lead you to focus exclusively on the massage department, remember the other staff who will make a profound impact

SPA PROFILE

Becky Zwickl, owner Becky's Day Spa, Scottsbluff, Nebraska

The Challenge of Building a Successful Spa Staff

Becky Zwickl has been a licensed massage therapist in Nebraska for over 10 years. She is an energetic and enterprising woman who is raising a family as well as running a thriving spa business that, so far, has beat out all the local competition, including a well-funded medical spa startup. Zwickl started as a massage practitioner working out of the back half of a garage (not even a whole garage, just half), and she kept growing her business until, in her own words, "I just couldn't take any new clients because I only had that small space and a fixed number of hours in the day. When it got to that point, I sought out other people to work with. A nail tech first, then another. I moved us first to a four-room office space with five people working there. And now in our current space I have 13 practitioners at 12 stations and treatment rooms, plus three receptionists. In addition, we've opened a second location in a nearby town with a total of 6,400 square feet, including a full salon."

All of this growth and success has been great for Zwickl, but along the way she has experienced challenges she never dreamed of when she first started. "One of the biggest problems I didn't see coming was internal competition among the employees," she says. "We as LMTs are into making people feel better, but when you open a spa and add cosmetologists, nail techs and estheticians into the mix, it becomes a completely different setting. I always thought the external competition with other businesses would be the big thing, but it was the internal competition among employees that ended up being the more serious problem.

"My big mistake was basing my success on the happiness of my employees at first. I always wanted to make them happy. Typical! Sometimes LMTs are the worst bosses because we want to make everything nice and smooth everything over. What have I done to counteract this tendency? I've gotten tougher! And I've gotten rid of my biggest delusion—thinking that all my employees were going to stay with me forever. I've found that you need to empower your own name, your own brand, not the names of the therapists working for you. Every time I promoted them in the local paper, etc. I was building their names, not my spa's name. I don't do that anymore."

There is no shortage of mistakes that Zwickl cautions other therapists to avoid when opening a spa of their own. "One of the dumbest things I did was hiring out of desperation when someone left the spa," she states. "Don't do it! Don't make decisions out of fear. If someone says, 'I'll leave if you don't do this for me,' then let them leave. And don't pay them too highly out of fear that they'll leave. Once you become clear about the value of your own business, people will stay anyway. I haven't lost anyone in three years, and some of the best therapists I have now are the ones I got after my so-called 'shining stars' left. I wouldn't have had these great employees if I'd been too afraid to say goodbye to people whom I once thought of as indispensable.

"Theft is another problem I didn't expect," says Zwickl. "Since I'm basically a trusting person, I didn't expect to have employees pocketing cash from my business. One way it happens is they make it look on the computer like they've canceled an appointment with someone who actually paid cash. With over a hundred people a day coming through our doors, it's hard for me to keep track of every appointment. But now I've found ways of preventing this, of putting up firewalls, and we've been able to catch someone red-handed doing this. To say the least, I was naïve to certain things."

Zwickl says that opening her spa has been a huge commitment in both time and money. "In fact," she

(Continued)

SPA PROFILE

Becky Zwickl, owner Becky's Day Spa, Scottsbluff, Nebraska continued

muses, "If I'd known everything I didn't know before opening a spa, I might not have done it in the first place! I've had many 80-hour weeks, and on top of it I take work home with me. When I used to work at another spa, I always wondered why the owner was so stressed out. Now I know! It's the overhead and unforeseen costs. When I first started, my overhead was $200 to $300 a month. My average now is $15,000 to $20,000. If I had known I would be spending this much when I started, it would have freaked me out."

Zwickl has a few last words of advice for therapists who would be spa owners. "Don't let your success go to your head immediately," she says, "because you have to maintain it over the long run. It could be all gone tomorrow. You have to stay constant and don't get too big for your own britches.

"And on the other hand, don't let your failures get you down. There were so many times something devastating happened and I wanted to quit, but I ended up finding out that your moments of weakness are when you find your strength. Don't quit. So many people don't realize how close they are to success. You just need to make that one last push to get over the hill. Then you're there!"

SPA TIP

Your employees are your best recruiters. Once you have a team with whom you work well, let them suggest new employees. Also, let them take part in the interview process on some level so they feel invested in each new hire.

on your guests' experience. Your receptionist, for example, will most likely speak to each and every guest who comes through the door. Doesn't it make sense to proceed slowly and wisely when it comes time to choose this key figure in your operation? Almost anyone can answer a phone and write an appointment in a book. A good number of people may be quick at entering information into a computer. But how many of them will have your customers' best interests at heart?

While it is important to find qualified people, you will do better all across the board, from janitors to front-desk staff to therapists, if you look at the person first and the skill set last. Skills can be taught. Personalities come as part of the package.

Do You Need a Spa Manager?

When they first open their spas, many therapist/owners attempt to do everything themselves, acting as lead therapist, accountant, supervisor, payroll expert, computer specialist, and several other roles. This may be necessary at first if the spa is not funded well enough, but you will soon need to make a choice. Are you going to be a manager? If so, you should cut back on the number of treatments you give or eliminate them altogether, focusing on your other duties. Or, you can opt to hire a manager and focus on what you do best, which is therapy. If the spa is large enough, you can hire a manager and other therapists. Then you will be able to focus on marketing, creating a vision, and growing your business. But you cannot do it all.

The decision is not an easy one. It takes money to hire a manager, but the money you spend may free you up to create more profits than you could if you were tied down all day managing things yourself. Ultimately, you are free to mold whatever situation works best for you. No law states that a spa manager must do one set of duties and no others. You can modify the position and find the right person to fill it, letting him handle all of those areas in which you are weak. This tactic has been successful for many therapists.

RESEARCH

Target a local spa and find out what their hiring policy has been. Do they advertise in the classified section of the newspaper? Over the Internet? At local massage, cosmetology, and esthetics schools? How do they find most of their best people? Through recommendations from current employees? Would you use the same strategy at your own spa? Devise your own hiring strategy for a day spa and write a paragraph summarizing it.

Leadership, Discipline, and Training

As a spa owner, you will be the one responsible for creating the rules and regulations that others must follow. If you have spent much of your career as an employee, this switch from being a follower to a leader can be difficult. People will not look upon you the same if you are a boss and an employer, and you will not be able to interact with employees in the same collegial way you have with co-workers in the past. It is essential, however, for your spa to have strong leadership in order to succeed, and you will benefit by following the five steps described below to create and maintain that leadership.

Step #1: Create an employee manual

Without clear, written guidelines that describe what is expected of them, employees are not likely to perform to their highest capacity. It is your job to create a comprehensive employee manual that outlines all details of the spa's operations, including job descriptions, procedures, standards, grooming, appearance, uniforms, etiquette, guest complaints, sanitation, gratuities, and more. You can purchase an employee manual template from the International Spa Association.

Step #2: Take charge

As with every business, each successful spa business has a distinct chain of command. As the owner, you will be at the top of this chain. In this position, you need to be willing to enforce discipline and even, at times, be less than pleasant if the situation warrants it. You need to get control of the spa's systems so that employees are not tempted to cheat those systems. You need to form strong alliances with employees but at the same time remain at a distance, clearly in charge.

Step #3: Ensure adequate training

Spa owners must make sure that their employees are adequately trained. This includes customer-service training, computer training, standards and procedures training, and, of course, hands-on training for therapists and estheticians. It will be up to you where this training comes from, whether from product vendors, outside CEU providers, or in-house trainers. Regardless of how it is obtained, training must take place on a consistent basis, and you must have in place adequate testing and feedback systems to ensure the training is effective.

Step #4: Commit to constant improvement

As owner, you are in charge of heading your business in the right direction. You must have goals in mind that you communicate to the other team members. Without constantly restating and reshaping those goals, and focusing attention toward their completion, your spa business becomes stagnant. Even if you are already successful, the spa still needs to focus on achieving better results, and you are the one responsible for making that happen. It is an ongoing process.

Step #5: Take ultimate responsibility

Although the proper delegation of authority is important, you need to let all staff members know that you are the one ultimately responsible for the quality of all services and guest experiences. By taking responsibility, you encourage those beneath you to take responsibility as well and to respect your leadership.

open-book policy

the practice used by many (spa) businesses of showing employees (especially therapists) actual income, expenses, and P&L statements so that these employees can better understand the expenses involved with running a spa business and why their own compensation needs to be kept at specific levels

overhead

the general, fixed cost of running a (spa) business, as rent, lighting, and heating expenses, which cannot be charged or attributed to a specific product or part of the work operation

SPA TIP

Start Compensation Levels Low

It is best to institute lower compensation models for practitioners in your spa right from the first moment you open for business. It is much more painful and difficult to change later, lowering wages, which often leads to therapists leaving. Do not make the mistake of thinking to yourself, as many neophyte spa owners do, "I will pay the highest rates around to attract the best practitioners." Almost always, this philosophy backfires a few months down the road, and you will end up with therapists who feel a sense of entitlement, rather than gratitude.

Compensation

As a spa owner, you will be on the other side of the compensation equation, and suddenly, things will be different. No longer will you be complaining that spa therapists' wages are too low, even at 40 percent, 50 percent, or higher. Now, you will understand firsthand how expensive it is to run a spa, and you will want to explain to your staff of therapists that you simply cannot afford to pay them as much as they think they deserve. When it comes time to have this conversation with your therapists, either individually or as a group, it is a perfect opportunity to practice the **open-book policy** used by many spas. Like Becky Zwickl, profiled in this chapter, many spa directors and owners have decided that their therapists need to see the business numbers in order to understand how much of the spa's income goes toward covering **overhead** expenses.

As far as what you should actually pay employees at your spa, opinions and practices vary widely. Across the entire spa industry, many experts counsel that anything over a 30 to 35 percent commission on services rendered by both massage therapists and estheticians is too high and may make it difficult or impossible for the spa to ever reach profitability. Some spas, especially those simple ventures with extremely low overhead and only a few employees, can afford to pay practitioners more than 35 percent, but that is usually a recipe for disaster. Other non-practitioner employees such as receptionists or spa attendants usually make $8 to $12 per hour. As noted earlier, employee compensation is by far the largest expense at every spa. You, as an owner, will find it crucial to keep this major expense to a minimum to provide a realistic chance for your spa's survival.

COMMON BUSINESS MODELS FOR SPA THERAPISTS

After assessing your preparedness level on the Spa Ownership Preparedness Profile, you may perhaps find that the wisest decision you could make as you pursue your goal to open a spa is to decide not to open a spa. After you take a long and realistic look at your situation, you may find it is better to stop before making an investment of time and money. This does not mean, however, that you have to give up your desire to help your clients and increase your income by offering spa modalities. You do not need to own a spa to personally offer spa services. Your massage practice can become a de facto spa with the simple addition of a few products and supplies. Also, you can offer spa services in someone else's place of business or in clients' homes.

Offering Spa Services in Your Own Place of Business

You can easily convert a one-room massage office into a spa dry room using the suggestions in this chapter. When it comes time to lay out your space, you'll need to configure the room for maximum effectiveness in the minimum square footage. In order to do that, you may want to take into consideration some of the suggestions in Figure 17–18. Note the following details in this figure:

- plenty of storage (below counters, under table, etc.)
- chair for clients to relax on
- hook to hang clients' clothing
- rolling cart upon which to place spa products, bowls, spatulas, brushes, etc.
- retail display area
- warming unit (hydrocollator, roaster, crock pot)
- music system
- therapist's stool
- sink (or other water source—does not necessarily have to be inside the room)
- **back bar** display for bulk spa products used in treatment room
- treatment table (ideally multi-purpose adjustable)
- a small fountain, candles, aromatherapy diffuser, white-noise generator

back bar

refers to the larger (compared to retail) spa product jars and bottles kept on the shelf and used in the spa treatment room; originally an esthetician's term

Your one-room spa treatment area will ideally be 10' × 12' at a minimum, and 10' × 14' is more comfortable. Remember that you will need more room for storage, linens, product, and equipment than you would need for a massage

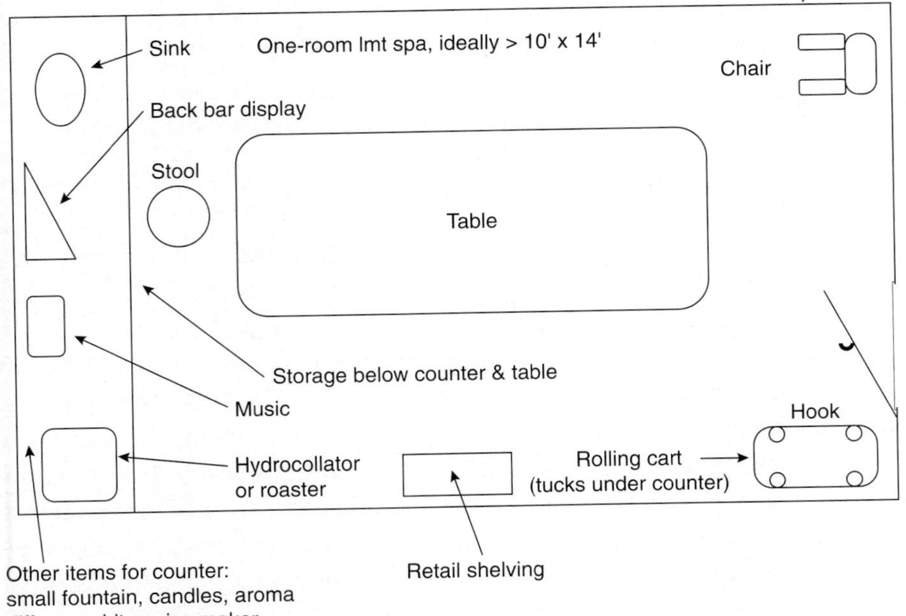

FIGURE 17–18 Note the details in a therapist's simple one-room spa setup.

room alone. There are many variations on the one-room spa. Some have a separate waiting area just outside the door. Others do not. Some have plumbing inside the room. Others do not. All of them, however, feature the basic elements listed above which, when used correctly, will create a true spa experience for your clients.

Offering Spa Services in Someone Else's Place of Business

Some therapists decide to build a mini–spa business inside of someone else's business. Most typically, this kind of spa setup is found in chiropractors' offices, massage clinics, and hair salons. While the arrangement works well in many environments, challenges sometimes arise between the various personalities involved. Usually, these challenges are a result of not having thought through the business model before embarking on the spa venture. The following illustrate some of the dilemmas that can develop in this situation:

- If a therapist agrees to build a spa business from the ground up, starting from scratch, in an empty, unused room in a chiropractor's office, does the chiropractor own the spa business, or does the therapist own the spa business?
- If a therapist offering spa services in a salon leaves to start her own business, is it ethical to take her spa clients with her?
- If a therapist working as part of a crew at a massage clinic begins offering spa services on his own initiative, who should buy the products, the therapist or the clinic owner?
- If a massage clinic owner decides to include spa services in her business, does she have to pay for training all of the therapists? Can she force her therapists to attend training without paying them? What if the therapists learn all they can, then leave to start their own spa businesses down the road?

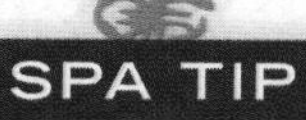

SPA TIP

Whenever embarking upon a spa practice within the confines of someone else's business, try your best to have a contract signed at the beginning of the relationship to avoid problems down the road.

These and other problems can and do arise when such potentially contentious issues are not clearly spelled out in advance. Many therapists have felt cheated after putting a great deal of time, effort, and sometimes even money into building a spa practice inside somebody else's business. Be careful.

The In-Home Spa Practice

If you set up a spa practice in your own home, one of the main concerns you'll have is to somehow separate the spa treatment area from your own living area. This is even more true for spa rooms than simple massage rooms because of the extra towels, linens, products, heating apparatuses, retail products, and possibly even hydrotherapy equipment that you will have in the area. Therapists take many creative approaches to solve this problem. Some therapists dedicate an attic or a basement to their spa setup. Others modify or create a separate entrance to the home so that clients can access the spa area without traveling through the living area. Some undertake new construction, creating walls or rooms to best suit the needs of their spa plans. And therapists in warmer climates have even set up spas outdoors (Figure 17–19). Whichever course you might choose to take

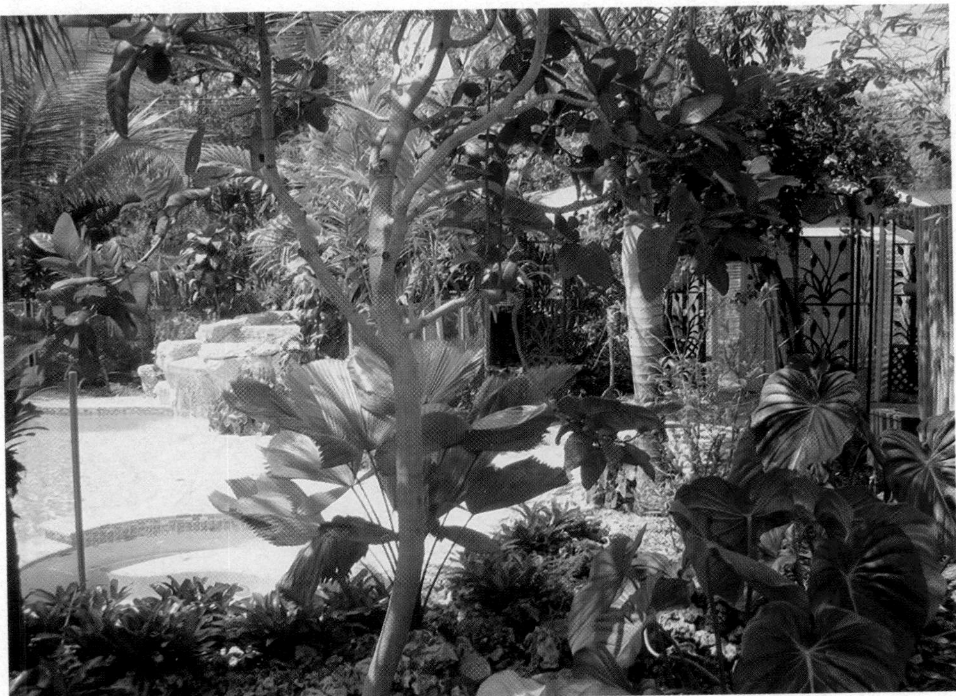

FIGURE 17–19 Therapists in warmer climates can set up spas outdoors (author's outdoor spa area with hot tub, massage deck, sauna and waterfall visible).

when setting up an in-home spa, remember these guidelines in order to avoid potential problems:

- Check local zoning laws.
  In some areas, it may be illegal to run a spa business out of your home. The applicable laws are the same as those for running a massage business in your home. Always check to make sure you are following local regulations.
- Stick with a theme.
  It is too easy for a therapist to blend the décor of his home with that of his in-home spa. The look and feel of the house can bleed unintentionally into the spa area, creating some unwanted effects. It is best to completely separate the spa and the home so that clients have a completely unique experience while visiting the spa. This can be accomplished simply and inexpensively through paying attention to the details mentioned above in the section on engaging the five senses.
- Maximize space use.
  Because space is at a premium, the in-home spa should feature only the most important equipment and supplies. It should also feature a "behind-the-scenes" area for preparation, cleaning, and storage that your clients will not see.
- Insulate the area.
  Determine which area of your home is going to be dedicated to your spa practice, and then insulate it from the rest of your living environment, creating a separate entrance if possible, as mentioned above.

Offering Spa Services in Clients' Homes

When clients do not have the time or the inclination to visit a spa, therapists can successfully bring the spa to them. This offshoot of the spa industry is growing quickly. With a minimum of equipment, therapists can recreate surprisingly elaborate spa experiences in clients' homes. This is an excellent offering for special occasions such as weddings, showers, birthdays, women's group meetings, and mother–daughter events. Some enterprising therapists have started their own **spa party** companies and have developed a substantial business in this manner. Exfoliation services, body wraps, hot stone massages, foot treatments, and more are all easily reproducible in this environment, but certain guidelines, once again, apply if you are to be successful.

spa party

an event held at a client's home where one or more therapists treat several invited guests to spa services

- Keep it simple.
  All you really need is your high-quality spa products, some towels, your massage table, and a heater to warm up towels and products. A stone roaster (turkey roaster) works well for this, and even a crock pot will suffice. Your business does not have to be too complicated, especially at the beginning. Other good portable options for the spa party include foot baths, robes, and slippers. If you want to invest in a more expensive portable piece of spa equipment, consider the Steamy Wonder table-top steam unit. It turns spa parties into truly therapeutic spa experiences.
- Arrive early.
  Setup is crucial in order to provide a seamlessly enjoyable spa experience in clients' homes or offices. You will need to arrive early in order to warm products, towels, water, etc. and create a spa-like atmosphere in the space you have to work with. Early arrival also allows you time to communicate thoroughly with the party hostess and iron out last-minute details.
- Concentrate on promotion.
  You will not have much overhead as a spa party provider, and some of the money you save on rent and utilities will be wisely spent in promoting your business. Internet promotion, local niche advertising, networking at health fairs, posting notices at local businesses, and providing press releases to bridal magazines and women's magazines are all good, inexpensive choices for marketing. See the section on marketing in Chapter 18 for information on promoting your spa business.

Actually performing spa treatments in clients' homes is not difficult. However, some therapists get carried away by the idea, thinking of it more as a party idea than a business idea, and they rush in to create their own mobile spa company without giving due consideration to the details. Just like any other business, this one should be approached with proper attention to detail.

SPA PROFILE

Blue Moon Body Treatments: Succeeding with Home Spa Services

Therese Jennings and Jane Irving live in the coastal village of Castine, Maine, where they offer spa services and massage to clients in homes and in many of the area's picturesque inns. They've dubbed their business Blue Moon Body Treatments, which has been in operation since 2001. What was the main motivating factor that got them involved with this specific niche? "We wanted to increase our incomes," says Therese. "It was as simple as that." And indeed, they have increased their incomes through this strategy. "In fact," says Therese, "we've increased our incomes as far as we can, considering where we live and the fact that there are only two of us. We're maxed out."

So, how do the pair of entrepreneurs make the contacts they need to garner all this business? Mostly through networking with local businesses. "We have business relationships with the owners of three or four local inns," says Jane. "They promote our services to their guests, then we come in and create spa parties for groups large and small. We also work with a local house rental business. The woman who owns it places a book of services in each rental property, and she sends this information to clients prior to their arriving as well. It really works. We're constantly getting calls. It's gotten to the point where we don't set aside certain days or times for anybody. The inns often wanted us to reserve certain days, like Mondays for example, in case their clients wanted to book. But we can't tie ourselves down to certain locations like that. Whoever gets us first, gets us."

Blue Moon Body Treatments also relies on the Internet to help drive business their way. "Our Web site has been good at bringing people to us," says Therese. "And some of the inns have links right to our home page. We've also had a few brushes with celebrity, and that's good as far as endorsements go."

When asked how they arrange the business end of the deal with the inns, Jane says it's simple. "We charge $75 per hour for each one of us. That's how much we decided we wanted to make, plus tips. So, if the inns want to make any money from the arrangement, they charge their guests something extra on top of that, and that's fine with us. If they choose not to, that's okay too. It's up to them. We're happy either way. We always make our $75.

"We have a 'we-can-do-anything' attitude," states Therese. "Though there are certainly a lot of little challenges that come up—we get to the site and there aren't enough plugs for our roasters, etc.—our secret is to act like we have the situation under control no matter what. Probably our biggest concern is the logistics of setting these experiences up for our clients. In order to make the whole thing appear seamless and easy, we spend a lot of time going back and forth on the phone making arrangements prior to each appointment. Who's going to mix up the salts and the butters and get all the stuff over there? Who's going to bring the hot stones? What about linens? What if we have two spa parties on the same day? How do we juggle things? Our biggest challenge is to create the time we need to cover our work load."

And make no mistake about it, states Jane, having a traveling spa business *is* a great deal of work. "We hear LMTs say they don't like to travel, that it's too difficult or it makes them feel a little less than professional, but we've found it to be not only profitable but fun. Not everybody would do spa massages on a sailboat. But if our clients want it, and we can do it professionally, we'll do it. There are a lot of LMTs out there, but many don't seem to want to put in the effort that we do. They say, 'I can only do 2 hours at a time.' Not us. We're all over the place. Give us the people, and we'll just keep going until we can't go any more. You have to be willing to work!"

"And it's not just hard work," adds Therese. "You need other qualities too in order to succeed in this market. Like patience, for example. At spa parties you

(Continued)

SPA PROFILE

Blue Moon Body Treatments: Succeeding with Home Spa Services *continued*

have to have extra patience because your clients don't want to feel rushed. They're there to chitchat, to have fun. We'll have five or six clients in a row to do, for example, and suddenly one of them will be missing. 'Betty went down the street to get more wine,' they'll say. So then we'll say, 'Sheila, get on the table.'"

"And you have to be flexible," chimes in Jane. "You have to be ready to change your methods when you see the need. For example, after we'd set up our spa party business, one of the biggest problems was women who would take one look at our tables and towels and say, 'Oh, but I didn't want to get undressed.' So, instead of banging our heads against the wall, we stayed flexible and ended up creating special fully-clothed spa experiences like our Head-to-Toe 75 minute package.

"All of our services, plus the time we end up spending between clients, setting up, etc., is all included in the price we charge: $75 per hour. The only thing we charge extra for is if we have to lug the heavy rocks for stone massage. We added $20 onto that service and nobody's blinked an eye. Really, the sky's the limit in this business. We've even created a DVD to show other therapists how to perform these treatments and be successful with it. All you've got to do is be smart about marketing, work hard, stay patient and be flexible. If you're willing, like we've been, to take this spa ball and run with it, you can go far."

THE GRAND OPENING

When it finally comes time to open your business, having a grand opening party for your spa is not only fun, but also quite important for the spa's overall success. Many challenges and much hard work lie ahead, but when you are finally ready to open your doors to the public, you have passed a real milestone, and the occasion merits a celebration. Also, your grand opening party will be a key part of your marketing plan as you go forward. The celebration allows you to contact local media and community leaders to let them know about your spa. It is also a way to kick-start your business, get a stream of customers through the door right off the bat, and allow you and your employees to get your hands on many people in a short period of time. The following suggestions will help you take advantage of all the opportunities for improving your business that a grand opening spa party presents.

- **Give mini-treatments.** Have your employees set up throughout the spa offering free 5- to 10-minute versions of your treatments. Make sure to keep them short, or some people will not get to experience them.
- **Offer food and drinks.** The spread does not have to be elaborate, but you should have snacks and beverages available. Wine and cheese are a popular option.
- **Make a short speech.** That's right. Stand up in front of people and thank them for coming. Also, tell them a little bit about you and your spa. It is appropriate as the host and business owner to say a few words. Toast to your guests' good health.
- **Give away promotional items.** Include small samples of your spa products as well as items with your name and logo on them in a little gift bag for each person who comes.
- **Hold a raffle.** Offer a door prize—a free spa day or similar prize—for the holder of the winning ticket.

ACTIVITY

Personal Budget Development

The objective of a business is to make a profit. While this may seem obvious, a surprising number of people get into business for other reasons and then forget that they need to make a profit to continue to do business. More than one massage therapist who has opened a spa has made this mistake. Do not let it happen to you.

Begin by looking at your own life. In a certain sense, one of the objectives of your life, just like your projected spa business, is to make a profit. If you do not make a profit (take in and keep more income than you put out in expenses) during your life, you will retire broke. So, start small with budgeting and see if you can work your way into profitability in your own life first before you engage in building the budget for an actual spa business.

1. In the income rows of Table 18–1, write in your average monthly earnings.
2. Total the incomes for each month.

PERSONAL BUDGET

		JAN	FEB	MAR	APR	MAY	JUN	
Income	Salary							
	Other							
Total Income								
Expenses	Mortgage/Rent							
	Insurance							
	Electric Bill							
	Phone Bill							
	Water Bill							
	Car Payment							
	Gas							
	Travel/Transportation							
	Groceries							
	Restaurants							
	Entertainment							
	Clothing							
	Maintenance/Upkeep							
	Work Tools/Supplies							
	Furniture/Appliances							
	Education							
	Loan Repayments							
Total Expenses								**GRAND TOTAL**
Profit (Deficit)								$

TABLE 18–1 Personal Budget Development Worksheet.

(Continued)

ACTIVITY

3. In the expense rows, list items that will have to be paid in the next six months. Estimate if you are not sure.
4. For each month, add up your total expenditures.
5. Subtract total expenses from total income for each month.
6. Write the result for each month in the profit/deficit row, then add up the grand total profit (or loss).

Note: If you have a deficit, or negative number, put parentheses around it, as is done in standard accounting practice. For example: –$185 is written ($185).

7. After completing your budget consider the following points:
   a. Are there any particularly difficult months ahead?
   b. At the end of the six-month period, will you be in debt, or will you be making a profit?
   c. What actions could you take to improve your budgeting and raise your profits?

Paying the Bills

If you have not had to deal with the financial aspects of running a business before, you may be surprised to learn how things work. For example, in order to receive professional discounts and credit terms on equipment, back bar supplies, spa products, and retail items, you will need to fill out a **business credit application**. As you can see in Figure 18–1, this application will require you to divulge your banking and credit information as well as past payment history with other vendors. If you do not have any established business credit history, you may have to pay with a credit card in the beginning until your spa's reputation and good payment history grows.

business credit application

form to fill out with information to be used for a company to determine whether to extend credit to a prospective customer

While filling out your first business credit application may be intimidating, it is well worth the effort because of the attractive terms such credit involves. Most vendors and suppliers will give you 30 days to pay your bills, with no interest or penalties of any kind, leaving you a little breathing room to fulfill your other obligations and receive income before you need to pay for the ongoing costs of outfitting your business.

Once your business credit application has been accepted and you are approved, you can begin ordering supplies. The way this is often done in business is through a **purchase order** (Figure 18–2). You fill out a purchase order and send it to the vendor in order for them to initiate the order, which is then sent to you with a packing slip inside the package. Only later will the vendor send you an **invoice**, which you have to pay within the allotted timeframe. This system is markedly different from the purchase and payment habits you have most likely used as a non–business owner.

purchase order

a commercial document used to request someone to supply something in return for payment

invoice

a statement of money owed for goods or services

Payroll

As a spa owner with employees, you will be responsible for the livelihoods of several other human beings. This can be a burden. When you are in charge of peoples' paychecks, they suddenly become very interested in you. You should be prepared to step into a quasi-parental role, because some employees may

Spa Therapy Supply Company, Ltd.

CREDIT APPLICATION FOR A BUSINESS ACCOUNT

BUSINESS CONTACT INFORMATION			
Title:			
Company name:			
Phone:	Fax:	E-mail:	
Registered company address:			
City:		State:	ZIP Code:
Date business commenced:			
Sole proprietorship:	Partnership:	Corporation:	Other:
BUSINESS AND CREDIT INFORMATION			
Primary business address:			
City:		State:	ZIP Code:
How long at current address?			
Telephone:	Fax:	E-mail:	
Bank name:			
Bank address:		Phone:	
City:		State:	ZIP Code:
Type of account	Account number		
Savings			
Checking			
Other			
BUSINESS/TRADE REFERENCES			
Company name:			
Address:			
City:		State:	ZIP Code:
Phone:	Fax:	E-mail:	
Type of account:			
Company name:			
Address:			
City:		State:	ZIP Code:
Phone:	Fax:	E-mail:	
Type of account:			
Company name:			
Address:			
City:		State:	ZIP Code:
Phone:	Fax:	E-mail:	
Type of account:			

AGREEMENT

1. All invoices are to be paid 30 days from the date of the invoice.
2. Claims arising from invoices must be made within seven working days.
3. By submitting this application, you authorize Spa Therapy Supply Company, Ltd. to make inquiries into the banking and business/trade references that you have supplied.

SIGNATURES

Title: Date:	Title: Date:

FIGURE 18–1 In order to receive professional discounts, you will need to fill out a business credit application.

Therapeutic Day Spa

PURCHASE ORDER

1234 Main Street
Any Town, NY 02101
Phone **[(509) 555-0190]** Fax **[(509) 555-0191]**

The following number must appear on all related correspondence, shipping papers, and invoices:
P.O. NUMBER: [100]

TO:
[Name]
[Company Name]
[Street Address]
[City, ST ZIP Code]
[Phone]

SHIP TO:
[Name]
[Company Name]
[Street Address]
[City, ST ZIP Code]
[Phone]

P.O. DATE	REQUISITIONER	SHIPPED VIA	F.O.B. POINT	TERMS

QTY	UNIT	DESCRIPTION	UNIT PRICE	TOTAL
			SUBTOTAL	
			SALES TAX	
			SHIPPING & HANDLING	
			OTHER	
			TOTAL	

1. Please send two copies of your invoice.
2. Enter this order in accordance with the prices, terms, delivery method, and specifications listed above.
3. Please notify us immediately if you are unable to ship as specified.
4. Send all correspondence to:
   Manager, Therapeutic Day Spa
   1234 Main Street
   Any Town, NY 02101
   Phone [**(509) 555-.0190**] Fax [**(509) 555-0191**]

Authorized by Date

FIGURE 18–2 Purchase orders facilitate the ordering of supplies.

Growing Financially

Did You Know?

Many therapists dream about bigger incomes. Few plan for bigger bills. The two, of course, often go hand in hand. It is only by expanding your operation that you can expand your profits. Unfortunately, many therapists get scared at the thought of spending thousands of dollars a month on overhead, payroll, and the myriad other expenses that crop up as part of running a successful spa.

In order to grow financially in the spa or massage business, you have to be willing to pay for it. Your investment must be a wise one—it is not, for example, a good idea to spend every last penny on a huge full-page newspaper ad—but you have to be willing to put your money where your mouth is. Each dollar that you do not reinvest into the business, especially in the beginning, could have a serious impact down the road and perhaps even force you to shut down.

It is going to cost you money to run a spa. But when people see the investment you've made and the time you've spent to create quality offerings, they will respond in kind. Thousands of massage therapists have been able to greatly enhance their careers through joining the "club" of spa owners, but every single one of them first had to be willing to pay the price of admission.

subconsciously cast you as a mother figure or father figure. The best way to handle this is to separate the emotional side of providing a living from the simple financial reality of cutting a paycheck. This is why it is important to have a good payroll system in place in the spa.

When you first start out, or if you have only one or two employees, you may be able to establish a system for calculating and distributing payroll on your own. However, you need to keep the following points in mind:

- You need to be able to determine the correct percentage of **withholding tax**, including federal, state, and social security, for each employee.
- Even if you pay your therapists as **independent contractors** instead of employees, and you believe you have no tax responsibility for them, you still need to consider taxes for receptionists and any other non-technician employees.
- You may also be responsible for additional payroll deductions of which you may not be aware, such as the unemployment tax.

Once the number of employees grows above five or six, doing payroll becomes more complicated, and the services of a payroll company are highly recommended. Payroll companies, for a fee, take care of paying all taxes, cut paychecks for all employees, handle the details of retirement plans like the 401(k), and offer many other services. As a spa owner, you should retain the services of a competent accountant to help you with your budgeting, payroll, and taxes.

Of course, when you first open a spa, it is crucial to have enough **cash flow** to cover payroll and pay all employees in a timely manner. Many therapists have run into trouble during the first year of operation when they overspent on construction, advertising, products, or equipment, and did not have enough left to pay everyone. When starting any spa operation, it is better to spend less on everything else and have enough left to pay ongoing operating expenses, including

withholding tax

money withheld (retained) by an employer and given directly to the taxation authorities in order to reduce tax evasion or failure to pay

independent contractors

workers who provides services to a company but are not employees or agents of that company

cash flow

the pattern of income and expenditures, as of a person or (spa) business, and the resulting availability of cash

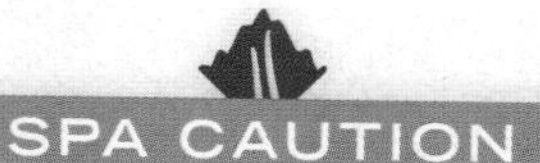

SPA CAUTION

Many therapists have become accustomed to being their own accountants and payroll experts over the years—especially those in private practice who develop an "I can do it all" attitude—and it often works in a massage practice or a sole-proprietor spa practice. When opening a spa, however, the professional services of an accountant and a payroll company are key to achieving success.

payroll. This is the bottom-up formula for success that many massage therapists have used. Some, like Becky Zwickl (profiled in Chapter 17), started with a bare-bones setup and only grew after becoming sure that they could meet payroll operations and keep the spa going month after month.

COMPUTER SYSTEMS MANAGEMENT

Few spas in operation today lack a computerized booking system. Many spas have expanded their use of spa software far beyond appointment booking to include inventory management, sales, employee scheduling, and even client-based marketing. Being familiar with computers and comfortable using them is essential if you want your spa to compete on equal footing with other modern, computerized spas (Figure 18–3).

The two main components of your spa's computer system with which you will need to become familiar are hardware and software. The hardware used to run spa businesses is exactly the same as that used by millions of people at home, though very few spas run Apple® (Mac®) computers. Hardware includes the computers themselves (Windows®-based PCs) plus monitors (touch-screen or regular), keyboards, mice, cables, printers, backup storage, routers, and phone lines. Software includes typical office-management programs like word processing and spreadsheet software, accounting software, and the specialized programs you use to run your spa business.

For a small spa with only one or two treatments rooms, one computer terminal is sufficient, but most spas have two or more computers networked together, either through wireless routers or over CAT-5 cables. The most obvious place for the spa's main computer is at the front desk, where a receptionist greets guests and uses the computer to sort out appointments, sales, and billing. This terminal can also be used for employee booking, resource scheduling, accounting, and

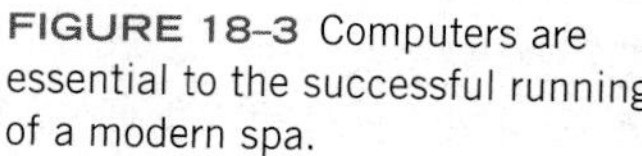

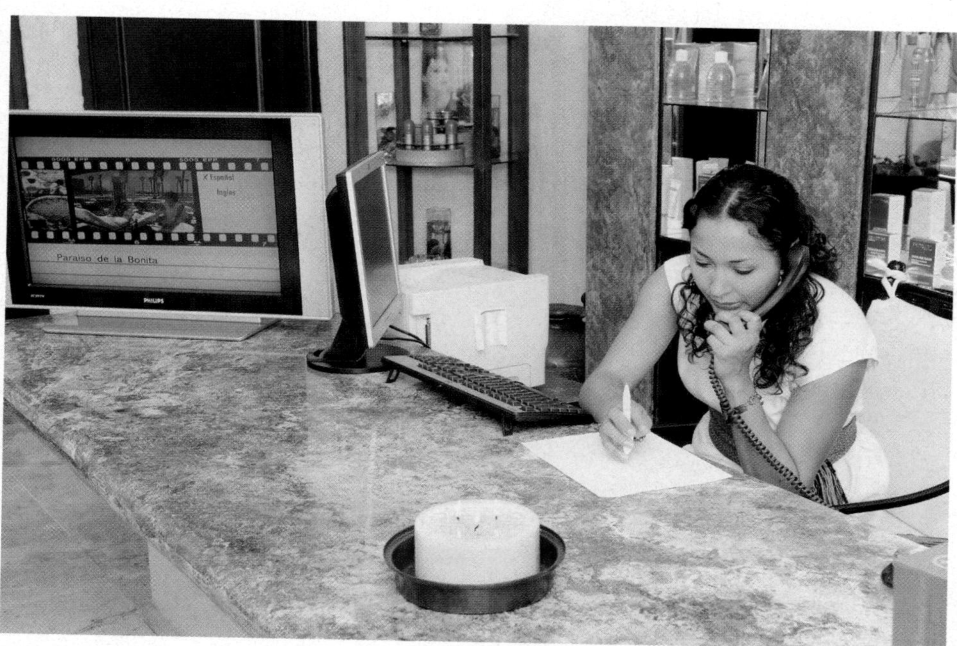

FIGURE 18–3 Computers are essential to the successful running of a modern spa.

even marketing purposes such as newsletter writing. However, if the spa has more than a handful of technicians, this computer can become overused very quickly, and a second terminal should be installed in the back of the house.

All computers in the spa are linked to a printer, usually located at the front desk also, which can generate receipts for sales as well as appointment reminders, reports for management, correspondence, and marketing materials. Most spa computer systems are also connected to the Internet in order to download current versions of the spa business software, connect with remote support, and stay in touch with clients.

There are many choices in spa software. Some of the programs are robust enough to run an entire resort hotel's booking system, and they would definitely be overkill for small, therapist-owned spas. They are also quite expensive. Because of this expense, some therapists choose to continue to use their massage business software when they open a spa, but this can be tricky. Most massage software does not allow for the wide range of treatments and room usage possibilities found in spas. A more common choice is one of the smaller day-spa software packages that can be purchased outright or paid for with an ongoing monthly fee. Choosing spa software is a highly personal matter. Some spa owners are looking for strong technical support because they do not feel comfortable with technology. Others want a clean, concise interface with few bells and whistles. Still others want their software to take care of every aspect of their spa business, and they are not intimidated at the thought of learning how to use it. Whatever your needs, it is wise to become familiar with several choices and receive personal recommendations from trusted colleagues before purchasing a program. The following sections outline the main components found in spa software and how they will affect a therapist-owned spa business.

SPA TIP

It is ideal to place an extra computer screen in the employee-only area. This screen does not necessarily need to have a keyboard attached to it for inputting data. Employees simply need to see their schedules and the schedule for each treatment room during the day. A mouse is sufficient to navigate to these screens, and the back-of-the-house computer can be configured to forbid any changes or modifications. Also, in larger spas, it is recommended to place a separate computer in a back office for making reservations so this function does not tie up the front desk, which should be dealing with clients who are already in-house.

Spa Appointment Scheduling

Appointment booking is what people think of when they think of spa software. They see rows of therapists and other technicians listed across the top of the page and time slots all down the left side. In each square, an appointment is booked.

SPA ETIQUETTE

Employees should be trained in proper "computer etiquette" to ensure that the use of computers makes guests' experience in the spa more comfortable, streamlined, and enjoyable rather than aggravating or unpleasant. Computer etiquette rules include the following:

- To avoid congestion at the front desk, no more than two employees at a time should view a single computer screen.
- Receptionists should make eye contact with guests and speak with them courteously for a moment prior to looking at the screen so as not to appear rude.
- A backup paper-based booking and billing system should be in place so that if the computer goes down for any reason, guests will not be inconvenienced. Employees need to be trained on this non-computerized system prior to any computer failure.

While it is true that this interface exists within every spa computer program, it is actually just the surface of the software. The real power runs invisibly in the background, and in order to make this invisible part work, you have to invest the time and effort needed to customize the software. The number of treatment rooms, types of treatments, and names of therapists must all be input into the system. In addition, the software must "learn" which types of treatments can be performed in which rooms and which therapists are qualified to do which treatments, as well as when they are scheduled to work. The price of each treatment must also be input, of course, along with any taxes, service charges, or other fees associated with it. Also, all the retail items, along with their prices, must be entered. Then, as each new guest visits the spa, their information must be entered as well. This is a complex process (Figure 18–4).

Once the data is entered, the software can integrate it all into a seamless experience at the computer terminal. Table 18–2 outlines the steps involved with booking a spa service using computer software. The column on the left is what the guest and employee experience in the spa, and the column on the right describes what happens in the background as the software makes it happen.

FIGURE 18–4 Spa software keeps track of the complex processes involved in running a spa.

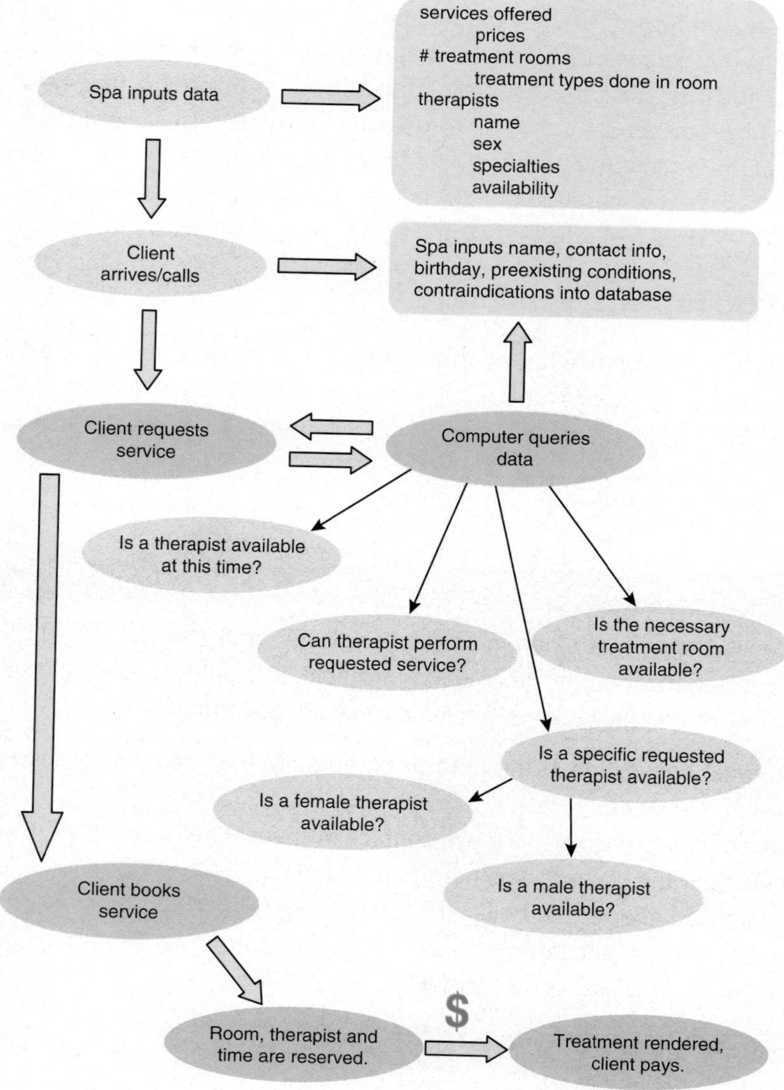

COMPUTERIZED SPA APPOINTMENT SCHEDULING TIMELINE	
WHAT HAPPENS IN THE SPA	**HOW THE SOFTWARE MAKES IT WORK**
1. CLIENT ARRIVAL A new client either calls or arrives in person at the spa to book a new appointment. A spa employee inputs the client's information, including name, address, contact information, birthday, and so forth. Note: before the first appointment, each client will fill out an intake card with more pertinent information, such as contraindications and pre-existing conditions, which will also be added into his file on the computer.	**1. DATA INPUT** The software places the new client's information into a **database** that can then be used by the rest of the software program to keep track of that person and to make this information available when creating appointments, remembering preferences, sending out reminders and marketing messages, etc.
2. SEARCHING FOR SERVICES The client then chooses one or more treatments from the menu and requests a time to receive them. The receptionist or other spa employee in charge of booking looks for open time slots on the requested day for the requested service (and sometimes for a particular requested therapist or a male/female preference).	**2. DATA QUERIES** The software searches through pre-installed data relating to treatment rooms, therapists, and time slots, and correlates matches between all three, which appears on the screen as availability.
3. BOOKING SERVICES The client accepts a particular time (and potentially a particular therapist or male/female choice) for the chosen treatment, and the receptionist enters the client's name in the appropriate time slot on the screen.	**3. SETTING A STATE** One of the many possible combinations of room/therapist/treatment/time is noted as occupied, and this "state" of unavailability is held for each resource.
4. CLIENT ARRIVES FOR TREATMENT Receptionist notes arrival and checks client in on the computer, sending him to the locker room or waiting area.	**4. MODIFYING THE STATE** Software records that specific resources are being used by client at the present time.
5. CHECKOUT/PAYMENT After the treatment, the client proceeds to the front desk to deliver payment. Retail sales can be recorded at this time also. Receptionist checks client out of computer system after receiving payment.	**5. GENERATION OF INVOICE** Software records that resources are no longer being used and generates an invoice based on the cost of resource use. Also, software records type of treatment and therapist preference for future marketing purposes.
6. REVIEWING TRANSACTIONS At any time after the treatment has taken place, the spa owner/director can review the transaction either separately or as part of a larger group categorized by time, treatment type, therapist, treatment room used, dollar value, or any combination of these over time.	**6. GENERATION OF REPORTS** Each detail of the transaction—from room usage to therapist preference to service type to amount paid for service or retail—is kept in a database and can be accessed at any time in any order to generate reports of sales, treatments given, hours worked, percent of retail sales achieved per transaction, etc.

TABLE 18–2 Computerized Spa Appointment Scheduling Timeline.

database
a comprehensive collection of related data organized for convenient access, generally in a computer

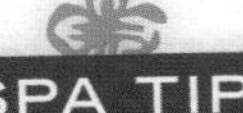

SPA TIP

Online appointment booking is increasingly common at spas. Online booking allows clients to book appointments via the spa's Web site. This does not have to be a complicated process, and several vendors sell products that allow spas to offer this option on their Web sites for a nominal fee.

SPA CAUTION

It is important to restrict access to your computer system with passwords so that only authorized personnel can make changes to employee schedules, guest bookings, and, most important, billing. Guard these passwords closely. Further, you can set administrative access to the software so that only you or your partner or spa director can make changes to key settings.

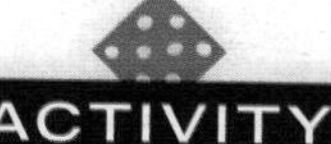

ACTIVITY

Spa Scheduling

Before computerization, all of the tasks outlined in Table 18–3 were taken care of manually, even at the largest of spas. Even though most scheduling now takes place on computers, it is still important to understand the basics of what those software programs are actually doing as they churn out the daily schedules for thousands of spas. In order to grasp the fundamentals of spa scheduling (and in order to be prepared to do it yourself in the event of a computer system failure), it is wise to practice juggling the intricacies of scheduling on a hard-copy version such as Table 18–3. Using the data listed in Table 18–4, fill in the schedule's empty

THERAPEUTIC DAY SPA					
	FRIDAY, JUNE 19				
DAILY SCHEDULE	SARAH	KAYLA	TOM	LORI ANNE	ROBERT
9:00					
10:00	Mr. Benjamin – M			Mrs. Stone – EX	
11:00	Mrs. Aston – M		Mr. Aston – SM	Mrs. Stone – SW	
12:00	LUNCH			LUNCH	
1:00			LUNCH	Mrs. Pierce – EX	Mr. Trent – M
2:00	Mr. Barnes – M		Mr. Barnes – HW Mr. Jones – HW	Mrs. Pierce – SW	
3:00		Mrs. Smith – EX		Mrs. Pierce – SM	Mr. Jones – SM
4:00	Mrs. Ferrer – M	Mrs. Smith – SW			Mrs. Leonard – M
5:00		Mrs. Stein – M	Mr. Stein – M	Mrs. Kaye – EX	Mr. Smith – EX
6:00		Mrs. Smith – M			Mr. Smith – SM
7:00		Ms. Chen – M			Ms. Lu – M

TABLE 18–3 Creating a Daily Schedule.

TECHNIQUE	SYMBOL	TIME	QUALIFIED THERAPISTS	ROOM NEEDED
Massage	M	1 hour	Tom, Robert, Lori Anne, Kayla, Sarah	Massage room 1, 2, 3, 4
Stone Massage	SM	1 hour	Tom, Robert, Lori Anne	Massage room 1, 2, 3, 4
Exfoliation	EX	½ hour	Lori Anne, Sarah, Kayla, Robert	Wet room
Seaweed Wrap	SW	1½ hours	Lori Anne, Kayla, Robert	Wet room
Herbal Wrap	HW	½ hour	Sarah, Kayla, Tom	Any room

TABLE 18–4 Spa Appointment Scheduling Data.

(Continued)

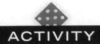

ACTIVITY

slots with appointments. The point is to avoid scheduling errors and conflicts and to become familiar with the important parameters involved with scheduling, parameters which are usually taken care of by software.

Notes:

- There are four massage rooms and one wet room.
- Herbal wraps, exfoliations, and seaweed wraps must be performed by a therapist who is the same sex as the client.
- Pay attention to the spa treatment order rules found in Chapter 17.
- Fill in the following appointment requests:
  - Mrs. Wagner – exfoliation and massage before 1:00 P.M.
  - Mrs. Alvarez – herbal wrap before 1:00 P.M.
  - Mrs. Connor – stone massage with a female therapist
  - Mr. Grant – herbal wrap and stone massage with a male therapist
  - Mrs. Labelle – herbal wrap and massage with a female therapist after 1:00 P.M.
  - Mrs. Taylor – massage with a female therapist
  - Mrs. Franklin – herbal wrap as late in the day as possible
  - Mrs. Leary – massage as late in the day as possible
  - Mr. Choudry – herbal wrap
  - Mrs. Fletcher – massage with Robert

As you fill in the remainder of the schedule, ask yourself these questions:

1. Why isn't it possible for Sarah to perform an exfoliation at 2:00?
2. Why isn't it possible to offer a stone massage at 9:00 A.M.?
3. What are the only two half-hour time slots left in which to offer an exfoliation?
4. Why can't Robert perform an herbal wrap at 5:00?
5. Where are the two half-hour time slots that cannot be filled with the current requests?

Show Me the Money

Did You Know?

Spa software plays a big role in keeping track of money so that spa directors can accurately monitor income, inventory, expenses, cash flow, and future projections. For this purpose, the **reporting function** built into all spa software is especially important. The software allows you to extract specific data in order to build charts, tables, and graphs depicting the spa's business health. For example, it can show the total number of massages performed in the month of February this year as compared to February the year before. It can chart that number month by month, year by year, and so on, and it can total the revenues in each time period, comparing them to all the other time periods (Figure 18–5).

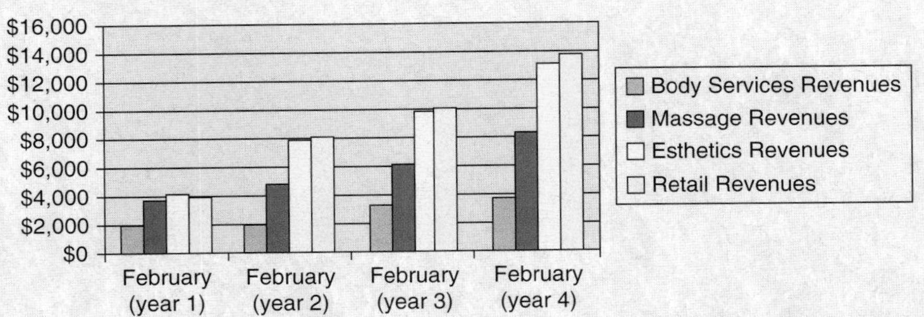

FIGURE 18–5 The reporting function built into all spa software is especially important.

reporting function
the specific ability of (spa) business software to arrange data such as sales, appointments, number of services provided, employee hours worked, etc. into reports, charts, and graphs in order to interpret past performance and forecast future trends

ACTIVITY

Deciphering Reports

THERAPEUTIC DAY SPA 12 MONTH SERVICE SALES REPORT - YEAR 4	JAN	FEB	MARCH	APRIL	MAY	JUNE	JULY	AUGUST	SEPT	OCT	NOV	DEC	ANNUAL TOTALS	PAST PERFORMANCE YEAR 1	YEAR 2	YEAR 3
Massage	112	113	129	106	91	88	95	102	77	95	110	140	1258	940	1020	1188
Sale price @ unit	75.00	75.00	75.00	75.00	75.00	75.00	75.00	75.00	75.00	75.00	75.00	75.00		65.00	70.00	75.00
M TOTAL	8,400	8,475	9,675	7,950	6,825	6,600	7,125	7,650	5,775	7,125	8,250	10,500	94,350	61,100	71,400	89,100
Stone Massage	82	75	80	81	70	58	54	42	53	78	80	89	842	475	520	695
Sale price @ unit	85.00	85.00	85.00	85.00	85.00	85.00	85.00	85.00	85.00	85.00	85.00	85.00		75.00	80.00	85.00
SM TOTAL	6,970	6,375	6,800	6,885	5,950	4,930	4,590	3,570	4,505	6,630	6,800	7,565	71,570	35,625	41,600	59,075
Exfoliation	32	33	20	40	44	50	56	59	41	40	32	30	477	99	212	306
Sale price @ unit	55.00	55.00	55.00	55.00	55.00	55.00	55.00	55.00	55.00	55.00	55.00	55.00		45.00	45.00	55.00
EX TOTAL	1,760	1,815	1,100	2,200	2,420	2,750	3,080	3,245	2,255	2,200	1,760	1,650	26,235	4,455	9,540	16,830
Herbal Wrap	53	49	49	51	41	42	37	33	41	52	58	61	567	218	321	437
Sale price @ unit	75.00	75.00	75.00	75.00	75.00	75.00	75.00	75.00	75.00	75.00	75.00	75.00		65.00	65.00	75.00
HW TOTAL	3,975	3,675	3,675	3,825	3,075	3,150	2,775	2,475	3,075	3,900	4,350	4,575	42,525	14,170	20,865	32,775
Seaweed Wrap	27	39	14	28	29	33	20	40	32	18	9	20	309	189	293	351
Sale price @ unit	110.00	110.00	110.00	110.00	110.00	110.00	110.00	110.00	110.00	110.00	110.00	110.00		95.00	95.00	95.00
SW TOTAL	2,970	4,290	1,540	3,080	3,190	3,630	2,200	4,400	3,520	1,980	990	2,200	33,990	17,955	27,835	33,345
HW/SM Package	18	16	12	22	8	12	14	7	14	21	27	25	196	89	140	152
Sale price @ unit	140.00	140.00	140.00	140.00	140.00	140.00	140.00	140.00	140.00	140.00	140.00	140.00		135.00	135.00	140.00
Pack1 TOTAL	2,520	2,240	1,680	3,080	1,120	1,680	1,960	980	1,960	2,940	3,780	3,500	27,440	12,015	18,900	21,280
EX/SW/M Pack	12	18	19	20	28	31	29	37	27	24	18	17	280	318	345	298
Sale price @ unit	220.00	220.00	220.00	220.00	220.00	220.00	220.00	220.00	220.00	220.00	220.00	220.00		175.00	175.00	195.00
Pack2 TOTAL	2,640	3,960	4,180	4,400	6,160	6,820	6,380	8,140	5,940	5,280	3,960	3,740	61,600	55,650	60,375	58,110
Monthly totals: All Treatments	29,235	30,830	28,650	31,420	28,740	29,560	28,110	30,460	27,030	30,055	29,890	33,730	357,710	200,970	250,515	310,515

TABLE 18–5 Deciphering Reports.

(Continued)

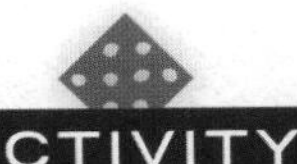

ACTIVITY

Spa software programs make it easy to generate a vast array of financial reports. Sometimes, the most difficult task faced by spa owners is figuring out what to do with all the numbers. Table 18–5 recreates one such report, giving the figures for total sales and income for an array of services at the Therapeutic Day Spa. Note the figures for previous years in the right-hand columns. Using the data provided in the report, answer the following questions.

1. Was there a change in the number of seaweed wraps sold in Year 4 as compared to Year 3? If so, can you speculate as to why this change occurred?
2. Which service brings in the most overall revenue?
3. At what time of year are stone massages most popular? What do you think causes this fluctuation? Do you think the same cause creates similar fluctuations in herbal wrap sales and Package 1 sales?
4. Based on the data, does it look like Package 1 (herbal wrap and stone massage) would still be popular with another $5 price increase?
5. What was the least popular single service in Year 4? How could knowing this answer help a spa director in promotional efforts?
6. Do exfoliation sales follow a similar or opposite pattern compared to stone massage and herbal wraps? What could explain this?
7. Which service saw the greatest increase in revenue from Year 1 to Year 4?
8. Which service saw the least increase in revenue from Year 1 to Year 4?
9. If the spa could somehow double its massage and Package 2 sales for Year 4, what would the total revenue be for all services?
10. In Year 4, which month brought in the highest number of total treatment sales? Which month brought in the least?

MOTIVATING A TEAM

One of the prime job descriptions of a spa owner is that of head visionary and inspirational leader. As an example of this, consider the owner of the Canyon Ranch spas. When he first opened his doors years ago, there were few customers. In order to inspire his team with a vision of what was possible, he signed up for and received a massage and a detoxifying herbal wrap almost every day for the entire first year. He believed in the results his own team was creating for him, which instilled confidence in each team member, and this confidence was eventually communicated to the guests, who started to arrive in ever-increasing numbers. Today, Canyon Ranch is one of the largest and most successful spas in the world.

Many therapists who open spas have not considered the fact that they will need to set motivational examples for other human beings. If you want employees to share your vision of what is possible for your spa, you first have to effectively communicate that vision. This can be accomplished through the "mission statement" discussed in Chapter 15 under the heading "A Team with a Mission." And then, in order to get your team to buy into that mission, you need to motivate them. Motivating a group of massage therapists is much different than working alongside them. In fact, massage therapists are not always the best ones to motivate their own colleagues, because it is difficult for them to step back and take a non-attached, objective view of what therapists want and what motivates

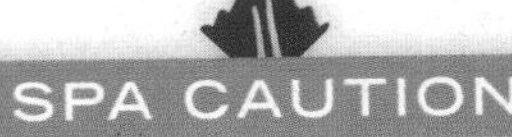

SPA CAUTION

Always, always, always have a backup storage device connected to your spa's computer to save data that might otherwise be lost in the event of a disk crash or other failure. Losing financial data or hard-won client contact information can be fatal to a spa business.

them. Therapists often refer to themselves as "artists," and it is true that their artistic healing talents are what makes spas work. It is instructive to consider for a moment how spa owners can best treat their own "artists" on staff in order to motivate them. The seven motivational techniques that follow work well for the hands-on staff at spas.

SPA TIP

Get your own team to teach you. Why not have your therapists give a class to the spa management and receptionists? Become a "coach" instead of a boss by allowing therapist employees to display their talents and shine. Then, share in their success.

As a spa owner, in order to motivate your team of hands-on experts, you should:

- Get to know your therapists better.
  Massage therapists speak their own lingo and have their very own "New Age" or "empathetic" or "therapeutic" way of looking at the world. They are, however, very social within their peer groups. Become a part of that community by continuing to take classes in order to stay current as a massage therapist. Also, stay interested in the current work of your therapists. What kind of modalities are they most excited about? How can they further help your clients?
- Learn what your therapists are looking for.
  Good pay and a reasonable compensation plan that has room for upward mobility are important, but as strange as it may sound, money is not the most important factor for most massage therapists. They believe in higher ideals and more than anything want to actually help the clients. They want to feel that they are making an impact. Plus, they like getting credit for their accomplishments. So, it is a good idea to create an incentive system based on bonuses for therapists who generate repeat business from clients who have been helped by them and request them repeatedly.
- Create new ways to promote your therapists.
  As a spa owner, you will need to find ways to promote therapists without turning them into managers. They need a forward career path, including recognition and more money, but they do not want to get bogged down behind a desk. Some spas create a dual career track, allowing therapists to partake in some supervisory decisions while still working hands-on most of the time.
- Let therapists create solutions for clients' problems.
  Therapists are trained to take care of people's problems, and if you can make them feel like they are helping to create true solutions for your clients, then they will be inspired to work hard for you. Especially when it comes to selling retail products, you have to show therapists how it is actually a way to help create therapeutic solutions for the clients. For therapists, selling must be seen as a personal crusade with meaning. Finally, each therapist needs some leeway when it comes to sales and service techniques. You can tell them what to do, but you cannot tell them how to do it.
- The best judges of therapists are other therapists.
  If you give therapists a forum within which to develop their own skills and hierarchy, you will find that they automatically weed out the poorer performers because they are very proud of their skills and their profession. They are very good at judging their own colleagues. You can also

have them make presentations to one another regarding skills they have learned elsewhere.

- Look for the natural leaders among your therapists.
  The natural leaders on your treatment staff will often not be the ones who are aching for that manager or supervisor position. You need to spot the therapists who naturally inspire and motivate the other team members and then make these people happy. Give them access to your ideas. Make them privy to your plans. Show them you appreciate their opinions.
- Be prepared for when therapists are discontent.
  Do not automatically intervene from the top down in therapist disputes. Consider bringing in outside "experts" to review the staff so judgments are not seen as coming from management. If you must make a negative change, frame it as a group decision or as a decision made by a respected therapist.

MANAGING A TEAM

Of course, owning and running a spa includes more than motivation and inspiration. The job is filled with nitty-gritty day-to-day realities that need to be taken care of: in a word, management. When it comes to spas, *management* can be defined as everything you do to keep the business running smoothly. Here are just a few of the issues you will have to deal with, which we will discuss further in this chapter:

- running staff meetings
- setting schedules
- recruitment and hiring
- giving promotions and raises
- disciplining and firing employees
- training

For a more exhaustive understanding of spa management principles, it is recommended that you pursue professional training after graduating from massage school.

Running Staff Meetings

When you run a staff, you need to hold staff meetings. These usually occur on a weekly or monthly basis, and although some therapist/owners are reluctant to hold meetings because they think it detracts from productivity or fosters resentment on the part of the staff, meetings are important for three main reasons:

- Morale
  No matter how bitterly some employees may complain about having to attend staff meetings, the morale is higher in spas where people communicate, where the goals of the business owners are made clear to everyone, and where employees can air their frustrations and suggestions.

- Structure
  People need structure, and they appreciate a cohesive work environment that has set routines and understandable guidelines. If everyone knows there is a staff meeting the first Thursday of every month, they will work it into their schedules and it will become an expected part of work life.
- Participation
  The nature of spa therapists' work means they spend a good deal of time with clients and not very much with fellow employees and management. For this reason, staff meetings are especially important in spas where group participation time is at a premium.

Theories differ on whether employees should be paid for attending staff meetings. Depending upon the legal status for your employees (as contracted laborers versus full-time employees with benefits), you may be required to pay for these meetings, so it is important to research applicable regulations. Usually, employees are paid something, even if it is less than their normal working wage. For example, some spas institute a minimum-wage rate for meetings. If you decide not to pay employees for staff meetings, it is more difficult to enforce attendance, and the meetings are usually shorter.

During a staff meeting, certain protocols should be followed consistently so every staff member knows what to expect and how to act. Normally, a staff meeting entails the following protocols:

1. Call to order at the beginning of the meeting
2. Attendance-taking or roll call
3. Review
   The spa owner/director reviews the previous meeting and updates attendees about any implemented changes that occurred as a result, in addition to other recent spa news.
4. Participation by recognized attendees
   Employees speak one at a time to update the entire staff about developments since the previous meeting.
5. Open discussion
   All participants are given an opportunity to vent concerns, offer opinions, or relate their own experiences.
6. Plan
   The spa owner/director agrees with each participant regarding plans to implement by the next meeting.
7. Closing

SPA ETIQUETTE

Spa staff meetings should not be free-for-alls, yet neither should they be dictatorial monologues by the spa owner. One successful day spa owner in Canada decides upon a topic and then lets one of her employees run the meeting each month based upon that topic. Often, the topic is a particular product or technique used by the spa, or a client issue that has been surfacing. The owner speaks privately with the employee before the meeting to agree upon an approach. This gives each employee a chance to run the show.

Setting Schedules

Setting employee schedules is a constantly recurring challenge for spa directors and managers. Because it is impossible to give every employee an ideal schedule, this issue often causes frustration among staff members. In order to make scheduling as streamlined and effective as possible, follow these general guidelines:

- Post schedules well in advance, at least two pay periods into the future. This allows employees to plan ahead and avoid last-minute conflicts in scheduling.
- Be stricter than you think you need to be. Most therapist/owners want to display a certain amount of flexibility when it comes to making and altering employee schedules. This usually creates a permissive atmosphere that therapists and other employees tend to take advantage of. A job is a job. A schedule is a schedule. If certain employees cannot make it into work when you need them, it is time for disciplinary action (see section on spa staff discipline below).
- Set a specific "sick day" policy, and then stick to it.
- Institute an official vacation request policy and post a sign-up sheet in the employee area of the spa (Figure 18–6).
- Furnish individual time records for each employee in each pay period so that every hour and all pay scale details are written down and agreed upon (Figure 18–7).

When it comes time to actually make the schedule, most spas work on a weekly system. Many tie their employee scheduling directly into their software system so there is no need for separate record keeping. The schedule itself is a table with hours, days, and employees clearly laid out (Table 18–6).

Recruitment and Hiring

When you have built your initial spa staff, trained them, and celebrated your grand opening, your job in recruitment and hiring is still far from over. In fact, it is never over. Spa owners need to be constantly on the lookout for resources, especially human resources, that can help them sustain high-quality service. During the first few years of operation, some shifts usually take place as the staff gets used to working together. Inevitable shakeouts occur. Sometimes, the people you thought were your prime players end up leaving for a competitive spa, or somebody you had written off as an underperformer turns out to earn top commissions every month and may even be management material. It is always something. Therefore, most spa owners find it beneficial to keep their fingers on the pulse of the local hiring scene. They forge relationships with local massage schools. They take referrals from current employees. And they interview people on a regular basis.

Many of the interviewing techniques used by spas were explained in the "Interviews" section in Chapter 14. If you open a spa and begin interviewing prospective employees yourself, it will be useful to review this section and use some of the techniques yourself, such as the staff review process and asking some of

Therapeutic Day Spa
Employee Vacation Requests

Employee vacations are allotted on a first-come, first-served basis. If an employee needs to change vacation dates, they rotate to the back of the line and need to reapply.

Vacation Requested For	Starting	Ending	Approved?
Salavaria, Sarah	09/25/12	10/06/12	yes

Therapeutic Day Spa
1234 Main Street
Any Town, NY 02101

2012

January						
1	2	3	4	5	6	7
8	9	10	11	12	13	14
15	16	17	18	19	20	21
22	23	24	25	26	27	28
29	30	31				

February						
			1	2	3	4
5	6	7	8	9	10	11
12	13	14	15	16	17	18
19	20	21	22	23	24	25
26	27	28				

March						
			1	2	3	4
5	6	7	8	9	10	11
12	13	14	15	16	17	18
19	20	21	22	23	24	25
26	27	28	29	30	31	

April						
						1
2	3	4	5	6	7	8
9	10	11	12	13	14	15
16	17	18	19	20	21	22
23	24	25	26	27	28	29
30						

May						
	1	2	3	4	5	6
7	8	9	10	11	12	13
14	15	16	17	18	19	20
21	22	23	24	25	26	27
28	29	30	31			

June						
				1	2	3
4	5	6	7	8	9	10
11	12	13	14	15	16	17
18	19	20	21	22	23	24
25	26	27	28	29	30	

July						
						1
2	3	4	5	6	7	8
9	10	11	12	13	14	15
16	17	18	19	20	21	22
23	24	25	26	27	28	29
30	31					

August						
		1	2	3	4	5
6	7	8	9	10	11	12
13	14	15	16	17	18	19
20	21	22	23	24	25	26
27	28	29	30	31		

September						
					1	2
3	4	5	6	7	8	9
10	11	12	13	14	15	16
17	18	19	20	21	22	23
24	25	26	27	28	29	30

October						
1	2	3	4	5	6	7
8	9	10	11	12	13	14
15	16	17	18	19	20	21
22	23	24	25	26	27	28
29	30	31				

November						
			1	2	3	4
5	6	7	8	9	10	11
12	13	14	15	16	17	18
19	20	21	22	23	24	25
26	27	28	29	30		

December						
					1	2
3	4	5	6	7	8	9
10	11	12	13	14	15	16
17	18	19	20	21	22	23
24	25	26	27	28	29	30
31						

FIGURE 18–6 Institute an official vacation request policy and post a sign-up sheet in the employee area of the spa.

the interview questions listed. Also, familiarize yourself with the "deal-breaker" words and phrases that can tip you off to poor candidates.

hiring procedures
standardized practices used by a (spa) business to seek out, interview, screen, vet, and train new employees

When hiring new employees, it is important to have established **hiring procedures** in place so that all applicants will receive an equal opportunity at employment and all people who take part in the hiring process have an agreed-upon set of guidelines to follow that are written down in the spa's employee manual. This system will vary from spa to spa, but every successful hiring system will include the following components.

- Create or adopt a standardized application form for all potential employees.
- Institute a thorough reference-checking system.
- Adopt a multi-step interview process and do not discuss compensation during the initial interview. More than one person at the spa should have input into the hiring of each new employee.

Therapeutic Day Spa

Therapeutic Day Spa
1234 Main Street
Any Town, NY 02101

Weekly Schedule

Employee: Salavaria, Sarah
Manager: Becky
Employee phone no.: 555 505-1212
Week ending: 21-Jun

Day		Regular Hours	Overtime Hours	Sick	Holiday	Total
Monday						
Tuesday						
Wednesday		4.00				4.00
Thursday		7.00				7.00
Friday		7.00				7.00
Saturday		6.00				6.00
Sunday		5.00				5.00
	Total hours	**29.00**				**29.00**
	Rate per hour	$25.00	$37.00	$8.00	$12.00	
	Total pay	**$725.00**				**$725.00**

Employee signature Date

Manager signature Date

FIGURE 18–7 Furnish individual time records for each employee.

THERAPEUTIC DAY SPA								
WEEKLY SCHEDULE		JUNE 15–JUNE 21						
	POSITION	MONDAY	TUESDAY	WEDNESDAY	THURSDAY	FRIDAY	SATURDAY	SUNDAY
Becky	manager	8:30 A.M.–9 P.M.	8:30–5	8:30–5	8:30–5	11–8	4–8	off
Marsha	receptionist	off	4–8:30	4–8:30	4–8:30	4–8:30	4–8:30	off
Monique	receptionist	off	off	off	off	12–8:30	off	11:30–6:30
Bertrand	receptionist	off	8:30–5	8:30–5	8:30–5	8:30–5	8:30–5	off
Beatrice	esthetician	10–5	10–5	9–4	9–4	9–4	off	off
Sylvia	esthetician	off	off	2–8	2–8	2–8	2–8	12–6
Sarah	therapist	9–5	9–5	9–5	off	9–5	off	12–6
Kayla	therapist	off	off	2–8	off	2–8	2–8	12–6
Lori Anne	therapist	10–6	10–6	off	10–6	10–6	10–6	off
Robert	therapist	off	4–8	1–8	1–8	1–8	9–2	off
Tom	therapist	11–8	off	off	11–8	11–7	11–8	12–6
Bill	spa attendant	off	11–8	11–8	11–8	11–8	11–8	off

TABLE 18–6 Weekly Schedule.

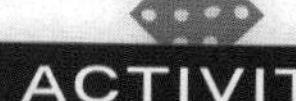

ACTIVITY

Setting Schedules

Using Table 18–6 as a guide, answer the following questions:

1. What day seems to be the busiest at the spa? How can you tell?
2. On which day are the fewest number of therapists scheduled to work?
3. With no receptionists scheduled for Monday, who is most likely going to take appointments and deal with clients at the front desk?
4. Which employees would be considered full-time (40 or more hours per week), assuming a half-hour lunch break? How might this impact scheduling decisions?
5. Judging by this schedule, which two therapists seem willing and able to work the most hours?
6. Using this schedule as a guide, draw a simple graph curve showing the amount of business expected throughout the week at the spa.
7. If Lori Anne requested a week off for vacation, would there be other female therapists available to cover her shifts? Could this present a problem?

- Have all new hires undergo the same initial training and familiarization period.
- Test new employees on their knowledge of spa policies and procedures after they have had the chance to study the spa's employee manual.
- Require all new employees to pass an initial probationary period during which employment can be terminated at any time.

SPA CAUTION

Checking references for spa employees is even more important than it is in most other industries because spa employees come into such intimate contact with clients. Even after receiving favorable references from past employers, there is still a potential for lawsuits if a therapist or other employee acts inappropriately or is even accused of acting inappropriately. Therefore, all favorable references received from past employers, even if they are taken verbally over the phone, must be documented and kept in the spa's written records.

Promotions and Raises

Monetary incentives, though not the prime motivator for many therapists, are still important. So, knowing that, how do you best structure promotions and raises? Many spa owners have found that the most effective technique is to tie the raise to performance and seniority, rather than just seniority alone, because therapists love to be recognized for their skills. Take a look at Table 18–7 for an example of tiered pay rates for therapists. You will see three pay levels that therapists can attain through:

- advanced training
- seniority
- a demonstrated ability to increase the spa's business through client requests and re-bookings

It is important to remember when promoting spa employees to always tie in their promotion to the spa's overall success. For example, holiday bonuses can be distributed to all employees if the spa makes its year-end goals. Entry-level employees such as receptionists and spa attendants will deliver improved performance if they know a bonus or a certain percentage of their pay raise is dependent upon the spa's financial success. Also, it is also important to note that the spa should always come first when it comes to recognition. Honoring employees in-house with such distinctions as "employee of the month" is fine, but do not make the mistake of promoting one employee over others to clients

			PAY LEVEL		
SERVICE	TIME	PRICE	THERAPIST	ADVANCED THERAPIST	MASTER THERAPIST
Basic Massage	1 hr	$75	$18.75	$22.50	$26.25
Advanced Massage (deep tissue, stone)	1 hr	$85	$21.25	$25.50	$29.75
Basic Spa Modalities (exfoliation, herbal wraps)	½ hr	$50	$12.50	$15	$17.5
Advanced Spa Modalities (body wraps, thalassotherapy, etc.)	1½ hrs	$120	$30	$36	$42
Package 2	2½ hrs	$220	$55	$66	$77
Therapist pay % of service price			25%	30%	35%

TABLE 18–7 Tiered Pay Scales for Spa Therapists.

or the general public. This can cause jealousy among co-workers. Also, clients begin to think it is more important to receive an appointment with a specific practitioner than with the spa in general.

Disciplining and Firing Employees

As part of your commitment to creating a solid workplace in which all participants know where they stand, it is necessary to set clearly defined rules for employees to follow. Consequences must result when those rules are broken. Otherwise, the staff will learn to disrespect those rules and the boundaries set by the spa.

The spa's rules should be clearly spelled out in the employee handbook, and all new employees should sign a form stating they understand those rules. Then, after the provisional employment period is over and full employment has begun, employees are given written warnings if they fail to observe the spa's guidelines (Figure 18–8). After a certain number of warnings—the most common number is three—the employee is terminated, and an employment termination form is filled out (Figure 18–9). If you have never had to fire anybody, you may find the first time you do so to be an unexpectedly powerful experience. You will become aware that the person's livelihood, or at least a part of it, is being determined by your decision. Firing an employee is never an easy decision to make, but it is often an obvious one. As the owner, you must take the overall soundness of the business into mind before all else. Do not let one employee's actions put other employees, or the spa business itself, at risk.

In order not to catch employees unaware, it is helpful to schedule periodic employment reviews to determine the level of performance and any needed improvements in particular areas. Typically, reviews in the spa setting are given once or twice a year, either by the spa director or the employee's direct supervisor. This review, like all interactions with employees, should be documented and kept on file (Figure 18–10). If for any reason an employee should sue or file a complaint against the spa, all relevant data will be available.

Training

Spa employees need to improve their performance on a consistent basis for the sake of the spa's success, and the most efficient way to accomplish this is through periodic training. Many spas offer some form of training in-house, and others offer partial or full compensation for employees who pursue trainings elsewhere. The two main forms of spa staff trainings are customer-service training and technique training.

Customer-service training can take many forms. Several companies offer standardized customer-service training modules that are applicable across the hospitality industry. Other companies specialize in customer-service training for spas. Some spas create their own customer-service trainings designed exclusively for their employees. Any customer-service trainings that you undertake should be standardized, and the results of such trainings should be measurable in terms of guest feedback and overall smoother operations at the spa. The following are the most common topics covered in spa employee trainings.

Therapeutic Day Spa
1234 Main Street
Any Town, NY 02101

Employee Warning Notice

Employee Information

Employee Name:
Employee ID:
Manager:

Date:
Job Title:
Department:

Type of Warning

☐ First Warning ☐ Second Warning ☐ Final Warning

Type of Offense

☐ Tardiness/Leaving Early
☐ Substandard Work
☐ Absenteeism
☐ Violation of Safety Rules
☐ Violation of Company Policies
☐ Rudeness to Customers/Coworkers
☐ Other: ____________________

Details

Description of Infraction:

Plan for Improvement:

Consequences of Further Infractions:

If this is your final warning, be advised that you need to take steps to correct your behavior by [date]. Your failure to do so will result in your termination.

Acknowledgement of Receipt of Warning

By signing this form, you confirm that you understand the information in this warning. You also confirm that you and your manager have discussed the warning and a plan for improvement. Signing this form does not necessarily indicate that you agree with this warning.

____
Employee Signature *Date*

____
Manager Signature *Date*

____
Witness Signature (if employee has heard or seen warning but refuses to sign) *Date*

FIGURE 18–8 Employees should be given written warnings if they fail to observe the spa's guidelines.

Therapeutic Day Spa
1234 Main Street
Any Town, NY 02101

Employment Termination Form

Employee Information

Employee Name:
Date:
Employee ID:
Job Title:
Manager:
Department:

Notice

Dear [**Employee Name**]:

We regret to inform you that your employment with **Therapeutic Day Spa** is being terminated, effective [date]. Your termination is the result of the following violations of company policy:

- **[Warning], [date]**
- **[Warning], [date]**
- **[Warning], [date]**

You were issued written warnings on [**date**], [**date**], and [**date**]. Copies of these warnings, signed by you, are in your personnel file. Your signature on each warning indicates that you discussed it with your manager, including steps you could take to correct the behavior cited in the warnings. As stated in your final warning, you needed to take steps to correct your behavior by [**date**]. Your failure to do so has resulted in your termination.

To appeal this termination, you must return written notification of your intention to appeal to [**Name**] on no later than [**date**].

Acknowledgement of Receipt of Termination Notice

By signing this form, you confirm that you understand the information in this termination form and that as a result of failing to correct behaviors cited during the warning process your employment is being terminated.

Employee Signature *Date*

Manager Signature *Date*

Witness Signature (if employee understands he/she is being terminated but refuses to sign) *Date*

FIGURE 18–9 If the employee is fired, an employment termination form is filled out.

Therapeutic Day Spa
1234 Main Street
Any Town, NY 02101

Employee Performance Review

Employee Information

Employee Name:
Employee ID:
Job Title:
Date:
Department:
Manager:
Review Period: to

Ratings

	(5) = Poor	(4) = Fair	(3) = Satisfactory	(2) = Good	(1) = Excellent
Job Knowledge	☐	☐	☐	☐	☐
Comments:					
Work Quality	☐	☐	☐	☐	☐
Comments:					
Attendance/Punctuality	☐	☐	☐	☐	☐
Comments:					
Initiative	☐	☐	☐	☐	☐
Comments:					
Communication/Listening Skills	☐	☐	☐	☐	☐
Comments					
Dependability	☐	☐	☐	☐	☐
Comments:					

Overall Rating (average the rating numbers above):

Evaluation

Additional Comments:

Goals (as agreed upon by employee and manager):

Verification of Review

By signing this form, you confirm that you have discussed this review in detail with your supervisor. Signing this form does not necessarily indicate that you agree with this evaluation.

Employee Signature *Date*

Manager Signature *Date*

FIGURE 18–10 Employee performance reviews should be documented and kept on file.

Telephone Etiquette

Receptionists and all other employees who answer the business phone need to be reminded how to best convey the spa's message. Without ongoing training, it is easy to fall into an overly informal manner.

Guest Interactions

Each and every circumstance under which employees interact with guests in the spa should be the subject of customer-service training. Effective techniques for such training are based largely on role playing and study of relevant scenarios (see activities in the "Customer Service on Steroids" section in Chapter 15).

Operational Protocols

Spa employees occasionally become lax regarding common procedures, and operational protocol trainings are used as a brush-up so that all employees perform duties in a uniform, excellent manner. Typical subjects covered in such trainings include front-desk protocols, opening and closing procedures, **inventory control**, and customer complaint management.

inventory control
supervision of the supply, storage, and accessibility of items in order to ensure an adequate supply without excessive oversupply

Product and Procedure Familiarization

Many times, spa employees will be asked by clients about products or procedures that are not within the realm of their expertise. While it is always possible to refer these questions to somebody else who knows the answer, it reflects well on the spa if all employees have at least some basic familiarity with many different facets of the spa's offerings. Therapists, for example, should be aware of the different types of facials offered by the estheticians, along with their benefits.

Vendor-Specific Technique Training

There is no shortage of spa product vendors that will offer hands-on training for your spa staff. This is often the simplest choice when you are first starting a spa and money is in short supply. Vendors can do a world of good for new, untrained therapists and estheticians, especially those who have never worked in a spa environment before. However, keep in mind that in order to receive the training, spas need to commit to purchasing a certain amount of product.

Spa-Specific Technique Training

Many spa owners and directors take technique training into their own hands and create a standardized format for each treatment that all technicians need to follow. In this way, they ensure a uniform experience for their guests based on their own standards rather than those of a vendor or other third party. In order for these trainings to be effective, they must be:

- Consistent—Each employee should receive the same training, no matter who is giving it or when it is offered.
- Repeated periodically—People need to be reminded about the spa's protocols on a periodic basis. Without that, many practitioners tend to

gradually slip into their own idiosyncrasies and offer clients a different experience than the one the spa promised to deliver.

- Updated—At least one protocol should be updated or one new service added each year.
- Mandatory—Although some employees will chafe at required trainings, they are necessary in order to offer clients superior service and therefore cannot be skipped.

SPA CAUTION

Some spas send one therapist out to trainings with the intention of bringing materials and knowledge back to co-workers at the spa so they can learn the technique as well. This practice is not recommended and may lead to substandard performance. Only qualified teachers should teach new techniques to spa staffs.

PROTECTING YOURSELF AS A SPA OWNER

When you run a spa, you need to take special precautions above and beyond those required by a traditional massage therapy business. There are many ways in which a spa business is particularly vulnerable to lawsuits, damages, and potential failure. Because of all the heat applications and the abundance of hot water, for example, clients are more likely to experience a scald or burn, and ample precautions must be taken to prevent this. Also, the presence of so much water makes the prevention of slippage especially important, and spas must invest in the proper flooring if they are to circumvent this problem. The high-tech equipment used in spas presents its own liability issues, and operators need to be especially cautious when using such techniques as microdermabrasion, body sculpting, and chemical skin peels, as well as during the application of exotic and/or organic materials to the skin.

Therapists working in a traditional massage practice have to be well-versed in ethical issues, draping, and boundaries, but spa therapists need to be even more vigilant about these same issues for three main reasons:

- The abundance of water
  The abundance of water used in spas, plus the multiple turns on the treatment table during services, plus the application and cleansing of products from the skin makes draping even more of a delicate issue than it is during massage, sometimes necessitating the use of disposal underwear products or other means to protect modesty. Spa therapists must be extra sure they are respecting clients' boundaries.
- The relaxed attitude of the clients
  Spa clients are told they are supposed to relax, and sometimes they take the message too far, leaving all inhibitions behind, disrobing inappropriately, becoming intoxicated before treatments (at resort spas) and becoming more likely to make sexual advances than they would in the clinical environment of a massage therapy practice. Spa personnel once again need to be extra-vigilant and steadfastly follow all proper procedures under these circumstances.
- Under-trained employees
  Many spas employ people as spa technicians, spa attendants, locker-room attendants, and others who come into contact with clients when they are disrobed before or after treatments. It is important that these employees be trained in boundaries and proper behavior, even if they are not working hands-on with the clients.

In spite of your best attempts to avoid it, at some point, a client might still feel justified in filing a complaint or even a lawsuit against you and your company. Whether the complaint has merit is of secondary concern. You may be absolutely in the right, but you need to be able to prove this to others, perhaps in a court of law, and this is why it is important to keep meticulous records of any incident, no matter how small, that may eventually trigger a problem. All spa directors and owners should encourage managers and employees to make a note of such occurrences with an **incident report** (Figure 18–11). An incident report should be filled out whenever a client complains to management, whenever an employee complains about a client or another employee, whenever somebody is injured or claims to be injured in the spa, whenever something in the spa breaks or becomes potentially dangerous, and whenever any outside authorities such as the police, fire department, or department of professional regulation are called for any reason.

incident report

official written, signed document outlining the details of an event that may potentially be cause for litigation or disciplinary actions

business liability insurance

insurance that covers businesses and business owners for claims related to allegations of negligent activities or failure to use reasonable care

Liability Insurance

It is essential for spas to have **business liability insurance** in order to protect themselves against potential claims. Each practitioner employed by the spa should ideally be covered by a liability insurance policy as well, either privately or through a professional association. But is such insurance enough to truly

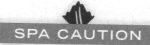

SPA CAUTION

Three True Cautionary Tales

The following three scenarios actually took place at operating day spas. Paying heed to the moral of each story will help you avoid similar liability issues in your spa business.

Tale #1: A client visited a spa for Endermologie, a cellulite treatment consisting of a machine with powerful rollers and a vacuum which glides over the skin. The woman had no adverse reaction to the treatment while at the spa, but afterward she noticed a large "pockmark" on the skin of her leg. She sued the spa and the manufacturer of the equipment for damaging her skin. Only later, after expensive litigation, did the truth come out: The pockmark was actually caused by a prior cortisone injection which weakened the tissues in the area. It had nothing to do with the spa treatment.

The moral: Even spas that follow every precaution and do no harm to their clients can still be sued. It is best to be prepared for that eventuality.

Tale #2: A paraplegic woman visited a spa in California to receive a massage. After the treatment, she complained to management that she had been molested by the therapist. The therapist admitted to the misconduct but claimed that the experience had been one of mutual consent. The client sued nonetheless, costing the spa thousands of dollars and almost closing the business down. The therapist was fired and prohibited from working as a massage therapist ever again.

The moral: Spas need to teach their therapists that only impeccably ethical behavior is acceptable in the treatment room. Shades of "mutual consent" do not matter in a lawsuit.

Tale #3: A spa in Florida hired an unlicensed man to perform Turkish hammam treatments that included exfoliation and massage. The man was accused of molesting a female client, and he fled the country. The owner claimed that the hammam was a distinct service that did not require a massage or cosmetology license to perform, but the spa was sued nonetheless.

The moral: No amount of creative interpretation and rationalization will keep people from suing. Be prepared by knowing all laws and regulations applicable in your area.

Therapeutic Day Spa
1234 Main Street
Any Town, NY 02101

INCIDENT REPORT FORM

(Incidents involving employees, clients, visitors)

Employee Information

Employee Name: Employee ID:
Job Title: Date:
Department:
Manager:

INFORMATION ABOUT THE PERSON INVOLVED IN THE INCIDENT:

Full Name:		Social Sec.#:
Home Address:		Gender: M F
Circle: Employee (Full-time, part-time, perm., temp.) Client Visitor		
Date of Birth:	Home phone:	Other Phone:

INFORMATION ABOUT THE INCIDENT:

Date of Incident:	Time:	Police notified: Yes No Case #:

Location of Incident:

Describe what happened, how it happened, factors leading to the event, substances or objects involved. **Be as specific as possible** (attach separate sheet if necessary):

Were there any witnesses to the incident? Yes No

If yes, attach separate sheet with names, addresses and phone numbers.

Was the individual injured? If so, describe the injury (laceration, sprain, etc.), the part of body injured and any other information known about the resulting injury(s):

Was medical treatment provided? Yes No Refused

If so, where (circle) : Emergency Room The Workplace Walk In Clinic Other

Will the employee miss time from work as a result of this incident? Yes No Unknown

INFORMATION ABOUT THE PERSON RECORDING THIS REPORT:

Full Name:	Position:
signature:	Date report completed:
witness signature:	

THERAPEUTIC DAY SPA

This is a confidential report and should not be made a part of an employee's personnel record. It is completed to allow us to obtain advice from legal counsel and for the protection of the spa and it's employees from potential liability.

FIGURE 18–11 It is important to keep meticulous records of any incidents in the spa.

cover a spa's liability? Increasingly, spas are faced with clients who are more than willing to file lawsuits and seek damages. There are two main reasons for this trend:

- Because of the dramatic rise in new spas being built recently, a small number of them inevitably have come to be run by people with low ethical and professional standards, and the stories that appear in the media regarding these spas taint the public's view of the overall industry.
- Spa businesses are now viewed as wealthy targets with deep pockets, worthy of being sued by people who are inclined to do so.

One of the most valuable things that spas can do to help protect themselves in the current legal environment is to invest in specialized trainings on the most common causes of lawsuits. These causes include:

- allegations of misconduct by hands-on practitioners while behind closed doors
- allegations of physical injury caused by substandard care or neglect on the part of the spa (failure to note contraindications, inappropriate treatment of medical conditions, lack of medical screening)
- allegations of injury caused due to spa facility (slip and fall, lack of sufficient safeguards and signage)

When spa businesses provide their employees with specific trainings that cover these issues in detail, they can significantly hedge their liability. All spas should maintain files with documents showing that their employees have undergone thorough training regarding contraindications, client boundary issues, sexual harassment, and workplace safety. Then, if a spa business is sued, the business owner can furnish proof that she has done everything possible to prevent such occurrences.

Licenses and Permits

Obtaining the proper licensing is essential for a spa business, and no spa should open its doors without all the licenses it needs to operate legally. Licenses and permits should be applied for well in advance of opening, because a delay in receiving the physical license could cause a delay in the actual opening date of the spa. This issue is covered here, rather than in the previous chapter—Opening a Therapeutic Spa—because licensing is an ongoing issue. Well beyond the date of your grand opening, maintaining current licenses for the facility, the business, and all practitioners will be a continuing managerial concern.

There are several different types of licenses and permits that may be necessary for a spa business. Generally, they are defined by local and/or state rules, referred to as **ordinances**. Once local authorities have determined that your business is in compliance with such ordinances, you will be issued the relevant permit(s) or license(s), enabling you to legally operate your spa. Local requirements vary by jurisdiction. Failure to have the proper permits may prevent your business from opening, and could result in fines or even being shut down.

ordinances

local and/or state rules that regulate the safety, structure, and operational practices of a (spa) business

Simply knowing which agencies to contact to obtain the right permits and licenses can be a very confusing task for the new spa owner. If you are confused, try contacting the SBA, your local chamber of commerce, trade associations, and even other businesspeople or attorneys working in the spa industry. Also, follow these five simple steps in order to obtain licenses:

1. Have your business paperwork in order, including any **fictitious name certificates**, **DBAs**, and your **employer identification number (EIN)**. You receive an EIN for your spa and reserve the name when you incorporate the business.
2. Contact your city hall, county, and/or state government offices to determine the kind of licenses you need and obtain necessary application paperwork. Libraries are a good source for state-specific licensing information.
3. Initiate proper application procedures and fill out all forms. In some cases, this step may require an on-site inspection.
4. File the application, along with any fees, with the appropriate government office. Sometimes this must be done in person.
5. Stay on top of annual renewals and/or other kinds of procedures as required by state law. Once granted, business licenses usually must be renewed (and renewal fees paid) annually.

fictitious name certificates

the same thing as a "doing business as" certificate, obtained by (spa) businesses through public announcement and filing, usually not necessary for spas that incorporate and receive an EIN

DBA

an acronym which stands for "doing business as," part of a filing that (spa) business can make with local authorities, banks, etc. in order to operate legally

employer identification number (EIN)

the taxpayer ID number for business, similar to a social security number for individuals, which is received upon incorporating the business

The three main types of licenses and permits needed by spas include: a local and/or state business license (also known as an *operational license*), retail license (also known as a *sales tax permit* or *reseller's permit*), and occupational license. There are also several specific permits that may be applicable to your spa business, including building permits, zoning permits, and home occupation permits.

Business Licenses

Nearly all spa businesses need a county or city business license, and most need some kind of state license or permit as well. These are general licenses that grant you, as the business owner, the privilege of legally operating a business within a certain city and/or county jurisdiction. Fees are typically low and these kinds of licenses are easy to obtain, but application procedures vary widely.

Retail Licenses

If your spa purchases wholesale merchandise for resale, your state will probably require you to register for a retail license (sometimes called a *seller's permit*, *reseller's permit*, or *sales tax permit*). This allows you to charge sales tax to customers on items purchased. Usually, your **state franchise tax board** grants seller's permits. Some counties and cities also require a separate resale permit of their own. You can inquire about this at the local city hall and seat of county government.

state franchise tax board

state government agency set up to collect personal and businesses taxes owed an individual state

Occupational Licenses

Each state has different agencies regulating the state licenses required for massage therapists, estheticians, cosmetologists, and other professionals, including ongoing continuing education requirements. As a massage therapist, in most states,

establishment license

a license, separate from the business license, generally granted by state boards of professional regulation, allowing (spa) businesses to offer specific services, such as massage, esthetic services, etc.

you will need an occupational license in order to perform massage on paying clients. All practitioners employed by spas in licensed states will need occupational licenses. Similar licenses are also issued to businesses that provide products or services regulated by law. This is referred to as an **establishment license**. In many locations, spa businesses will need such a license to operate legally. It is wise to contact the state boards of massage, cosmetology, and esthetics for information about establishment licenses.

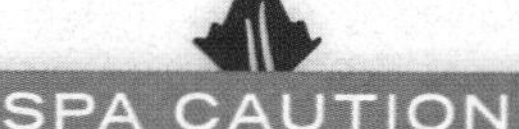

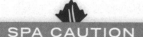

SPA CAUTION

Of course, spa owners need to make sure the practitioners they hire are licensed and fully legal. In addition, spa employees need to confirm that the spa where they work is legal, with the appropriate establishment license for each profession represented in the business, including massage, esthetics, and cosmetology. Authorities at state departments of professional regulation have the power to discipline therapists working in an unlicensed facility. Even though you may be fully licensed and legal, if the spa is not, you may be liable for penalties. Make sure to check on the spa's license status before accepting employment.

Building Permits

If your spa plans include remodeling or building, you will need to get a building permit. Make sure as well that your business space is in compliance with other local ordinances as well, such as access and facilities for the disabled.

Zoning Permits

You must make sure that the space in which you operate your spa is properly zoned for the use you have in mind. Some cities require that each new business gets a zoning compliance permit before it opens. If you plan on having accommodations for clients to spend the night, you may also need a lodging permit. You can research the details through your local zoning board, planning department, or library.

Home Occupation Permits

If you create a home-based spa therapy business, some local governments will require you to obtain a home occupation permit. The best way to find out if this is necessary is to call your city hall and ask for zoning information. If you rent your apartment or home, check with the manager or owner of your building. In some communities, the local homeowners' association should be consulted as well.

Variances

If for some reason you feel a certain ordinance is being unjustly enforced, you can petition the authorities for a special permit, called a **variance**, which would allow you to, in effect, violate the ordinance. Variances are not granted easily, and they can be expensive to obtain, especially in terms of attorneys' fees. Be sure you really need the variance before you try to obtain it.

variance

a special permit allowing a (spa) business to effectively violate a local ordinance, such as zoning or building

SPA MARKETING

No spa can be successful without an influx of new clients and a strategy in place to keep current clients coming back. You cannot assume that just because your techniques and products are good, people will automatically seek you out or return once they've found you. Consumers have a vast number of choices when it comes to spas, and there is a strong temptation to try something new or experience the latest exotic treatment at a competitor's spa. This is why you need to have a marketing plan. The term **marketing** as it is usually applied to spas can be described as any technique that is used to promote

marketing

all activities a company undertakes to acquire customers and maintain relationships with them, with the ultimate goal of matching products and services to the people who need and want them, in order to ensure profitability

lockers, and free product samples. Membership dues bring up-front money to the spa and create a sense of community and loyalty.

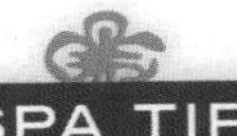

SPA TIP

Spas can apply for inclusion on Spa & Salon Wish, which enables people from around the world to buy gift certificates that are good for use at the local spa. A person in California, for instance, who wants to buy a massage and body wrap for her sister in New York, can do so by purchasing a Spa & Salon Wish gift certificate. The sister receives the certificate and takes it to any participating New York spa. Visit http://www.salonwish.com, or call (888) 772-9474.

Stay in Contact

Spa businesses need to stay in contact with clients by sending out periodic e-mail or direct-mail messages regarding seasonal promotions, discounts, new services, and changes at the spa. Also, personalized contact for anniversaries and birthdays creates extra loyalty, and a quarterly newsletter keeps clients informed and feeling like they are part of the spa's family. Thank-you cards sent to clients after they refer new clients are a nice touch too. Some spas also make calls each day to clients who they know may be interested in last-minute openings at the spa.

Join a Spa Gift Certificate Service

Many spas take advantage of nationwide services that offer people the opportunity to buy gift certificates that are redeemable at thousands of spa businesses, regardless of location. In order for a spa to be accepted by such services, they have to be more extensive than a one-person private spa practice.

Web Site

Even small private-practice spas need to establish a Web site in order to compete effectively with other spas (Figure 18–13). Without a Web site, spas miss out on the growing number of people who search for spa services on the Internet. A spa Web site should reflect the look of the spa's collateral and the physical spa itself in order to create a consistent image. Many spas offer Web site-only specials to entice visitors. Others offer online booking or gift certificates, while others increase their marketing reach by including an e-mail list sign-up box on the home page so visitors can choose to be contacted in the future.

SPA TIP

Spas can enhance the marketing power of their Web sites by using e-mail contact managers such as Constant Contact (http://www.constantcontact.com), or by incorporating online scheduling and gift certificates offered by companies such as Spa Boom (http://www.spaboom.com). Also, you can send out periodic do-it-yourself e-mails to your mailing list.

Spa Marketing Collateral

Spas depend heavily upon their image in the public eye. People want spas to have a certain feel and a certain look. Even small, single-therapist spas need to exercise care in creating the right atmosphere as explained in the "A Consciously Created Spa Environment" section of Chapter 17. Equal care should be given to projecting the right image in the spa's **collateral**. Collateral material includes everything a spa sends out to represent itself in the public eye. The most typical items include brochures, newsletters, postcards, menus, business cards, and letterhead (Figure 18–14). A spa's Web site can also be considered part of its collateral. The overall success of a spa, even a small, single-therapist spa, is often highly dependent on the look and quality of its collateral materials. Therefore, you as a spa owner or practitioner should not skimp when it comes time to invest in these materials. High-quality paper, meaningful verbiage, and attractive images and layout are all important. Refer to Table 18–8 for descriptions of specific types of collateral material along with their purpose in the spa and typical mistakes that therapists make when first creating these materials for their new spa practices.

collateral

any (spa) marketing items that are distributed directly to individual customers or can be viewed by those customers in person, including brochures, letters, cards, presentations, displays, e-mails, Web pages and more

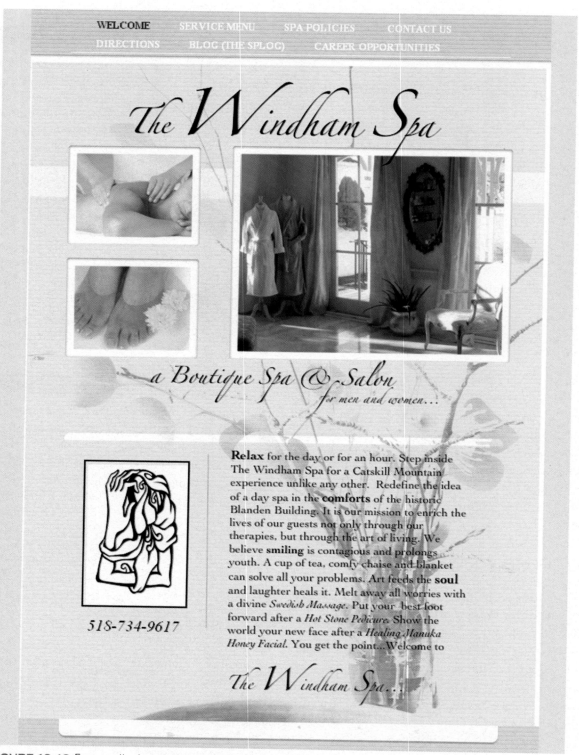

FIGURE 18–13 Even small private-practice spas need to establish a Web site.

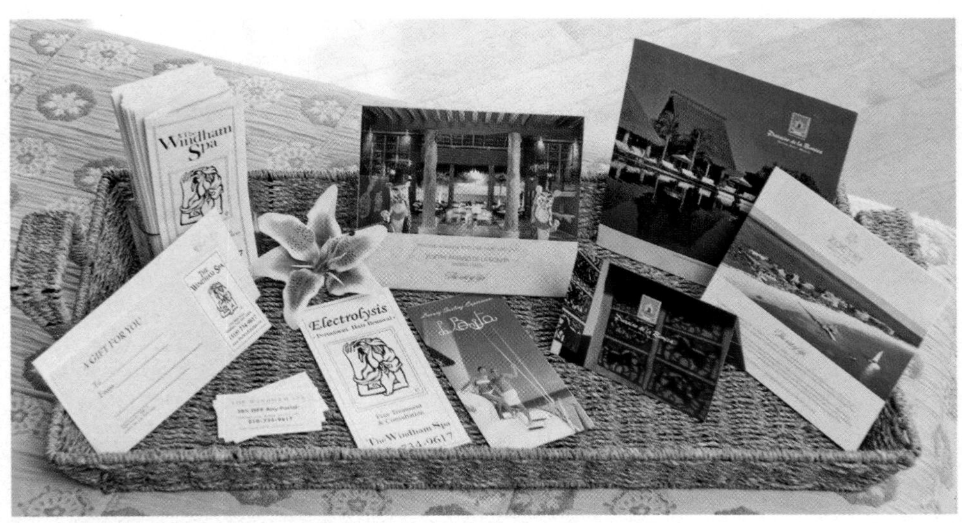

FIGURE 18–14 Collateral material includes everything a spa sends out to represent itself in the public eye.

call to action

a direct request to the potential client at the end of a marketing piece, requesting him or her to pick up the phone or come to the (spa) business in order to purchase products or services

COLLATERAL	DESCRIPTION	PURPOSE	TYPICAL MISTAKES
Spa Newsletters (Figure 18–15)	should have four main sections: 1. owner's message 2. latest news about the spa, events, employees, etc. 3. one treatment highlighted and put on special 4. coupons and descriptions of retail	to stay in touch with clients and keep them informed about events, new treatments, personnel changes, and other news	therapist/owners underestimate the curiosity clients have about the spa and leave out interesting information, making the newsletter one big ad instead
Brochures (Figure 18–16)	attractive pieces suitable for mailing featuring photographs, descriptions, philosophy, and overview of services	to entice new clients and reassure existing clients about the stature and quality of the business	not enough emphasis placed on making the brochure a work of art, turning the brochure into a glorified menu
Postcards	targeted mailings about specific specials or services, or simply to keep in touch	to remind customers of your offerings and gain new customers through direct mailing	a lack of specific information about particular products, services, or events, with no **call to action** at the end
Menus	a thorough description of all the services offered at the spa in easy-to-understand language, often with graphics for esthetic purposes and as an aid in description	to help clients decide which service to choose and to entice potential clients with rich descriptions of the services	overly flowery wording, overly succinct wording, assumption of familiarity with spa etiquette and services
Business Cards	can include color and/or photographs, logo, tag line, graphic designs, and list of service types along with contact information	to provide prospective clients, vendors, partners, and employees basic information and a general image of spa	inconsistent look divorced from theme of other collateral and the spa itself
Letterhead	stationery with spa's logo and contact information	to provide a consistent image for everyone who receives letters from the spa	low-quality paper or printing, inconsistent with rest of collateral
Web Site	pages on the Internet where clients can view the spa's information, be linked to other spa resources, engage in e-commerce, and feel connected to the spa without actually being there	to provide clients information, updated news, and descriptions of the spa and its services, to gather names for mailing list, and also potentially to offer products for sale and online booking	inconsistent look with rest of spa's collateral, not enough interactivity, infrequent updating, lack of user-controlled options such as printing out gift certificates

TABLE 18–8 Important Collateral Materials for the Spa.

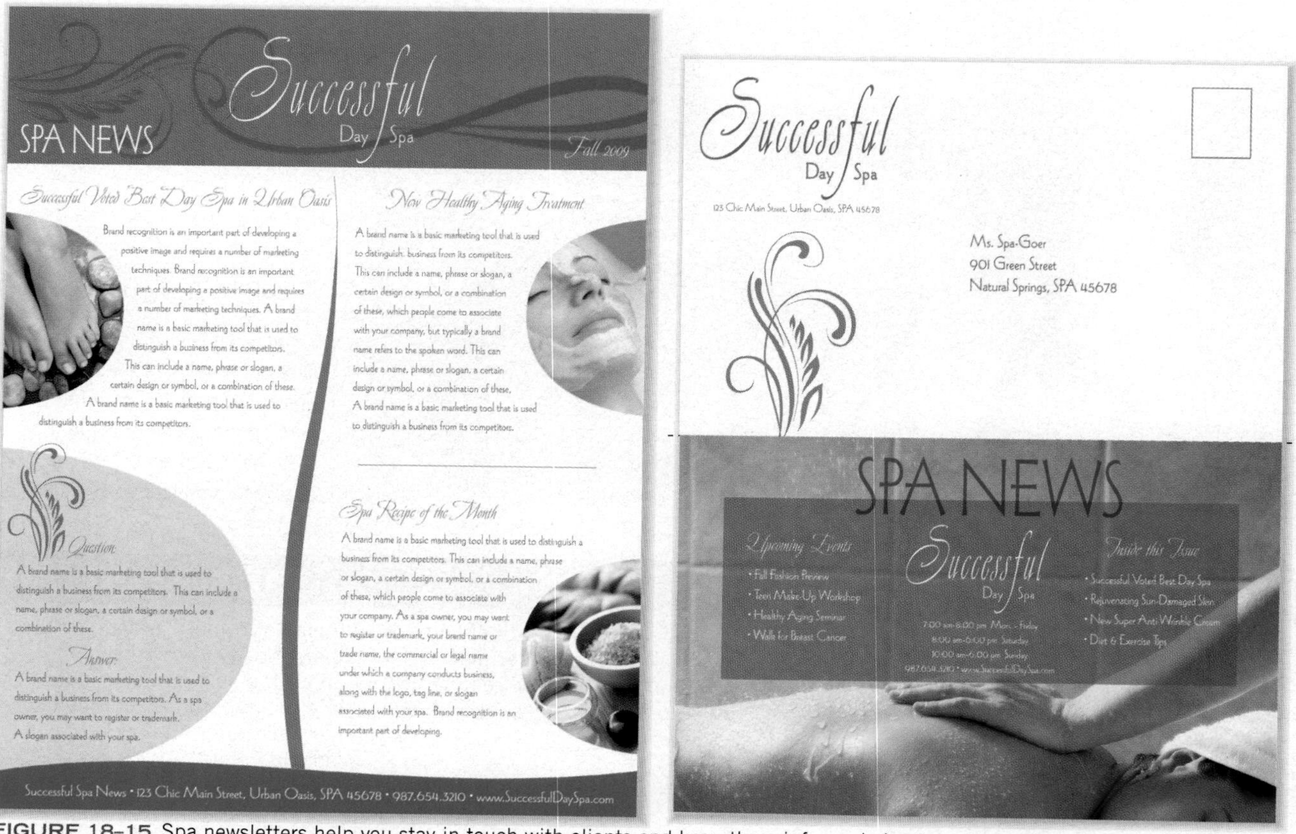

FIGURE 18–15 Spa newsletters help you stay in touch with clients and keep them informed about events, new treatments, personnel changes and other news.

> **SPA TIP**
>
> Do not embed the prices for your spa services in the wording of your brochure or menu, because it will then be difficult to change prices on these important (and expensive) collateral items. It is wiser to insert the prices on a separate sheet of paper or card, called a **tariff card**, that can be changed periodically at minimal expense.

tariff card

insert to a spa menu or brochure that lists prices for services, used so that prices can be changed periodically without the expense of reprinting collateral

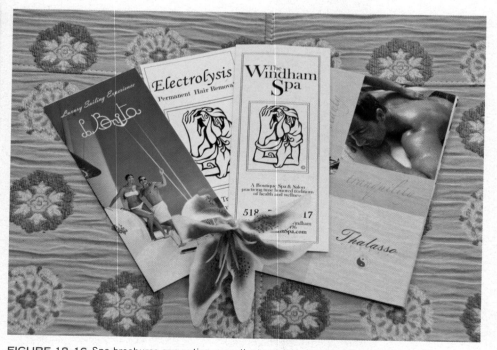

FIGURE 18–16 Spa brochures can entice new clients and reassure existing clients about the stature and quality of the business.

SPA OPERATIONS CHECKLIST

Mastering all the tasks and responsibilities required of a successful spa owner may seem burdensome at first, but over time you will find yourself naturally focusing your attention on those items that call for it most at any given moment. To make sure that you do not let any of these important duties slip through the cracks, create a checklist similar to the one provided here to remind yourself of what needs to get done, and when.

✓	TASK		FREQUENCY
	scheduling clients		daily
	order supplies and interface with vendors		daily
	payroll		weekly
	scheduling staff		weekly
	review budget projections		monthly
	order staff uniforms		annually
	manage client complaints		ongoing
staff training		motivational training	monthly
		write in-house newsletter	bi-monthly
		customer-service training	semi-annually
		hands on training	quarterly
marketing advertising		contacting clients	daily/as needed
		public relations	as needed for special events and promotions
		writing collateral	semi-annually
	risk management		prepare incident reports in advance and check monthly
	recruit		ongoing (to have a pool of recruits from which to choose)
	hire		as needed
	licensing and permits		quarterly

It is important not to get bogged down by the ongoing stream of chores that inevitably arise during spa operations and to avoid spending all of your time "putting out fires." For this reason, it is a good idea for you to have checklists of daily items that need to be taken care of, preferably by a staff member rather than yourself. Here, for example, is a list of daily opening tasks for a typical spa:

- ✓ turn on computer
- ✓ turn on spa equipment, heaters, steam room, etc.
- ✓ check schedule for the day, confirm therapist availability
- ✓ check treatment rooms – fully stocked? clean?
- ✓ check spa common areas – clean? orderly?
- ✓ check to make sure all paperwork—intake forms, retail order forms, receipts—are prepared and available
- ✓ turn on spa sound system and treatment room music options
- ✓ turn on water features, fountains, lighting
- ✓ check restrooms and showers – sanitary? tidy?
- ✓ set temperature controls for optimum spa environment, different for treatment rooms and common areas

SPA PROFILE

Monica Roseberry – Marketing Massage

Monica Roseberry knows a thing or two about marketing massage therapy. In fact, she has written a book on the subject: *Marketing Massage: From First Job to Dream Practice*. Her book first helps therapists market themselves to potential employers (especially spas) for jobs, and then gives practical marketing skills and tools to help therapists build or expand their private practices. She also offers advice that can be applied by therapists who are expanding into the spa marketplace.

"I wrote a book about marketing," says Roseberry, "because too many of the massage students in my business classes still couldn't make a living even after learning so much about practice-building. Many of them worked out of their homes, or did outcall to clients' homes, which made it unsafe to use traditional marketing and advertising. In addition, many therapists were working in a hostile environment with vice squads harassing legitimate therapists as if they were prostitutes. A lot of cities would not issue therapists business licenses, or their zoning laws required crazy things like having a drain in the floor of the massage room so the therapist could 'hose down the room.' In those circumstances, many therapists chose to work 'under the radar,' which meant that normal marketing options weren't available to them. There was no resource out there that honestly addressed what it took to build a practice, or that dealt with all the many details of marketing massage."

What started out as a simple desire to help her students became quite an odyssey. "First," says Roseberry, "I called other massage schools and talked to their business teachers to see what they were doing to teach their students marketing. Most of what I heard was about marketing techniques for other businesses being transferred to the massage industry, but that just doesn't work. Massage has unique issues that traditional marketing doesn't address, especially the issues of trust, value, and how people perceive massage. When I didn't get satisfying answers from the business teachers, I called massage association leaders, massage school owners, and people I had met at massage conventions to ask how they marketed their practices. I got answers that I didn't think would help my students, and so I decided to do my own field research to find those answers. I packed up my truck and pop-up tent trailer and drove through 25 states over 5 months, stopping along the way and visiting massage schools, calling local therapists who were listed in the phone book, and most important, talking with non-massage people I met along the way. I learned more about marketing massage listening to comments from the general public about massage and complaints from former massage clients than from any other source."

Roseberry came away from all this research with some simple but important discoveries. "I found the most important key to success was the desire to serve others," she says. "If this factor was not in place, no amount of marketing could override it. Another crucial factor I found was what I call marketing through the 'Ethernet.' This is basically using focused intention and clear desire to draw people to you. It may sound 'woo-woo,' but quantum physics proves that we are all connected energetically, and if you radiate out the message that you want clients, they show up from the strangest places. On the flip side, if your intention is not clear, or you have fears or negative beliefs that interfere with your message resonating out to others, people will subconsciously know it and not find you or book with you. Of course, at the same time you also need to be doing the work to be seen and heard so that people can find you when they are ready for massage."

Roseberry also found that many massage therapists make some practical errors when trying to attract new clients. "One of the biggest problems therapists face when trying to market their services is the inability to see themselves through their clients' eyes," she states. "If therapists could switch places with their clients and look at their business cards, brochures, Web sites, conversation topics, and personal presentation like clothes and hairstyles, all through the needs, fears, concerns, and hopes of

(Continued)

SPA PROFILE

Monica Roseberry – Marketing Massage *continued*

the massage client, they would make choices that are client-centric, not self-centric. Therapists often market using what they like, understand, and value, but their potential clients often can't relate to or understand what the therapist is talking about, or they aren't convinced that what they are being offered will have much value for them or be worth the price."

As far as marketing a spa as compared to a massage practice, Roseberry believes there are some important differences. "Spas have a reputation," she states, "which they are working hard to dispel, that massage in their venues is primarily for pampering and beauty enhancement. Spas need to overcome that perception through effective marketing that shows potential clients that the spa has multiple therapists trained in many skills that can meet many needs. In this way, they can build a reputation for being the one-stop shopping place for health and wellness, as well as beauty and relaxation."

Roseberry has one concrete tip for therapists heading into the spa market, and she has one typical mistake she counsels against. "For a therapist offering spa services in a private practice," she says, "the best tip I can offer is to develop, script out, and practice a short and sweet conversation you can have with your clients that gets them excited to try your new services. And the number-one mistake for massage therapists to avoid when marketing a spa practice is not identifying a target market *before* creating a marketing plan and putting together marketing materials. The market should determine everything, but most massage therapists create marketing materials that they like and that appeal to them, and decorate their offices or design their spaces based on their preferences. Therapists need to know what appeals to and attracts their ideal customer, and only then should they create marketing that does that."

As for learning more about marketing, Roseberry thinks that the best source of information isn't from marketing professionals. "Therapists need to remember that their clients are their best resources to understanding if their marketing is effective or not," she says. "Therapists need to ask their clients what attracted them to working together, or to their space, or to their marketing materials. Marketing professionals could be hired and they could guess at what would attract the right kind of clients, but only clients really know what made them book a massage or spa treatment in the first place. Finally, if therapists really want to know how to market massage, they should start a casual conversation about massage with anyone within 10 feet of them, and then be quiet and listen. Many people have had massage, and often are happy to talk about what they liked and didn't like about their prior massage experiences. Smart therapists will especially listen for complaints so they can avoid them, or really happy experiences so they can re-create them."

INTO THE FUTURE

The spa industry continues to expand and change, with new trends emerging every year and old trends resurfacing over and over again. Throughout it all, one thing has remained consistent: Spas are becoming more popular, more accepted, and more demanded as an essential part of the lifestyle for a large and growing number of people. It is impossible to know for certain what this industry will look like in 10 or 20 years, but regardless of the details, massage therapists will be able to grow into positions of increased authority and success because the spa industry in a way "belongs" to them. It belongs to you.

You, as a professional massage therapist, come into direct contact with spa guests, making an impact on their lives one at a time, and if you choose to grow into other aspects of the spa industry, you may be able to impact exponentially more people. It is surprisingly common for therapists to move into allied aspects of the spa world, taking a big step outside the treatment room and into the supervisor's room, the director's room, and even the board room.

As you continue to expand your possibilities in the spa industry, numerous options will present themselves, and it is important to understand what each entails in order to make an informed decision. The five main directions therapists branch into as they pursue careers in the spa field are supervising, directing, training (in-house or your own workshops), consulting, and providing allied services.

Growing Within the Spa Industry

How do you know which path to pursue and how to put your plan into action? The best way is to follow a five-step process that will occur naturally throughout your career in the spa industry. These steps are *experience*, *inspiration*, *refocusing*, *goal setting*, and *persistence* (Table 18–9).

Experience

You will, as a matter of course, have a wide range of experiences when working in the spa industry. Some of these experiences will inspire you. Others will not. Take careful note of these experiences as they arise. When you are dealing with the spa director or the treatment supervisor, do you wish that you could be in his shoes in order to do a better job? When you watch one of the fitness instructors teaching a class, do you wish you could help people get in shape that way? When you sit in on a lecture at the spa given by a nutritionist or physician, do you experience a strong craving to have the same knowledge yourself and share it with others? Pay attention to all your experiences while working in the spa industry, and at one point a magic moment may arrive.

Inspiration

The magic moment comes when you realize you are inspired to pursue an entirely new direction in your life. When you first started massage school, you may have thought you would be a therapist throughout your career, but after seeing that spa director in action, you knew that is the course you wanted your life to

STEP 1	EXPERIENCE	⇒	work hard as a spa practitioner or owner and gain experience
STEP 2	INSPIRATION	⇒	identify the experience that most inspires you
STEP 3	REFOCUSING	⇒	refocus your career and work intentions based on your inspiration
STEP 4	GOAL SETTING	⇒	set new goals to pursue your new inspiration
STEP 5	PERSISTENCE	⇒	persist through challenges as you pursue your goals

TABLE 18–9 Growing Within the Spa Industry.

take. This exact scenario has happened to hundreds of massage therapists. Or you experience an outside trainer who comes in to work with the staff, and you are inspired to become a trainer yourself. It happens all the time. Pay attention to this inspiration, and then make a change.

Refocusing

After realizing you have found a new inspiration, the first step to take is to begin shifting your perceptions and your self-definitions. Begin to study what it would take to become the person you want to be. How, for example, could you make the switch from being a therapist to a fitness trainer? What schooling would you need? What certificates? What experiences? Or what would you have to do in order to be considered for the spa treatment supervisor's position? How would you have to act? What would you need to learn? At this stage, the only thing you are changing is your mind, but it still takes courage to change, even mentally. If you are sufficiently inspired to make this kind of change in your career, then *not* changing will feel painful and restrictive.

Goal-Setting

Once you have decided upon a direction and refocused your intentions, it is time to make concrete goals, benchmarks you can reach incrementally along the path toward realizing your new self-image. Many therapists find that they are inspired to help build spa therapy programs and staffs from the ground up, for example, and they pursue a path in spa consulting. Others find that they want to be in charge of their own spas, and so they set goals that will take them step by step toward that dream.

Persistence

Once a new inspirational direction has been chosen and goals have been set, the most important quality for any therapist to cultivate is persistence. It is not always easy to shift a personality from that of an empathetic one-on-one therapist to that of a proactive take-charge owner, director, trainer, or consultant. But it has been done by many therapists. You can do it, too.

Becoming a Supervisor of Spa Services

The most obvious initial progression for a spa therapist is to become a supervisor of other spa therapists. Many therapists have taken this as a first step up the corporate ladder in larger spas or as a learning experience with an eye toward ownership of their own spas one day. If you choose to follow this path, however, you must be aware that in the short term, you may experience some subtle unpleasant shifts in your relationships with co-workers as a result of your new position of authority. Even so, if you find yourself with even the slightest inspiration to explore this avenue, you should take any opportunity that arises to become a supervisor in order to find out how it really feels. You may find that you are born to lead others and organize a department full of your colleagues. On the other hand, you may find that you have no interest in scheduling, disciplining, and supervising others. Many therapists have ended up feeling this way after a switch to a supervisory role and then chose to go back to their former role of spa therapist.

Becoming a Spa Director

No precise statistics are available regarding how many massage therapists have moved on to become spa directors, but the number is assuredly high. Most spa therapists feel comfortable working for a director who understands their point of view and their concerns firsthand, from personal experience. Also, therapist/directors are often better at communicating with guests, because they know the guests' expectations regarding spa therapies better than anyone else. Finally, the general managers and spa owners who oversee spa directors usually appreciate having someone who can "translate" between themselves and a staff of therapists whom they often find difficult to understand.

On the other hand, many therapists-turned-spa-directors have found it difficult to deal with the corporate bureaucracy that comes with the position. They do not like sitting in meetings for hours, dealing with office politics, or being expected to reach certain quotas, benchmarks, or revenue goals. Spa directors need to be able to compromise with the leaders of other departments in large spas, sometimes putting the good of the entire enterprise before the good of the therapists who count on them. It can be a tricky position.

The position of spa director is a relatively new one. Enough experienced, qualified candidates cannot be found to fill all the positions that become available as new spas are built. If you are a person with a desire to greatly enhance your economic opportunities while also staying within a field that you feel passionate about, the job of spa director is well worth exploring.

Becoming a Spa Trainer and Workshop Teacher

It is a great goal of many therapists to teach what they know to others. Fortunately, spas offer many opportunities for therapists to do exactly that. Every spa of any size needs to keep its staff of hands-on professionals current with technique and product usage. Spas often have in-house trainers, or they use the spa treatment supervisor as the trainer, building that responsibility into the job description. The position of trainer or teacher brings with it many opportunities for advancement. Spa product companies and distributors, as well as spas themselves, are looking for enthusiastic trainers with good presentation skills.

If you consider becoming a trainer, work on the communication aspect of the job as well as the technique and product knowledge. Thousands of therapists know how to effectively apply Dead Sea salts, but only a small percentage know how to teach specific protocols, benefits, and contraindications in an engaging manner that will be remembered by students. Therapists with strengths in this area will be wise to pursue training opportunities either in their own spas or with other companies.

SPA TIP

If you pursue the path of becoming a spa trainer or workshop leader, be prepared to start out small. In fact, plan on it. Even the most popular and successful trainers in the field started training just a handful of people at a time. Rather than feeling frustrated, be happy about that; it allows you time to build your skills gradually on a strong foundation.

Becoming a Spa Consultant

A growing number of therapists are choosing to become spa consultants. Spa consultants are people who help others open or manage spas. The barriers to entry into this field are quite low. Mostly, what therapists need to get a successful start in spa consulting are self-confidence and good communication skills. Thousands of businesspeople, dreamers, and investors are actively seeking professionals who can help them in a business they know very little about. Getting one or two spa consulting contracts is not the most difficult part of the job, however. The only way a therapist can develop the type of résumé that will get other investors to take a risk with him is by successfully completing multiple spa projects that become revenue-generating businesses.

One good way to start in the consulting business is to help with an already-established consultancy, and the best way to network with such consultancies is by attending trade shows and other spa industry events. Also, some enterprising therapists, after learning about the rigors of spa setup through their own experience, write manuals and books that others can follow to do the same thing, and this becomes their calling card. Good information is always valuable, regardless of how many other people have written on similar topics. If you have the ambition and have paid some dues by working in the spa industry in several capacities, spa consulting may be for you.

> **SPA CAUTION**
>
> No rules, regulations or certification boards control the field of spa consulting. Some people get into the field before gaining enough experience and understanding to do the job well. Some massage therapists have been guilty of this over-ambition. Before hanging out your spa consultant shingle, ask yourself if you bring sufficient knowledge and expertise to the table to really help prospective clients.

Becoming an Allied Service Provider

Some therapists, once they are exposed to the wide range of services provided for guests in spas, decide to pursue a career path entirely out of the massage therapy field. The two most common areas of interest are nutrition and fitness (Figure 18–17). Becoming a certified fitness instructor, an aerobics teacher, a sports nutritionist, or a registered dietician means that you will have to go back to school, but the rewards for doing so can be substantial. Many spas are seeking employees with talents and certification in multiple fields, and if you decide to one day open your own spa, the more information you have about overall health

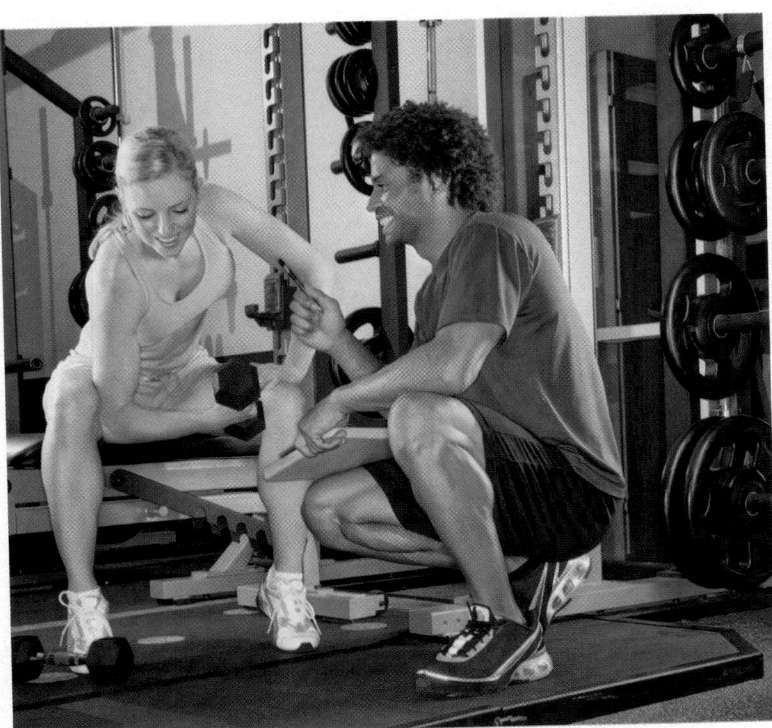

FIGURE 18–17 The rewards for becoming a personal fitness instructor or an aerobics teacher can be substantial.

and well-being, the better you will be able to serve your clients. Some therapists have been able to combine two or more disciplines in their spa careers, offering nutritional supplements and personal training in addition to massage and spa services, for example.

RESEARCH

Choose another position in the spa industry other than massage therapist in which you are interested—supervisor, director, owner, trainer, consultant, or allied professional. Use magazines, books, or the Internet to research information about how other people have enjoyed or been challenged by work in those positions, then write one page about why you would like to explore that line of work yourself and what you might experience when you do so.

CONCLUSION

You now have a wide array of new skills and knowledge at your disposal. You know the history of spas and how they have developed in the modern age. You are familiar with all the equipment and products used by top professionals doing the most sought-after spa therapies. You have learned the protocols for many spa services, including therapeutic benefits, safety precautions, contraindications, and more. And you have learned what it takes to work in a real spa environment or even to open a spa practice of your own. Your dream spa job or spa business can now become a reality. Opportunities in this field continue to expand, but competition is making it more important than ever to be as prepared as you possibly can before taking your initial steps into this exciting field. Use the resources you discovered in this book and in this course wisely. Study. Practice. Continue to learn. Then, when you are prepared, go out and seek your niche in the spa industry, constantly testing the limits of your abilities and your ambitions along the way. A career as a massage therapist in the spa industry can be much more than a job. It can be an adventure.

REVIEW QUESTIONS

1. Name some reasons why it is a good idea to make a pro forma budget for your spa startup.
2. In essence, what two things does every kind of budget track?
3. Name at least four of the tasks involved with the day-to-day management of a spa.
4. Therapists working in a spa setting need to be extra-vigilant about ethical issues, draping, and boundaries for what three main reasons?
5. What is the best way, in addition to insurance, that spa business owners can protect themselves from lawsuits and hedge their liability?
6. Name the three main types of licenses needed by spas.
7. Marketing a spa therapy practice is different than marketing a straight massage therapy practice for what three main reasons?
8. What are the four key components, or "4 Ps," of marketing?
9. What are the five main directions therapists branch into as they pursue a career in the spa field?

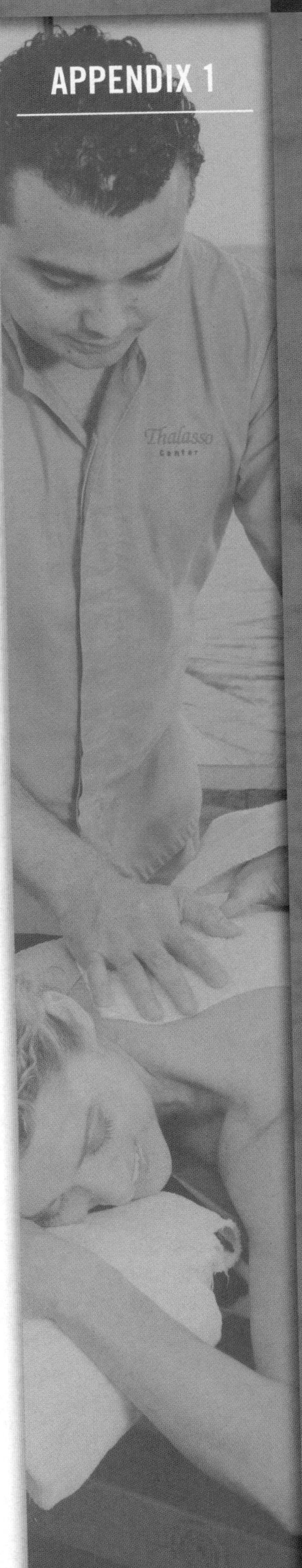

APPENDIX 1

Answers to the Review Questions

Chapter 1

1. Explain the origins of the word "spa."
   ANSWER: Came from the Belgian town of Spa, named after its hot spring waters. In 1596, English physician Dr. Timothy Bright called a healing spring in the United Kingdom the "English Spaw," beginning the use of the word as a general description of a place with healing waters.
2. What is the difference between an acronym and a "backronym," and how does it apply to the word "spa"?
   ANSWER: An acronym is a word formed by putting together the first letters of other words, such as SPA for "sanitas per aqua" (health through water). A backronym is a word thought to be originally coined as an acronym but in reality its source was different and the acronym was applied later. This is true for the word "spa."
3. What did the ancient Greeks develop as forerunners to more modern spas?
   ANSWER: Greeks developed basic hot water tubs and hot air baths known as *laconica*. Built next to a gymnasium, they were round with a high, tapering roof that could be closed or opened to permit the escape of hot air and steam.
4. How did the Roman balneum and thermae differ?
   ANSWER: Balnea were smaller, neighborhood, less elaborate bath houses, while thermae were larger, elaborate, and ornate, commissioned by emperors.
5. Briefly describe the typical massage practitioner in a Roman thermae.
   ANSWER: The typical Roman masseur was a skilled slave, likely known as an *unctor*. These slaves either belonged to the owner of the bath house, or to a particular wealthy patron who would bring them along to the baths for his own private use.
6. How were the Roman thermae heated?
   ANSWER: The entire indoor area was kept perpetually warmed by means of a furnace-like room below the floor called the *hypocaust*.
7. Give a brief description of a typical day for a Roman citizen at one of the thermae.
   ANSWER: Bathers visited a series of different rooms, some with baths, heated to various temperatures. They also could engage in exercise, massage, and exfoliation, as well as eat, drink, listen to music and poetry, and simply visit with friends.

8. What were some of the defining characteristics of a Turkish hammam?
ANSWER: The Turkish hammam was originally built as part of a mosque in the Ottoman Empire and gradually became a stand-alone entity. They included a large communal room with a marble slab upon which bathers were exfoliated and scrubbed. Massage attendants in the baths were known as *tellaks*. In the West, the hammam is known as a "Turkish bath."
9. What does it mean when European spa goers "take the cure"?
ANSWER: European spa goers follow a more medically oriented spa philosophy, and spa visits are often prescribed by physicians. These visits include immersions and ingestions of therapeutic waters, as well as undergoing several spa therapies, in the treatment of disorders.
10. Who was Sebastian Kneipp, and what were his major contributions to the world of spa therapies?
ANSWER: A German priest born in 1821, Sebastian Kneipp cured himself of tuberculosis with natural methods he called *the kur.*
Known as "the father of modern hydrotherapy," he wrote books and developed a five-part program for others to follow. The five pillars of his method are hydrotherapy, phytotherapy (plant therapy), exercise, nutrition, and lifestyle.
11. Name two examples of early American sweat lodges.
ANSWER: The kiva from the American Southwest and the temazcal from Mexico.
12. Which Asian country developed the most extensive bathing culture? What are their bathing facilities like?
ANSWER: Japan developed an extensive bathing culture, building many "onsen" at hot spring sites across their volcanically active country. These are found in natural settings and include massage and hydrotherapy. The Japanese observe special customs while using the onsen in order to maintain their tranquil healing atmosphere.

Chapter 2

1. Name some trends in the spa industry.
ANSWER: Trends include more men using spas, mothers and daughters enjoying spas together, weight loss, and paying top dollar for the once-in-a-lifetime luxury of going to a spa.
2. Approximately how many people were working in the spa industry in 2008?
ANSWER: Approximately 303,719 people were working in the spa industry in 2008.
3. What is the main difference between a destination spa and a day spa?
ANSWER: At a destination spa, guests generally stay overnight and focus their entire stay on spa services, spa food, exercise, and spa lifestyle. At a day spa, guests visit for an hour to several hours to receive treatments but do not generally partake in an overall spa lifestyle while there.
4. What are the five general categories of spa goers, and how can therapists positively affect their experiences in the spa?
ANSWER: The five general categories of spa goers are: non–spa goer, novice, opportunistic, enthusiastic, and seasoned. Therapists can positively affect their experiences by adapting to the special needs of each spa goer.
5. Which professional spa associations are most relevant to therapists working in the spa industry? Why?
ANSWER: The Day Spa Association and the International Spa Association are relevant for therapists because they offer trade shows and other opportunities for networking, purchasing, and education.
6. How do those therapists who are not directly employed by the spa industry

stand to benefit greatly by the popularity of spa modalities?
ANSWER: Therapists not directly employed by the spa industry can benefit from the popularity of home spa visits by offering spa modalities to their private clients.

7. What are some of the member codes of ethics of the International Spa Association that directly affect massage therapists who work in spas?
ANSWER: The member code of ethics of the International Spa Association governs the quality of service offered by spa staff members, including massage therapists. The code outlines rules for courtesy, respect, anticipating guests' needs, believing in and adhering to the spa's philosophy, and guarding guests' privacy and modesty, among other points.
8. Why is it important for massage therapists to be familiar with companies that are related to the spa industry?
ANSWER: Massage therapists in the spa industry need to be familiar with such companies and their products in order to understand spa guests' overall experiences and help them achieve their desired goals.

Chapter 3

1. What are the main differences between a wet room and a dry room?
ANSWER: A wet room has plumbing, usually a shower and sometimes a hydrotherapy tub, and tiles to protect surfaces from water. A dry room can be carpeted and have a water source outside the room, though equipment and products are available to perform spa services such as exfoliations and body wraps.
2. What are the advantages and disadvantages of a wet room versus a dry room?
ANSWER: Wet rooms offer more high-tech luxurious hydrotherapy services with an abundance of water, but they are expensive. Dry rooms are inexpensive, include more hands-on care, and can be easily incorporated into a massage practice, but they offer no high-tech hydrotherapy and it is sometimes difficult to clean spa products from the skin without a shower.
3. What piece of equipment is the centerpiece for any successful spa dry room?
ANSWER: The centerpiece for any successful spa dry room is the treatment table. Ideally, this should be a multi-purpose table, meaning it can be used for a number of spa services plus massage in a manner that is comfortable for clients and ergonomically effective for therapists.
4. The equipment used in spa wet rooms or wet areas can be broken down into four main categories. What are they? Give examples of each type.
ANSWER: The four main categories of equipment used in spa wet rooms are: showers, tubs, tables, and chambers. Examples of showers include regular, Vichy, Swiss, and Scotch. Tubs include hydrotherapy tubs, hot tubs/whirlpools/Jacuzzis, soaking tubs, and mud/enzyme baths. Examples of tables include wet table, pedestal, and soft pack. Examples of chambers include steam rooms, hammams, Rasuls, and spa suites.
5. What are some general guidelines for dealing with all the laundry generated in a spa treatment area?
ANSWER: Whenever possible, hide laundry concerns from clients. Wash linens in hot water for sanitation reasons. Use storage wisely. Conserve on the number of towels and sheets used in each service.
6. What risk factors do spas pose that are not found in such abundance in other environments where massage therapists work? What problems may arise because of them?

ANSWER: The risk factors are the pervasive use of heat and water, which can lead to a number of potential dangers, including fainting, heart attacks, slips and falls, drowning, burns, and scalds.

7. Therapists who perform spa treatments hold two key advantages regarding self-care, as compared to those who perform massage therapy alone. What are they?
ANSWER: The products, hydrotherapy, and heat that spa therapists apply to clients have an equally therapeutic effect on their own bodies, and many spa modalities require less effort on the part of therapists to perform.
8. Why is it a good idea to keep your spa treatment room (and your practical spa classroom) neat and organized?
ANSWER: If all spa products, plus the equipment and supplies needed to prepare them, are within easy grasping distance in the treatment room, this will eliminate the need to reach, bend, and lift unnecessarily.
9. What are the three main categories of risk management issues faced by spa businesses?
ANSWER: Employment issues, sexual harassment issues, and tort liabilities issues.
10. When should spa equipment, from the smallest brush to the largest hydrotherapy tub, be sanitized? What are some of the implements used for sanitizing in the spa?
ANSWER: Equipment should be sanitized after each and every treatment. Sanitizing implements include germicidal solution, germicidal cabinet, and autoclave.

Chapter 4

1. Name and explain the three main types of effects produced by hydrotherapy.
ANSWER: The three main types of effects produced by hydrotherapy are thermal, mechanical, and chemical. The thermal effects are the most important; they are caused by heat and cold in water of different temperatures. The mechanical effects are caused by the impact of water on the surface of the body, and the chemical effects are caused when water is ingested or used for colonic irrigation.
2. Explain the workings of the hypothalamus. How does it relates to spa therapies?
ANSWER: The hypothalamus gland regulates temperature and the transference of blood from one part of the body to another through the hydrostatic effect. For this reason, the functioning of this gland, also known as the "master gland" because it has so many vital functions, is crucial to the effectiveness of hydrotherapy treatments.
3. What are the five methods of heat transference in the body and which one is most important to the majority of spa therapies?
ANSWER: The five methods of heat transference in the body are conduction, convection, conversion, radiation, and evaporation. Most hydrotherapy treatments use conduction to transfer heat to or from the body.
4. Explain the basic effects of hot water versus cold water.
ANSWER: Hot water has a stimulating effect, which changes gradually into a relaxing effect. Cold water causes shivering, goose flesh, constricted blood vessels, higher pulse rate, and faster respiration, plus increased metabolism and muscle tone. Heat creates an atonic effect, while cold creates a tonic effect. Effects vary according to the duration.
5. What is the RICE technique, and when is it appropriate to use in spas?
ANSWER: RICE stands for Rest, Ice, Compression, and Elevation, and it is used in case of acute injury. If a spa client requests treatment for an acute injury,

spa therapists need to know that heat should normally not be applied for at least 72 hours because increased blood flow caused by the heat application makes swelling and pain worse, and may cause tissue damage to the injured area. Acute injuries are contraindicated for many spa services, but the RICE method is appropriate.

6. Why can clients remain in therapeutic baths longer than Jacuzzis, hot tubs, hot springs, and whirlpools?
   ANSWER: Maximum time for hot baths (100°F or above) is usually 15 minutes, but therapeutic baths cool down over time, as compared to Jacuzzis, hot tubs, hot springs, and whirlpools, which maintain a constant high temperature. Therefore, clients can remain in therapeutic baths longer.
7. Describe a typical high-tech hydrotherapy tub used in top spas.
   ANSWER: Hydrotherapy tubs have several zones with multiple jets in each zone through which air and water is directed at clients' bodies during baths. Also, they feature high-powered underwater massage hoses that therapists use to massage clients during treatments. Therapeutic ingredients are typically added to the water for increased effectiveness.
8. What are the benefits of a cold plunge?
   ANSWER: The cold plunge offers a quick way to close the pores and to refresh the body. It is also said to improve immune functioning, decrease blood pressure, decrease heart rate, and increase circulation.
9. Name and describe the three main types of therapeutic showers used in spas.
   ANSWER: The three main types of therapeutic showers used in spas are the Swiss shower, a walk-in shower with multiple jets on each wall that can alternate between high pressure/low pressure, hot water/cold water; the Vichy shower, a horizontal shower bar with several nozzles that spray water over clients lying on table below; and the Scotch hose, which is a high-pressure hose that sprays water at clients from a distance of approximately 10 feet.

Chapter 5

1. Describe the three main types of effects created by both heat and cold.
   ANSWER: The three main types of effects created by heat and cold are local, systemic, and reflex. Local effects are present on the skin at the site of application, plus a few centimeters deep into the tissues. Systemic effects are found throughout the body, and reflex effects are found in organs inside the body, away from the application site.
2. Explain the processes of derivation and retrostasis, and how they can work together.
   ANSWER: Derivation is the drawing of blood or lymph away from one part of the body by increasing the amount sent flowing to another area. Retrostasis is using cold to drive blood and lymph away from an area. Both principles of derivation and retrostasis can be applied simultaneously, as when heat is applied to the feet and cold to the head at the same time to treat headaches.
3. What are the five major heat contraindications for spa therapies?
   ANSWER: The five major heat contraindications for spa therapies are high or low blood pressure, cardiovascular conditions, diabetes, fever, and pregnancy.
4. What is the difference between an affusion and an ablution?
   ANSWER: An affusion is the pouring of water onto the body through a hose. An ablution is a sponge or towel bath.

5. What are the origins of the sauna? What are some of its traditions?
ANSWER: The sauna derives from ancient Finland, and saunas are sometimes called *Finnish steam baths*. For hundreds of years, people in Finland have built these special structures for the purpose of heating and cleansing the body. The Fins believe you should act the same way in a sauna as you would in a church. Whole families go together, and afterward they head outside to take a roll in the snow or jump into a freezing lake, which, they claim, refreshes them and strengthens the immune system.
6. Describe what it is like to receive a spa treatment in a Rasul chamber.
ANSWER: Rasul chambers are a variation on the Turkish bath. They are small chambers with beautiful mosaic tiles, which clients enter alone or with a partner to spread muds on themselves. Steam and moisture wash the muds away. The experience is often followed by a massage.
7. Why is paraffin important for spa therapies, and what are its three main beneficial properties?
ANSWER: Paraffin is important for spa therapies because of its ability to store heat, and as an emollient; its three main beneficial properties are occlusion, lubrication, and humectation.
8. Why would a wet sheet wrap be beneficial?
ANSWER: Being wrapped in a cold sheet stimulates the body's heat-producing mechanisms so that, after an initial few minutes of cold, the interior of the wrap goes through a warming period until it eventually becomes hot. The wet sheet wrap has three distinct stages—cooling, neutral, and heating—each with its own benefits.
9. What are the traditional reasons for administering a cold mitten friction treatment?
ANSWER: Cold mitten friction is a traditional hydrotherapy treatment used for building immune resistance and helping clients recover from fevers.
10. What is the hydrosphere, and how do we human beings fit into it?
ANSWER: The hydrosphere is the Earth's self-contained watery environment, of which we humans are an integral part. Every 20 days we lose 100 pounds of water, and we have to bring that back in somehow from the outside world. In this way, we have a symbiotic relationship between our bodies and the planet.

Chapter 6

1. What are the three main objectives of exfoliation services used in spas?
ANSWER: The three main objectives of exfoliation services are to cleanse the pores and prepare skin for absorption of products, to help the skin perform its natural processes, and to leave the client's skin texture and appearance improved.
2. What are the two main types of exfoliations used in spas, and how do they differ?
ANSWER: The two main types of exfoliation are mechanical and chemical. Mechanical exfoliations scrub the skin with abrasive products or tools, while chemical exfoliations contain ingredients that dissolve dead skin cells.
3. Where do most of the salts come from that are used for exfoliation in spas? Why?
ANSWER: They come from the Dead Sea in Israel. They are chosen because of the size of the granules, which range from fine to semi-coarse, and for their high concentrations of magnesium chloride, potassium chloride, and calcium.
4. What is the difference between sugar and salt, used as exfoliants?

ANSWER: Sugar is less abrasive than salt. Sugars do not contain the minerals that salts do and therefore do not offer the mineralizing benefits of salt, but they do contain naturally occurring glycolic acid to create a chemical exfoliation action.

5. Can massage therapists use alpha hydroxy acids to do exfoliation in spas?
ANSWER: Therapists can only use those exfoliants with AHAs that are sold to the public over the counter because they have not been trained in the safe use of professional-strength levels of these products.
6. What layer of the skin does exfoliation directly affect? How does it change this layer?
ANSWER: Exfoliation affects the outer layer, the epidermis. Spa exfoliation procedures are a type of therapist-aided desquamation (naturally occurring skin-renewal process) in which dead keratinocytes (skin cells) are purposefully swept away from the stratum corneum.
7. What are the main contraindications for spa exfoliation?
ANSWER: The main contraindications are sunburn, cuts, abrasions and sores, eczema, recent shaving, allergies, and delicate skin.
8. Why should you not apply moisturizing cream to the skin if you are moving from an exfoliation procedure directly to a body wrap with seaweed, mud, clay, or herbs?
ANSWER: The cream will block the freshly cleaned pores, slowing absorption of therapeutic products.
9. What type of spas feature stand-alone dry bristle brushing services? Why are they offered in this type of spa?
ANSWER: Dry bristle brushing is a technique primarily used in spas that have a focus on natural health and detox programs because it stimulates the elimination of the toxins.

Chapter 7

1. Who was René Quinton and what was his contribution to thalassotherapy?
ANSWER: French biologist René Quinton published *Seawater: Organic Medium* in 1904. His work using seawater to treat dogs and human patients showed dramatic results and became an underpinning for thalassotherapy.
2. What is required in order to be considered a true thalassotherapy facility?
ANSWER: The seawater at the facility should be warmed to approximately 98°F, the water itself must be pumped directly from the sea, the facility must be located on the shore or very near it, and the facility must be supervised by a physician and use seawater and sea product treatments exclusively.
3. What is photosynthesis, and why is it important in the application of thalassotherapy?
ANSWER: Photosynthesis is a process in which absorbed sunlight goes through a chemical transformation, converting it into potential energy to be stored for later use. Through photosynthesis, algae becomes rich in oxygen and nutrients, making it powerfully therapeutic.
4. What is the most often cited benefit of thalassotherapy treatments? Why is it so important?
ANSWER: Remineralization is the most often cited benefit of thalassotherapy treatments, and it is important because our foods and environment are mineral-depleted, and seaweed is a way to reintroduce those lacking minerals into our bodies.
5. What are the two main types of plankton found in seawater, and what is the difference between them?
ANSWER: Phytoplankton and zooplankton are the two main types of plankton

found in seawater. Phytoplankton is made up of algae, and zooplankton is made up of minuscule crustaceans and fish larvae.

6. What are some of the specific conditions treated by thalassotherapy?
ANSWER: Some of the specific conditions treated by thalassotherapy include stress, depression, obesity, cellulite, rheumatism, peripheral circulatory problems, and recovery from surgery or illness.
7. What are the contraindications for thalassotherapy treatments?
ANSWER: The contraindications for thalassotherapy treatments are claustrophobia caused by wrapping in seaweed wraps and sensitivities to essential oils and additives.
8. What are the seaweed and seawater treatments performed most by massage therapists?
ANSWER: The treatments are seaweed baths, seaweed wraps, and cellulite services.
9. What seaweed ingredient has been found to have potential beneficial effects on weight loss?
ANSWER: A Japanese professor found that fucoxanthin, a pigment found in brown algae, promotes fat burning within white adipose tissue by increasing the action of the protein thermogenin, resulting in weight losses of up to 10%.
10. If we came from the oceans, why don't our bodies have the same salt content as the oceans?
ANSWER: Cellular life originated in the oceans at a time when the oceans' salinity was much lower (0.9% versus 3.5% today), and the salt content in our cells reflects the salt content of the oceans at the time life was first formed.
11. Are seaweed wraps considered heat treatments? Why or why not?
ANSWER: Seaweed wraps are not considered heat treatments because they do not include the application of heat to the body. However, clients may become warm because body heat is being trapped by the layers of blankets, sheets, and plastic.
12. Traditional thalassotherapy centers offer baths in fresh seawater. How do average spas re-create that experience for guests without actual seawater?
ANSWER: Most spas add seaweed or seawater extracts to a municipal water source to introduce the benefits found at traditional thalassotherapy centers.
13. Which spa treatment is most frequently used to eliminate cellulite?
ANSWER: No spa treatment can eliminate cellulite, but vigorous massage, stimulating topical products, hydrotherapy, and thalassotherapy can help in the *temporary* reduction in the *appearance* of cellulite.
14. Who is the best candidate for a spa cellulite service?
ANSWER: The most appropriate candidate, who has the best chance at experiencing noticeable results, is a woman who is willing to lead a healthy lifestyle during the program and who is slightly overweight, with a moderate amount of cellulite.

Chapter 8

1. Ideally, what should therapists be doing while a client is wrapped in seaweed, mud,
or clay?
ANSWER: Therapists should offer something extra, such as spa reflexology or a scalp massage, while the client is enveloped in a full-body wrap. Clients pay well for this service and feel shortchanged if they are left alone for 20 to 30 minutes while the therapist attends to other matters.
2. What are some of the things that all body wrap services have in common?

ANSWER: All body wraps are similar in that they envelop the client inside various layers while products are acting upon the skin, and within that enclosed environment, they all provide a sense of comfort, security, and warmth.

3. What is the best way to overcome some clients' sense of claustrophobia during a full-body wrap? Why does it work?
   ANSWER: To avoid claustrophobia in most cases, it is best to instruct clients to leave their arms outside all layers of the wrap except the very top one. This allows clients to exit the wrap by themselves whenever they wish.
4. In what way is the skin typically prepared for a full-body wrap? Why is this technique used?
   ANSWER: Usually, some form of exfoliation is applied prior to a full-body wrap. The purpose of the exfoliation is to allow the skin to more readily absorb the benefits of the products that are applied.
5. Do you know or can you guess if a massage is usually applied before or after a body wrap service? Why are the services typically offered in this order?
   ANSWER: Massage is usually given after a body wrap, sometimes as a part of the services itself, turning the application of finishing product into a longer massage. The services are offered in this order because applying massage with a cream, oil, or other product before the wrap would block the pores and hinder the body from absorbing the product applied to the skin during the wrap.
6. All the different types of muds used in spas are classified under what heading? Name some of the types typically found on spa menus.
   ANSWER: Muds come under the heading of peloids, and typical types found in spas include clay, peat, moor, and fango.
7. What is the main active substance in most muds used in spa therapies, and what is its specific therapeutic action?
   ANSWER: One of the main active substances in mud is humic acid, which is known to aid in the purification of the body through the process of chelation.
8. Why can muds be applied to the body at hotter temperatures than water?
   ANSWER: Muds have a lower specific heat and do not conduct heat as well as water, and their point of thermal indifference is 100°F as compared to 93°F for water.
9. The main contraindications to any mud therapies are caused by what factor?
   ANSWER: The contraindications are caused by the application of heat to the body in the form of heated mud. The chemical constituents of mud do not normally present any significant contraindications.
10. What are the most common herbal applications used in spas?
    ANSWER: The most common herbal applications are herbal wraps and herbal compress therapy. Herbal baths and herb-based exfoliations are also applied, but not as commonly.
11. What kind of benefits would an herb with antipyretic qualities offer to spa clients?
    ANSWER: Such herbs help lower fever and reduce heat production in the body. They are good for clients who are overheated.
12. How do herbal wraps work? What is the underlying mechanism that makes it possible for these wraps to help purify the body?
    ANSWER: Herbal wraps induce a "false fever" in the body, triggering a release of impurities through the pores, just like the body does in a real fever.
13. What are some of the other potential benefits of herbal wraps in addition to purifying and cleansing the body?

ANSWER: In addition to purifying and cleansing the body, herbal wraps can help with weight-loss programs, smoking cessation programs, and purely for relaxation.

14. What four distinct types of therapeutic benefits are offered to clients through application of herbal compresses?
ANSWER: Aromatherapy, herbal therapy, heat therapy, and massage are all experienced by spa clients who receive herbal compress therapy.

Chapter 9

1. How could low expectations regarding the treatment on the part of a spa client contribute to a less-than-optimal massage?
ANSWER: Many spa clients arrive with no particular complaints or pains, and they do not expect the massage therapy session to help them very much beyond simple relaxation.
2. Why is the term "relaxation massage" not completely accurate when it comes to describing a massage in a spa?
ANSWER: Many spas describe their Swedish massage as a "relaxation massage," as compared to an advanced modalities, but Swedish massage can also be invigorating, stimulating, therapeutic, and downright intense.
3. What are some of the techniques that can put clients at ease during the first few moments after the therapist greets them in the spa?
ANSWER: Therapists can help put spa clients at ease quickly with a reassuring touch on the shoulder, an explanation of draping procedures, use of the client's name, and a firm handshake with eye contact.
4. What are some of the ways in which a sense of timelessness can be created in a spa massage?
ANSWER: A timeless sense can be created by slowing down, internalizing one's timing, and focusing on the moment while giving the massage.
5. What are some of the ways in which massage can help pregnant women who visit a spa?
ANSWER: Massage can soothes pregnant clients' tired legs and sore lower back muscles. It can also be very nurturing and complement an overall wellness program for women at a time when they need to remain healthiest.
6. What is the name of the theory upon which reflexology is based? What is the theory?
ANSWER: The theory of zone therapy states that the entire body can be divided into various zones, and anything that affects the body in one area affects other parts of the body within the same zone. Thus, pressure to the feet can bring relief to a distant part of the body that lies within the same zone.
7. What is "spa reflexology"? What are some of the advantages of performing it for clients?
ANSWER: Spa reflexology is a simplified, shortened version of the full reflexology technique. It can be completed in 10 minutes, and its maneuvers are condensed so that several points are stimulated at once. Both feet are treated at the same time, rather than consecutively. Benefits are that clients can receive the treatment while still dressed, in a waiting room or other public area, thus freeing up valuable treatment room space; the technique is targeted to just one easily accessible area, but addresses the entire body; and it can be performed while the client is wrapped during spa services.
8. Why is the inclusion of "deep tissue" massage on spa menus sometimes confusing to clients?

ANSWER: The term "deep tissue" may be confusing because there is little consensus among spa patrons as to what they can expect from such a treatment once they sign up for it. The true definition of deep tissue massage refers to techniques that affect the deeper tissue structures of the muscles and especially the fascia, but many spa clients sign up for it thinking it is simply a deep Swedish massage.

9. According to spa industry experts, are couples massage rooms overused or underused?
ANSWER: They are greatly underused, averaging just 7% usage industry-wide.

10. Is chair massage typically on the menu at most spas?
ANSWER: Chair massage is not typically on the menu at most spas, but it is often used for promotional purposes. Some spas in heavily trafficked locations such as airports do use massage chairs extensively.

Chapter 10

1. What are the three primary forms of rock, and from which are massage stones sourced?
ANSWER: The three primary forms of rock are igneous, sedimentary, and metamorphic. Most massage stones are sourced from the most plentiful form of igneous rock, basalt.

2. What is the main factor that determines any particular basalt stone's heat-retaining capacity?
ANSWER: The concentration of iron in any particular stone will most determine its ability to retain heat.

3. How would a therapist create "blood pumping" action through stone massage?
ANSWER: By alternately applying hot and cold stones, therapists induce contrast therapy, which can create the blood pumping action.

4. Which massage modality is most frequently used with stones?
ANSWER: Swedish is most often used with stones, but stones can be effective as an addition to all massage modalities.

5. What is the general temperature range for the use of hot stones? Why?
ANSWER: The water for heating stones should be between 110°F and 140°F. Below 110°F doesn't generate enough warmth, and above 140°F makes it difficult to handle the stones.

6. Why do therapists need to monitor the pressure they exert on clients more closely during stone massage than during Swedish massage?
ANSWER: Stones penetrate forcefully, magnifying the force of therapists' fingers or thumbs and potentially causing damage.

7. Are varicose veins a contraindication for stone massage?
ANSWER: Varicose veins are not contraindicated. However, the application of hot stones over the affected areas should be avoided. Cool stones may be used gently.

8. What are the two broad categories into which stone massage techniques can be broken down?
ANSWER: Placing stones on the body and holding stones while applying massage maneuvers.

9. Describe a good way to keep from shocking clients when a hot stone or cold first comes into contact with the skin.
ANSWER: Introduce stones gradually by touching the back of the hand to the client's skin first and slowly letting the stone come into contact.

10. What does it mean to "flip" and "pin" massage stones? Why are these techniques used?
ANSWER: Flipping a stone means to turn it over at the end of a massage stroke so

the opposite side comes into contact with the client's skin on the subsequent stroke. Pinning means to hold the stone with one's palm fully against the body instead of grasping it with the fingers. These techniques are used primarily to save wear and tear on therapists' hands and arms and also to make the massage more pleasant for the client.

Chapter 11

1. Who coined the term "aromatherapy," and what prompted this person to do so?
   ANSWER: René-Maurice Gattefossé, a French chemist, coined the term after a laboratory accident allowed him to experience firsthand the healing properties of essential oils on his own body.
2. What is the difference between the French and the British models of aromatherapy? Which are you more likely to practice in a spa yourself?
   ANSWER: The French model is more medically oriented and includes intensive use of full-strength oils both externally and internally, while the British model is more spa-like and focuses on the use of diluted oils in massage and other therapies. Spa therapists in North America follow the British model.
3. What is it called when the plant materials used to create essential oils are found in nature as compared to cultivated?
   ANSWER: Wildcrafting.
4. What is considered by many therapists the "classic" and most authentic way to distill essential oils from plant materials?
   ANSWER: Steam distillation.
5. Why do some people feel that carbon dioxide extraction is the most efficient method for creating essential oils?
   ANSWER: After extraction, which does not involve heat, the CO_2 evaporates into a gas and leaves no chemical residues. In this way, almost all of the plant's compounds are preserved.
6. How should essential oils be added to a carrier oil to attain the correct dilution?
   ANSWER: Usually, essential oils should be added drop by drop for complete control of the dilution process. Most aromatherapy bottles have openings that facilitate this.
7. What are the three different categories of essential oils that are referred to when blending them?
   ANSWER: Top notes, middle notes, and base notes.
8. Why do essential oils have such a profound impact on memory and emotion?
   ANSWER: The molecules of oil land on receptors of the olfactory epithelia, which has neurons protruding directly from the brain's limbic system, and this system controls memories and emotions.
9. What is photosensitivity, and which oils are most likely to cause it in a client?
   ANSWER: Photosensitivity is a heightened degree of sensitivity to sunlight. Several citrus peel oils extracted through cold pressing are called *photosensitizers*, such as bergamot, grapefruit, orange, and Neroli.
10. What is the most effective form of essential oil diffusion?
    ANSWER: Nebulization forms the smallest particles, which penetrate deepest into the lungs, creating the greatest therapeutic effect.

Chapter 12

1. What is the name of the Ayurvedic lifestyle program that is included at some spas? What does it include?
   ANSWER: The Ayurvedic lifestyle program is known as *pancha karma*, and is meant to cleanse and rejuvenate the body. It can include massage, specialized body treatments, purgative therapies that clean

out the body, herbal medicines, meditation, chanting, and other techniques.

2. What is abhyanga?
ANSWER: Abhyanga is a special massage in the Ayurvedic system, usually given by two therapists who focus on specific circulatory channels and marma points, 107 of which are located on the body at the junction of different types of tissues, such as muscles, ligaments, bones, joints, or veins. The main purpose of this massage is to unblock energy, or *chi*.
3. Practitioners of craniosacral therapy tune into the pulse of what bodily fluid?
ANSWER: Practitioners tune into the natural pulse of cerebrospinal fluid in the spine and skull, the subtle effects of which can be felt throughout the body.
4. The Javanese Lulur procedure offered in some spas is based upon what ancient tradition?
ANSWER: The Lulur is based upon a seventeenth-century ritual from the royal palaces of Central Java, in Indonesia, during which, every day for 40 days prior to a marriage celebration, the bride-to-be would receive treatments and counseling from other women in the family.
5. Traditional lomilomi sessions include what other components in addition to the forearm massage with which we have become familiar?
ANSWER: Traditional lomilomi includes chiropractic manipulation, physical therapy, stone therapy, bone setting, hydrotherapy, herbal medicine, dietary advice, prayer
(Pule), and heartfelt communication (ho'oponopono).
6. Why is manual lymphatic drainage an important advanced modality practiced at spas?
ANSWER: MLD helps the body eliminate impurities and improve appearance, which are goals of many spa services. It is incorporated into some spa services, such as cellulite treatments.
7. Why might myofascial therapy be more effective when provided at a day spa as compared to a resort spa?
ANSWER: This type of therapy is usually more effective when applied in successive sessions over time, and day spas with local repeat clientele are better-equipped to provide this type of continuity than resort spas.
8. What two body systems is neuromuscular therapy primarily designed to treat?
ANSWER: The nervous system and the musculoskeletal system are the two body systems neuromuscular therapy is primarily designed to treat.
9. Which two advanced modalities commonly found on spa menus originated in Japan?
ANSWER: Two advanced modalities commonly found on spa menus that originated in Japan are Reiki and shiatsu.
10. What are some of the common characteristics of spas' signature services?
ANSWER: Most spas' signature services share the characteristics of singularity, elaborateness, expense, exotic ingredients, and location specificity.

Chapter 13

1. Instead of diagnosing skin conditions and using skin-specific products, what can massage therapists apply to the skin during face treatments?
ANSWER: Therapists can apply generic products that are good for all skin types, including cleansers, exfoliants, and moisturizers.
2. How is paraffin typically applied to the face by massage therapists?
ANSWER: Therapists usually spread the paraffin atop a layer of gauze, which keeps the paraffin in place so the wax can harden over the contours of the skin.

3. What is the most popular natural enzyme exfoliant used by massage therapists in spas?
ANSWER: The most popular natural enzyme exfoliant is papaya enzyme.
4. What is a common term for the back treatments offered in spas? Why are they called this?
ANSWER: Back treatments are commonly called "back facials" because these services usually focus on cleansing and skin rejuvenation featuring products that are sometimes applied to the face.
5. When performing scalp treatments in the spa, therapists are not allowed to choose specific protocols for particular hair types or scalp conditions. Why not?
ANSWER: Determining specific conditions or hair types is what cosmetologists are trained to do and is outside massage therapists' scope of practice.
6. What is the condition most commonly benefited by spa scalp treatments? What causes this condition? How do spa scalp treatments help?
ANSWER: Dry hair and scalp is the condition most commonly benefited by spa scalp treatments. It is caused by inactive sebaceous glands, and the treatments help it by introducing moisture through natural products and increasing local circulation.
7. What procedures are massage therapists not allowed to perform when giving a hand or foot treatment?
ANSWER: The procedures therapists are not allowed to perform include cutting, filing, shaping, or buffing the nails, applying or removing nail polish, and trimming or shaping cuticles.
8. What are some of the benefits of performing foot treatments in a spa's waiting area?
ANSWER: Performing foot treatments in the waiting area frees up the treatment rooms so they can be generating more revenue. Also, other clients see the service being performed and want to sign up for one themselves. Finally, offering services out in public view creates a tranquil atmosphere.

Chapter 14

1. What are some of the benefits specific to working in a larger spa? Explain your answers.
ANSWER: Some of the benefits to working in a larger spa include:
Larger spas offer a proving ground in which to hone new skills by doing a large volume of massage.
Larger spas offer a low barrier to entry to new therapists fresh out of school without much experience.
Larger spas offer camaraderie for therapists who spend much of their time alone with clients.
Larger spas offer you a chance to gain valuable experience in how spas are run so you will be able to move up the ranks in the spa or open a spa of your own one day.
Larger spas often offer training to faithful employees.
Larger spas offer an automatic clientele with no need to spend the time and effort to build a clientele of your own.
2. What are the three key traits for which spas will be looking in all of the therapists they hire?
ANSWER: The three key traits spas look for in therapists are: (1) a positive attitude and pleasant appearance, (2) a history of success/longevity in positions, and (3) a well-put-together résumé.
3. What are the main components of a successful spa therapist's résumé, and what are some ways to enhance the information contained in it?
ANSWER: The main components of a résumé are objectives, experience,

education, references, and skills, and ways to enhance its effect include: customizing the résumé, calling yourself a therapist, emphasizing your strengths, emphasizing customer service skills, and choosing references wisely.

4. What guidelines should be followed when filling out a spa employment application form?
ANSWER: When filling out a spa employment application, you should follow the instructions on the application carefully, be neat and thorough, provide plentiful information, be truthful but not negative, do not mention specific salary requirements, provide good references, and check your application before turning it in.
5. What guidelines should be followed during a job interview at a spa?
ANSWER: During job interviews at spas, therapists should be flexible regarding schedule, speak up about their own attributes and skills, be prepared to answer questions, and watch out for negativity.
6. Name three "deal-breaker" words or phrases that may hurt your chances when applying at a spa.
ANSWER: Deal-breaker words and phrases include "backstabbing," "unfair," "in my last spa," and "it would be so relaxing to work here."
7. Why do some spas administer personality tests as part of the hiring process?
ANSWER: With these tests, spas seek to categorize potential employees so they can understand them in order to better use their innate strengths while minimizing the adverse impact of their weaknesses.
8. What are the four personality types according to the Social Styles model? Under which type do massage therapists usually fall, and why?
ANSWER: The four personality types according to the Social Styles model are *analytical*, *amiable*, *driver*, and *expressive*. Massage therapists usually fall under the *amiable* type because they tend to be cooperative, compassionate, warm, and good listeners, while at the same time being undisciplined, independent, rebellious, and overly creative, which can make it difficult for spa directors and owners to manage them.
9. Define "interview massage" and state its purpose.
ANSWER: An interview massage is a massage given to staff personnel to determine eligibility for employment as judged by hands-on techniques, customer-service skills, and other qualities.
10. Why is it a good policy for spas to have a provisionary employment period?
ANSWER: It is a good policy to have a provisionary employment period in place because spas have found through hard experience that some therapists who look good during the interview process turn out not to be such good employees after all.
11. Name some factors that influence therapist compensation in the spa.
ANSWER: Factors that influence therapist compensation in the spa include the spa's overhead expenses, the locale, therapist seniority, benefits offered, seasonality, and spa policy.
12. Name some places to search for spa therapist job opening announcements.
ANSWER: Spa therapist job opening announcements can be found in the local newspaper, at local massage schools, on spa Web sites, and online at job posting sites such as spajobs.com and experienceispa.com.

Chapter 15

1. Define *customer service*.
ANSWER: *Customer service* can be defined as the ability of an organization or individual to take care of the needs, wishes,

questions, requests, and complaints of its clientele. Excellent customer service consists of doing these things consistently, to a very high standard of satisfaction, and in a largely transparent manner, which means that the customer often does not even notice the efforts being made on his or her behalf.

2. What are the seven main customer-service skills for a spa therapist?
ANSWER: The seven main customer-service skills for a spa therapist include:
Sensitivity – the strength of compassion
Flexibility – the strength of adaptability
Positivity – the strength of hope
Humility – the strength of self-confidence
Responsibility – the strength of respect for others
Maturity – the strength of experience
Connectivity – the strength of communication
3. Define how spas offer therapists "professional career management."
ANSWER: Professional career management consists of a number of valuable services spas offer that many therapists take for granted, such as scheduling, billing, payroll, medical benefits, marketing, rent, supplies and equipment, and more.
4. Define "spa stress."
ANSWER: Spa stress is created by the juxtaposition of the calm, cool, collected image spas create and the "back of the house" point of view of the staff, which often feels like a battleground.
5. Proper comportment in the spa can be defined as __________.
ANSWER: Proper comportment consists of the dignified way you handle yourself in all situations, day to day, minute by minute, at the spa.
6. Name some typical grooming rules for spa therapists.
ANSWER: Typical grooming rules for spa therapists include:
    - No visible piercings except for one on each earlobe for women
    - No facial hair on men
    - Hair must be neat and tidy
    - Hair off the shoulders for men
    - Hair tied back or in a bun for women
    - No visible tattoos (or only small, inconspicuous ones)
    - Shorts must be mid-thigh or longer
    - Shirts must have sleeves
    - Shirts must be tucked in
    - Uniforms must be kept clean and wrinkle-free
    - Shoes must be clean and new-looking
    - No sandals
    - No gum chewing
7. Name some of the top behavioral characteristics of a successful spa therapist as listed by spa directors.
ANSWER: Top behavioral characteristics of a successful spa therapist as listed by spa directors include:
    - Team player
    - Responsible
    - Caring and open-hearted
    - Open-minded
    - Mature
    - Good communicator
    - Positive
    - Calm under pressure
    - Honest/trustworthy
    - Able to follow instructions
    - Passionate about doing spa work and massage
    - Healthy/leading a healthy lifestyle
    - Customer-service–oriented
    - Sales-oriented
    - Common sense
    - Ability to accept change
    - Humility

- Desire for continuous improvement—how many classes have they taken?
- History of success/longevity in positions
- Neatness/tidiness

8. Why are professional ethics especially important in spas?
ANSWER: Professional ethics are especially important in spas because few professions allow so much private time to be shared between client and provider. The lines between familiarity and professionalism must be drawn and redrawn again and again by therapists in their treatment rooms with their clients. And while ethics are a vital part of the massage profession as a whole, they play an especially crucial role in the spa because spas become by default liable for any questionable ethical behavior on the part of the therapists who work in them.
9. Which major massage association's code of ethics states that it is *not* permissible for therapists to sell products to their clients?
ANSWER: No major massage association's code of ethics states that it is not permissible for therapists to sell products to their clients.
10. Define "etiquette."
ANSWER: *Etiquette* can be defined as the rules governing socially acceptable behavior in a particular situation.
11. What are the three main settings in which etiquette must be considered in the spa?
ANSWER: The three main settings in which etiquette must be considered in the spa are in the treatment room, outside the treatment room, and outside the spa.
12. Name some ways in which an effective job description will help you be a better therapist.
ANSWER: An effective job description will help you be a better therapist by:
    - Guiding you into a new awareness of precisely what it is you are doing while working as a spa therapist.
    - Serving as a guidepost for all of those moments when you are not giving treatments and need to stock, refill, replenish, clean, and prepare the treatment space.
    - Instructing you in "relationship management," which is a crucial part of working in any spa, showing the proper patterns of interaction between you and other employees, clearly laying out who has authority over you and in what ways you are autonomous.
    - Giving concrete guidelines regarding your responsibilities in other areas of the spa outside the treatment room, locker room, and front desk, outlining behavioral requirements and other duties while on the property at large.
    - Offering guidance regarding dress, deportment, and grooming.
    - Describing the proper role you will play for guests and what to do if improper conduct is encountered at any time by a guest or another employee.
13. Name several components of an effective job description.
ANSWER: Components of an effective job description include:
    - what you do
    - what you do ***not*** do
    - who your supervisor is
    - whom you supervise
    - the special ways in which you focus on guests
    - the elements of customer service emphasized in your position

- those duties beyond your core responsibilities you should learn to master
- your proper interactions with all levels of co-workers
- an understanding of how your efforts contribute to the overall mission of the spa
- an understanding of how your efforts on the spa's behalf influence your progress along your own personal life and career paths

14. Name some core points that must be mentioned in a good spa mission statement.
ANSWER: Core points that must be mentioned in a good spa mission statement include:
    - **Philosophy:** What are the strengths, beliefs, core values, aspirations, and philosophical priorities of the spa?
    - **Customers and market:** Who are the spa's customers, and from what demographic market do they primarily come? How is this market reached?
    - **Products and services:** What are the spa's most important products and services?
    - **Commitment to success:** What plans does the spa have to achieve profitability tempered with sustainability?
    - **Larger community:** What image and impact does the spa wish to project into the community at large?
    - **Employees:** What is the spa's attitude toward employees?

Chapter 16

1. Why do massage therapists often find it easier to sell MLM products than retail spa products?
ANSWER: Massage therapists usually believe deeply in the effectiveness of products they sell through MLM. In comparison, they often do not believe in the health benefits of the products they are told to sell in the spa. This is the fault of spa owners, spa directors, and product vendors.
2. What are the three main types of fear that sales elicit in massage therapists?
ANSWER: The three main types of fear that sales elicit in massage therapists are the fear of rejection, the fear of change, and the fear of success.
3. Define *sales commissions*.
ANSWER: *Sales commissions* can be defined as a percentage of the total dollar amount sold given in compensation for making the sale.
4. What factors can influence the sales commission levels given to therapists, estheticians, and cosmetologists in the spa?
ANSWER: Seniority, the type of product sold, and the amount of product sold by a particular employee in a certain time period can influence sales commission levels in the spa.
5. What are the two main commission structures used in most spas? Describe them.
ANSWER: The two main commission structures used in most spas are "straight" and "sliding." In a straight sales commission structure, therapists are given a specific percentage of the sales price of each item they help sell. In a sliding commission structure, therapists receive a lower percentage at first, then a higher percentage as they sell more products in a specific sales period.
6. What are private label products, and why can therapists often earn higher commissions for selling them?
ANSWER: Private label items are manufactured by companies that specialize in creating products to sell under the brand name of other businesses. Therapists can receive a higher commission on these spa products because they often have a higher markup and profit margin.

7. What is soft selling, and what are three of its main components?
ANSWER: Soft selling means non-aggressive selling, and it can be broken down into three basic components: relation, education, and cooperation.
8. Name some verbal and non-verbal communication techniques that help promote successful sales in the spa.
ANSWER:
Verbal techniques: diction, clarity, brevity, uniqueness
Non-verbal techniques: neatness, grooming, composure, posture, eye contact, firm handshake
9. What are the steps in the Three-Step Spa Sales Rule? Why are they important?
ANSWER: The steps are (1) show the product, (2) describe the product, and (3) offer the product. They help sales and make therapists' sales efforts more natural and honest.
10. List several types of retail spa products that could be sold by massage therapists.
ANSWER: Moisturizers, exfoliants, body wash, herbs, clays, seaweeds, muds, weight loss and cellulite reduction, supplements, massage tools, sunscreens, and non-treatment items.
11. In what area of the home are spa clients most likely to use a retail exfoliation product sold to them by a therapist?
ANSWER: Spa clients are most likely to use a retail exfoliation product in the shower.
12. What non-treatment items might spa therapists suggest to guests as retail items?
ANSWER: Non-treatment items can include neck pillows, eye pillows, candles, water, snacks, incense, cards, clothing, logo items, CDs, books, and sundries.
13. What is the FIFO system, and why is it important for spa retail?
ANSWER: This stands for First In, First Out, and it means that when items are stocked on the spa shelf, the ones that have been there longest should be moved to the front of the shelf. Newer items should be placed on the back of the shelf, behind the older items.
This is important because many spa items such as creams, lotions, muds, and herbs have an expiration date when they begin to lose effectiveness or go bad.

Chapter 17

1. What four basic ingredients are needed to create a true spa experience for your clients?
ANSWER: The four basic ingredients necessary to create a true spa experience for your clients are hands-on therapeutic skills, high-quality products, a few essential pieces of equipment (table, warmer, water source), and a consciously created environment.
2. Name four or more resources appropriate for therapists who are considering opening a spa.
ANSWER: Some resources appropriate for therapists who are considering opening a spa include books, magazines, videos, DVDs, workshops, and trainings.
3. Name at least two conferences appropriate to attend for therapists who are committed to building a spa.
ANSWER: Conferences appropriate to attend for therapists who are committed to building a spa include:
    - Day Spa Expo
    - International Salon & Spa Expo
    - Cosmoprof North America
    - Spa & Resort/Medical Spa Expo & Conference Exhibition
    - International Esthetics, Cosmetics & Spa Conference
    - International Spa Association (ISPA) Convention Spa Evolution
    - Spa Evolution (Canada)

4. Name the three main categories of spa consultants.
   ANSWER: The three main categories of spa consultants are trainers, full-service consultants, and vendors/suppliers.
5. How do you know when you can ethically and legally use the term "spa" as part of your business name?
   ANSWER: You can ethically and legally use the term "spa" as part of your business name when you have incorporated three ingredients into your business:

   1. a dedicated space
   2. the therapeutic use of water
   3. a well-developed spa services menu

6. Define SWOT analysis.
   ANSWER: A self-assessment tool that provides insight into your current real-world potential for building or growing a (spa) business. SWOT stands for *strengths*, *weaknesses*, *opportunities*, and *threats*.
7. What are the six main sources of financing for therapists who are opening up a spa?
   ANSWER: The six main sources of financing for therapists who are opening up a spa include cash, bank loan, home equity line of credit, SBA loan, credit cards, and lease.
8. Define the word "demographics."
   ANSWER: *Demographics* can be defined as the characteristics of human populations and population segments, especially when used to identify consumer markets.
9. What is the key element you will want to keep in mind when making decisions about the layout and plan of your new spa space?
   ANSWER: The key element you will want to keep in mind when making decisions about the layout and plan of your new spa space is revenue-generating space.
10. Name the five key elements of spa retail area design.
    ANSWER: The five key elements of spa retail area design are accessibility, ubiquity, quality shelving, touchability, and lighting.
11. What is rule number one regarding pricing spa services in your own spa?
    ANSWER: Rule number one regarding pricing spa services in your own spa is: Do not undersell yourself.
12. When a client receives a package of three treatments—massage, exfoliation, and body wrap—in which order should they be applied?
    ANSWER: When a client receives a package of three treatments—massage, exfoliation, and body wrap—they should be applied in the following order:

    1. exfoliation
    2. body wrap
    3. massage

13. How does creating a removable price sheet that can be inserted into the menu help spas save money?
    ANSWER: Removable price sheets can be changed periodically without going through an expensive reprinting of the entire spa menu.
14. What do you need in order to create a conscious spa environment?
    ANSWER: To create a conscious spa environment, all you need are some items that engage the five senses: lighting, sound, aroma, taste, and texture.
15. What is a white-noise generator?
    ANSWER: A white-noise generator is an inexpensive machine used in some spas to generate a mixture of sound waves extending over a wide frequency range (low-level background noise), making unwanted noises and voices less audible and the atmosphere in the treatment room more enjoyable.
16. Of what does the aroma known as the "spa smell" primarily consist?
    ANSWER: The "spa smell" primarily consists of sea-based products, boiling herbs,

and essential oils, either in pure form or burned in candles.

17. What four guidelines should a therapist follow in order to avoid potential problems when setting up an in-home spa?
ANSWER: The four guidelines a therapist should follow in order to avoid potential problems when setting up an in-home spa include:
    1. Check local zoning laws
    2. Stick with a theme
    3. Maximize space use
    4. Insulate the area
18. What are the three basic options regarding whether to hire a spa manager?
ANSWER: (1) You can focus on being a manager and cut back on the number of treatments you give. (2) You can hire a manager and focus on doing therapy. (3) You can modify the position and find a manager who handles all of those areas in which you are weak.
19. What are some of the tasks a spa owner must take care of in order to assume a position of leadership in the business?
ANSWER: To show leadership, spa owners should create an employee manual, take charge of the business, provide adequate training, commit to constant improvement, and take ultimate responsibility for everything that happens at the spa.
20. What are the three guidelines for offering spa services in a client's home?
ANSWER:
To successfully offer spa services in clients' homes, therapists should keep the operation simple, arrive at the job site early, and concentrate on promoting their businesses.

Chapter 18

1. Name some reasons why it is a good idea to make a pro forma budget for your spa startup.
ANSWER: It is a good idea to make a pro forma budget for your spa startup because:
    1. It forces you to concentrate on the financial realities of your proposed venture.
    2. It allows you to share your financial projections with others who may be able to help you.
    3. It gives you a starting place and a benchmark against which you can judge future progress.
    4. It gives you a clear picture of who will be responsible for each expense and each unit of income, allowing you to asses performance.
2. In essence, what two things does every kind of budget track?
ANSWER: Every kind of budget tracks income and expenditures.
3. Name at least four of the tasks involved with the day-to-day management of a spa.
ANSWER: Some of the tasks involved with the day-to-day management of a spa are running staff meetings, setting schedules, recruitment and hiring, giving promotions and raises, disciplining and firing employees, and training.
4. Therapists working in a spa setting need to be extra-vigilant about ethical issues, draping, and boundaries for what three main reasons?
ANSWER: The three main reasons therapists working in a spa setting need to be extra-vigilant about ethical issues, draping, and boundaries are the abundance of water, the relaxed attitude of the clients, and under-trained employees.
5. What is the best way, in addition to insurance, that spa business owners can protect themselves from lawsuits and hedge their liability?
ANSWER: In order to hedge their liability, spa business owners should provide their employees with specific trainings that

cover contraindications, client boundary issues, sexual harassment, and workplace safety, then maintain files with documents showing that their employees have undergone such training.

6. Name the three main types of licenses needed by spas.
ANSWER: The three main types of licenses and permits needed by spas include a local and/or state business license, retail license, and occupational license.
7. Marketing a spa therapy practice is different than running a straight massage therapy practice for what three main reasons?
ANSWER: Marketing a spa therapy practice is different than running a straight massage therapy practice because of higher expectations, higher overhead, and higher number of offerings.
8. What are the four key components, or "4 Ps," of marketing?
ANSWER: The four key components, or "4 Ps," of marketing are *product*, *price*, *place*, and *promotion*.
9. What are the five main directions therapists branch into as they pursue a career in the spa field?
ANSWER: The five main directions therapists branch into as they pursue a career in the spa field are supervising, directing, training, consulting, and providing allied services.

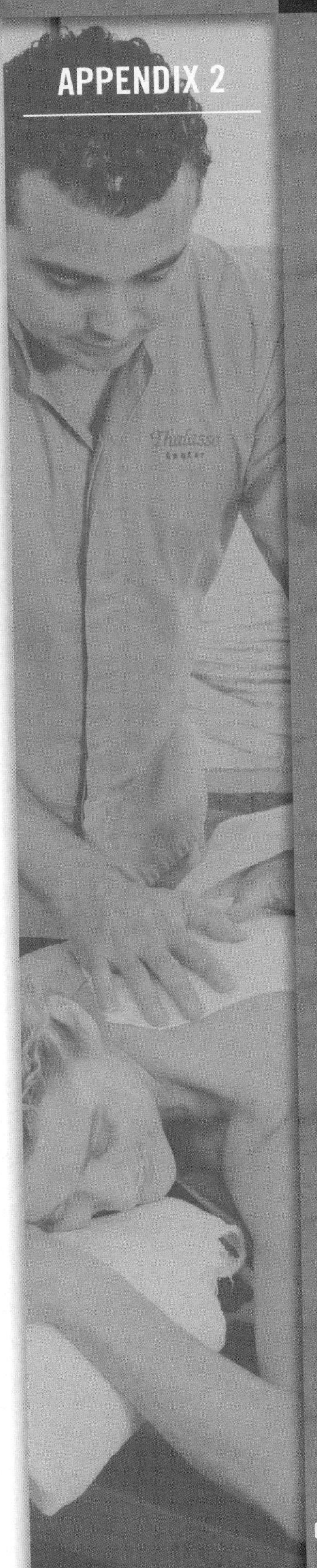

Bibliography

Aaland, M. (1978). *Sweat: The illustrated history and description of the Finnish sauna, Russian bania, Islamic hammam, Japanese mushi-buro, Mexican temescal, and American Indian and Eskimo sweatlodge.* Capra Press.

Alexandra, S. (2003). *The art of stone healing.* Sonia Alexandra Inc.

Arvigo, R. (2003). *Spiritual bathing: Healing rituals and traditions from around the world.* Celestial Arts.

Barron, P. N. (2003). *Hydrotherapy theory & technique.* Pine Island Publishers.

Batmanghelidj, F. (1992). *Your body's many cries for water.* Global Health Solutions.

Beck, M. (2006). *Theory and practice of therapeutic massage.* Cengage Learning.

Bergel, R. R., and Leavy, H. R. (2003). *The spa encyclopedia: A guide to treatments & their benefits for health & healing.* Cengage Learning, 2003.

Born, B. A. (2005). *The essential massage companion: Everything you need to know to navigate safely through today's drugs and diseases.* Concepts Born.

Brue, A. (2003). *Cathedrals of the flesh: My search for the perfect bath.* Bloomsbury.

Burt, B., and Price, P. J. (2006). *100 best spas of the world*, 3rd ed. GPP Travel.

Carcopino, J. (1940). *Daily life in ancient Rome.* Yale University Press.

Chai, M. R. (Ed.). (2005). *Na Mo'olelo Lomilomi: The traditions of Hawaiian massage and healing.* Bishop Museum Press.

Chaithavuthi, J., and Ranchanoo, M. (2007). *Thai massage the Thai way: Healing body and mind.* Thai Massage Book Press.

Croutier, A. L. (1992). *Taking the waters: Spirit, art, sensuality.* Abbeyville Press.

D'Angelo, J. M. (2006). *Spa business strategies: A plan for success.* Cengage Learning.

Davis, P. (1988). *Aromatherapy: An A–Z.* Verimilion.

Davis, W. (1972). *A day in old Rome.* Biblio.

Eidson, R. (2008). *Hydrotherapy for health and wellness.* Cengage Learning.

Emoto, M. (2004). *The hidden messages in water.* Beyond Words.

Farrer-Halls, G. (2005). *The aromatherapy bible: The definitive guide to using essential oils.* Sterling.

Fowlie, L. (2006). *Heat and cold therapy.* Curties-Overzet Publications.

Gattefossé, R.-M. (1937). *Gattefossé's aromatherapy.* Saffon Walden.

Green, L., and Goggins, R. W. (2008). *Save your hands! The complete guide to injury prevention and ergonomics for manual therapists.* Body of Work Books.

Grimal, P. (1963). *The civilization of Rome.* New York: Simon.

Hembry, P. M. (1990). *The English spa, 1560–1815: A social history.* Associated University Press.

Howard, P. J., and Howard, J. M. (2004). *An introduction to the five-factor model of personality.* Charlotte, NC: Center for Applied Cognitive Studies.

International Spa Association. (2007). *2007 spa industry study: A profile of the spa industry in the United States and Canada.* Association Resource Center.

Lad, V. (1984). *Ayurveda: The science of self healing.* Lotus Press.

Levinson, J. C. (2007). *Guerrilla marketing: Easy and inexpensive strategies for making big profits from your small business,* 4th ed. Mariner Books.

Menen, A. (1973). *Cities in the sand.* Dial.

Merrill, D. W. (1981). *Personal styles & effective performance,* CRC.

Mertz, B., and Mertz, R. (1968). *Two thousand years in Rome.* New York: Coward.

Miller, E. (1996). *Day spa operations.* Milady.

Moor, F. B., Peterson, S. C., Manwell, E. M., Noble, M. C., and Muench, G. (1964). *Manual of hydrotherapy and massage.* Pacific Press Publishing Association.

Moren, S. A. (2005). *Spa & salon alchemy: The ultimate guide to spa & salon ownership.* Cengage Learning.

Nelson, M., and Scrivner, J. (2004). *The official LaStone therapy manual.* Piatkus.

Nikola, R. J. (1995). *Creatures of water: Hydro and spa therapy textbook.* Europa Publishing.

Payne, R. (197). *Ancient Rome.* American Heritage.

Phillips, C. (1995). *In the bag: Selling in the salon.* Milady.

Rojas Alba, H. (1996). "Temazcal, the traditional Mexican sweat bath." *Medicinas Tradicionales y Alternativas,* 2.

Roseberry, M. (2002). *Marketing massage: How to build your dream practice.* Cengage Learning.

Salguero, C. P. (2007). *Traditional Thai medicine.* Hohm Press.

Scrivner, J. (2003). *LaStone therapy: The amazing new form of healing bodywork that will transform your health.* Piatkus.

Slavin, S. (1997). *The art of the bath.* Chronicle Books.

Smith, B. (2001). *The Japanese bath.* Gibbs-Smith.

Stillerman, E. (1992). *MotherMassage.* Dell.

Stillerman, E. (1996). *The encyclopedia of bodywork.* Facts On File.

Stillerman, E. (2008). *Prenatal massage: A textbook of pregnancy, labor, and postpartum bodywork.* Mosby.

Stobart, J. C. *The grandeur that was Rome.* New York: Praeger, 1961.

White, J. E. M. (1979). *Everyday life of the north American Indian,* Dover Publications.

Yegül, F. (1995). *Baths and bathing in classical antiquity.* MIT Press.

Yilmazkaya, O. (2003). *Turkish baths: A guide to the historic Turkish baths of Istanbul.* Citlembik.

Resources

One of the most comprehensive Web sites for spa industry information of all kvhttp://www.discoverspas.com. Julie Register, the owner of Spa Quality, who is profiled in Chapter 2, has created a resource listing spas, spa software, spa philosophy, spa consultants, spa reviews, soap consultants, and much more.

Spa Software: The Discover Spas Web site lists several professional spa software options here: http://www.discoverspas.com/spa_business_resources/spa_software.shtml.

Online Spa Gift Certificates: Spa Boom offers the ability to pay for and print out spa gift certificates online. http://www.spaboom.com.

The Touch Research Institute, headquartered in Miami, Florida, has conducting numerous studies on the clinical effects of massage and allied spa modalities such as aromatherapy. The main Web address is: http://www6.miami.edu/touch-research/. The aromatherapy study can be found here: http://www6.miami.edu/touch-research/Aromatherapy.htm.

The International Spa Association is dedicated to connecting and enhancing all professionals working within the spa industry. They produce the largest international gathering for the industry each year and have many educational offerings as well. http://www.experienceispa.com.

Elaine Stillerman's special insights into working with pregnant spa clients has been featured throughout this book. Visit her Web site (http://www.mothermassage.net) for information about her classes, seminars, and books. She is very helpful.

Peggy Wynn Borgman and Lisa Star hold some of the best "Real World Spa Startup/Expansion Workshops" anywhere. And they also offer first-class consultation. They can be found at http://www.wynnebusiness.com.

Douglas Preston has created some top-notch training and product programs for the spa industry, including one of the very few spa consultant trainings available today: http://www.prestoninc.net.

Destination Spa Vacations (http://www.destinationspagroup.com) lists information for people interested in the full-immersion experience found at destination spas, where all guests are focused on the spa program.

SpaFinder (http://www.spafinder.com) is a spa travel agency, spa travel portal, purveying of spa gift certificates, publisher of spa magazines, and much more.

Celsius-to-Fahrenheit Conversion Chart: to translate any of the temperatures mentioned in this book from Fahrenheit to Celsius, see chart on following page. Alternately, you can use the following formula: °C = (5/9) × (°F − 32)

°C	°F	°C	°F	°C	°F
50	122.0	27	80.6	4	39.2
49	120.2	26	78.8	3	37.4
48	118.4	25	77.0	2	35.6
47	116.6	24	75.2	1	33.8
46	114.8	23	73.4	0	32.0
45	113.0	22	71.6	−1	30.2
44	111.2	21	69.8	−2	28.4
43	109.4	20	68.0	−3	26.6
42	107.6	19	66.2	−4	24.8
41	105.8	18	64.4	−5	23.0
40	104.0	17	62.6	−6	21.2
39	102.2	16	60.8	−7	19.4
38	100.4	15	59.0	−8	17.6
37	98.6	14	57.2	−9	15.8
36	96.8	13	55.4	−10	14.0
35	95.0	12	53.6	−11	12.2
34	93.2	11	51.8	−12	10.4
33	91.4	10	50.0	−13	8.6
32	89.6	9	48.2	−14	6.8
31	87.8	8	46.4	−15	5.0
30	86.0	7	44.6	−16	3.2
29	84.2	6	42.8	−17	1.4
28	82.4	5	41.0	−18	−0.4

To convert any of the measurements in this text from ounces or tablespoons to metric, use the following chart:

U.S. MEASUREMENT	METRIC MEASUREMENT
1 teaspoon	5 milliliters
1 tablespoon	15 milliliters
1 fluid ounce (2 tablespoons)	30 milliliters
2 fluid ounces (1/4 cup)	60 milliliters
8 fluid ounces (1 cup)	240 milliliters
16 fluid ounces (2 cups = 1 pint)	480 milliliters
32 fluid ounces (2 pints = 1 quart)	950 milliliters (.95 liter)
128 fluid ounces (4 quarts = 1 gallon)	3.75 liters

ablution: a treatment that involves washing the skin of a spa client, usually with a coarse linen cloth and cold water, either over the entire body or a certain area such as the legs or abdomen

absolute: a highly concentrated aromatic extract derived from plant material which has undergone at least two extraction processes by chemical solvent and is free from waxes and other by-products; similar to a regular essential oil but more highly concentrated

abhyanga: four-handed Ayurvedic oil massage

acne: chronic inflammation of the sebaceous glands caused by retained secretions; in severe cases cysts and nodules can form, resulting in scarring

ADA compliant: in conformance with regulations of the Americans with Disabilities Act, usually used in reference to physical facilities of a (spa) business being set up to accommodate people in wheelchairs and with other physical restrictions

affusion: spa treatment popularized by Kneipp featuring a stream of water of specific temperatures over the entire body or certain areas; an affusion under pressure is the same but with water directed at high pressure at the body to produce more pronounced mechanical effects

aleipterion: warmed room for applying oil in an early Roman bath

alga: singular form of algae, refers to aquatic plants or plantlike chlorophyll-containing nonvascular organisms

algology: the science and study of algae; see phycology

alopecia areata: a condition in which hair is lost, usually from the scalp, creating bald spots, especially in the first stages; certain essential oils have been shown to have a positive impact on the condition

alpha hydroxy acid: a wide range of exfoliants such as glycolic acid and malic acid derived from fruit and milk sugars; they unglue dead skin cells from the surface, allowing them to slough off; best used on thickened, sun-damaged skin without oily buildup

amenity spa: located within a larger resort setting which caters to guests on vacation and business travel, these spas are often looked upon as secondary to the guest experience and are therefore not expected to make much profit or offer superlative therapies.

analgesic: a substance that relieves pain

analgesic: a technique or substance capable of relieving pain, such as application of ice

antipruritic: a substance that relieves or prevents itching

antipyretic: preventing or alleviating fever

apocrine sweat glands: scent glands that develop in puberty, responsible for sweat's odor

apodyterium: changing room in a Roman bath

arteriosclerosis: hardening of the arteries

asteatosis: diminished or arrested action of the sebaceous glands caused by advanced age and exposure to cold, resulting in dry scaly skin

atonic effect: response produced by exposure to heat in hydrotherapy, in which the body exhibits a lack of muscle tone

attunement wand: an oblong piece of crystal, often of quartz or rose quartz, used unheated in stone massage to align and balance client's subtle energies.

autoclave: device for heating substances above their boiling point, used to sterilize (spa) instruments

ayate: fiber from the agave cactus used to make exfoliating cloths for spa services, see sisal

Ayurvedic: referring to the holistic alternative medicine that is the traditional system of medicine of India

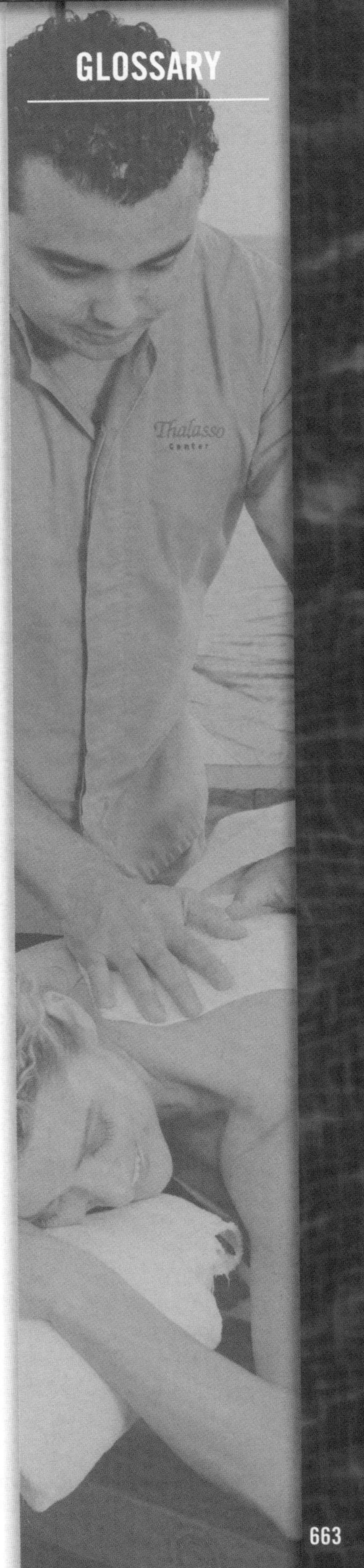

back bar: refers to the larger (compared to retail) size spa product jars and bottles kept on the shelf and used in the spa treatment room, originally an esthetician's term

balance sheet: a summary of a company's financial condition at a specific point in time, including assets, liabilities and net worth

balneotherapy: the use of baths to induce health benefits, often utilizing thermal waters with specific therapeutic ingredients such as essential oils, herbs and minerals

balneum: smaller neighborhood communal bathing facility of the Roman Empire, precursor to the much larger and more grand Thermae

banya: traditional Russian communal steam bath

basalt: a dark-gray to black, dense to fine-grained igneous rock of volcanic origin

base note: an essential oil used in a blend; fragrance lasts longer than middle or top notes and is heavy, sweet-smelling and calming

bath sheet: extra large bath towel, especially appropriate for draping clients during spa treatments or to preserve modesty while disrobing for bath treatments

beta hydroxy acid: salicylic acid, a lipid-soluble exfoliant able to penetrate into pores which contain sebum in order to dislodge the dead skin cells there, best used on oily skin with blackheads and whiteheads

bian stones: stones refined into fine needles and used as instruments of healing in ancient China

Bindegewebsmassage: a type of myofascial release massage that uses light strokes to affect the superficial fascia, rarely offered in spas

biocompatible: compatible with living tissue or a living system, not toxic, injurious, reactive or causing immunological rejection; said of whole spa products such as seaweed which have similar properties as human tissues

blood pump: action created by contrast therapy whereby alternating heat and cold bring in fresh blood to an area and help flush out wastes

body masque: French spelling of the word "mask;" an application of seaweed or other spa product to the body, usually entailing wrapping of the body as well

booth rental: (taken from the salon industry where it means renting a hair styling booth from a business owner) the practice of paying a business owner for the right to operate a massage or spa practice within her facility for a set weekly or monthly rental fee with all other proceeds retained by the practitioner

Botox®: trademark name for a highly purified preparation of botulinum toxin Type A, injected under the skin to smooth wrinkles and to treat certain muscle conditions

breakeven analysis: a calculation of the approximate retail and service sales needed to cover costs, below which the spa business would be unprofitable and above which it would be profitable

budget: estimate or plan of expenditure in relation to income or a periodic estimate of a (spa) business's revenue and expenditure

Bumbu: meaning to add "spice," a skin rolling massage technique incorporating all four fingers opposite the thumb, used in Javanese Lulur treatments

burnout: the fatigue or injury suffered by therapists as a result of an excess workload

business credit application: form to fill out with information to be used for a company to determine whether or not to extend credit to a prospective customer

business liability insurance: insurance that covers businesses and business owners for claims related to allegations of negligent activities or failure to use reasonable care

business plan: a written document outlining the details of a proposed business venture, including information such as financial strategies, products and services to be provided, estimated market, profits, key team members, and return for investors

caldarium: main hot room in Roman baths

call to action: a direct request to the potential client at the end of a marketing piece, requesting them to pick up the phone or come to the (spa) business in order to purchase products or services

camekan: changing room in a hammam

carbon cycle: the cycle of carbon in the earth's ecosystems in which carbon dioxide is transformed through photosynthesis into organic nutrients, like oxygen, then ultimately turned back into an inorganic state, as through human respiration

carrageenan: a colloid extracted from various red algae (as Irish moss) used as a thickener or stabilizer in ice cream, medicines, cosmetics and spa products

carrier oil: oil appropriate for massage therapy, such as sweet almond, grape seed and others, into which drops of essential oil are added, thus diluting the strength of the essential oils and making them easy to apply in massage and body treatments

cash flow: the pattern of income and expenditures, as of a person or (spa) business, and the resulting availability of cash

cellulite: dimpled appearance of the skin created by deposits of

intake form: a series of questions related to health, allergies, spa experience and general information (address, birthday, etc.) asked of clients when they first visit the spa, sometimes includes a waiver or disclaimer

intake specialists: also referred to hospitality specialists in some spas; see 5; these employees are responsible for helping clients decide which programs and treatments to experience while at the spa

International Spa Association (ISPA): most visible and widespread worldwide professional spa association, founded in 1991 by a small group of North American spa professionals, headquartered in Lexington, Kentucky, now with branches in Europe and Asia, and holder of the largest annual international spa convention

interview massage: massage given to staff personnel to determine eligibility for employment as judged by hands-on techniques, customer service skills, and other qualities

intrusive: igneous rock that has crystallized from molten magma while still below the surface of the Earth, solidifying underground before reaching the surface

inventory control: supervision of the supply and storage and accessibility of items in order to insure an adequate supply without excessive oversupply

invoice: a statement of money owed for goods or services

job description: document containing written guidelines and requirements for employees who are performing a particular job

kahuna: Hawaiian healer skilled in the full spectrum of lomilomi techniques that extend beyond massage, including diet, herbal medicine, counseling, elements of chiropractic, and more

keratinization: the process of changing into keratin, the hardened protein substance that makes up hair, nails, claws, etc.

keratinocyte: skin cells found in the epidermis, generated in the stratum basale and eventually moving up to the stratum corneum where they are shed through natural means or through exfoliation services

kese: a coarse mitten carried in the soap case, it not only scoured the dirt out of the pores, but also served to deliver a bracing massage; it was specially woven out of hair or plant fibers

kiva: a large chamber, often wholly or partly underground, in a Pueblo Indian village, used for religious ceremonies and other purposes, sometimes heated to create a sauna-like environment

kur: German word meaning (course of) treatment, or cure, often used in conjunction with "wasser" meaning water; Wasserkur can mean "hydrotherapy" and specifically that type taught by German healer Sebastian Kneipp

La'au: sticks used as therapeutic massage tools in lomilomi treatments

laconicum: hot, dry chambers in Roman baths, similar to today's sauna, named after the more ancient Greek hot air bath (singular laconica)

laser skin resurfacing: procedure in which a laser is used to remove areas of damaged skin, scaring, uneven pigmentation, wrinkles, and fine lines

laser skin resurfacing: sometimes used in medical spas, the process of using laser light to remove damaged or wrinkled skin, layer by layer, to minimize fine lines, especially around mouth and eyes and also for treating facial scars or uneven pigmentation

LaStone Therapy: original form of stone-based treatment developed by Arizona massage therapist Mary Nelson in 1993, including energy work, deep tissue stone work, sage smudge stick purification and the application of hot and cold stones

latent heat: the quantity of heat absorbed or released by a substance undergoing a change of state, such as ice changing to water or water to steam, at constant temperature and pressure

leukocyte: blood cells that engulf and digest bacteria and fungi; an important part of the body's defense system

limbic system: area of the brain consisting of the olfactory bulb, hippocampus, amygdala, hypothalamus and related structures that support emotion, behavior and memory; strongly affected by aroma and thus aromatherapy

lipolysis: the breakdown of fat stored in fat cells during which free fatty acids are released into the bloodstream; said to occur during spa cellulite treatments

lithification: the process through which sediments compact under pressure, lose fluids and gradually turn into stone; the final stage in the process of petrification and creation of sedimentary rocks

loess: a fine-grained unstratified accumulation of clay and silt deposited by the wind

löyly: word used by Finns to describe the particular attributes of the heated air in a sauna room

luk pra kob: Thai name for therapeutic herbal compresses used in traditional Thai medicine for centuries and recently in spa therapy

Lulur: type of spa service that recreates an Indonesian pre-nuptial ritual, including exfoliation, massage, yogurt application, and bath

lymphedema: swelling caused by lymph accumulating in the tissues;

often treated with manual lymphatic drainage (MLD), which complements many spa therapies

lymphocytes: a leukocyte that normally makes up a quarter of the white blood cell count but increases in the presence of infection

lypossage: non-mechanical massage treatment intended to reduce the appearance of cellulite

maceration: softening by soaking or steeping a substance in a medium such as water or oil; used for making herbal-infused massage oils

mafic: of, relating to, or being a group of usually dark-colored minerals rich in magnesium and iron, as are basalt stones used in stone massage

magnetite: a black isometric mineral that is an oxide of iron and an important iron ore

malic acid: a colorless crystalline solid acid found in fruits such as apples, used in some chemical exfoliants, one of the alpha hydroxy acids

manager on duty (MOD): manager on site after hours, sleeping over at (spa) facility to handle all concerns or emergencies should they arise when no other managers are present

marketing: all activities a company undertakes to acquire customers and maintain a relationship with them, with the ultimate goal of matching products and services to the people who need and want them, in order to ensure profitability

markup: the amount above the wholesale cost of a product charged to retail customers

marma points: a total of 107 specific points on the body that are stimulated as part of an ayurvedic massage

mastoid process: prominence of the temporal bone behind the ear at the base of the skull

mesotherapy: injection of fat-dissolving compounds into the skin to treat cellulite and sculpt the body

metamorphic: of rocks that have been formed under great pressure and heat

microdermabrasion: technique using a high pressure stream of abrasive crystals against the skin for exfoliation, usually performed only on the face by licensed estheticians

micronized: pulverized into particles a few micrometers (millionths of a meter) in diameter

middle note: an essential oil aroma that lasts longer than a top note, offering body to oil blends; aromas are usually warm and soft rather than strong

milia: small white or yellowish nodules resembling millet seeds, produced in the skin by the retention of sebaceous secretion

mission statement: a summary describing the aims, values, and overall plan of an organization or individual

Mohs scale: a scale of relative hardness devised by Friedrich Mohs in 1812, used as an aid to identify minerals

moor: nutrient-rich black silts formed by the decomposition of excess plant life in eutrophic lakes, used in spas for its purifying and chelating properties

muslin: a type of finely-woven cotton fabric, used in spa treatments and specifically the herbal wrap

myristicin: a pharmacologically active compound found in various essential oils such as nutmeg

Na'au: the word for large intestine or colon Hawaiian; also means "soul" or "heart"

nalins: the wooden clogs, often ornate, worn in the hammam to help avoid slipping

natir: a female version of the tellak, traditional hammam worker

neat: by itself, at full strength; said of 100% pure essential oils that have not been blended with a carrier oil or diluted in any other way

nebulizer: a dispenser that turns liquids, such as essential oils, into a fine mist

nervine: having the quality of acting upon or affecting the nerves; quieting nervous excitement, as do several herbs and oils used in spa treatments

Nurnberger–Muller scale: breakdown of the visible signs of cellulite into four distinct stages, 0–3, ascertainable by self-testing

occlusion: closure or blockage, used when describing paraffin wax, which creates an occlusive barrier that retains moisture in the skin

Ohashiatsu: derivative style of shiatsu developed by Wataru Ohashi in the U.S.

olfactory bulb: the most forward structure of the brain, transmits smell information from the nose into the brain's limbic system; necessary for the perception of smell

olfactory epithelium: area of tissue inside the nasal cavity, approximately one inch by two inches in size, located on the roof of the nasal cavity and connecting to the olfactory bulb; directly responsible for detecting odors

olfactory system: the body's system of smell, including all the structures and processes through which that happens

on call therapist: a contracted worker (usually receiving no benefits) who is not guaranteed a particular number of work hours per week but rather called only when the spa is busy and in need of extra therapists

onsen: hot springs, and especially the bathing facilities and resorts around them, in Japan

onychosis: any disease or disorder of the nails

open book policy: the practice used by many (spa) businesses of showing employees (especially therapists) actual income, expenses and profit & loss statements so these employees can better understand the expenses involved with running a spa business and why their own compensation needs to be kept at specific levels

ordinances: local and/or state rules that regulate the safety, structure, and operational practices of a (spa) business

osmosis: diffusion of molecules through a membrane from a place of higher concentration to a place of lower concentration until the concentration on both sides is equal, a process that can take place through the skin when substances such as seaweed are applied to it

overhead: all costs of running a (spa) business not including or related to labor, materials or administration

owner/slave syndrome: tendency for therapists and other hands-on practitioners who open spas to rely upon their own work to support the business rather than build their spa's brand through the work of employees

P&L (profit and loss) statement: a financial document published by a company, showing earnings, expenses, and net profit

palaestra: exercise area found at many early Roman bath houses, modeled after the ancient Greek wrestling schools

paleomagnetism: science that studies the intensity and direction of residual magnetization in ancient rocks

palpate: examine by feeling an area to determine the state of the tissues there

Pancha Karma: meaning "five actions" in Sanskrit, this is a cleansing and rejuvenating program for the mind and body, known to benefit overall health and stimulate self-healing; often applied in spas featuring Ayurvedic treatment programs

parabens: a group of chemicals widely used as preservatives in cosmetics and personal care products, including some spa products; because they are synthetically produced, some spa clients and therapists avoid them

paraspinal: adjacent to the spinal column

peat: partially carbonized vegetable matter saturated with water

peloids: mud prepared and used for therapeutic purposes

pesternal: ornate cloth or silk wrap worn around the body while at a hammam

petrissage: The application of lifting, squeezing, and kneading strokes to tissues of the body

petrology: the branch of geology that studies rocks, their origin, formation, and composition

phenols: any of a class of weakly acidic organic compounds; many phenols occur in the herbs used in spa treatments and are a contributor to their effectiveness

phlebitis: inflammation of a vein, most commonly in the legs

phonolite: compact igneous rock containing; thin slabs of which give a ringing sound when struck; a primary source of fango for spa treatments

photosensitizer: any substance that creates sensitivity to the influence of radiant energy, especially light

photosynthesis: the conversion of light energy into chemical energy by certain living organisms such as algae

phycology: the science and study of algae; see algology

phytohormones: plant hormones that regulate physiological processes, found in seaweeds

phytoplankton: plant constituent of plankton; mainly unicellular algae

phytotherapy: the use of plants or plant extracts for medicinal purposes, especially plants that are not part of the normal diet

piezoelectricity: electricity produced by mechanical pressure on certain crystals, notably quartz, or a change in the linear dimensions of the crystal caused by electrostatic stimulation

pinch test: self-examination to determine degree of cellulite present in the body

pitting edema: edema in which pitting results in a depression in the edematous tissue which disappears only slowly

polysaccharides: complex carbohydrates found in seaweeds that help skin absorb moisture

pooled commission: a percentage of income from the sale of certain items that is pooled together then split evenly among front desk and reception staff members; usually consisting of non-therapy items such as candles, books, etc.

preeclampsia: a serious condition developing in late pregnancy that is characterized by a sudden rise in blood pressure, excessive weight gain, generalized edema, severe headache, and visual disturbances; may result in convulsions and possibly coma if untreated

prep area: space in which to mix ingredients, heat towels, wring sheets and also store products and supplies, either inside the treatment room, ideally curtained off, or outside the room in a hallway, closet, etc. (same as staging area)

private label: items manufactured by one company for sale by another, with the label of the retailer on the item and no sign of the manufacturer visible to the purchaser

professional career management: a number of valuable services that therapists receive as spa employees including scheduling, billing, payroll, medical benefits, marketing, rent, supplies, and equipment

proforma: used to describe elements of a financial plan that are estimated or projected and not expected to be completely accurate, such as budget projections and P&L (profit and loss) statements in advance of the opening of the business

provisionary employment: period immediately after hiring during which the spa monitors performance and can terminate the therapist's employment at will with no need for an explanation

Pule: Hawaiian for prayer, traditionally part of lomilomi healing sessions

purchase order: a commercial document used to request someone to supply something in return for payment

radiation: heat transfer to a body through direct exposure to infrared rays

raw space: unfinished interior of a building, often with no walls or flooring, that will need a good amount of construction to render into a usable (spa) business environment

reductionism: a theory that complex systems can be completely understood in terms of their components; as regards spa treatments, the use of specific constituents found in a substance such as seaweed or herbs, rather than the whole substance itself

remineralization: the process of supplying the body with minerals that have been depleted through lifestyle and/or environmental factors; the main benefit of thalassotherapy treatments

reporting function: the specific ability of (spa) business software to arrange data such as sales, appointments, number of services provided, employee hours worked, etc. into reports, charts and graphs in order to interpret past performance and forecast future trends

retrostasis: the driving of blood and lymph away from an area of the body by applying cold to that area

return on investment (ROI): the income that an investment provides

revenue-generating-space (RGS): the square footage inside a (spa) business that generates revenue—examples include treatment rooms and retail displays—as compared to those spaces such as hallways, relaxation areas, and waiting rooms that do not normally produce revenue

RICE: an acronym that stands for rest, ice, compression, and elevation, the recommended preliminary treatment within the first 72 hours after an acute injury

risk management: the technique of assessing, minimizing, and preventing accidental loss to a (spa) business through the use of insurance and safety measures

Rolfing: type of deep structural alignment body work developed by Ida Rolf in the 1950s, not often offered in spas because if its intensity and the need for several consecutive sessions in order to be optimally effective

rosacea: a skin disease in which blood vessels of the face enlarge, resulting in a flushed appearance and sometimes pustules

Russian steam cabinet: small, usually fiberglass chamber in which a person sits, head outside, while bathed with steam generated from a unit in the base

sales commissions: a percentage of the total dollar amount sold given in compensation for making the sale

sales to service ratio: the percentage of money that comes into the spa in relation to the amount coming in from actual treatments. It can be measured per-therapist or over the entire spa per unit of time. For example, if a therapist sells $10 worth of products for each spa treatment given, and the treatments cost $100, then the sales-to-service ratio is 10%.

salicylic acid: the only beta hydroxy acid, common in many plants and willow bark, causes dead cells to slough off and the top layer of skin to be removed, unclogging pores

sanatoriums: also spelled sanitariums, resorts for improvement or maintenance of health, especially for convalescents, early examples of which, such as the Kellogg Sanatorium in Battle Creek, Michigan, are thought of as precursors to the modern health spa

saponin: an agent, found in several herbs used in spa treatments, that forms soapy lather when mixed with water

sarsen: a type of dense, hard sandstone; the prehistoric builders of Stonehenge used the substance to erect their monument

savusauna: sauna in which wood smoke is allowed to permeate the room before bathers enter

seasonality: the tendency for a business to be more popular in certain times of the year than others, which especially affects spas in summer resort and winter resort areas

sebaceous glands: a small gland in the skin which secretes a lubricating oily matter called sebum into hair follicles to lubricate skin and hair